Family-Focused Nursing Care

Sharon A. Denham, PhD, RN, CNE

Sandra Eggenberger, PhD, RN

Norma Krumwiede, EdD, RN

Patricia Young, PhD, RN

Family-Focused Nursing Care

Sharon A. Denham, PhD, RN, CNE

Professor Emeritus, Ohio University, School of Nursing, Athens, OH
Professor, Houston J. & Florence A. Doswell Endowed Chair in Nursing for
    Teaching Excellence, Texas Woman's University, College of Nursing, Dallas, TX

Sandra Eggenberger, PhD, RN

Professor
Minnesota State University, Mankato, MN

Norma Krumwiede, EdD, RN

Professor
Minnesota State University, Mankato, MN

Patricia Young, PhD, RN

Professor
Minnesota State University, Mankato, MN

F.A. Davis Company • Philadelphia

KH

F. A. Davis Company
1915 Arch Street
Philadelphia, PA 19103
www.fadavis.com

Printed in the United States of America

Last digit indicates print number: 10 9 8 7 6 5 4 3 2 1

Publisher, Nursing: Joanne Patzek DaCunha, MSN, RN
Acquisitions Editor, Nursing: Megan Klim
Content Development Manager: Darlene Pedersen
Content Project Manager: Christina L. Snyder
Manager of Art and Design: Carolyn O'Brien

As new scientific information becomes available through basic and clinical research, recommended treatments and drug therapies undergo changes. The author(s) and publisher have done everything possible to make this book accurate, up to date, and in accord with accepted standards at the time of publication. The author(s), editors, and publisher are not responsible for errors or omissions or for consequences from application of the book, and make no warranty, expressed or implied, in regard to the contents of the book. Any practice described in this book should be applied by the reader in accordance with professional standards of care used in regard to the unique circumstances that may apply in each situation. The reader is advised always to check product information (package inserts) for changes and new information regarding dose and contraindications before administering any drug. Caution is especially urged when using new or infrequently ordered drugs.

Library of Congress Control Number: 2014960188

9/23/16

The purpose of *Family-Focused Nursing Care* is to help nursing students and practicing nurses identify ways to bring a family focus into all individuals' care. A major theme of this book is the emphasis on *thinking family* anywhere and anytime nursing care is given. This book provides a theoretical background for understanding that nursing practice involves realizing that individuals belong to family units that cannot be separated and should not be ignored. However, every chapter emphasizes application of knowledge and skills. *Thinking family* is an attitude tied to intentional actions. Communication and relationships are key to the individual-nurse-family partnership and important to the provision of coordinated care that extends beyond settings, practitioners, and time. Each chapter begins with objectives and key terms that are discussed in the chapter. Unique features include case studies, evidence-based examples, and recognition of leaders in family nursing. Chapters include figures and tables newly constructed for this book and provide aids to conducting practice so that the family is always viewed as the unit of care.

Skills and knowledge to assess families and address the connectedness of health and illness to the communities where they live have great significance. As emergencies are addressed and acute or chronic conditions managed, nurses can advocate for family members, family households, and community needs. Professional accountability, safety, care needs across the life course, and high-quality valued outcomes need attention. Medical care delivery occurs in hospitals, physician offices, clinics, urgent care centers, community centers, and public health settings. However, people live in family households and family units care for and coach each other. They share and make decisions about finite resources to address valued needs. Too often the individual and family stories are overlooked or ignored.

ACKNOWLEDGMENTS

We would like to acknowledge the support provided to us by F. A. Davis and the many staff members we worked with during the writing and production processes. We want to especially recognize Joanne DaCunha, MSN, RN, a now retired long-time nursing acquisitions editor at F. A. Davis. She believed in us and in the merits of this book. We thank Lynn Kuechle, Coordinator of the Glen Taylor Nursing Institute for Family and Society at Minnesota State University, Mankato, for her assistance in obtaining the photography for the book's artwork. We are grateful for the work of the chapter authors who contributed their insights. We acknowledge the family nurses who have worked diligently and developed the scientific evidence about the strengths and importance of addressing family units when meeting individual care needs.

TABLE OF CONTENTS

CHAPTER **10** Family-Focused Care in Acute Settings   **253**

CHAPTER **11** Family-Focused Care and Chronic Illness   **293**

CHAPTER **12** Family-Focused Care to Meet Population Needs   **325**

In 1980, Dr. Jean Miller and Ellen Janosik published a nursing text called *Family-Focused Care*, which aimed to address the artificial gap between physical and mental health care. Nursing care is about meeting the needs of whole people. This new textbook suggests some 21st century alternatives for nursing practice. Instead of merely caring for patients, the focus is on needs tied to life in a family unit, a family household, and a community. When persons are ill, families are usually their primary care providers. Families provide support and are intimately linked with their members. The dominant form of care has used the medical model and traditional practices focused on episodic problems. However, families teach members about health and illnesses and offer caregiving supports. Family is the source of both strengths and liabilities. The family transmits genetic traits to individuals, but also contributes to strengths and vulnerabilities as their health and illness conditions are managed (Feetham & Thompson, 2006).

Nurses can intentionally care for individuals as they *think family*. Yet, health and illness have implications beyond clinical settings. Daily routines or habits of multiple family members influence health and illness of individuals within the household. Family is important throughout the life course, not just when parenting children or teens. Families manage disabilities, addictions, mental health conditions, and care at the end of life. Nurses can assist family units in gaining knowledge and skills for managing health and illness.

Families share some similarities, but they also have unique qualities. Professional nurses need therapeutic communication skills and family care knowledge. Nurses need to know ways to be collaborative and form partnerships with families and interprofessional teams. *Thinking family* calls for a relationship-based practice in which nurses go from just "doing for" patients to "being with" them in ways that consider their values and satisfy their concerns. This family care meets individuals and family units where they live, listens to their stories, and addresses their concerns. Care needs reach beyond the medical unit, surgical ward, and clinic. Home and community are tied to well-being and self-management. Evidence indicates that when self-management includes individuals and families, health outcomes are improved (Ryan & Sawin, 2009).

The nursing profession is relevant to society, and advocacy roles are enhanced when we embrace the needs of families attached to individuals receiving care. This book weaves empirical knowledge about family concepts and theories and ties them to the art of nursing practice. Synthesis of knowledge combined with effective use of technologies is needed. Family-focused nursing requires skill competence, critical thinking, clinical judgment, intentional actions, prioritizing, decision making, delegating, evaluating, and other nursing roles. Nurses need self-confidence as they manage some of the best and most critical moments of human life. Assumptions, biases, and prejudice must be examined. Social influences evolve, technologies change, knowledge grows, policies get reshaped, but individuals and families always require nurses' attention.

Florence Nightingale is an enduring symbol of what nurses can be as they give care. Observation and assessment, use of scientific principles and knowledge, and attention to human factors influencing health and illness are paramount. In *Notes on Nursing* (pages 54–59) Nightingale discusses communication, providing information about practical actions, the importance of spending time with individuals, and the value of pets. Holistic care addresses personal needs. Nightingale's values and opinions are still important. Relationship-based care includes responses to tragedies, crisis, uncertainties, difficulties, and challenges faced as families experience member needs. Nurses can recognize and commend strengths, support resilience, and address care needs that are continuous. Nurses who *think family* use presence and human connections, not just medical diagnostics and treatments, to address health and illness. Knowing what to say, how to say it, and when to say it are part of caring connections. The question "Does anyone really care about me, about my family?" often goes unanswered. Florence Nightingale's wisdom, insight, and principles still remind us that we must care for individuals, embrace family units, and safeguard community health. The idea of *thinking family* is used to communicate, assess, set goals, strategize, and evaluate outcomes.

This textbook has five sections and 15 chapters. Theoretical underpinnings and evidence suggest ways for *thinking family* and taking action. Section 1 identifies differences between individual and family-focused care. Chapter 1 explores health care needs for the 21st century. Chapter 2 discusses ideas about moving practice from primarily individual focused to one where family unit care needs are explored. Chapter 3 describes ways *thinking family* can be used to guide and deliver nursing care. Section 2 examines key nursing practices (i.e., communication, family assessment, cultural diversity) and describes ways they are linked with family care. These topics are often addressed in nursing courses, but this chapter helps one move from merely thinking patient to *thinking family* unit needs.

Section 3 introduces several theoretical viewpoints to examine health and illness care. Chapter 7 introduces family theory and its relationship to nursing practice. Chapter 8 explains family-focused nursing practice and describes evidence about the knowledge, skills, experiences, and intentional actions needed to develop individual-family-nurse relationships. Chapter 9 defines concepts around nurse presence and family presence. Section 4 encourages readers to rethink acute, chronic, and population care delivery. Finally, Section 5 includes three chapters that identify strategies for taking action with families. Chapter 13 differentiates between "doing for" and "being with" as nursing care is provided. Chapter 14 explains the core processes of the *Family Health Model* and describes ways to use them as intentional caring practices. Chapter 15 discusses various forms of support needed by families and suggests ways nurses can identify and implement the form of support needed. Each chapter includes a case study, presents information about evidence-based practice, and recognizes two international family nursing leaders. We hope this book initiates spirited dialogue in classrooms and clinical practice as the implications of family as the unit of care are thoughtfully considered.

Sharon A. Denham

References

Feetham, S. L., & Thompson, E. J. (2006). Keeping the individual and family in focus. In S. M. Miller, S. H. McDaniel, J. S. Rolland, & S. L. Feetham (Eds.), *Individuals, families, and the new era of genetics*. New York: W. W. Norton & Company, Inc.
Ryan, P., & Sawin, K. J. (2009). The individual and family self-management theory: Background and perspectives on context, process, and outcomes. *Nursing Outlook, 57,* 217–225.

CONTRIBUTORS

Kathryn Hoehn Anderson, PhD, RN, ARNP, LMFT
Professor
Georgia Southern University
Statesboro, GA

Sue Ellen Bell, PhD, RN, PHCNS-BC
Professor, Graduate Programs
  Coordinator
Minnesota State University, Mankato
Mankato, MN

Mary Bliesmer, DNSc, RN
Emerita Professor, School of Nursing
Minnesota State University, Mankato
Mankato, MN

Angela Christian, DNP, RNC
Clinical Practice and Education Specialist
Allina Health, Nursing
Minneapolis, MN

Jennifer M. Demma, MSN, RN, CNM
Clinical Faculty Director
Nurse-Midwifery/Women's Health Nurse
  Practitioner Program
Georgetown University, Washington, DC

Hans-Peter de Ruiter, PhD, RN
Associate Professor
Minnesota State University, Mankato
Mankato, MN

Patricia Earle, PhD, RN
Professor Emerita
Minnesota State University, Mankato
Mankato, MN

Julia Hebenstreit, EdD, RN, CNE
Associate Professor, School of Nursing
  Chairperson
Minnesota State University, Mankato
Mankato, MN

Marianne Kriegl, RN, Mag. phil.
Professor, Dean, Department Health
  Sciences
Programme Director, Advanced Nursing
  Practice
University of Applied Sciences, Krems
Krems, Austria

Kelly Ann Krumwiede, PhD, RN, PHN
Assistant Professor
Minnesota State University, Mankato
Mankato, MN

Susan Lampe, MS, RN

Nancyruth Leibold, EdD, RN, PHN, LSN
Assistant Professor
Minnesota State University, Mankato
Mankato, MN

Linda L. Lindeke, PhD, RN, CNP, FAAN
Associate Professor
University of Minnesota, School of
  Nursing
Pediatric Nurse Practitioner, NICU
  Follow-up Program
University of Minnesota, Masonic
  Children's Program
Minneapolis, MN

Wendy Sue Looman, PhD, RN, PNP
Associate Professor
University of Minnesota, School of
  Nursing
Minneapolis, MN

Sonja J. Meiers, PhD, RN
Professor and Director, Graduate
  Programs in Nursing
Winona State University, Rochester
Rochester, MN

Colleen Royle, EdD, RN
Assistant Professor, Learning Resource
    Center, Simulation Coordinator
Minnesota State University, Mankato
Mankato, MN

Joachim Schulze, RN, Dipl. - Pflegewirt FH
Professor, Programme Director General
    Nursing
University of Applied Sciences, Krems
Krems, Austria

Laura Marie Schwarz, DNP, RN, CNE
Assistant Professor
Minnesota State University, Mankato
Mankato, MN

Marcia S. Stevens, PhD, RN
Professor
Minnesota State University, Mankato
Mankato, MN

Stacey Van Gelderen, DNP, RN
Assistant Professor
Minnesota State University, Mankato
Mankato, MN

REVIEWERS

Laura Blank, RN, MSN, CNE
Assistant Clinical Professor
Northern Arizona University
Flagstaff, AZ

Shannon Burton, MS, APRN
Assistant Professor (Clinical)
University of Utah College of Nursing
Salt Lake City, UT

Barbara M. Carranti, MS, RN
Clinical Associate Professor, Department
    of Nursing
Le Moyne College
Syracuse, NY

Maryanne Davidson, DNSc, APRN, CPNP
Associate Professor
Southern Connecticut State University
New Haven, CT

Laura Dulski, RNC-HROB, CNE, MSN
Assistant Professor
Resurrection University
Chicago, IL

**Kay Foland, PhD, RN, PMHNP-BC,
    PMHCNS-BC, CNP**
Professor
South Dakota State University College
    of Nursing
Rapid City, SD

**Patricia Frohock Hanes, PhD, MSN, MAED,
    RN, CNE**
Associate Professor
Azusa Pacific University School of Nursing
Azusa, CA

Brenda L. Hage, PhD, CRNP
Associate Professor, Nursing
Director of Graduate Nursing Programs
Misericordia University
Dallas, PA

Susan Haussler, EdD, RN, CNE
Associate Professor, Retired
University of Massachusetts, Boston
Boston, MA

Deborah S. Janssen, MS, RN
Assistant Professor
Capital University Department of
    Nursing
Columbus, OH

Lee-Ellen Charlotte Kirkhorn, PhD, RN
Professor of Nursing
University of Wisconsin–Eau Claire
Eau Claire, WI

Heather Meyerhoff, RN, MSN
Associate Professor, Nursing
Trinity Western University
Langley, British Columbia, Canada

Treva V. Reed, BScN, MSN, PhD
Professor of Nursing
Collaborative BScN Program
Canadore College/Nipissing University
North Bay, Ontario, Canada

Dawn Rigney, PhD, RN
Assistant Professor
University of Virginia
Charlottesville, VA

Joy Shewchuk, RN, BSc, BSN, MSN
Professor, Nursing
Humber College
Toronto, Ontario, Canada

Linda D. Wagner, EdD, MSN, RN
Professor, Chairperson, Department of
    Nursing
Central Connecticut State University
New Britain, CT

Vita Wolinsky, RN, BS, MA, CNS:BC
Assistant Professor of Nursing
Dominican College
Orangeburg, NY

CHAPTER 1

Health Care Needs for the 21st Century

Patricia K. Young • Linda L. Lindeke

CHAPTER OBJECTIVES

1. Identify global trends linked with nursing practice.
2. Describe changes in global demographics and how they influence health.
3. Define vulnerable population, health disparities, health equity, and social determinants of health.
4. Analyze gaps between current health care trends and individual, family, and societal health and illness needs.
5. Explain links among individual, family, community, and population health and illness experiences.
6. Explain the role of the nurse in family care coordination.

CHAPTER CONCEPTS

- Environments of care
- Globalization
- Health disparities
- Health equity
- Population health and illness
- Social determinants of health
- Urbanization

Introduction

Change is inevitable. Florence Nightingale, the founder of modern nursing practice, was a nonconformist who challenged a man's world. In the mid-1850s, nurses were largely drawn from the poor, were unskilled, and were often viewed as immoral persons. Refined, well-to-do, and educated women did not put themselves in situations in which their character might be called into question or do work viewed as beneath their societal class. Nightingale was willing to forfeit her family's support, if necessary, in order to do the work she believed she was called to do. She cared for the social good, and is described as a reformer working to redesign the way nursing was practiced and a leader who questioned the status quo of the day. Everywhere she went, change followed. In fact, her work might be viewed as a fight for change.

Have you ever wondered about the forces that drive nursing practice today? Have you questioned whether current procedures and methods might in future generations appear foolish or even wrong? It can be uncomfortable to question tradition. Nursing has focused on patient needs and built practice around the individual. As care became more complex, seeing the needs of the whole person became difficult. Individual medical professionals concentrated on their part of the human system rather than the whole. Who sees the whole person as they really are? Who tends to the holistic care needs of the person? Where does family fit into this picture?

Sometimes students and nurses agree that family is important but are not sure how to approach these connected relationships in their practice. Sometimes families are viewed as disruptive, in the way, or extra burdens in already too busy days. Throughout this book the ideas of thinking family and family-focused care are explored and some new ways of thinking are introduced. This first chapter provides background to help identify some reasons why families need to be respected and included in the care of individuals.

Understanding Global Trends and Their Health Effects

Because the care of individuals and families does not occur in a vacuum, nurses need to be informed about the bigger world systems that influence where they work and the ways health care costs get paid. For instance, nurses often lack clear understandings about the costs of health care services and about the laws and guidelines that influence reimbursement or payments. They seldom consider the limits of various health care payment systems (e.g., Medicare, Medicaid, private insurance, universal health care) as a student or in practice.

Nurses must fundamentally understand—at their nursing core—that health and illness are a family affair and that where individuals live and who they live with influence health status and illness or disease management. Unique sets of individual circumstances give meanings to every situation. Individuals are situated in families that provide background, history, and lived stories that reflect their lives. Families are situated in social groups or networks that make up communities—these provide the lenses for understanding the larger world's similarities and differences. These provide individuals with ways to view their health and illness. Health professionals are learning more about ways in which these larger contexts or worlds or environments influence wellness and disease. Things that shape or impinge on the family (e.g., resources, time, relationships, culture) affect health and illness of individual members. Nurses have unique opportunities to help others understand these global influences on local life.

Science and Technology

Science and technology are huge drivers of global change and have greatly developed our understanding of health and illness. Health professions science, including nursing science, has generated multiple perspectives about health and illness. Florence Nightingale was the original champion of nursing science, focusing on the effects of environment on health. Box 1.1 provides a brief biography of Florence Nightingale. Starting with Nightingale's work, research has shown us that health is determined not only genetically but also by the environment, which has considerable influence. Her work greatly revolutionized ideas about the ways nursing should be practiced. Maybe we should ask: What would Florence Nightingale do if she faced the science and technology of this time? Would she accept things as they are or would she challenge those in leadership and suggest some innovative approaches to the care needs of today's populations?

Health care–related knowledge has greatly influenced health care professionals' education—shifting the focus from memorization and merely becoming informed to being

---

BOX 1-1

Florence Nightingale

Florence Nightingale (1820–1910) is considered to be the founder of the nursing profession and sets a fine example for nurses and all who wish to improve world conditions. She used scientific thinking to lead changes in health and illness care. Unusual in Victorian times, she considered the environmental effects on health and emphasized hygiene and good nutrition. During her long life she looked at poverty and disease scientifically and holistically, laying the foundation for modern methods of education and practice. She used statistics to prove her theories and was highly skilled in working with community and political leaders for social reform and public policy advocacy. In her day much of the sick care took place at home and she wrote letters, articles, and books containing detailed instructions for creating nutrition and healing environments. She continues to be a powerful role model, especially because of her effective ways of promoting the empowerment of women to activism for the poor and neglected in society.

---

able to access information, analyze it, and make critical decisions about its use (Frenk et al., 2010). Nurses need skills to search for scientific evidence about the effectiveness of care or interventions and identify the best ways to alleviate problems. Evidence-based practice is the language used as nurses and others determine the best course of action to care for a particular disease. Table 1.1 provides the progression of steps used in implementing evidence-based practice.

TABLE 1-1   *Moving Forward in Evidence-Based Practice*

The first step is always to develop a clear question about what you want to know. Without a question to clearly guide your investigation, you will not be able to secure the forms of evidence needed to identify the best nursing practices. A search must consider differences between good and bad information and identify the highest level of evidence.

1. Define and clearly articulate the information needed to answer a specific question. If your question pertains to family nursing, then you must be sure to include the word *family* in your search.
2. Identify and choose appropriate sources of information relevant to the identified question. You may limit your search by years, journals, language, or other factors. A reference librarian can assist you.
3. Develop and use clear and effective search strategies using predetermined terms. These terms need to be linked with your question.
4. Locate and retrieve all information that appears relevant to your question. At first you gather everything that seems connected to the question you have asked.
5. Appraise the information retrieved and evaluate its usefulness. You will usually want the latest information that comes from the most credible sources.
6. Organize and analyze the information pertinent to your specific question.
7. Determine if any important facts relevant to the question asked are still missing (e.g., economics, legal, social, policy). If important aspects are missing, then you will need to do additional searches.
8. Synthesize or combine all of your findings in ways that best answer the initial question asked.
9. Determine the strength of the evidence used to answer the question asked. The strength of evidence rests in the quality and type of research efforts used.
10. Decide whether evidence identified is strong enough to alter practice or if more information is still needed.

Today nurses cannot simply know the steps of a procedure or intervention; they also need to know the intended effects and outcomes. Advances in communication, technologies, and global knowledge can help nurses consider the best ways to use evidence to solve problems. They need to consider several factors that can influence health:

- Environmental or geographical influences
- Where care is delivered (e.g., home, hospital, nursing home, health department)
- The places where individuals and families live

The knowledge and information explosion has not only advanced science and technology, but also influenced the ways individuals and families seek health care services and interact with health care professionals. Medical knowledge is no longer isolated, but is readily available to all persons through the Internet. Some people are very knowledgeable about health and illness, but others are clueless. Many know their rights, ask questions, make demands, have high expectations, and want to be partners in their health care experiences. Nurses need effective communication, collaboration, and advocacy skills to partner effectively with those seeking care (Hook, 2006; McCloughen, Gillies, & O'Brien, 2011; Mitchell, Chaboyer, Burmeister, & Foster, 2009).

Natural Resources and Environment

Environmental changes, whether natural or produced by civilization, are increasingly being linked with health and illness. A new awareness of humankind's effect on the planet's food, water, energy, and environmental resources is emerging. According to the Natural Resources Defense Council (NRDC, 2011), a nonprofit environmental action group, climate change affects health in six ways: air pollution, extreme heat, infectious disease, drought, flooding, and extreme weather. Children, the elderly, and the poor are most vulnerable to health problems due to climate change (United States Global Change Research Program, 2009). Where people live matters! For example, air pollution is worsened in rising heat. When the number and intensity of "bad air" days are increased, threats for persons with asthma and other respiratory tract conditions are also increased. Box 1.2 provides information about ways families can protect themselves against air pollution health threats.

BOX 1-2

Tips to Protect Against Air Pollution Health Threats

- Check news reports on the radio, TV, or online for pollen reports or daily air quality conditions. Or visit the Environmental Protection Agency's Air Now Web site [http://www.airnow.gov/] for air quality information.
- If you or someone in your family has allergies or asthma, on days when pollen or ozone smog levels are high, minimize outdoor activity and keep your windows closed.
- Shower after spending time outdoors to wash off pollen that may have collected on your skin or hair.
- Wash bedding and vacuum frequently to remove pollen that may settle in sheets and carpets.

Source: Natural Resources Defense Council (n.d., Air pollution). Adapted from Hunter, A., & Crabtree, K. 2011. Global health and international opportunities. In J. M. Stanley (Ed.), *Advanced practice nursing: Emphasizing common roles* (3rd ed., pp 327–350). Philadelphia: F. A. Davis.

Global Infectious Disease Threats

According to the World Health Organization (WHO, 2011), in 2008, 4 of the top 10 causes of death in low- and middle-income countries were infectious diseases compared to 1 of the top 10 in high-income countries. New and reemerging infectious diseases pose threats to human health globally and cause costly periodic disruptions in trade and commerce, political instability in developing nations, and tensions in developed nations (National Intelligence Council [NIC], 2000). The threat of increased infectious diseases is influenced by several factors:

- Food contamination, potentially from worldwide importation of food products
- Infections acquired while hospitalized (nosocomial infections)
- Increased use of antibiotics causing resistant organisms
- Increases in international travel
- Immigration
- Return of military or other personnel from overseas assignments (NIC, 2000)

Infectious Illness

The most common infectious illness to affect travelers is diarrhea from foodborne or waterborne organisms (WHO, 2012a). Some vaccines are available that can be taken before travel to prevent an infection. In the past decade, increased travel resulted in national concerns about epidemic bedbug infestations at low-budget and upscale hotels. However, bedbugs are found everywhere (e.g., airplanes, subways, movie theaters, locker rooms, stores, even hospitals). They reproduce quickly, can live for a long while without feeding, and even the cleanest persons are susceptible. These bugs can be transported into households in luggage and then affect entire families.

New strains of influenza get introduced through exposure to infected individuals. Those with severe influenza and coexisting chronic illnesses may require admission to the intensive care unit and are at increased risk of dying. Nurses need to be prepared to identify and intervene with those at greatest risk for poor health outcomes and consider implications for family, household, and community risks.

Use of Antibiotics

A longtime concern is the inappropriate use of antibiotics to treat infections that have resulted in the growth of microorganisms resistant to drug therapy (Lehne, 2013). One example is multidrug-resistant tuberculosis (TB). According to the WHO (2012b) Tuberculosis Fact Sheet, about 8.8 million new and relapsed cases of TB were reported in 2010. In 2010, an estimated 1.4 million people died from TB. Dr. Paul Farmer details his experience of the TB epidemic among the people of Haiti in the book *Mountains Beyond Mountains* (Kidder, 2003). Rather than base his treatment of drug-resistant TB on the approach of utilitarianism (i.e., what is good for the many outweighs what is good for the one), he focused on treating TB one case at a time—working with the individual and the family living with the infected person. Evidence showed that caring for the one person and those sharing the dwelling, rather than the many, positively influenced health outcomes. His results altered conventional thinking about the best way to treat TB when resources are limited.

Proper use of antibiotics includes the following recommendations:

- Use antibiotics when prescribed.
- Complete the full prescription.
- Throw away unused drugs.

- Do not share medicines.
- Use antibiotics only for bacterial illnesses, not viral infections.

It is estimated that as many as 50% of prescriptions written for antibiotic use may be unnecessary (Hicks, 2013) and that antibiotics are so widely prescribed because patients demand them. The result is the growth of antibiotic-resistant bacteria. For example, infection with MRSA (methicillin-resistant *Staphylococcus aureus*) has long been known to be a threat to the sick and the elderly and continues to be a growing problem. A new form of superbacteria known as CRE (carbapenem-resistant Enterobacteriaceae), a life-threatening bacterium resistant to most antibiotics, is also a growing problem (Centers for Disease Control and Prevention, 2013). CRE appears to have the capacity to transfer resistance to other bacteria that normally would not be much of a threat. This bacterium is easily transferred through physical contact, is often found in hospitals and long-term care facilities, and is a risk for those in compromised physical conditions. Family members can introduce infectious diseases to each other if they are not aware of good hand washing and isolation techniques.

The spread of infectious diseases results from changes in human behavior—lifestyle changes, such as those occurring at the individual and family level. Nurses, as educators, can play huge roles in facilitating lifestyle changes linked with wellness and prevention.

The Global Economy, Globalization, and Health Care

We often hear the term *global economy* in the world of business and learn about its influence on the daily lives of people from various nations. The term *globalization* refers to the increasing commercial trade among countries and includes exchange of ideas, language, peoples, and popular culture. Globalization implies that human exchanges occur in ways that are increasingly more integrated, open, and without borders.

Global threats from infectious diseases are serious world health concerns. For example, ebola has been known since the 1970s but recent outbreaks have spread and have had high mortality in low-resourced countries. However, in countries with good health care systems, early identification, tracking contacts, targeted isolation precautions, and excellent care of infected individuals has produced good results. Disease spread is no longer just confined to small communities, but presents global and international challenges.

Globalization and the Medical Workforce

Globalization in health care is also occurring. The U.S. Bureau of Labor Statistics recently reported that the job growth in the health care sector accounts for one out of every five jobs created. In 2010, about 209,000 primary care physicians or about one third of all U.S. physicians managed 51.3% of all clinical visits (Agency for Healthcare Research and Quality [AHRQ], 2011). About half the business went to one third of the physicians—those in primary care. According to the American Academy of Family Physicians, primary care is defined as the care provided by physicians specifically trained for and skilled in comprehensive first contact and continuing care for those with undiagnosed symptoms, signs, or concerns. This care form includes health promotion or maintenance, disease prevention, education, diagnosis, and treatment of acute and chronic illness. Primary care occurs in a variety of settings (e.g., physician office, inpatient care, long-term care, ambulatory care). Others also provide primary care (i.e., nurse practitioners, physician assistants). The need for registered nurses is expected to grow from 2.74 million in 2010 to 3.45 million by 2020 (Squires, 2012). In 2011, the number of nurse practitioners reached 180,233 and some projections expect that number will double by 2025 (Pearson Report, 2011). Likewise, the number of physician assistants is likely to continue to grow, with projections reaching 127,821 by 2025 (Hooker, Cawley, & Everett, 2011). Geographical distribution of primary care providers is uneven, with far more of these primary care professionals practicing in urban than rural regions.

Nurses share similar educational standards, but such factors as educational preparation, regulation, credentials, licenses, entry into practice, and clinical practice vary considerably among nations. Across nations, pathways for becoming a nurse, practice expectations, and care delivery vary. For example, midwifery is viewed as a separate profession in Australia, but it is a nursing specialty in the United States. Foreign-educated nurses often face huge challenges as they transition into U.S. health care employment settings (e.g., differences in practice, language barriers, procedures for medication administration, use of technology).

Levels of Nursing Education

Interest in having nurses attain higher levels of education continues to grow with the aim that the nursing force's knowledge and skill level will keep increasing. Dr. Catherine Gilliss was one of the first nurse leaders to sound the alarm that nursing practice should include the family unit and not just the individual (Box 1.3). Yet, little research has been done to determine the presence of family nursing in nursing programs. An older U.S. study of Bachelor of Science in Nursing (BSN) programs found that students were inclined to study some things about family nursing, but the amount, type, and content varied widely (Hanson, Heims, & Julian, 1992). A Canadian study (Wright & Bell, 1989) had similar findings with gaps found in family intervention and interview skills. A more recent study of graduate education for family nurse practitioners found that while these students obtained some education about family in their core courses, students were not usually expected to complete family assessments or plan interventions for the family unit when taking clinical practicum courses (Nyirati, Denham, Raffle, & Ware, 2012).

BOX 1-3

Family Tree

Catherine Gilliss, DNSc, RN, FAAN (United States)

Catherine Gilliss is the Helene Fuld Health Trust Professor, Dean of Duke University School of Nursing, and Vice Chancellor for Nursing Affairs at Durham, North Carolina. She is a graduate of Duke's undergraduate nursing program and is the first alumna from the School of Nursing to hold the position of Dean. Dr. Gilliss earned a Bachelor of Science in Nursing degree from Duke and a Master of Science in Nursing degree from the Catholic University of America. After earning an adult nurse practitioner (ANP) certificate from the University of Rochester, she went on to the University of California at San Francisco, where she earned a Doctor of Nursing Science (DNSc) degree and completed a postdoctoral fellowship. Dr. Gilliss also holds honorary degrees from Yale University and the University of Portland. Her illustrious career has been devoted to graduate nursing education, with a scientific focus on the family and chronic illness. Her research has investigated the experience of family members in the context of illness; the impact of innovative models of nursing intervention on situations that affect the family and its members; and the development and synthesis of scientific work in this area of nursing science. She has received many awards, including the Yale School of Nursing Medal, and has been recognized by the International Society for Family Nursing with its Lifetime Achievement in Research Award. Dr. Gilliss's contributions to the science of family nursing have revolutionized research in this field and have strongly influenced care for chronically ill patients and their families. Her scholarly works are considered groundbreaking and several are preeminent resources for junior and senior nurse scientists.

Global Spending for Health Care Costs

Worldwide health care costs continue to accelerate, and the distribution of resources is not always equitable. But how much money is truly spent, what goods and services are bought, and what characterizes the real quality or value of what is bought are not easy to determine. In economics, usually scarce quantities produce high demands and high costs, but adequate or abundant supplies decrease demand and cost. These principles do not work when it comes to health care costs. Even though the health market keeps increasing availability, costs have not been reduced. Health care spending and costs are a result of millions of private, corporate, employer, and government decisions. The cost-benefit ratios of medical expense compared to clinical outcomes are difficult to evaluate. The supply and use of diagnostic imaging devices are important, but the cost and use of technologies vary greatly (Squires, 2012). Table 1.2 provides a view of the use and cost for two machines.

Growing evidence shows that well-educated nurses have an impact on health care outcomes and costs, but nurses are often at risk for being cut during an economic downturn (Kavanagh, Cimiotti, Abusalem, & Coty, 2012). Hospital care is a large part of the U.S. health care system and nurses are the largest direct care providers. Adequate nurse staffing improves safety and quality, decreases infection rates, lowers mortality rates, and decreases adverse events, length of stay, and other things. Despite these savings, nurses are a large expense to hospitals. Models that demonstrate the value of nursing care as a financial incentive need to be implemented and effectiveness of nursing care made visible to society (Kavanagh et al., 2012).

Global Changes in Demographics

Major demographic changes are occurring worldwide, especially in the more advanced nations. Population growth is slowing, numbers of youth are decreasing as a result of lower fertility rates, and numbers of elderly are rising as people live longer. Migration, immigration, and global travel are part of this picture. Families are moving away from the villages and cultures of their youth. Global changes not only affect the workforce, economics, and politics of individuals living in different geographical regions, but they also influence the health and illness concerns of families and the larger society.

TABLE 1-2	Diagnostic Imaging Device Use and Cost for Selected Countries		
COUNTRY	NUMBER OF MACHINES PER 1 MILLION POPULATION	NUMBER OF EXAMINATIONS PER 1,000 POPULATION	AVERAGE COST PER EXAMINATION
United States	25.9 MRI machines	91.2	$1,080
France	6.5 MRI machines	55.2	$281
United States	34.3 CT scanners	227.9	$510
Canada	13.9 CT scanners	125.4	$122

CT, computed tomography; MRI, magnetic resonance imaging.
Source: Adapted from Squires, D. A. (2012, May). Explaining high health spending in the United States: An international comparison of supply, utilization, prices, and quality. Issues in international health. The Commonwealth Fund pub. 1595, Vol. 10. Retrieved May 6, 2012 from http://www.commonwealthfund.org/~/media/Files/Publications/Issue%20Brief/2012/May/1595_Squires_explaining_high_hlt_care_spending_intl_brief.pdf

Changing World Demographics

Trends in birth, death, migration, and immigration patterns point toward population growth in Asia and Africa that will result in those places becoming the "youthful" areas of the world. The population in developed parts of the world (e.g., United States, Canada, European countries) will effectively age so that people under age 30 will make up less than one third of the population (NIC, 2008). Populations of India, China, and countries in sub-Saharan Africa are expected to grow the most (NIC, 2008). Countries such as the United States, Canada, and Australia, with high immigration rates, will also grow, but at lesser rates. Generally, life expectancy at birth has increased steadily over past decades so that, in 2009, the average life expectancy at birth for the global population was 68 (WHO, 2011). In 2009, the lowest life expectancy at birth was 47 years (in Malawi) while the highest was 83 years (Japan and San Marino). Aging populations can also mean decreased family incomes as huge numbers of people retire (NIC, 2008). More resources will likely be needed to support pensions and health care costs of the elderly. This expense could mean fewer dollars are available for education, care of the environment, and national defense. Furthermore, an implication of a "youth bulge" in many parts of the undeveloped world is increased risk for the emergence of political violence and civil conflict (NIC, 2008). The World Health Organization (2009) predicts that men between the ages of 15 and 60 years have much higher risks of dying from injuries, violence, conflict, and heart disease than women in this age category.

Effects of Place on Health and Illness

Where people live matters. Living and working conditions such as overcrowded housing, lack of adequate sanitation, and unsafe working conditions are called social determinants of health. These factors arise from the social or physical environment and can lead to health problems. Living conditions influence not only individual health and illness but also health of the family unit. Young adults from rural communities keep moving into urban dwellings. Small rural communities are often populated with the very old and very young, groups more susceptible to ill health and identified as vulnerable populations.

Urbanization partly contributes to a widening gap between the rich and the poor. Poverty is extensive throughout the world with major concerns still linked with Africa, Asia, and other places. Over half the world's people live on $2.50 or less per day, and 27% to 28% of children in southern Asia or sub-Saharan Africa are underweight or stunted in growth (Shah, 2010). According to the WHO (2011c), around the world, 33 countries have more than 80% of their people living in urban areas. Worldwide, one in three urban dwellers lives in slums or poor settlements that can lead to increased health inequities and broad health disparities. As population demographics change, the risks for various health problems affecting individuals and families also change. For instance, morbidity and mortality rates from infectious diseases (e.g., pneumonia, diarrhea) are higher in undeveloped countries. As countries develop, more improvements in medical care, fewer deaths from easily curable diseases, and public health interventions (e.g., immunizations, clean water, sanitation) occur (WHO, 2009). This change often means that morbidity and mortality statistics in developed countries are most likely the result of noncommunicable diseases (e.g., cardiovascular disease, cancers).

Traditional risks for disease tend to affect low-income populations and are linked with poverty, inadequate nutrition, unsafe water, poor sanitation and hygiene, unsafe sex, and indoor smoke from solid fuels (WHO, 2009). These risks are in sharp contrast to problems that threaten health in higher-income countries, where modern disease risks include overweight, obesity, physical inactivity, tobacco, and substance abuse. Some nations are fighting both traditional and modern disease risks as length of life increases and noncommunicable

---

BOX 1-4

Family Tree

Shirley Hanson, PhD, RN, ARNP/PMHP (United States)

Dr. Shirley Hanson is professor emeritus from Oregon Health Sciences University, School of Nursing. Dr. Hanson has written, coauthored, and edited more than 150 books, chapters, articles, CDs, and various other reports pertaining to families and nursing. Her work centers on fathers/fatherhood, single-parent families, and family assessment and intervention. Her work on the future of family nursing in the United States has been critical to the development of family nursing as a discipline and has contributed to the body of knowledge in family social science. Dr. Hanson's co-authored textbook for undergraduate and graduate nursing students, *Family Health Care Nursing: Theory, Practice and Research*, first published in 1996, is now in its fifth edition. The text has been translated into Japanese and Portuguese and has been adapted by a group of family nurses in Scotland. Dr. Hanson's many contributions to nursing in the area of family were recognized when she was inducted in 1984 as a fellow in the American Academy of Nursing (FAAN), one of the highest honors for nursing leaders in the United States. In 2001, Dr. Hanson was inducted as a fellow of the National Council on Family Relations in recognition of her many contributions in service, publications, research, and practice with families and family social science. In 2007, Dr. Hanson was recognized by the International Family Nursing Conference in Bangkok, Thailand, with the Lifetime Achievement Award for her distinguished contribution to family nursing.

---

diseases become a major cause of death (WHO, 2009). Risks exposure can be addressed with public health interventions. For example, enacting strong tobacco-control policies or air pollution public health policies helps avoid high levels of disease. Nurses who understand large environmental and place-linked risk factors are prepared to improve population, family, and individual health. Dr. Shirley Hanson authored one of the leading nursing textbooks used by students around the world to study family nursing (Box 1.4).

Changing Family Demographics

Observing diverse families provides insight into the ways families and relationships change over time. Some changes are now seen in mother and extended family roles, the time children spend in school, the age at which retirement is expected, and the years lived alone. Issues such as fewer two-parent families, high divorce rates, cohabitation, remarriage, mixed-race marriages, and civil unions have altered some family foundations that stood for generations. Family alterations could cause both negative and positive results. New ideas about family households, intergenerational care forms, housing and living arrangements, more integrated family values, benefits of intergenerational households, and wider sustainable networks arising from different partnerships could arise. Societal changes often evolve from the needs of individuals and families. Family responses to societal trends influence social and public policies. Factors such as taxation, education, social institutions, travel, and housing are linked with families. A nation's health is solidly vested in its people and families.

Presently, a definition of the family from an international perspective is not available. This inability to define family in global terms presents problems in terms of immigration, migration, and even health care. Understanding family offers a way to understand the larger units of societies. Today, many family units do not live under the same roof. Growing numbers of people are living alone (e.g., single room occupancy hotels, assisted living facilities, nursing homes). Social isolation for those who are frail, elderly, poor, and vulnerable presents concerns. In the United States, more adult children currently live with their parents than at any time since the 1950s. The term *accordion families* is used to describe the ways members move in and out of households. The 2010 census data found that 27% of people live in one-person households compared to 25% in 2000 and only 13% in 1960, trends not seen in less developed countries with families that are primarily traditional extended family households.

Racial, ethnic, gender, and other factors linked with family types are important considerations when considering demographics. In 2012, in the United States, Child Trends (2013) reports that 33% of black children lived with two parents as compared to 85% of Asian children, 75% of white children, and 60% of Hispanic children. However, 2010 census data indicate that 66% of all children under 18 years are living with two parents, down from 69% in 2000. Data show that 40.4% of co-resident grandparents had primary care responsibility for grandchildren with 20.2% of these grandparents living in poverty and about 14% having English language challenges (Murphey, Cooper, & Moore, 2012). The 2010 census identified that the median age at first marriage for men was 28.2 and women 26.1, a long-time upward trend noted since the mid-1950s. Additionally, the overall percentage of those married was 48.4% in 2010 compared with 51.7% in 2000. Finally, recorded same-sex households increased from 0.3% in 2000 to 0.6% in 2010, a small percentage increase, but this growing sector raises questions about the ways people identify family. In the United States, family type often has profound effects on the family's income and each member's access to health insurance.

Family Migration

Families have always migrated in one sense or another. Today's families often relocate for similar reasons as in the past. Employment opportunities, income, and the need to care for an ill family member are often leading reasons. Migration may vary based upon personal factors, but most people move where increased opportunity seems likely. It is common to find committed couples or families that live apart from each other. The geographical proximity of family has implications across the family life cycle, as nearness and distance are important factors for child and elder care. An interesting factor linked with parental and elder care has to do with siblings; siblings are more likely to live further away from parents than only children (Rainer & Siedler, 2010). This factor could influence parental caregiving roles.

International Families

Changes in international families suggest trends to be considered. For example, fertility rates are a key aspect of family structures and are declining worldwide (Central Intelligence Agency [CIA], 2012). Birth rates indicate that total population is increasing to more than replace the parental generation. Births range from an estimated high of 7.5 children per woman in the country of Niger to a low of 0.78 births per woman in Singapore. The United States has an estimated fertility rate of 2.06 children per woman (CIA, 2012). Many humanitarian projects aim to support child spacing to improve maternal and child health outcomes and potentially create more stable families. Marriage rates, cohabitation, and divorce can affect their adequacy in meeting member health and illness needs. Population customs and characteristics influence unique family needs. Religious beliefs, personal values, and international traditions also affect families (Fig. 1.1).

Wealth and Health

Growing evidence suggests that wealth and health go together (Braveman, Egerter, & Barclay, 2011), and it is widely accepted that higher incomes mean longer lives. Therefore, families

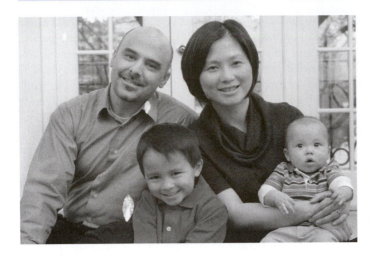

FIGURE 1-1 An international family.

with greater economic resources are most likely to have greater health and a higher quality of life. For example, in 2009, persons in families living in the poorest communities had 1,420 hospitalizations per 10,000 population for all ages combined, compared with 1,189 of those living in wealthier communities (Healthcare Cost and Utilization Project [HCUP], 2011). Being able to afford health insurance and medical care is not the only factor that influences health and well-being. Family income influences the neighborhoods where families live, level of safety in daily lives, access to good education, availability of nutritious food, access to various forms of leisure activities, and member health. Standards of living vary from place to place across the globe. In 2012, the Department of Health and Human Services Poverty Guidelines identified that an annual income below $23,050 for a U.S. family of four is below the poverty level. In 2007, the richest 1% of U.S. households held one-third of the nation's total wealth and the richest 5% held more than half (Kennickell, 2009). Links between wealth and health begin early in life. Low birth weight is linked to developmental delays and challenges and chronic conditions. Children born in lower income families have higher rates of asthma, heart conditions, hearing problems, and digestive disorders (Braveman et al. 2011). Health equity is a concern when some have so much and others so little. Thus, it is important to realize that equality can be more of a myth than a reality for many individuals and families.

Health Care Trend Influences on Nursing Practice

Current health care trends have critical implications for individuals and families; those of concern to the larger society or population also affect individuals and families. Trends also shape the ways in which health care services are made available, how these services are provided, and the clinical practices of the workforce. Even without being aware of personal connections, we are all more closely related than we realize. People in small towns or rural communities easily recognize these connections as extended family lives nearby, but those living in urban settings may not. In today's global society, the lives of all people and places are interconnected, interdependent, and complex. Nurses need to be aware of these relationships and identify the health and illness implications of an intricately linked world even when things do not appear directly related at a point in time.

Gender and Health Risks

Gender is an issue of concern when it comes to health. Women's rights are an important way to understand personal well-being. In the United States, women's suffrage fought for and only gained the right to vote in 1920. An affirmative action policy that covered discrimination based on gender was added to a previous 1964 Civil Rights Act in 1967. This policy ensured American women and minorities the same educational and employment opportunities as white males. During the 1960s and 1970s, the feminist movement waged war for women's rights in the workplace. By the late 20th century and early 21st century, greater equality has spread with pay for men and women becoming more equal. In the United States, the American Civil Liberties Union continues to fight for equal opportunity for women in areas of education, the workplace, gender-based violence, and harms to women in the criminal justice system. Nursing, a largely female discipline, has also been affected by these long and continued battles.

It is now widely understood that when nations lack health care infrastructure and opportunities for a full education, the poor and women suffer the most. For thousands of years, gender roles have been socially constructed and beliefs aligned with biology have driven religious and traditional practices. Gender inequality often means that women are unable to overcome poverty and have less ability to raise healthy and well-educated sons and daughters. Women worldwide are often the targets of physical and sexual violence, genital mutilation, and many other forms of cruelty. Poverty is often the fate of women, who represent two thirds of the world's poor. Across the globe, gender equality is a battle still being fought in many places. The battle to improve women's rights to live full and productive lives, decrease maternal health risks, increase choice in family planning, and combat issues linked with HIV/AIDS and other diseases is still being fought. Nurses can advocate for gender equality.

Noncommunicable Disease

The focus for many nursing students and nurses has largely been acute care, in which they attend to patient problems or diseases. In addition, the Hollywood depiction of a nurse as rescuer in times of critical need doesn't address the complex family stories linked with health and illness. According to the United Nations (2012), noncommunicable diseases cause 36 million deaths worldwide in a decade, a number that accounts for 63% of all deaths. These conditions often result from cumulative lifestyle factors (e.g., tobacco use, lack of adequate nutrition, physical inactivity, substance abuse). When individuals and family units have unhealthy lifestyles, then it is likely that they will have a disproportionate number of deaths from noncommunicable diseases. Growing numbers of elderly persons are at risk, 20% or more of the population in developed countries is 60 years of age or over, and 80% of all deaths are currently attributed to noncommunicable diseases (United Nations, 2012). If nurses fail to focus on individual and family lifestyles, then the care needed to support their health and wellness will likely be neglected.

Taking a Proactive Stance

Nurses can take action before something goes wrong. A proactive nurse is concerned about wellness, health promotion, and prevention, which are strong predictors of health and illness outcomes, and can help influence the daily lives of individuals and family members. Proactive nurses can use nursing actions to not only address critical acute needs, but think beyond the present and help individuals and families prevent future problems. They ask questions and think outside the box of usual care to address family household, adequacy of supports, availability of needed resources, and access to needed information during care delivery and they use evidence and competencies to satisfy patient and family needs. Nurses can help individuals and families by listening, answering questions, becoming partners in care, and addressing home and community needs.

Noncommunicable diseases should challenge the way nurses think about how nursing care is organized and delivered. These diseases are linked with lifestyle changes, urbanization, and globalization. Costs of these diseases pose economic burdens for individuals, families, and larger societies related to absenteeism, disability, lost income, and even bankruptcy. Medication costs for some conditions can be equivalent to several days' wages. Those without health insurance or with inadequate finances might forfeit the medications and increase their risks for catastrophic illness or even early death. Thoughtful nurses see beyond the acute phase, note possible causative factors, and weigh potential needs and risks linked with discharge. Proactive nurses know that families can greatly influence the ways individual members manage needed lifestyles at home.

Practicing Nursing and Thinking Family

Nursing practice applies science and art to everyday real-life problems that influence health, wellness, illness, and disease. It is more than just identifying problems and fixing them; it is also recognizing that problems exist in larger systems (e.g., households, worksites, social domains). Nurses help those seeking care find ways to prevent, manage, and resolve problems. Nurses treat, educate, counsel, coach, minister to, advocate for, direct, assist, and support. Some of the work of skilled nurses can get done without requiring much critical thought. However, other nursing actions must be intentional and should include reflection that evaluates whether what was accomplished is most desirable. Holistic nursing care considers unique needs and values. Nurses help those seeking care find ways to prevent, manage, and resolve problems (Box 1.5).

Families as Allies

To communicate effectively with multiple family persons about the needs of a member, nurses need skills that prepare them to facilitate care that involves the whole of individuals' lives. Too often, family support persons are merely handed a patient handbook with a reading level too high for them to understand or information is given in impersonal ways without considering specific recipient needs. Family members do not always know what they should ask or expect as they may have never experienced this situation before. Families do not expect errors or mistakes because they want to believe things are under control and everyone knows what they are doing. However, family members are often fearful, extremely stressed, unclear about the complexities linked with a condition, and unclear about what should happen or when. Telling individuals and families what to expect and when things will happen can create allies who may be helpful in preventing mistakes along the way and delivering care that better meets needs.

Throughout this textbook, you will find the idea of *thinking family* is continually used as a form of reference for caring for every individual met in a health care delivery setting or system. Nurses who *think family* understand ways in which the larger social context and current trends affect individuals, family lives, and family health. These relationships can be used to inquire about needs, connect with persons, listen, and respond in valued ways as care is received (Doane & Varcoe, 2005). An important aspect of nursing care is the time given to hear the voiced needs. Nurses who *think family* seek the voices of others and take time to listen.

BOX 1-5

Evidence-Based Family Nursing Practice

Illness Beliefs Model

Creating a context for changing beliefs about illness can be difficult, and these concerns constitute the foundation of the Illness Beliefs Model. The first thing to consider is the way in which the nurse meets an individual and the impression formed within the first few minutes of the meeting. Show genuine interest and desire to collaborate by taking the temperature of the relationship while preparing for a therapeutic conversation. Knowing the diagnosis alone is not enough; the nurse must also understand the ways illness has affected lives. It is useful to learn about illness suffering, beliefs about diagnosis, causative factors, and beliefs about healing and prognosis. Many things can enter into the experience of living with an illness. An important role of the nurse is to ask questions that identify actions to be taken. Nurses can also speak the unspeakable, offer alternative ideas, and offer commendations. If it is possible to use a reflective clinical team, they may offer additional ideas for families to consider. The family can then respond to the new ideas and identification of any new beliefs that emerge can be recognized. Recognizing family strengths and acknowledging their suffering can invite new energy and a positive direction. Immersion in practice with families needs to be observable. Two things stand out about family practice:

- Expert practice with families needs to be visible, measured, synthesized, and mentored.
- Processes and outcomes of family nursing practice are messy and complicated.

Through intensive immersion at the Family Nursing Unit at the University of Calgary, clinical scholarship allowed many nurse researchers to examine and describe the family practice. Over the years, many masters and doctoral students completed practicums in the family unit and seven doctoral students, one post-doctoral fellow, and two visiting scholars working with faculty conducted research about family nursing practice. Study findings, in turn, reflected changes in practice. The term *family systems nursing* was coined to signify care for the family unit as opposed to the term *family nursing*, which had mainly focused on individuals.

The Illness Beliefs Model strongly identifies the strength of beliefs to influence behaviors and responses to them when it comes to suffering. Beliefs of individuals, family members, health providers, and society all come into play when an illness diagnosis occurs. Knowledge creation and knowledge transfer for family nursing practice are still needed. Recommendations for change require action in several areas: create innovative opportunities for systems changes from the top down, create family nursing teams and harness their energy for practice changes, learn from the practice knowledge already identified, and keep your eye on what you as a nurse bring to nursing practice. Family nursing is first about change in nurses as they become more curious, less judgmental, and more open to others' realities.

_____

Source: Bell, J. M., & Wright, L. M. (2011). The Illness Beliefs Model creating practice knowledge in family systems nursing for families experiencing illness. In E. K. Svavarsdottir & H. Jonsdottir (Eds.), *Family nursing in action* (pp 15–51). Reykjavik, Iceland: University of Iceland Press.

Individuals Are Family Members

When nurses isolate individuals from families, it is like taking an amputee's prosthesis and asking him to walk. As students, nurses spend much time learning the science of nursing and ways to use evidence and become experts at delivering nursing care. But they need to guard against believing that they are also the experts on what individuals and families perceive that they need. Nurses need to be willing to hear from individuals and families about their bodies, lives, and experiences. Great inequities exist and not everyone, even those with the same diagnosis, seeks or needs care in the same way. Expectations differ and if all care is delivered in uniform ways without respect for unique needs then critical concerns can be overlooked.

Health and illness occur within the context of daily life, lives that are outside the view of nurses and other health care providers. A brief visit of 10 to 15 minutes with health care providers is often inadequate to ascertain all the issues linked with complicated lives and problems. When nurses *think family*, they reflect about the connections between individuals and families. They realize that any health alteration of a member, young or old, affects the family unit. Nurses who *think family* recognize that people live connected and interdependent lives and support by family members can vary. Nurses' attitudes and actions have potential to shape experiences in negative and positive ways. Families require skills, information, and answers to questions to successfully care for individual needs.

Recognizing Family and Community Links in Nursing Care

The culture, tradition, and history of a geographical place influence the lives of those living there in health and illness. Nurses living or employed in particular geographical areas must be attuned to the benefits and risks of place that might impinge on health and create risks.

Coordinated Care: An Important Family Nursing Role

Care coordination ensures that individual needs and preferences for health services and information are met (National Quality Forum, 2010). While not the same, care is sometimes used interchangeably with terms such as case management and disease management. Table 1.3 shows the differences in these terms and nurses' roles. Nurses who *think family* assume important roles with individuals and families and can take leadership in three important caregiving areas:

- Care management
- Disease management
- Care coordination

BOX 1-6

Family Circle

While working as a care coordinator in an inner city community clinic, Nurse Jones has been caring for Maria and her 2-year-old daughter Natalie for more than a year. Natalie has been admitted to the hospital three times in the past 6 months because of asthma that did not resolve with ongoing medications and nebulization treatments at home. These hospitalizations are very costly for Maria, who has to miss work when Natalie is ill. They are also very frightening for both mother and child. Nurse Jones has worked with Maria and Natalie to be sure that the medications are correct. Nurse Jones decides to arrange for a home visit to assist this family in preventing further episodes. When Nurse Jones arrives at Maria and Natalie's apartment, she sees that a city bus stop is located right outside. When looking around the windows in the apartment, Nurse Jones observes that Natalie's room is at street level. Maria explains that the noise of the busy street sometimes disturbs their sleep.

1. What do you notice in this situation?
2. Provide two or three alternative explanations for Natalie's current situation of frequent admissions.
3. Discuss the case with a peer and compare interpretations. Discuss actions Nurse Jones can take as she works with this family. Decide on next steps to be taken by the care coordinator.

What resources are available in your community for Maria and Natalie?

As they navigate health care systems to locate and obtain needed care, individuals and families can become frustrated with the barriers they meet. Nurses who *think family* are able to anticipate these needs and provide guidance about needed resources that might be in the community. Review the Family Circle case study and use it as an opportunity to begin thinking about the ways you can include families in your nursing care (Box 1.6)."

Care coordination makes sure that individuals in health care settings get the right care, at the right time, by the right persons. Care coordination involves assessment, planning, implementation, evaluation, monitoring, support, and advocacy so that care is not duplicated, safety is promoted, and medical errors are prevented (Lindeke, Leonard, Presler, & Garwick, 2002). Coordinated care, which includes physician support, health literacy, prevention, and emotional and social support, is most widely used in work with children, especially those with chronic conditions and special care needs, and to a lesser degree with older adults. However, family needs to be included in the care of all sick members, regardless of age. Coordinated care is important to families for all chronic conditions, advanced illness, and end-of-life care and can promote planning, improve satisfaction, and lower costs (Englehardt et al., 2006).

Family-Centered Care Coordination

Models and guidelines to specifically describe cycles of care coordination activities that ensure appropriate and well-coordinated health care have been developed (WHO, 2000). The WHO proposes that a family health nurse, who works with individuals and families in primary health care and public health, be a key contributor to a multidisciplinary health care professional team for the 21st century. The project, called HEALTH21, has three basic values:

1. Health as a fundamental right
2. Equity in health and solidarity in action between countries, between groups of people within countries, and between genders
3. Participation by and accountability of individuals, groups, and communities and of institutions, organizations, and sectors in health development

TABLE 1-3	Comparing Nurse Roles for Care Coordination, Case Management, and Disease Management		
NURSING ROLE	**CASE MANAGEMENT**	**CARE COORDINATION**	**DISEASE MANAGEMENT**
Focus	Care planning, monitoring referrals, resources, risks	Assess, connect, educate, communicate	Engage individuals in appropriate symptom management
Typical techniques	Episodic oversight of care related to illness or disability	Comprehensive ongoing integrated care planning	Disease-specific clinical guidelines, formularies, focused patient education programs, symptom monitoring
Examples	Hospital-based discharge planning	Patient/family-centered medical or health home	Immunization education and tracking; smoking prevention and treatment

The Institute for Healthcare Improvement (IHI) is a vast, multifaceted health care organization improving systems worldwide through a creative range of projects and coalitions. They have established what they broadly refer to as the Triple Aim initiative to pursue three critical objectives for health care design:

- Improve the health of the population.
- Enhance the patient experience (i.e., quality, access, and reliability).
- Reduce or control the per capita cost of care.

Nurses who *think family* ensure that individuals and families are told about the types of support they will need, attend to specific coordinated health care needs, and assist with personal care decisions as needed. The Presler Model of Family-Based Care Coordination (Box 1.7) was tested with 83 families whose children received specialty care for complex health conditions (Nolan, Orlando, & Liptak, 2007). Findings indicated that parents given this form of care greatly appreciated it, became responsible for most aspects of care coordination, and were very satisfied. Nurses who *think family* realize that adults offered similar care would likely respond positively as well.

BOX 1-7

Presler Model of Family-Based Care Coordination

Step 1. Identifying and engaging families that lack care or experience fragmented care

Step 2. Assessing families regarding:

- Needs, concerns, priorities
- Strengths and resources
- Current health/functional status, including health records review
- Need for symptom management, services or resources to improve quality of life
- Access to primary and specialty health services
- Access to health care insurance (public or private)
- Access to therapies, nursing services, durable medical equipment or supplies
- Technology or environmental supports or modifications currently used or needed
- Access to basic resources such as food, housing, transportation, respite
- School/employment placement and satisfaction
- Community inclusion and satisfaction
- Perceived need for care coordination services and desired role of the care coordinator

Step 3. Developing family-centered interdisciplinary/interagency plan of care

- Identifying family preference for care coordinator activities and roles
- Identifying current and future goals and priorities
- Developing comprehensive health services plan that includes:
  - Medical/health care home
  - Specialty care referrals and integration
  - Home health care needs and services
  - School/daycare/employment health services needs
  - Emergency services

Step 4. Implementing the plan of care

- Teaching the family about the importance of health promotion, health condition management and prevention of secondary disabilities
- Teaching the family essential skills for self-advocacy, self-management and care coordination
- Providing resource information

BOX 1-7

Presler Model of Family-Based Care Coordination—cont'd

- Facilitating interdisciplinary and interagency referrals
- Arranging for and coordinating services
- Advocating for and with the family as needed
- Working with third party payers to ensure appropriate access and payment
- Promoting information exchange with community agencies, schools/employers and health systems providers including appropriate health care providers at times of transition
- Preparing for and facilitating transition to systems of care, roles and responsibilities as developmentally appropriate at each encounter

Step 5. Monitoring and evaluating the plan of care

- Assessing individual and family outcomes
- Assessing systems-related outcomes
- Advocating for systems change to improve outcomes
- Providing resource information

Step 6. Disengaging from active care coordination

- Determine individual and family desires and abilities to coordinate care
- Maintain care coordination records
- Periodically assess individual and family's desires or needs for care coordination

If care coordination services are needed, return to Step 2.

Source: Used with permission of B. Presler, PhD, RN, CPNP, APRN.

Families are usually interested in and willing to take part in care delivery but they often lack the knowledge of what to do. Too often, nurses and other health care providers assume they will do what is needed. In the case of both children and adults, if families aren't informed about what needs to be done, the individual and family are inadequately prepared to manage the illness or prevent complications. Rethinking the ways individuals and families are included in care situations should improve service delivery, reduce complications and errors, save money, and increase satisfaction. Family and friends are usually primary care providers for young and old individuals and need nurses prepared to *think family* (Fig. 1.2).

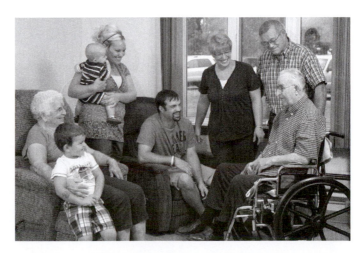

FIGURE 1-2 Nurses include individuals and families in care situations.

Shared Decision Making

Nurses often have competing demands with many decision points during a single workday or shift. Some tasks are purely administrative and others are process decisions about care needs. Nurses who *think family* thoughtfully decide what are the most efficient and optimal ways to spend their time. Nurses who *think family* form therapeutic relationships and advocate for policies and practices that can best address needs of the family unit. For example, policy says an assessment must be completed on every new admission. This generally means a form must be completed that details assessment findings and observations. Nurses who *think family* will effectively use this time to listen to find out the greatest needs of the individuals and families, to see that questions are answered, to give needed support as care is delivered, and to set priorities.

This shared decision making with the families occurs within therapeutic relationships that honor unique individual and family preferences and circumstances. Care options use "decision aids" based on the best available evidence that is presented in clear language so the best choices can be made. An international collection of high-quality decision aids is now available for nurses and others to use, thanks to collaboration between stakeholders from 14 countries in the International Patient Decision Aids Standards Collaboration (IPDAS). IPDAS goals guide individuals and families as they engage in "values clarification" around health, a process integral to the Presler Model of Family-Based Care Coordination and consistent with a family-focused nursing care approach.

When nurses *think family*, multiple members are included in the discussions. The intent is to reach a conclusion whereby individual rights are weighted highly, but consensus from family members who individuals regard as important are included. A number of organizations and agencies offer Web sites and tools for use in shared decision making (e.g., Agency for Healthcare Research and Quality, Cochrane Collaboration, Center for Shared Decision Making, Choosing Wisely, Health News Review, Informed Medical Decisions Foundation, Kaiser Health News, U.S. Preventive Services Task Force). Use of decision-making aids can be helpful for making decisions and helping families make difficult choices.

Chapter Summary

Health care is driven by many factors. Natural disasters, economic disparities, political upheavals, and many other things affect health. Social issues such as poverty, housing, and education along with growing scientific evidence and technology are just a few things that affect health and illness treatment. In a continually changing world picture, nurses are challenged to stay abreast of global influences on current trends. The relationships and interdependence of many factors, social determinants of health, influence health and illness. Individuals live in families and are part of communities. Health care delivery is not always equitable. The places people live have implications for nurses to consider as care is given. Where families live, learn, work, play, and pray influences health needs and illness risks. This chapter introduces some initial ideas about thinking family and why a family-focused approach in nursing is needed. Proactive nurses identify ways to coordinate care between acute care settings, homes, and communities. Florence Nightingale responded to the concerns of her time; what would she do if she were here now?

REFERENCES

Agency for Healthcare Research and Quality. (2011, October). Primary care workforce facts and stats no. 1: The number of practicing primary care physicians in the United States (AHRQ Publication No. 12-P001-2-EF). Rockville, MD: Author. Retrieved from www.ahrq.gov/research/pcwork1.htm

Bell, J. M., & Wright, L. M. (2011). The Illness Beliefs Model creating practice knowledge in family systems nursing for families experiencing illness. In E. K. Svavarsdottir & H. Jonsdottir (Eds.), *Family nursing in action* (pp 15–51). Reykjavik, Iceland: University of Iceland Press.

Braveman, P., Egerter, S., & Barclay, C. (2011, April 1). How social factors shape health: Income, wealth, and health. Princeton, NJ: Robert Wood Johnson Foundation. Retrieved from http://www.rwjf.org/en/research-publications/find-rwjf-research/2011/04/how-social-factors-shape-health1.html

Bureau of Health Professions. (2008). National sample of registered nurses. Washington, DC: Health Resources and Services Administration.

Bureau of Labor Statistics, U.S. Department of Labor. (2012). *Occupational outlook handbook*, 2012–13 ed., Registered nurses. Retrieved from Bureau of Labor Statistics, U.S. Department of Labor Web site: http://www.bls.gov/ooh/healthcare/registered-nurses.htm

California Healthcare Foundation (2012). California Health Care Almanac: Health care costs 101. Retrieved January 7, 2013 from http://www.chcf.org/publications/2012/08/health-care-costs-101

Centers for Disease Control and Prevention. (2013). New CDC vital signs: Lethal, drug-resistant bacteria spreading in U.S. healthcare facilities. Retrieved April 11, 2013 from http://www.cdc.gov/media/dpk/2013/dpk-vs-hai.html

Central Intelligence Agency. (2012). *The world factbook*. Washington, DC: Author. Retrieved on May 8, 2012 from https://www.cia.gov/library/publications/the-world-factbook/rankorder/2127rank.html

Child Trends. (2013). Family structure. Retrieved from Child Trends Data Bank Web site: http://www.childtrendsdatabank.org/alphalist?q=node/334

Doane, G. H. & Varcoe, C. (2005). *Family nursing as relational inquiry: Developing health promoting practice*. Philadelphia: Lippincott Williams & Wilkins.

Englehardt, J. B., McClive-Reed, K. P., Toseland, R. W., Smith, T. L., Larsen, D. G., Tobin, D. R (2006). Effects of a program for coordinated care of advanced illness on patients, surrogates, and healthcare costs: A randomized trial. *The American Journal of Managed Care, 12,* 93–100.

Frenk, J., Chen, L., Bhutta, Z., Cohen, J., Crisp, N., Evans, T., ... Zurayk H. (2010). Health professionals for a new century: Transforming education to strengthen health care systems in an interdependent world. *Lancet, 376,* 1923–1958.

Hanson, S., Heims, M., & Julian, D. (1992). Education for family health care professionals: Nursing as a paradigm. *Family Relations, 41*(1), 49–53.

Healthcare Cost and Utilization Project (HCUP). (November, 2011). HCUP facts and figures 2009. Rockville, MD: Agency for Healthcare Research and Quality. Retrieved May 6, 2012 from http://www.hcup-us.ahrq.gov/reports/factsandfigures/2009/exhibit1_5.jsp

Hicks, L. A. (2013, April 11). U.S. outpatient antibiotic prescribing, 2010. *The New England Journal of Medicine, 368,* 1461–1462. doi: 10.1056/NEJMc1212055

Hook, M. L. (2006). Partnering with patients—A concept ready for action. *Journal of Advanced Nursing, 56*(2), 133–143. doi: 10.1111/j.1365-2648.2006.03993.x

Hooker, R. S., Cawley, J. F., & Everett, C. M. (2011). Predictive modeling in the physician assistant supply: 2010–2025. *Public Health Reports, 126,* 708–716.

Hunter, A. & Crabtree, K. (2011). Global health and international opportunities. In J. M. Stanley (Ed.), *Advanced practice nursing: Emphasizing common roles* (3rd ed., pp 327–350). Philadelphia: F. A. Davis.

Kavanagh, K. T., Cimiotti, J. P., Abusalem, S., & Coty, M. B. (2012). Moving healthcare quality forward with nursing-sensitive value-based purchasing. *Journal of Nursing Scholarship, 44*(4), 385–395.

Kennickell, A. B. (2009). Ponds and streams: Wealth and income in the U.S., 1989 to 2007. Report #2009-13. Washington, DC: Federal Reserve Board. Retrieved from http://www.federalreserve .gov/pubs/feds/2009/200913/200913pap.pdf

Kidder, T. (2003). *Mountains beyond mountains: The quest of Dr. Paul Farmer, a man who would cure the world.* New York: Random House.

Lehne, R. A. (2013). *Pharmacology for nursing care* (8th ed.). St. Louis: Elsevier Saunders.

Lindeke, L. L., Leonard, B. J., Presler, B., & Garwick, A. (2002). Family-centered care coordination for children with special needs across multiple settings. *Journal of Pediatric Health Care, 16*(6), 290–297.

McCloughen, A., Gillies, D., & O'Brien, L. (2011). Collaboration between mental health consumers and nurses: Shared understandings, dissimilar experiences. *International Journal of Mental Health Nursing, 20,* 47–55. doi: 10.1111/j.1447-0349.2010.00708.x

Mitchell, M., Chaboyer, W., Burmeister, E., & Foster, M. (2009). Positive effects of a nursing intervention on family-centered care in adult critical care. *American Journal of Critical Care, 18,* 543–552. doi: 10.4037/ajcc2009226

Murphey, D., Cooper, M. C., & Moore, K. A. (2012). Grandparents living with children: State-level data from the American Community Survey. Child Trends Research Brief (Pub. #2012-30). Retrieved January 7, 2012 from http://www.childtrends.org/Files/Child_Trends-2012_10_01_ RB_Grandparents.pdf

National Intelligence Council. (2000). The global infectious disease threat and its implications for the United States. Retrieved from National Intelligence Council Web site: http://www.dni .gov/nic/special_globalinfectious.html

National Quality Forum. (2010). Quality connections: Care coordination. Washington, DC: Author. Retrieved from National Quality Forum Web site: http://www.qualityforum.org/Publications/ 2010/10/Quality_Connections__Care_Coordination.aspx

Nolan, K., Orlando, M., & Liptak, G. (2007). Care coordination services for families with special health care needs: Are we there yet? *Families, Systems and Health, 25,* 293–306.

Nyirati, C. M., Denham, S. A., Raffle, H., & Ware, L. (2012). Where is family in the Family Nurse Practitioner Program? Results of a U.S. Family Nurse Practitioner Survey. *Journal of Family Nursing, 18*(3), 378–408.

Pearson Report. (2011). The American Journal for Nurse Practitioners, NP Communications CC. Retrieved January 7, 2013 from http://www.pearsonreport.com

Pittman, P. M., Folsom, A. J., & Bass, E. (2010). U.S. based recruitment of foreign-educated nurses: Implications of an emerging industry. *American Journal of Nursing, 110*(6), 38–48.

Rainer, H., & Siedler, T. (2010). Family location and caregiving patterns from an international perspective. (Discussion paper 4878.) Bonn, Germany: Institute of Study of Labor. Retrieved May 5, 2012 from http://ftp.iza.org/dp4878.pdf

Shah, A. (2010). Poverty facts and stats. Global issues. Retrieved January 7, 2012 from http:// www.globalissues.org/article/26/poverty-facts-and-stats

Squires, D. A. (2012, May). Explaining high health spending in the United States: An international comparison of supply, utilization, prices, and quality. Issues in International Health. The Commonwealth Fund pub. 1595, Vol. 10. Retrieved May 6, 2012 from http://www.commonwealthfund .org/~/media/Files/Publications/Issue%20Brief/2012/May/1595_Squires_explaining_high_hlt_care_ spending_intl_brief.pdf

United Nations. (2012). Population ageing and the non-communicable diseases (No. 2012/1). Department of Economic and Social Affairs. Population Division. Retrieved May 5, 2012 from http://www.un.org/esa/population/publications/popfacts/popfacts__2012-1.pdf

United States Global Change Research Program. (2009). Global climate change impacts in the United States. Retrieved from United States Global Change Research Program Web site: http://www .globalchange.gov/publications/reports/scientific-assessments/us-impacts

World Health Organization. (2000). The family health nurse: Context, conceptual framework, and curriculum. Retrieved May 8, 2012 from http://www.see-educoop.net/education_in/ pdf/family_health_nurse-oth-enl-t06.pdf

World Health Organization. (2002). WHO assembly report: Millennium development goals and targets. Retrieved from World Health Organization Web site: http://www.who.int/mdg/en

World Health Organization. (2009). Global health risks: Mortality and burden of disease attributable to selected major risks. Geneva, Switzerland: WHO Press. Retrieved from World Health Organization Web site: http://www.who.int/healthinfo/global_burden_disease/global_health_risks/en/index.html

World Health Organization. (2011). Causes of death 2008: Data sources and methods. Retrieved from World Health Organization Web site: http://www.who.int/gho/mortality_burden_disease/causes_death_2008/en/index.html

World Health Organization. (2012a). International travel and health. Geneva, Switzerland: WHO Press. Retrieved from World Health Organization Web site: http://www.who.int/ith/en/

World Health Organization. (2012b, March). Tuberculosis fact sheet No. 104. Retrieved from World Health Organization Web site: http://www.who.int/mediacentre/factsheets/fs104/en/index.html

World Health Organization Working Group for Risk Factors for Severe H1N1pdm Infection. (2011). Risk factors for severe outcomes following 2009 Influenza A (H1N1) infection: A global pooled analysis. Retrieved from World Health Organization Web site: http://www.who.int/influenza/surveillance_monitoring/Risk_factors_H1N1.pdf

Wright, L., & Bell, J. (1989). A survey of family nursing education in Canadian universities. *The Canadian Journal of Nursing Research, 21*(3), 59–74.

CHAPTER 2

Moving to Family-Focused Care

Sharon A. Denham

Sharon A. Denham

CHAPTER OBJECTIVES

1. Differentiate between individual care and family-focused care.
2. Define key terms involved in family-focused care.
3. Describe differences between family as the context of care and family as the unit of care.
4. Compare and contrast a systems model and an ecological model.
5. Discuss some of the ecological dimensions of family health.
6. Introduce some ways in which family-focused care influences individual and family health.

CHAPTER CONCEPTS

- Ecological model
- Family
- Family as the context of care
- Family as the unit of care
- Family-centered care
- Family-focused care
- Family health

- Family Health Model
- Healthy family
- Individual care
- Patient
- Patient-centered care
- Systems Model

Introduction

Nursing practice is large in scope and often considered both an art and a science. Throughout this chapter you will see how ideas linked with thinking family and family-focused nursing care can improve the ways you care for patients. Those ideas outlined here will be more fully explained in following chapters. The term *thinking family* is an attitude or way to approach nursing and use a family-focused perspective. Some of the literature introduced in this chapter has served as a foundation for family nursing.

Understanding Family Health Terminology

Concepts are ideas that persons in a shared culture understand. Terms and concepts can be familiar and have specific meanings; however, because everyone does not share the same vocabulary, ideas are often understood differently. This section focuses on the art of nursing and provides terms and definitions related to family-focused care.

Individuals and Their Health

Nurses mostly attend to individuals in clinical practice. The word *individual* suggests ideas of separateness, distinct needs, and differences. The word *person* is also used to refer to an individual. Nurses care for people; some share characteristics, values, beliefs, attitudes, and actions, but all have unique, distinct qualities, and diverse behavioral patterns.

Patient Versus Person

In health care, the term *patient* is used to refer to those looking for and receiving medical and nursing care. For some, the word suggests dependence, lack of individuality, and even anonymity. Nurses and other health care professionals often view patients as dependent with needs to be fixed, repaired, or healed. When a person becomes a patient, he sometimes loses individuality and unique needs may be overlooked or ignored. Being a patient often means inability to be a free agent. Patients are often acted upon by others, by professionals they usually do not know. Nurses say "my patient" or "our patient," suggesting ownership. But people seeking care do not belong to nurses, other health professionals, agencies, or institutions. Sometimes the term *client* is used to describe those seeking medical care. This word has some similar connotations to *patient*, but it also refers to a customer or consumer of care. This term might imply choice and the right to have a voice in care, and in the business world "the customer is always right." Some health care providers like the idea of client, but some say it sounds too business-like and prefer the word patient. Regardless of the terminology used, these persons are care seekers needing professional help. They enter a care delivery setting like foreigners going to an unfamiliar country.

Differentiating Among Individuals

People want to be seen as individuals who are different and unique even though most still see themselves as parts of groups. People get classified based on many qualities: gender, age, race, sexuality, culture, ethnicity, economics, education, vocation, and social network. Personality, motivation, wisdom, values, beliefs, character, and attitudes are other differences. Yet, they also want to show their uniqueness with clothing, hairstyles, tattoos, and piercings. In addition, most want to determine their own fate and be treated with respect. They want personalized, not generic, health care. Failure to see persons as part of a family and household unit can create unintentional barriers to optimal care (Table 2.1).

Family

Family is the basic unit of society. The word *family* refers to two or more people related biologically, legally, or emotionally. For generations, families followed what was considered a traditional pattern—two parents who reared and launched children, a nuclear family. Some argue that families should never have been characterized this way (Coontz, 1992, 1997), that this ideal comes from white middle-class American families and is not representative of the diversity that defines families (Coontz, 2006). Current marriage and cohabitation patterns seem radically different from those of the past.

    The term family is prone to misinterpretation. Authors, policy makers, educators, and health care providers use the word, but may fail to describe what they mean. Terms such as family values, family health, family practice, and family care mean various things to

TABLE 2-1	*Changing Patient Roles*
OLD PATIENT ROLE	**NEW PATIENT ROLE**
Defer to authority of others.	Become a partner in health and illness care.
Expectations of medical practitioners are primary concern in care.	Expectations of individual seeking care and medical practitioner should be mutually shared.
Respect the expertise of the medical practitioner.	Respect is mutually shared between medical practitioner and person seeking care.
Seek solutions of problems or get "fixed" by medical practitioners.	Be actively engaged in self-management and personal care of health or illness.
Depend upon the expertise of others.	Identify different medical choices or diverse care options and participate in choosing.
Accept information as provided and not ask questions.	Expect to have information presented to you in clear, easily understood language.
Answer questions when asked.	Come prepared with own questions and receive answers.
Give only information asked for by others.	Share beliefs, values, and preferences.
Adhere to instructions of others or become labeled noncompliant.	Choose plan of care based upon wisdom of expert and personal preferences.
Rely upon medical experts to solve problems.	Seek expert medical support and actively engage in solutions to personal care needs.
Expect the health care practitioner to tell you everything you need to know.	Obtain additional information from a variety of external sources.
Assume medical practitioners to tell you how you are doing.	Assume responsibility for own care and monitor progress between care visits.
Expect others to prescribe medicine and treatments needed.	Consult with others and take personal responsibility for knowing whether what is prescribed is what is needed.

different people. Religious activists, local politicians, physicians, and even nurses have ideas about families. These ideas may not match the thinking of peers, teachers, or those to whom they provide care. "No traditional [family] arrangement provides a workable model for how we organize family relations in the modern world" (Coontz, 1992, p 5). Marriage definitions have been hotly debated and are viewed in divergent ways by ethnic and cultural groups (Coontz, 2006). Shared ancestry, who lives under a single roof, or a common head of household may provide instructive guides. However, these distinctions are just guides and do not exhaust the ways family is defined.

Family has long been identified as "a group of people, connected emotionally and/or by blood, who have lived together long enough to have developed patterns of interaction and stories that justify and explain these patterns" (Minuchin, Lee, & Simon, 1996, p 29). Dr. Suzanne Feetham has contributed greatly to our understandings about family as the 'unit of care' needing nurses' attention (Box 2.1). In this textbook, family is loosely defined as a collection of persons who call themselves family and have a general commitment to the care and well-being of one another. Although this is not a legal definition, it allows nurses to identify persons who see themselves connected as a family unit. This imprecise definition also offers flexibility in characterizing family units.

BOX 2-1

Family Tree

Suzanne Feetham, PhD (United States)

Dr. Suzanne Feetham, RN, PhD, FAAN, has held clinical, research, and leadership positions in academia, health systems (Children's National Medical Center, Washington, D.C.), the federal government (U.S. Department of Health and Human Services [DHHS], National Institutes of Health (NIH), National Institute of Nursing Research (Deputy Director and Chief of the Office of Science Policy, Planning and Analysis), and Health Resources and Services Administration (HRSA). Her work has focused on health care for families, underserved populations, and health policy. She is recognized nationally and internationally for her research and scholarship in nursing research of families and the integration of genetics and genomics in national education, practice, and policy. Dr. Feetham has a program of research in the care of children with health problems and their families. She has numerous publications on nursing research about families, using research to effect change in practice, families and health policy, health and urban families, genetics education, and genetics and families. In 1977, she developed the Feetham Family Functioning Survey (FFFS). Currently, this survey instrument is used in research of families across disciplines and has been translated into several languages including American Sign Language, Spanish, Russian, Bosnian, Chinese, and Japanese and has reported application in more than 70 research publications. She was co-editor of the first state of the science *Handbook of Clinical Nursing Research* in 1999, and in 2001, she edited a volume of *Nursing and Genetics—Leadership for Global Health* for the International Council of Nurses, Geneva, Switzerland. From 1996 to 2001 at the University of Illinois at Chicago, she was co-investigator on federally funded family studies, including a family intervention for Bosnian torture survivors, and was principal investigator for a funded interdisciplinary project to develop a Web-based course on clinical genomics for health professionals. As holder of the H. H. Werley Endowed Research Chair at the University of Illinois at Chicago, she was principal investigator on a study of families considering genetic testing for cancer susceptibility; she was also co-investigator on four family studies funded by the NIH. She has also served as a Visiting Professor at University of Wisconsin–Milwaukee, a research consultant at Children's National Medical Center, Washington, D.C., and a board member for the International Family Nursing Association. In August 2011, the American Academy of Nursing announced that Dr. Feetham was a recipient of the Living Legends Award for her notable accomplishments.

Thinking Family

Thinking family is an attitude nurses use in clinical practice situations. Nurses who *think family* know that individuals value members of their family unit, and even when members are not present in the care delivery setting, they still need to be considered. Nurses who *think family* know individuals are influenced by a family point of view. Nurses often lack the time needed to clarify relationships of linked persons. But nurses can ask who are the important persons the individuals connect with in daily life. Some family members give important support; some create conflicts and burdens.

The Family Household

Family is a context that links members over the life course. Families have different expectations of their members. Some encourage individuation and originality, and others insist upon conformity. Some have tight boundaries. Others have no boundaries. The family household has many implications (e.g., a structure, shelter, neighborhood, tangible or intangible resources) for unique family units (Denham, 2003). The household is more than just the space the family inhabits; it is linked to place and social networks, things that affects members' lives (e.g., power of one's name, finances, access to health). Understanding the difference between the healthy family and family health concepts is useful for nurses.

Healthy Family

Individuals initially learn about health and illness in their family households. The household is where people first deal with the basic facts of life, such as conflict, comfort, care, adversity, and suffering. Early experiences of health and illness (e.g., injuries, accidents, illness, disease, disabilities) occur at home. Many household experiences become health and illness determinants, because the household is the place where habits, routines, and responses to health and illness are learned.

The term *healthy family* has been identified with nurture and care that members offer one another; healthy family traits (e.g., good communication, respect, shared responsibility, balance of interactions, shared religious core) have long been described (Curran, 1984). Healthy family suggests that members come together for the common good and that they support one another's growth and maturity. They share time, interests, traditions, and resources. A healthy family is vibrant, has a sense of stability, has access to needed supports, provides its members emotional support, and balances individual needs against those of the family unit (Denham, 2003). A healthy family is one that effectively balances competing aspects of the household that have health and illness consequences for its members' well-being and is successful at accomplishing needed tasks. Members care for one another's needs as resources are acquired and equitably distributed to individuals. The idea of healthy family does not always include a health-illness perspective or factors relevant to biomedical concerns.

Being an Unhealthy Family

An unhealthy family is one in which pain, biophysical symptoms, or emotional problems prevent or limit an individual's self-efficacy and the family unit is unable to perform needed tasks linked with concerns. An inability to effectively complete needed tasks, fulfill roles, or meet social obligations might indicate a family is unorganized. Even though this situation could lead to being less healthy, the family might not see their circumstances as unhealthy. Judgments from the outside are not always aligned with what families view as reality. When physical pain, symptoms, or emotional suffering interfere with abilities to complete self-care or family care, an unhealthy situation might exist. If members are unable to perform roles, fulfill obligations, or complete duties, outsiders might call them unhealthy. When social expectation are unfulfilled, one might be tempted to place an unhealthy label. For example, a family using or dealing illegal substances or a home where neglect or abuse occurs might be labeled an unhealthy family. Social values often influence what is or is not viewed as healthy. Thus, labeling a family healthy or unhealthy should occur with great caution.

Making Health Judgments

Nurses need to be careful about making judgments about what is and is not healthy. Some health care providers use the terms dysfunctional and noncompliant, referring to individuals or families that do not follow what is prescribed. To ensure a therapeutic relationship, nurses need to avoid judgmental attitudes. Families have ideas about what they need, and these ideas can differ from what nurses think.

For example, a nurse might meet a person with type 1 diabetes based upon laboratory results. A 36-year-old man presents with a blood glucose level of 198 mg/dL on a routine physician visit. The high blood glucose level might mean this person has failed to follow doctor's orders, lacks personal motivation, or is irresponsible. However, before lecturing this man about the problem, be sure that fact finding is complete. The nurse may only know part of the story. He may think that he is working very hard on daily management efforts. He might lack family support. Maybe he has inadequate health insurance coverage and can't afford the medical supplies. Maybe he doesn't know how to manage his diet or has not been adequately instructed about needs for physical activity. The high cost of test strips might prevent regular daily glucose checks. He might be focused on pressing personal problems. A family assessment might reveal that he has great emotional and financial stress about a child with a serious and worsening disability. Nurses who *think family* know that individuals seldom have one problem at a time. They learn about holistic needs before making judgments.

Family Health

When terms like family as a system, family system, and family nursing practice are not defined, confusion about what is implied can occur. Medical professionals often focus on medical care for single persons. Implications for the family unit are largely ignored. A lack of conceptual clarity about family health contributes to this neglect. Nursing students often learn about family care needs when infants or children are involved. Families are largely ignored when adults need care unless they are disabled or need end-of-life care.

The term *healthy family* speaks to attributes of interacting members. It refers to ways members support and care for one another. The idea of family health is somewhat fuzzy. It is often referred to in the literature and identified as a goal of nursing, but it is seldom defined (Loveland-Cherry, 1996). Family health is a phenomenon that explains the complex interactions and relationships of a family household unit as they collaborate to maximize individual abilities for wellness and maintain what they view as healthful (Denham, 2003). Family health is connected to the whole family unit. Family health aims to maximize potentials of member actions (e.g., resilience, organization, adaptation, stability, support, caregiving) that contribute to the family unit's health and well-being. Family health occurs when household resources are used to enhance member and unit well-being.

Families uniquely organize their lives. Some live in disorganized fray. It is useful to consider ways members relate and possible implications on health and illness. Family health refers to the health status of the whole family unit and how well the group is functioning. How well do members use their actions, abilities, and resources for the good of the whole, but also meet unique individual needs? A family focused on wellness will likely instill ideas about good nutrition and physical activity from cradle to grave. At the same time, individual factors can alter the family unit. Early work on addictions demonstrates that an individual member can radically alter the family health of the entire unit by using enabling behaviors (Steinglass, Bennett, Wolin, & Reiss, 1987). A child born with a severe disability places great demands on family resources over a lifetime. Thus, family health is strengthened or damaged based upon the family unit's abilities and willingness to satisfy the needs for its members (Fig. 2.1).

Family Health Patterns

The family household is where members' shared lifestyles produce uniquely constructed health patterns and routines. It is where health behaviors are taught, learned, and practiced (Denham, 2003.) Households are the basic units of analysis for collecting U.S. census data.

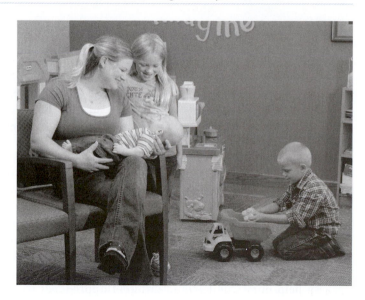

FIGURE 2-1 Nurses *think family* health and individual health.

The census defines a family household as: where two or more persons related by birth, marriage, or adoption, but unrelated people live. Non-family households are places where people live alone or share the place with unrelated individuals. Members of non-family households are connected to other households where they are still viewed as immediate or extended family members. Less than half of Americans are currently married, and similar reductions have been noted in other advanced postindustrial societies. Social class, culture, age, and race often influence family forms. Households members experience a continuum of wellness-illness care needs. This continuum is influenced by many things (e.g., genetics, culture, religion, peers, beliefs, values, attitudes, available resources). Developing individuals respond to things that threaten or support health and care management daily. The scale and forms of family influence upon individuals differ. Nurses can ask individuals about family priorities in caring for health and illness.

Individual Health

Research about family health identified that being healthy is more than merely the absence of disease (Denham, 1999a, 1999b, 1999c). Health is often described as holistic, but it is often viewed in terms of the presence or absence of disease or illness. Ask someone you know about her health. She might tell you about an illness or disease or say that she is not sick. She might describe her inability to be active, complete activities, care for basic needs, or do things for herself. Few will answer the question in terms of well-being.

Health could be described as the ability to have an active life. It might include things like taking part in family life, having emotional strength, feeling spiritually connected, or doing meaningful tasks. Some might think of health in terms of routines (e.g., eating a nutritious diet, being physically active, refraining from risky behaviors). Those living with a serious disease or a terminal illness might see themselves as healthy if basic self-care needs (e.g., take part in valued daily living activities, fulfill usual roles, do meaningful things) can be completed. Health is an adaptive state experienced as persons seek meaningful ways of being and wrestle with personal, family, household, and environmental liabilities across the lifespan (Denham, 2003). Family nurses help persons and family units clarify their expectations and engage in healthful activities they value.

Models for Understanding Family Nursing

Ideas about family nursing have been evolving for decades. Many nursing scholars have contributed to a growing body of evidence about the value of family nursing. Yet, the question remains: How should family nursing be defined? In this textbook, we define family nursing as clinical practice approaches that address the person and family unit even when only one individual is present for care. Family nurses focus on families and their home settings where health problems are addressed and endeavors to create a healthy family are targeted (World Health Organization, 2000). Family nurses assist individuals and families to manage all aspects of wellness, health, illness, disease, and chronic disabilities. Family nurses realize that care needs exist beyond health care settings and aim to deliver coordinated care to family households.

In nursing, the application of a variety of theories and models offers different ways to define and deliver nursing care. Some grand nursing theories (e.g., Orem, Roy, Neuman) have been generated by nurses to guide nursing practice. Many of these frameworks have had several revisions and were updated so family perspectives were better addressed. Theory can help nurses understand different approaches to clinical care. Theories directly linked with family nursing have emerged over the past several decades. These family theories offer distinct ways to think about how individual health is influenced by the family unit and household. Ideas about family systems nursing have been advanced through the Calgary Family Assessment Model and the Calgary Family Intervention Model (Wright & Leahey, 2013). These models are discussed later in this textbook. In many of the following chapters, a variety of middle-range theories useful in family-focused nursing practice are introduced.

A Systems Perspective

A non-nursing theory often used by nurses is *general systems theory* (von Bertalanffy, 1950). It can be used to think about care of individuals and families and encourages the nurse to consider the whole as more than the sum of its parts. Systems thinking provides ways to understand the connectedness and feedback responses as individuals interact with family members and their environment. Systems theory suggests that too much focus on the whole can result in overlooking the importance of the parts and too much attention to the parts risks the possibility of overlooking the whole.

Systems theory has been influential, but critics say it tends to emphasize some perspectives and ignore others. Systems theory can help one understand some aspects of family member interactions, but influential historical, cultural, and political factors are often ignored. Understanding about equilibrium might cause one to assume that individuals and families seek balance, but this assumption is not always true. Using systems theory, one might think that experiences or conditions are linear or circular in progressing from causation to outcomes, but life more often is random and chaotic. Systems thinking can help nurses understand that multiple interacting forces are in play when an illness occurs or when needs to promote wellness arise. However, nurses might find some implications vague or difficult to apply in a practical way.

No clear-cut rules govern the ways family members interact with each other. The family is more than the sum of its members. How can one explain family health without taking into consideration the complexity of multiple member interactions outside the family unit? Is the family even fully explained by the members? Do other things also need to be taken into account? The uniqueness of family units, their discrete traits, and the roles of members need consideration. Systems theory aims to explore the whole, but the number, type, and magnitude of multiple member interactions and their implications for individual and family health can be overlooked. In systems thinking, ideas about environment are often vague and clear distinctions about values and relationships ignored.

An Ecological Perspective: The Family Health Model

There are different ways to consider individual and family health. Research findings about family health suggested that an ecological perspective could be a better model to describe family health, one with a household and community lens to better understand the family unit (Denham, 2003). The Family Health Model moves the focus away from acute episodic clinical care to more mindful thoughts about an individual's relationships with the family unit, household, lived spaces, and the needs posed by daily life. An ecological model is a good way to think about multiple factors relevant to health such as:

• Relationships of shared and separate events and contexts
• Individual and collective experiences
• Interactive behaviors within and outside the family household
• Effects of social networks, larger communities, and environmental circumstances
• Perceived meanings, beliefs, values, or interpretations tied to health and illness
• Multiple personal and family interdependent factors linked with health or illness

The Family Health Model suggests ways to identify interconnecting events and circumstances. Nurses can use these interrelated ideas to complete assessments and complete nursing actions or interventions. This model views family health as a socially constructed phenomenon. The Family Health Model has three domains: context, function, and structure. Each domain provides a way to understand factors linked with individual and family health and to identify nursing practice actions (Fig. 2.2).

The Family Health Model provides a framework for thinking about nursing practice that includes relationships, needs, connectedness, and environment (Fig. 2.3). It is a way to think about the many obscure, interacting, and conflicting factors associated with health and illness. Family health is influenced by the family's internal and external environments. Box 2.2 provides some explicit points about the Family Health Model. This model includes ways individuals view themselves in connection to their family unit and household, but also offers ways to consider how these and other relationships or environments influence health and illness. This model suggest that things be considered over time and place. The lived shared experiences of multiple household members and their shared internal and external environments have potential to affect their well-being, life quality, and illness or disease potentials.

Ecological thinking implies that multiple interacting, dynamic, and enduring factors across the life span are important. Family nurses can use these varied factors to see that intrinsic and extrinsic factors are assessed. When first using ecological thinking, one can be overwhelmed. New terminology is introduced. This thinking offers many different areas to assess—so many ways care might be delivered. Keep in mind that nurses do not address all factors with every person. Instead, these ideas can be used in conjunction with presenting clinical problems. Consider the following questions: What is most important at this time? Are there other factors that should be considered? What features about this person's family unit and household might be relevant to this situation? Answers to these questions give directions for assessment areas that might lead to needed nursing actions.

Family Context

The Family Health Model also suggests that health and illness are influenced by the family context, which is the first domain to consider when conducting an assessment. The term

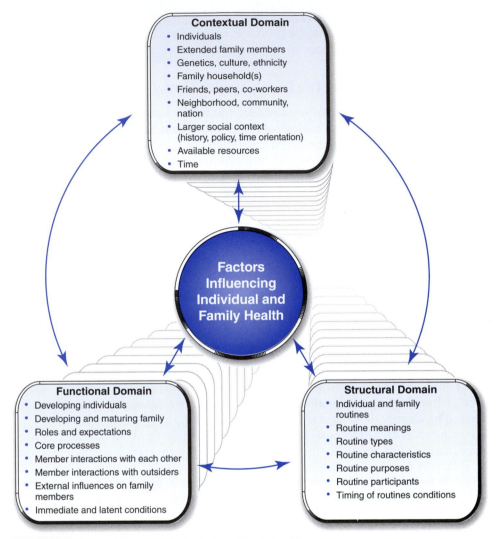

FIGURE 2-2 Factors influencing individual and family health.

family context explains the deeply connected experiences that family unit members share over a lifetime. While the family unit is the context for its members, this unit is embedded into other complex systems (e.g., neighborhoods, communities, nations). These larger systems have other factors that influence health and illness (e.g., institutions, organizations, political milieu). Family members have discrete and shared viewpoints and often experience things differently. It is paradoxical that while families are somewhat predictable, they are also dynamic. Members and families evolve; they change over time. Nurses who *think family* know that family socialization and experience are critical factors when it comes to health and illness. The larger cultural, social, and physical environment exerts negative and positive potentials.

Family context mirrors some aspects of the larger societal systems. It is the stage for relationships and social discourse. The household is the place internal and external environments meet and exchange ideas that influence behaviors. The household is where many unique identities, values, beliefs, and attitudes are formed. It is where genetics, religion, culture, traditions, history, and behaviors, among other things, are shared. Care

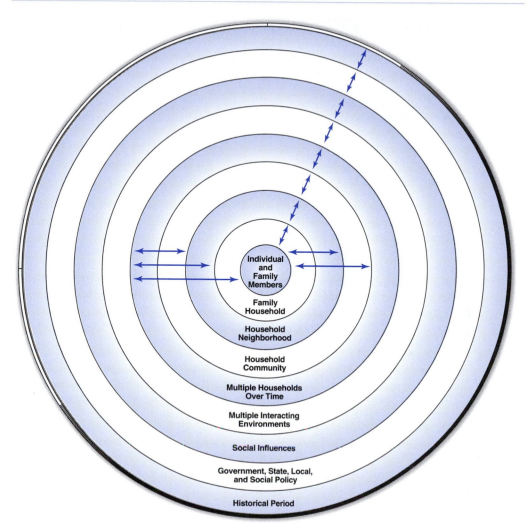

Individual
and
Family
Members

Family
Household

Household
Neighborhood

Household
Community

Multiple Households
Over Time

Multiple Interacting
Environments

Social Influences

Government, State, Local,
and Social Policy

Historical Period

FIGURE 2-3 Ecological influences on individual and family health.

given to individuals in clinical environments seldom reveals the complexities of family unit and household needs. Nursing assessment findings that take families into consideration help the nurse figure out the best ways to address care needs.

Family Function

In the Family Health Model, the functional domain is used to explain the interactive processes that occur as family members develop, mature, share time and experiences, and change within their household (Denham, 2003). The functional domain pertains to ways members interact, communicate, and relate within and outside the household and it helps explain roles, processes, and behavioral interactions. Members use many forms of relational processes to meet personal and collective needs.

Parents and others give social cues to developing children about ways to respond to health and illness. Family members often test these experiences as they engage the larger community (i.e., for work, play, school, faith, social or public policy). Ways to respond to wellness or disease are learned behaviors over time. Some ideas are steadfast, and others can be altered, but basically those ideas are formed as members interact with family. Some

---

BOX 2-2

Key Principles of the Family Health Model

1. Developing persons experience individual and family health in relationship to all aspects of their lives; both can be either stable or dynamic over time.
2. Individual and family health are inextricably tied to the family household and communities. These influences can be positive and negative aspects of individual health and the health of the family unit.
3. Individual and family health are affected by the ecological relationships that connect family members within the family household to the larger environments with which they directly or indirectly interact.
4. The family is a microsystem that includes those viewed as part of the family and encompasses all the interactions occurring among individuals as they interact with external environments in everyday life.
5. The family and its members interact with multiple external environments (e.g., home, work, school, peer groups) that have the potential to affect individual and family health both negatively and positively.
6. The family and its members interact with diverse environments (administrative decisions by parent's employer, boards governing school policies, etc.) that have the potential to affect individual and family health even when members are not direct participants.
7. Larger societal systems that represent the ideologies of the evolving world (e.g., legislation, social policy, culture, media, history) can potentially affect individual and family health.
8. Time and historical experiences have the potential to influence the family, its members, and their health in positive and negative ways.
9. Family health results from the complex interactions of the family, its members, and larger environments over time as the multiple interacting factors have potential to maximize or minimize the health and illness of individuals and the family unit.
10. Family health routines are important ways to discuss, describe, assess, intervene, and evaluate interventions and outcomes pertinent to individual and family health.

Source: Adapted from Denham, S. A. (2003). *Family health: A framework for nursing*. Philadelphia: F. A. Davis.

---

families encourage healthy lifestyle behaviors, but others do not. Some factors (e.g., resilience, identity, adaptation, accommodation) are influenced by family, but peer groups also play roles. Time alters some behaviors, but others change little. Some life events (e.g., mental illness, disability, crisis, tragic death) can have dire effects on family units. Nurses who *think family* consider how these functional factors pertain to an individual's health and illness.

Nurses need to know ways to interact with both well-functioning and troubled families. In clinical practice, nurses meet and aim to help people from all walks of life; some have multiple troubles that extend beyond the reason for currently seeking care. Nurses often meet people facing distressful life situations, critical incidents, and long-standing troubling predicaments. The Family Health Model suggests ways that nurses can use core processes (e.g., communication, cooperation, coordination, caregiving) to address functional aspects of health and illness (Denham, 2003). These processes are described in Chapter 14. Each indicates ways nurses can use caring, treatments, education, counseling, and other nursing actions. Dr. Peri Bomar, in the late 1980s, published the first book to address health promotion with families (Box 2.3).

Family Structure

The third aspect of the Family Health Model is the structural domain (Denham, 2003). This domain focuses on patterns of behaviors, which includes habits and family health

---

BOX 2-3

Family Tree

Perri Bomar, PhD

Dr. Perri Bomar's first degree was a nursing diploma from a hospital school in Canton, Ohio. Subsequently she earned a BSN, MSN, and PhD. Her career took her to various institutions, the U.S. Department of Health and Human Services, the University of San Diego, and the University of North Carolina Wilmington (UNCW). At UNCW she served as Associate Dean and was instrumental in establishing the first master's degree program in nursing, which began in 1998. Her first edition of *Promoting Health in Families*, in 1989, was recognized as the *American Journal of Nursing* Book of the Year and the Nursing Outlook Book of the Year. Two follow-up editions of this text were published. This book has been used by nurses in the United States, Canada, Japan, Thailand, and other nations. As an African American nurse, Dr. Bomar has been instrumental in modeling the value of graduate education and has mentored many students who have sought her guidance and support. A number of her graduate students have progressed to doctoral studies with a focus on family or health disparities in underserved populations. Her most recent research is focused on describing and developing family nursing interventions that incorporate community-participatory research methods using evidence-based research focusing on self-management, spirituality, and the rural environment to improve health promotion with African American families.

---

routines. These patterns develop as members interact within the family household and with other larger environments. Family health routines have distinct traits: they are recognized by others, are shared in some instances, and have the potential to affect the health-illness continuum (Denham, 2003). These patterns, while not static, seem firm or stable over time. Routines may not be visible or of concern until something conflicts with them. Family members can often describe each other's behaviors with great accuracy.

Family health routines are relevant to behaviors with disease risks. Nutrition and dietary routines are one category with great significance for wellness or disease management. For example, food consumption has many linked routines (e.g., meal plans, shopping, label reading, food preparation, meal patterns). Diets often include sugary drinks and chemical-laden processed foods with large portion sizes and high-calorie snacks. Despite the relevance of habitually shared behaviors in family households, questions about them are rarely asked. Nurses who *think family* know that family routines influence individual risks and can include these concerns when doing assessments and planning nursing actions. A person diagnosed with type 2 diabetes needs to modify his diet. What needs to be known about current individual and family dietary routines? How can long-standing family behaviors be changed? What are the goals or outcomes to measure?

Nurses who *think family* assess linked individual and family behaviors. They consider the family unit and household resources in goal setting. Strategies for change identify meaningful, achievable, and measurable outcomes. A dietary assessment (e.g., proximity of grocery store, food costs and availability, preparation time, nutritional knowledge, literacy level) that considers contextual, functional, and structural factors is an important step toward change. One needs to know what is currently happening before real change can be planned. Things like mealtime interactions of young children with asthma have been found to influence the quality of life (Fiese, Winter, & Botti, 2011). Disease management for young and older persons almost always involves family in some way. Family-focused care requires collaborative planning and decision making. Deconstructing risky routines and constructing new ones takes planning and intentionality. Nurses who *think family* begin by learning what is valued. They identify members' cooperative spirit. They evaluate motivation or readiness for change. Medical care often involves needs for change that are not easy. Family-focused care includes multiple members who either support or thwart behavioral changes.

Nurses who understand the importance of shared routines linked with health and illness use them during assessment, planning care interventions, and evaluating outcomes. Six areas of family health routines are identified in the Family Health Model (i.e., self-care, safety and prevention, mental health behaviors, family care, illness care, family caregiving). Families organize daily routines in ways viewed as meaningful and replacing old routines with new ones is difficult. Nurses who *think family* assist them in identifying goals and action steps that are Specific, Measurable, Attainable, Realistic, and Timely (SMART goals). Changing routines takes planning, strategies for making changes, and steps to evaluate along the way.

Moving Toward Family-Focused Care

Providing family-focused clinical care takes forethought and reflection. Nurses who *think family* plan care that considers the family unit needs. The frantic pace of daily work does not make it easy to always be thoughtful about what will be done, but taking the time to consider family needs can pay a big return. This next section describes differences between family-centered care and family-focused care.

Family as Context of Care Versus Family as Unit of Care

Nurses need to plan the ways in which they approach clinical care. One can see family as the context of care or the unit of care. These terms were initially coined by Dr. Suzanne Feetham (1991), an internationally recognized family scholar and researcher (see Box 2.1). Family as the context of care implies that family is connected to individuals seeking care but is in the background. Family members might be viewed as directly relevant, but be seen as visitors, an afterthought, and not essential to immediate care.

On the other hand, when family is viewed as the unit of care, family members are in the forefront. They are viewed as fundamental to individual care. Individuals and family members are viewed as perpetually connected or inseparable. Individuals are inherently tied to others even when they are not physically present. When nurses recognize family as the unit of care, they understand that shared lives, resources, and identities play active roles in one another's health or illness. Family is an abiding presence and not a transitory aspect of life. Attachments formed in the household are ties that bind even when we wrestle against them. As the unit of care, nurses think about individual care in terms of deep, intricate, entangled, and inseparable household member bonds. The family shares resources, provides caring relationships, and gives support for members. Thinking family means meeting holistic care needs of the individual in ways that include family involvement. Table 2.2 compares the ideas of family as the context of care and family as the unit of care.

Patient- and Family-Focused Care

The terms patient-centered and family-centered care are not often used consistently and therefore are poorly understood. Disease-centered care largely uses a biomedical focus with individual attention mainly given to clinical expertise, diagnostic tests, episodic care, and medical management. Patient-centered care requires health care providers who think about patient needs and focus attention on the individual receiving care.

TABLE 2-2	*Families as the Context of Care or the Unit of Care*

FAMILY AS THE CONTEXT OF CARE	FAMILY AS THE UNIT OF CARE
Individual is the care focus	Family is the care focus
Family is in the background	Family is in the forefront
Family is composed of individuals	Family is a unified whole
Individual data reflect family	Family data also reflect individuals
Care of solitary persons	Care of individuals and family

Patient-Centered Care

The Institute of Medicine (2001) suggests that patient-centered care implies that a respectful and responsive partnership among practitioners, care seekers, and their families to address patient values, wants, needs, and preferences is available. This model assumes that individuals actively seek care and take part in identifying needed services. Many people have limited knowledge about health care systems or the business of medicine. Identifying needed services in timely ways is not always easy. Individual needs are the target, but family involvement needs to be encouraged. Many are uncertain about how care should look in practice. Care consumers often make quick decisions. Technology and the Internet make access to medical information easy, but wading through Web sites when you have no medical background is difficult. Medical terminology and explanations are hard to decipher. The general public is often unsure about what is reliable or accurate. Too often, the first information accessed can be biased, confusing, incomplete, or not supported by scientific evidence.

Primary Care

Primary care is recommended whenever treatment is non-life-threatening and choices exist. Primary care begins when the person meets a health–care professional in a medical practice setting. Most people seek care infrequently over the life course. When the visit ends, the care recipient is expected to follow through on the prescribed treatment. Because care delivered is often limited to 8 to 15 minutes per visit, pertinent questions go unanswered. In addition, people seldom receive a follow-up call to ask if everything is going well. A national study of 1,837 physicians who practiced at least 3 years past residency found that only 16% communicated via e-mail with patients, only 36% get patient feedback, less than 50% use patient reminder systems, and only 14% of those in solo practices have adopted half of the patient-centered care practices (Audet, Davis, & Schoenbaum, 2006). Technology is available, but links between primary care providers and care consumers is lagging. Box 2.4 provides a list of patient-centered practices that can be used in primary care.

Questions remain about how much power and control are truly shifted to patients or families. The quality of care we currently have in the United States might be far from the quality we could have (Berwick, 2009). Patient-centered care needs to be linked with an experience in which individuals are informed in ways they desire (Berwick). This care should be transparent, individualized, and provided in respectful ways in which the dignity of persons is upheld. Personal choice and family involvement would make this care form superior to current delivery systems (Box 2.5).

BOX 2-4

Patient-Centered Care Practices

Examples of practices that incorporate actions sensitive to individual needs and evidence-based practices that can be used effectively in the clinical setting:

- Schedule same-day appointments.
- Exchange e-mail with patients.
- Text appropriate disease management reminders.
- Use reminder notices for preventive or follow-up care.
- Keep registries of individuals with chronic conditions.
- Update patient medication lists regularly.
- Store information in electronic medical records.
- Make information from referral physicians available promptly.
- Ensure that medical records or test results are readily available when needed.
- Feed back patient survey data into practice.
- Be aware that patient ratings of care affect compensation.
- Make information on quality of care about the referral physician available.

BOX 2-5

Providing Patient-Centered Care With a Family Focus

Care that is patient centered implies that individuals who are patients have more autonomy, share in decision making, and have a voice in what, where, when, and how things are done. For this form of care to truly become family centered, then the following changes need to occur:

- Hospitals would not have visitation restrictions, except those chosen by and under the control of patients.
- Patients determine the food selected to eat and what clothes they wear in hospitals (to the extent health status allows).
- Patients and family members participate in rounds and are included in reports.
- Patients and families participate in the design of health care processes and services.
- Medical records belong to patients. Clinicians, rather than patients, would need to gain access to them.
- Shared decision-making technologies would be used universally.
- Operating room schedules would minimize waiting time for patients rather than follow the convenience of the clinicians.
- Patients physically capable of self-care would, in all circumstances, have the option to perform it and have family assist.

Source: Adapted from Berwick, D. M. (2009). What "patient-centered" care should mean: Confessions of an extremist. *Health Affairs, 28*(4), 555–565.

Integrative Care

Integrative medicine is defined as patient centered, healing oriented, and a care form that embraces both conventional and complementary therapies (Maizes, Rakel, & Niemiec, 2009). It is different from the dominant biomedical model in that it is more focused on holistic needs. It recognizes that high-tech medicine is not always useful in addressing chronic health problems. Addressing health promotion and disease prevention needs by including other methods such as nutrition and stress management could be more viable options but are out-of-pocket costs. Nurses' education about integrative medicine is often limited (Box 2.6).

Origins of Family-Focused Care for Children

Family-centered care was first described by former Surgeon General C. Everett Koop at an American Academy of Pediatrics conference in 1987. He spoke about care access and quality of life for children with special care needs. He called for commitment to establish a national agenda for families and professionals to work together through an initiative to focus on family-centered, community-based, coordinated care for children and their families (Box 2.7).

Many children's hospitals include parents in care delivery. About 15 years ago, it was suggested that pediatric practice would be improved when nurses and other health professionals approached care in intentional ways in which needs, cultures, resources, and strengths were included (Dunst & Trivette, 1996). Care needed to be delivered with efficiency, flexibility, quality, confidentiality, and privacy. Enlisting family members to teach nursing students and hospital staff about family needs has been suggested. Since 1998, family advisory councils have been in place in many children's hospitals to improve customer service.

Family-centered care assures the health and well-being of children and their families through respectful family-professional partnerships (National Center for Family-Centered Care, 1989). This care focuses on the best interests of the child and family respecting the skills and expertise that each person brings to the care setting. Care hallmarks include trusting relationships, meaningful communication, cooperative decision making, and

---

BOX 2-6

Principles of Integrative Medicine

- Individuals and practitioners are partners in the healing process.
- All factors that influence health, wellness, and disease are considered (e.g., body, mind, spirit, community).
- Appropriate uses of conventional and alternative methods are used to assist the body's innate healing response.
- Natural and less invasive interventions should be used whenever possible.
- All practice should be based upon the best scientific evidence available, open to inquiry or questions, and allow for new practice forms.
  - Individuals must decide on what treatments to have based on their personal values, beliefs, and available evidence.
- Treatment alone is not enough; broad ideas of health promotion and prevention must also be included.
- Integrative medicine practitioners should be exemplars of the practices they suggest and be committed to self-exploration through reflection and continued development.

Source: Adapted from Maizes, V., Rakel, D., & Niemiec, C. (2009). Integrative medicine and patient-centered care. Commissioned for the IOM Summit on Integrative Medicine and the Health of the Public. Retrieved January 29, 2012 from http://www.iom.edu/~/media/Files/Activity%20Files/Quality/IntegrativeMed/Integrative%20Medicine%20and%20Patient%20Centered%20Care.pdf

BOX 2-7

Elements of Family-Centered Care for Children

More than 20 years ago, Surgeon General Koop identified some critical aspects of family-centered care for children with special health care needs. Ideas suggested then also appear relevant to needs of adult family members seeking health care services. These ideas include the following:

- Recognize that the family is the constant in a child's life, while the service systems and personnel within those systems continually change and fluctuate.
- Share complete and unbiased information with parents about their child's condition on an ongoing basis in an appropriate and supportive manner.
- Recognize that families have strengths, individuality, and different methods of coping.
- Encourage and make referrals so parents facing challenging situations with children can gain support from other parents facing similar concerns.
- Facilitate parent/professional collaboration at all levels of health care (e.g., care of an individual, program development, implementation, evaluation, policy formation).
- Ensure that health care delivery system design is flexible, accessible, and responsive to individual needs and families.
- Implement appropriate policies and programs that provide emotional and financial support to families.
- Understand and incorporate the developmental needs of children and families into health care delivery systems.

Source: Adapted from Surgeon General Koop (1987).

willingness to negotiate. Research supports these ideas. For example, highly cohesive families with low internal family conflict and a child with type 1 diabetes respond positively to a family-centered care approach (Hanson, DeGuire, Schinkel, & Kolterman, 1995). While family has been included into thinking, planning, and delivery of children's care, adult care has been ignored.

The Institute for Patient- and Family-Centered Care (2010), created in 1992, was originally focused on advancing family-centered care in pediatric, maternity, and newborn care. Their philosophy is grounded in thinking family members should play important roles on the care team. Now, because they realize that family is important in all care processes, too, their mission also includes adult and geriatric care. This vision acknowledges the profound changes needed in health care delivery. Nurses and other health professionals need to build on individual and family strengths, enhance their confidence, and build their competence. Family is indispensable to collaborative partnerships. Empowered relationships matter. Family can serve as advisors.

Origins of Family-Focused Care for Adults

Family participation in health care is essential to nursing practice (Williams, 2006). Since ideas about family participation have primarily targeted children, there is little evidence of progress in actively including family in the care of all people regardless of age. Family-centered care for adults has been occurring during end-of-life care (hospice). Yet, while decades of results indicate positive outcomes of end-of-life care at home, some still die in institutions where poor communication between family and staff, inadequate support, and rude treatment still occur (Teno et al., 2004).

Challenges to Family-Focused Care

Clearly, a lack of appreciation for family-centered care by many still exists. Numerous constraints continue to occur:

- Overly demanding provider-patient staffing ratios
- Restricted family visitation
- Health care systems focused on a provider-centric model of care
- Unequal distributions of power
- Lack of time to provide adequate information and support
- Communication difficulties
- Limits of fiscal resources

Many providers still restrict family visitation. Family care is ineffectively integrated, and information and education are provided without regard for unique needs, literacy level, or culture. Coordinated care still falls short during inpatient stays and is mostly disregarded when it comes to discharge home and the needs of those self-managing home care. Technologies keep evolving and conversations about needs for cost reduction continue. Reduced length of acute care stays and growing numbers of those with chronic illnesses mean caregivers face greater burdens for longer time periods. Caregiver burden, stress, role fatigue, spousal burnout, and inadequate access to needed information are growing concerns. The inability to navigate the breadth of options in an unsystematic health care industry is often neither family driven nor caring. This evidence points to needs for different forms of care.

Nurses face stress from practice roles that make it difficult to separate professional expectations and personal values. Nurses still take directions from the institutions, organizations, and agencies that employ them. They observe the gaps between needed care and what is provided. They often sense they are powerless to make needed changes. Institution-based supports, adequate education for individual care needs, empathetic supervision, nonpunitive workplaces, and safe work environment where nurses can discuss and be included in the resolution of dilemmas are needed. Nurses need knowledge and abilities to be leaders in health care delivery and advocate for sensitive and supportive work environments that attend to individual and family unit needs.

Realizing Family-Focused Care

Adding another title to describe nursing care might seem superfluous or unnecessary, but the term *family-focused care* is used throughout this textbook to claim caring ideas that nurses can call theirs. The terms *patient-centered* and *family-centered care* are useful terms, but groups outside nursing largely control them. The term family-focused care is proposed to describe a care form that uniquely belongs to nursing. This practice is characterized by intentional actions and deliberate supports aligned with the wishes and needs of individuals and those they identify as their family unit. Family-focused care uses mindful relationships to meet holistic health and illness care needs; it is a care attitude conveyed through *thinking family* that intentionally and purposely guides nursing actions. This care values and respects the unique needs of individual and family units. Regardless of the care system or situation, family is always viewed as the unit of care. Coordinated care identifies needs beyond the immediate ones. Nurses who *think family* look beyond episodic care and identify the preventive actions needed to protect health and encourage wellness for the family unit. Clear communication is a hallmark of every nursing care encounter. Health education relevant to care management is provided in clear language and culturally appropriate ways. While providing family care, nurses ensure that adequate resources are available and interventions respect family household and environmental concerns. Family nurses use theories and scientific evidence to guide practice.

Implications of Family-Focused Care

In family-focused care, the individual and family are the unit of care. When single persons are seen in caregiving settings and family members are absent, nurses still identify the family household unit as the focus of nursing care. Because family-focused care is relationship-based, it fosters collaboration or partnerships. Nurses bring initiative, authenticity, and responsiveness to the care situation (Doane & Varcoe, 2005). Nurses who *think family* listen and hear the voices of those seeking care as well as those they recognize as family.

The nurse is aware that some ambiguity and uncertainty will always be found in caring situations. Family nurses avoid biased opinions, assumptions, prescriptive solutions, easy answers, and quick fixes. These nurses understand that many factors shape experience (e.g., culture, ethnicity, language, policy, systems). Family nurses notice personal strengths and use them in empowering ways. These nurses aim to understand the implications of the family household on individual care needs. Finally, family-focused nursing allows space for personal reflection, examination of biases and prejudices, and promotion of self-care and knowing oneself.

Usefulness of Family-Focused Perspective

People are connected to others through family and their social networks and nurses who *think family* know that. Even when some family members are not physically present, they have personal meaning and influence. Those who seek medical care services are still attached to the values, fears, and stresses linked with their personal lives. Individuals may never give voice to these concerns unless invited to share them and perceive a caring person willing to listen. Influences beyond the immediate interaction may have great relevance to care. When nurses *think family*, they approach individuals judiciously and respect unspoken needs and concerns. Whenever you are involved in a clinical situation, it is good to take time and reflect about the skills required to effectively interact with individuals and their family members (Box 2.8).

As nurses deliver care, they are aware that other relevant factors beyond the immediate situation might need consideration. For example, a middle-aged gentleman is alone in the hospital room after a surgical procedure and says he is unable to sleep. An immediate response might be that he is awake from discomfort related to the earlier surgery. A nurse who thinks family understands that the sleep difficulties might have their foundation in family or household concerns. He might be worried about missing work and the income it represents. He could be concerned about the extra burden his wife bears for their disabled adult child. He could be anxious about his hospital bill and payment without insurance coverage. Although sleep medicine might resolve the immediate problem, it will not likely solve the more complex family-related hurdles. Family nurses look beyond the immediate and inquire about other possiblities.

Nurses' Roles in Family-Focused Care

Family-focused care addresses young and old, healthy and sick, and dependent and independent. Varied needs are treated with sensitivity and the understanding that a larger underlying story exists. Family members are seen as tangible supports. On the other hand, nurses also realize that sometimes families can be barriers. Some even sabotage the needed care. Family-focused care is used to assess family needs and assets. Outcome evaluation considers what is possible in a given family situation. Nurses build trusting relationships in which they

---

BOX 2-8

Evidence-Based Family Nursing Practice: Trilogy Model of Family Systems Nursing

Use of family systems nursing knowledge in clinical practice has been a challenge in the United States and many other parts of the world. Problems primarily occur in two areas. One is the concerns of nurses about their relationships with those seeking health care and beliefs about their roles. The second area of concern has to do with ways to bring nurse educators, researchers, and practitioners together as partners. These researchers have noted that the prevalent biomedical perspectives may be at odds with family systems nursing (FSN). Their findings suggest that the FSN approach uses a partnership perspective and competencies involve creating space for family members to participate in goal setting and identification of solutions. A study examined different forms and time lengths of education to prepare for practice in a variety of clinical settings. Findings indicated that nurses progressively incorporated FSN in practice as they received positive feedback from colleagues and families. The authors concluded that students and nurses need more time in supervised practicums to develop needed skills (e.g., family interviewing, therapeutic conversations, fears linked with family suffering and emotions, uncertainty). It seems that nurses seek the same level of direction and support for relational skills as they do for technical ones. Findings indicated that educators' personalities and capacity to comfortably apply FSN skills influenced students use of knowledge. Messages about the potential use of FSN need to be shared among researchers, educators, and practitioners to demonstrate ways these three areas are interlinked.

Source: Duhamel, F., & Dupuis, F. (2011). Towards a trilogy model of family systems nursing knowledge utilization: Fostering circularity between practice, education and research. In E. K. Svavarsdottir & H. Jonsdottir (Eds.), *Family nursing in action* (pp 53–68). Reykjavik, Iceland: University of Iceland Press.

---

can be respectfully curious about things not discussed and experiences not shared. The fused lives of multiple persons can enhance or threaten quality of life and wellness potentials.

Transforming the Nursing Perspective

A biomedical model is a common way students learn about nursing practice. Students are taught using biological, anatomical, and physiological aspects of human function and disease processes. Learning about body systems can be difficult. However, gaining proficiency in responding to the complex interacting biological and social systems can be even more challenging. As the science of care is taught, the art of nursing care (e.g., process, emotions, consciousness, presence) is often relegated to the background. A reductionist perspective, in which individuals are viewed as separate parts or systems, can be shortsighted. It is like not seeing the forest for the trees! Wellness, health, disease, and illness situations have underlying stories that are unlikely to be easily or quickly told. Medical diagnosis is important, but it explains only part of the story connected to personal and family lives.

Nurses are usually taught to relate to single individuals. Education and experience communicating with families or groups can be limited for many students. Often a sick model of care is internalized, with care being sought by an individual only when he senses or observes a malfunction or problem. Most people report physiological problems. Those of an emotional, psychological, or social nature are often ignored or discounted. Immediate acute care needs get the most attention. Chronic disease management, prevention, and lifestyle behaviors to promote health often get overlooked. Family nurses know that coordinated care also includes wellness, health promotion, prevention, community, and population-based care needs. Take some time to review the case presented in Box 2.9 and consider ways the content of this chapter might fashion your thinking about care needs.

BOX 2-9

Family Circle

As you begin your early morning clinical experience in the medical unit today, you walk into a room and see Mrs. Cattrell, a frail older woman resting in a rumpled bed. Alongside the bed is a man who appears to be in his mid-30s; he is sleeping, reclining in a chair about halfway covered with a blanket. On closer examination, you notice that two IV lines are on one side of the bed. A large bag of normal saline is dripping steadily into a right arm site and a blood transfusion is dripping slowly into the left arm. The Foley catheter bagging hanging at the end of the bed looks as if it was recently emptied. You were told that her diagnosis is adult acute lymphocytic leukemia. She was diagnosed several months ago, and her condition has steadily declined over the past few weeks. She had experienced severe symptoms for several months before going to her medical doctor and being diagnosed. In morning report, you heard that Mrs. Cattrell has not been eating, slept poorly last night, seems somewhat agitated, and makes frequent demands on the nursing staff. Nothing was said about the man in the chair beside her. You were instructed to obtain her vital signs and assess her condition.

1. Using what you have previously been taught about completing traditional assessments, write a four- to five- sentence summary to describe the approaches you would take and identify the various things you would consider.
2. Now, use what you have learned from reading this chapter and think about ways a family-focused approach might be different from a traditional assessment. Write four to five sentences that describe the different kinds of things to include in a family-focused assessment.
3. Next, compare and contrast your ideas with three to four others in a small-group discussion. Make a list of the pros and cons of each approach to care.
4. Finally, come to group consensus about the best forms of nursing care for Mrs. Cantrell.

Chapter Summary

This chapter introduces many ideas and terms nurses link with family-focused care. The idea of *thinking family* is used to introduce different ways to provide nursing care. An ecological model—the Family Health Model—is described as a useful way to view the complex lives of individuals and families. More about ways this model can be used in delivering nursing care will be discussed throughout this book. The varied places individuals and family units live influence health and illness. Nurses who *think family* acknowledge that influences on health and illness can be assessed and this information offers opportunities for nursing interventions. Family units and their households give important clues about resources, supports, strengths, and hurdles to overcome when it comes to getting healthy or well. Nurse who *think family* know that family is always present to individuals, even when members are not physically visible. This presence has meaning and direct implications for nursing care in all settings. The following chapters explore many implications of family-focused care and thinking family.

REFERENCES

Audet, A., Davis, K., & Schoenbaum, S. C. (2006). Adoption of patient-centered care practices by physicians: Results from a national survey. *Archives of Internal Medicine, 166,* 754–759.

Berwick, D. M. (2009). What "patient-centered" care should mean: Confessions of an extremist. *Health Affairs, 28*(4), 555–565.

Coontz, S. (1992). *The way we never were.* New York: Basic Books.

Coontz, S. (1997). *The way we really are.* New York: Basic Books.

Coontz, S. (2006). *Marriage: A history.* New York: Penguin Books.

Craft-Rosenberg, M., & Pehler, S. (2011). *Encyclopedia of family health*. Thousand Oaks, CA: Sage Publications.

Curran, D. (1984). *Traits of a healthy family*. New York: Ballantine Books.

Denham, S. A. (1999a). The definition and practice of family health. *Journal of Family Nursing, 5*(2), 133–159.

Denham, S. A. (1999b). Family health: During and after death of a family member. *Journal of Family Nursing, 5*(2), 160–183.

Denham, S. A. (1999c). Family health in an economically disadvantaged population. *Journal of Family Nursing, 5*(2), 184–213.

Denham, S. A. (2003). *Family health: A framework for nursing*. Philadelphia: F. A. Davis.

Doane, G. H., & Varcoe, C. (2005). *Family nursing as relational inquiry*. Philadelphia: Lippincott. Williams & Wilkins.

Duhamel, F., & Dupuis, F. (2011). Towards a trilogy model of family systems nursing knowledge utilization: Fostering circularity between practice, education and research. In E. K. Svavarsdottir & H. Jonsdottir (Eds.), *Family nursing in action* (pp 53–68). Reykjavik, Iceland: University of Iceland Press.

Dunst, C. J., & Trivette, C. M. (1996). Empowerment, effective helpgiving practices and family-centered care. *Pediatric Nursing, 22*(4), 334–337.

Feetham, S. L. (1991). Conceptual and methological issues in research of families. In A. L. Whall & J. Fawcett (Eds.), *Family theory development in nursing: State of the science and art* (pp 55–68). Philadelphia: F. A. Davis.

Fiese, B. H., Winter, M. A., & Botti, J. C. (2011). The ABCs of family mealtimes: Observational lessons for promoting healthy outcomes for children with persistent asthma. *Child Development, 82*(1), 133–145.

Hanson, C. L., DeGuire, M. J., Schinkel, A. M., & Kolterman, O. G. (1995). Empirical validation for a family-centered model of care. *Diabetes Care, 18*(10), 1347–1356.

Institute of Medicine. (2001). *Envisioning the National Health Care Quality Report*. Washington, DC: National Academies Press.

Institute for Patient- and Family-Centered Care. (2010). Institute's new name. Retrieved July 30, 2011 from http://www.ipfcc.org/about/name-change.html

Loveland-Cherry, C. (1996). Family health promotion and health protection. In P.J. Bomar (Ed.), *Nurses and family health promotion: Concepts, assessment, and interventions* (pp 13–25). Baltimore: Williams & Wilkins.

Maizes, V., Rakel, D., & Niemiec, C. (2009). Integrative medicine and patient-centered care. Commissioned for the IOM Summit on Integrative Medicine and the Health of the Public. Retrieved January 29, 2012 from http://www.iom.edu/~/media/Files/Activity%20Files/Quality/IntegrativeMed/Integrative%20Medicine%20and%20Patient%20Centered%20Care.pdf

Minuchin, S., Lee, W. Y., & Simon, G. (1996). *Mastering family therapy: Journeys of growth and transformation*. New York: John Wiley.

National Center for Family-Centered Care. (1989). *Family-centered care for children with special health care needs*. Bethesda, MD: Association for the Care of Children's Health.

Nationwide Children's Hospital. (n.d.). Family-centered care. Retrieved July 30, 2011 from http://www.nationwidechildrens.org/family-centered-care

Steinglass, P., Bennett, L. A., Wolin, S. J., & Reiss, D. (1987). *The alcoholic family*. New York: Basic Books.

Teno, J. M., Clarridge, B. R., Casey, V., Welch, L. C., Wetle, T., Shield, R., & Mor, V. (2004). Family perspectives on end-of-life care at the last place of care. *JAMA, 29*(1), 88–93.

von Bertalanffy, L. (1950). The theory of open systems in physics and biology. *Science, 111*, 23–29.

Williams, W. (2006). Advanced practice nurses in a medical home. *Journal for Specialists in Pediatric Nursing, 11*(3), 203–206.

World Health Organization. (2000). The Family Health Nurse: Context, conceptual framework, and curriculum. Retrieved November 26, 2011 from http://www.see-educoop.net/education_in/pdf/family_health_nurse-oth-enl-t06.pdf

Wright, L. M., & Leahey, M. (2013). *Nurses and families: A guide to family assessment and intervention* (6th ed.). Philadelphia: F. A. Davis.

CHAPTER 3

Thinking Family to Guide Nursing Actions

Sharon A. Denham

CHAPTER OBJECTIVES

1. Identify various perspectives linked with health and illness.
2. Differentiate among the terms healthy, unhealthy, and societal health.
3. Describe ways in which nurses *think family* to deliver family-focused care.
4. Discuss ways in which thinking family improves individual, family, and societal health.

CHAPTER CONCEPTS

- Biomedical model
- Health care
- Illness
- Interdisciplinary practice
- Nursing roles
- Public health nursing
- Scope of nursing
- Social Policy Statement
- Societal health
- Theoretical perspectives

Introduction

The world of health care is changing. Health care costs keep rising and many argue about the best approach for health care reform. The Affordable Health Care Act continues to be debated. Health care programs based on need rather than ability to pay, as practiced in Canada and Europe, are continually being reformed as these countries wrestle with the growing costs. Nursing practice the world over is influenced by each nation's health care policies. If nursing is to reach a place where practice can confidently meet societal health care needs, then changes are needed in some of the care approaches nurses use. Nurses have primarily been taught to focus on individual care needs. This perspective too often ignores the at-home family and household experiences and the societal linked health and illness risks. This chapter provides some ways to consider societal health and its meanings for individuals and families. New directions for thinking family in care delivery are described (Fig. 3.1).

Differentiating Among Health and Illness Perspectives

Health is a value or a desirable quality that allows a person to be capable of activities that add worth, quality, and enjoyment to daily life. We all want to avoid illness, health

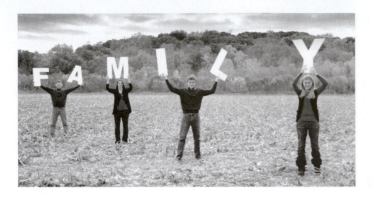

FIGURE 3-1 Thinking family.

threats, and injuries that lead to disease. Being healthy allows us to accomplish many meaningful things. It can be difficult to agree on health norms when a single standard for evaluation is unavailable. We live in a perplexing time with changes coming rapidly from every direction, a time of need for radical innovations that offers great opportunity. An amazing array of health enhancements (e.g., braces, glasses, contact lenses, cataract surgery, plastic surgery, gastric bypass) is available, yet many of these advances were unimaginable less than 50 years ago.

Health care is often considered to entail diagnosis, treatments, tests, and drugs. Important things that might help avoid being ill, such as sleep, dietary changes, physical activity, and stress management, are often ignored. We might say that health and disease begin at a level difficult to see. Are our bodies really like a 3D print of how we live? What does it mean to live a full, joyful, and authentic life? Some think spirituality and faith are important for the body and the mind. Some say that being physically able is important but then drive around a parking lot several times to get the closest parking place. Many engage in risky behaviors (e.g., tobacco use, overeating, sedentary lifestyle). People often think that disease or illness can be fixed. Nurses mostly see people with medical problems.

Health allows us to be active and do many things. However, the meaning of normal or excellent health is not always clear. Health care consumers often hear confusing media messages. Ideas about norms differ, and it is often difficult to establish a single standard. In 1947, the World Health Organization (WHO) defined health as a state of complete physical, mental, and social well-being and not merely the absence of diseases. Capabilities that have a continuum of function (e.g., vision, sleep, and mobility) are difficult to measure. Some attributes are naturally altered with age. How does one measure a dynamic quality such as health? Even wellness has variability—optimal wellness to lower level wellness. Persons afflicted by the same disease do not suffer in the same ways. People with disabilities are not equally impaired. Healing and rehabilitation occur at various paces. It is not always easy to discuss disease rates, mortality, quality of life years, or environment. Persons in one geographical region may have health advantages not enjoyed by others. Genetic factors differ. Many health alterations are only identified over time. Some cultural and ethnic groups have norms viewed as abnormal in other places. We must take care not to confuse happiness and well-being with longevity and health. Good health does not guarantee a longer or better life. Living longer does not equal good health.

Rethinking the Ways We Define Health

Health and illness have multiple dimensions. Nurses might ask, Who is healthy? Who is sick? How do we decide who is and who is not healthy? Advanced technology (e.g., imaging, genetic screenings) is used to identify medical conditions that we cannot always cure. Diagnosis confirms that someone is ill, but when did the sickness begin? If a person has a chronic condition (e.g., diabetes, hypertension, heart disease, cancer), does this mean he is unhealthy? What factors cause people to see themselves as sick or well? A medical problem might imply that a special diet is needed, but is this person ill? Someone with a common cold might say she is sick and unable to attend school, go to work, or complete usual tasks. Ways in which individuals and family units interpret symptoms differ. These points of view can be extremely different from those of nurses or other health professionals. Judgments about who is sick or well differ widely.

Perhaps nurses need to discuss health and illness in different terms. What would happen if we spoke less about things related to medical care delivery (e.g., hospitals, physicians, technology, pharmaceuticals) and more about social determinants of health (e.g., environment, water, sanitation, employment, housing, social justice)? Suppose issues were discussed in more measurable terms. For example, would it be better to spend less on repairing people after they are ill and more on keeping people healthy? It is good for nurses to understand some things about the ways money is spent for health care and its implications for families (Box 3.1).

Nursing Actions Related to Societal Health

What does health mean to large groups or broad populations? People often attend to their activities of daily living without giving great thought to health. Yet many actions relate to individual, family, and societal health. Some needs are basic (e.g., food, shelter, sleep, mobility). Others are aligned with quality of life (e.g., stress, hope to fulfill dreams, achievement, self-worth). In the United States, the aging populations have Medicare hospice benefits for end-of-life care. Growing numbers of aged persons over the next decade may need long-term care for chronic disorders that meets care needs at home. Caregivers will be needed more than ever. Older adults have different concerns than younger ones, and more attention will be needed for geriatric care and alternative care arrangements that include family (Scitovsky, 2005). Providing for the costs and needs of family members as they care for dependent family members 24 hours a day, 7 days a week, might be more critical than payment for brief primary care visits. Eight essential care dimensions have been identified that primarily relate to acute care settings (Box 3.2). Five

---

BOX 3-1

Evidence About Changing Costs for Medical Care

A decade-old study that examined Medicare outlays in the last year of life in 8,000 deaths found that little change had occurred over the prior 20 years, as 27.4% of medical expenditures were incurred in the last year of life (Hogan, Lunney, Gabel, & Lynn, 2001). Most persons had at least four significant health problems in the year of their death. Medicare expenditures largely included persons with heart disease, cancer, stroke, chronic obstructive pulmonary disease, pneumonia, or dementia. A surprising finding from this study was that minorities living in high poverty areas or factors viewed as social determinants of health were likely to have 28% per capita higher Medicare spending costs than those who did not. In this study, about 50% of those diagnosed with cancer were likely to use hospice care, yet only 10% of all others used it. However, 40% of the Medicare beneficiaries spent some of their last life year in a nursing home, where many deaths occurred. These findings indicate that the high cost of death largely has to do with caring for severe illness, dealing with functional impairment, and covering nursing home expenditures.

BOX 3-2

Patient-Centered Care

In the late 1980s, the Picker Commonwealth Program for Patient-Centered Care and the Picker Institute identified important care dimensions: care access; respect for values and preferences; care coordination; information, communication, and education; physical comfort; emotional support; involvement of family and friends; appropriate preparation for discharge and care transition. Care needed includes the following things:

- Effective treatments provided by trusted staff
- Patient involvement in decisions and respect for their preferences
- Rapid access to reliable health care advice
- Clear and understandable information that supports self-care
- Physical comfort in a safe and clean environment
- Emotional support and empathy
- Involvement of family and friends
- Continuity of care with carefully managed transitions

Source: Gerteis, M., Edgman-Levitan, S., Daley, J., & Delbanco, T. L. (Eds.). (2002). *Through the patient's eyes: Understanding and promoting patient-centered care.* San Francisco: Jossey-Bass.

---

primary drivers of exceptional family-centered inpatient hospital care experiences are identified as follows (Bailey, Conway, Zipper, & Watson, 2011):

- Leadership demonstrates a culture focused on patient- and family-centered care.
- Staff and care providers are fully engaged in patient- and family-centered care.
- Respectful partnerships among care providers enable them to anticipate and respond to needs (e.g., information, comfort, emotional, spiritual).
- Health care delivery is reliable and competent.
- Evidence-based care is practiced.

When physicians discuss end-of-life choices with cancer patients, their health care costs are much lower in the last week of life (Zhang et al., 2009). Yet, many dying persons never get referred to hospice. More than a third of those referred spend only 7 days enrolled, and many would benefit greatly from aspects of care management lasting longer (Jennings, Ryndes, D'Onofrio, & Baily, 2010). Hospice care offers several things that families desire:

- Response to human consequences of profound illness (e.g., comfort, safety, support, choice)
- Continuity of caregiving among settings and providers
- Response to evolving community needs (e.g., multiple diseases, children, prisoners, rural residents, bereaved)

Dying persons and their families want autonomy and dignity. Things like responses to suffering, compassion, and vigilance at the end of life are important.

Concerns about societal health might consider what forms of care delivery are most cost effective in supporting family needs. What does society need when it comes to such problems as cognitive dysfunction, mental illness, long-term disability, genetic disorders, or the homeless? Political leaders' debates should include pressing family and societal health needs. For example, the obesity crisis is of great concern. About 33.8% of U.S. adults are overweight or obese (Centers for Disease Control and Prevention [CDC], 2011). Obesity is a growing problem for other countries as well. Growing numbers of young children are at risk for becoming obese and even morbidly obese. Obesity is linked with heart disease, stroke, hypertension, type 2 diabetes, and some forms of cancer. Medical costs linked with obesity are in the billions, with obese persons spending $1,429 more annually for health care than those of normal weight (Finkelstein, Trogdon, Cohen, & Dietz, 2009). Others have found that obesity raises medical costs even higher ($2,826 in 2005 dollars), with estimates that annual treatment costs are about 16.5% of the national spending budget on medical care (Cawley & Meyerhoefer, 2010). Another study about relationships between middle-aged individuals, Medicare costs, and mortality found that obese persons at 45 years of age had a smaller chance of surviving to age 65 (Cai, Lubitz, Flegal, & Pamuk, 2010). Obese persons had lifetime Medicare expenditures of $163,000 compared to $117,000 for those at normal weight. Left unchecked, by 2030, it is predicted that obesity-related medical costs could rise to $48 billion to $66 billion a year in the United States (Wang et al., 2011). This is a great deal of money! Increased lifetime costs will substantially increase the overall Medicare expenditures for today's middle-age population. We are still learning about the full magnitude these costs will have on employment, disability, and health insurance.

In the 1990s, the World Health Organization began warning that the growing burden of obesity was becoming a global epidemic for industrialized nations and developing countries. More still needs to be known about a global food system of processed, inexpensive, and commercially marketed items to children and adults. Nurses and the general public are often unaware of public health measures that might be used to reverse this still-growing epidemic. Some solutions rest outside the health care industry, but clinicians might make important differences. For example, lifestyle choices, the built environment, leadership capacities, prevention, public policy, and government interventions offer alternative approaches to the obesity problem. Coordinated actions are needed to solve a problem of this magnitude. Nurses who *think family* can help by looking beyond primary care settings and finding ways to address this concern.

While concerns grow about obesity, malnutrition and starvation are also growing problems. Inadequate nutrition affects physical, cognitive, and behavioral development. It can also cause irritability, lead to fatigue, and lessen the ability to concentrate. Not only is hunger a concern for people who are homeless and unemployed, but it is faced daily by families with inadequate incomes. Families often must choose between food and other basic needs (e.g., rent, utilities, and medical care). In 2014, *Feed the Children* reports that more than 17 million U.S. households face not having enough food for everyone in the family. Nurses who *think family* consider the health and illness of family units and the larger society, not merely individuals.

Think Family and Improve Societal Health

Health has many points of view. Physical health is usually discussed, but mental and societal health are often ignored. Societal health includes wealth distribution, equal opportunity, human rights, and ways people get along with each other. Health can be discussed as motivation, attitude, moral principles, or availability of care providers, systems, or programs. Societal health has been defined by such terms as employability, marital satisfaction, sociability, and community involvement (Renne, 1974). Evidence shows relationships between social networks and health status (Haas, Schaefer, & Kornienko, 2010; Song, 2011; Umberson & Montez, 2010). Societal health has effects on individual and family health.

American veterans from the Iraq and Afghanistan wars number 2.3 million; 20% or more of them suffer from post-traumatic stress syndrome (PTSD) or depression, 19% of them might have traumatic brain injury (TBI), and perhaps 7% or more have both. Alcohol and drug abuse are problems for others (U.S. Department of Veterans Affairs, 2014). These injuries are often accompanied by other physical disabilities. Veteran families from many wars experience trauma, suffering, and challenges that last a lifetime. Homelessness and suicide are other factors faced by many veteran families.

Philosophy can provide other ways to consider social aspects of health. For example, health can imply abilities to adapt to changing environments, social situations, or surroundings (Dubos, 1987). Health is linked with relationships; it is an adaptive process, and is a socially constructed reality (Illich, 1975). Social groups attend to things they prize, things viewed as needed or attainable (e.g., car seat belts, infant seats, drug, alcohol, or tobacco use). Health can be discussed in terms of suffering and recovery. Some find individual suffering valuable, others don't. Health can be medicalized with prescribed treatments that ignore the potentials of things the human spirit can accomplish.

People live interdependent lives with connections to social institutions. Do we really act on our own volition? Or are we continually influenced by household, neighborhood, and societal factors? So, what health indicators should we measure? What social factors are linked to family and individual health? Individuals and families are bound to the places where they live, learn, work, play, and pray. Social determinants influence thinking about health and are linked with life experiences (e.g., birth, development, live, work, age). Access to nutritious foods, quality housing, health care services, physical activity, workplace environment, and educational opportunity are social determinants of health. They affect everyday lives. An ecological point of view encourages one to see connections between society, individual, and family health.

Financial Costs of Health Care

Health factors can be influenced by one's culture or nation. For example, even though Canada is part of North America some cultural perspectives differ from those in America (Box 3.3). The United States is one of the wealthiest nations in the world and spends more money on health care than any other country. Yet, the United States has growing health disadvantages with higher mortality rates and inferior health from birth (Woolf & Laudan,

---

BOX 3-3

Canadian Perspective of Societal Needs for Medical Care

The Royal College of Physicians and Surgeons of Canada (2011) agrees that when it comes to medicine, societal needs have both quantitative and qualitative perspectives. Quantitative needs are addressed by having the appropriate type and mix of physicians. These characteristics largely represent the public's interest and role of educational institutions. Qualitative needs have to do with the adequacy of the physicians' knowledge, skills, attitudes, and willingness to assume the roles needed by diverse societies. Similar observations can also be made about nurses and other health care professionals. Professional competencies needed by population groups are often culturally specific responses to societal needs, social determinants of health, and the burden of illness. Although health systems play roles, policy choices that influence distribution of money, power, and resources at local, national, and global levels are extremely influential. Social concerns often result in legislation or laws that greatly influence the health of a society.

2013). When compared with peer countries, the United States fares worse in nine areas of health (birth outcomes, injuries and homicides, teen pregnancy and sexually transmitted infections, HIV and AIDS, drug-related deaths, obesity and diabetes, heart disease, chronic lung disease, disability) than some other nations. These health problems affect all age groups until after 75 years and are of particular concern for persons up to 50 years. Several reasons for the concerns were found:

- Fragmented health care; weak public health and primary care; and a significant segment of uninsured people
- High-calorie consumption; abuse of prescription and illicit drugs; traffic accidents; more firearms; more sexual activity (earlier, more partners, riskier practices)
- Higher poverty rates; pace of education is falling behind
- Stark differences in land use (distance from food sources, residential segregation by socioeconomic status)

Although U.S. health care spending is almost 2.5 times higher than that of other nations, adoption of health information technology has lagged behind (Organization for Economic Cooperation and Development, 2011). In the United States, the government plays a large role in financing health spending and spends more than any other developed country.

Some might say that the United States is an illness profit industry. Health care and hospital cost finances have evolved without clear pricing formulas or attention to wide cost variations across geographical settings (Reinhart, 2006). Few Americans truly understand the complex payment systems. Nurses and other professionals are uncertain about the ways costs are derived and have a difficult time making sense of medical expenses. Some people pay far more for medical care than others. Health care spending involves more than just making everybody's insurance cheaper; it is also pertains to cutting unnecessary spending and paying for needed things in equitable ways.

Health Care Reform

Health care reform is needed. Dissatisfaction with current processes abound, yet the best ways to restructure things continue to be argued. The Affordable Health Care Act was intended to hold insurance companies more accountable, lower health care costs, offer health care choices, and improve care quality (Box 3.4). The Affordable Health Care Act is intended to improve quality of care and the population's health, but also to reduce costs of quality care. Yet, this reform does little to alter the ways care services are delivered. Family nurses can lead the change in ways care is provided. Nurses who *think family* can

---

BOX 3-4

Affordable Health Care Act

The Affordable Health Care Act established a National Strategy for Quality Improvement in Health Care (U.S. Department of Health and Human Services, 2011) that has set these priorities:

- Make health care safer by reducing harm caused in care delivery.
- Ensure that patients and families are engaged as partners in their care.
- Promote the most effective prevention and treatment practices for leading causes of death (e.g., cardiovascular disease).
- Enable communities to promote wide use of best practices to enable healthy living.
- Make quality care more affordable for all by developing and using new health care delivery models.

identify needs of family units and plan care to truly satisfy unique care needs. A culture of health innovation is essential if acute and home care is to support safe practice, health equity, and comprehensive needs. Nurses who *think family* can provide leadership in rethinking the ways coordinated care is delivered across care settings.

Nurses' Roles in Societal Health

Nurses who *think family* can ask: What forms of health care are most needed to promote societal health? A compelling body of evidence suggests that some old ideas need to be reexamined to meet present and future needs. Are biophysical needs the only concern? How can psychological and emotional needs also be considered? What can be done to provide better care for families and society? How can nurses use integrative medicine? What roles can nurses play in partnerships and interprofessional care? How can nurses better evaluate whether quality care has been delivered? Many things are of great concern, but which are within the scope of nursing practice? What would society consider effective nursing practice? In what ways can nurses use critical thinking, clinical judgments, and moral reasoning to set priorities for nursing care delivery?

As one thinks family, nurses must be able to gather, analyze, and synthesize information from a variety of sources. Options and implications need to be weighed. What happens if you act one way instead of another? Thinking family employs intentional actions, evaluates needs, and weighs costs and benefits of actions taken. Societal health is linked with the places people live and what they do in their households. Increasing evidence shows that geography matters and needs are influenced by where people live (Behringer & Friedell, 2006; Cummins, Curtis, Diez-Roux, & Macintyre, 2007). Noting where people live (e.g., rural, suburban, urban) and related concerns (e.g., isolated, dangerous, natural disasters) gives important information.

Reform in moving from a disease management focus to a sustained healing network is needed. Nurses have long had a social contract with the public (Box 3.5). The Social Policy Statement suggests that nurses need to lead in some care processes and be therapeutic collaborators in others (American Nurses Association, 2010). Collaborators can assist individuals, families, and communities in ways that satisfy care needs outside traditional medical delivery sites. Nurses who *think family* might seek answers to these questions: How can I be prepared to meet individual and family needs? As a nurse, what does society expect from me? What does the social contract imply about nursing roles? Proactive responses to these questions can lead in new directions.

BOX 3-5

American Nurses Association Social Policy Statement

As early as 1995, the American Nurses Association's Social Policy Statement described family as a target for nursing care. The Social Policy Statement is a contract that acknowledges the care mechanisms to be incorporated into practice. Ideas included in this contract are public accountability, professional social responsibilities, appropriate stewardship, and a valued scope of practice dedicated to meeting the needs of the society served. The 2010 revision of this contract reaffirms the importance of social roots and nursing's societal commitments at all levels of practice and educational settings. The scope of nursing practice includes concerns about educational content of nursing programs, clinical practice experiences, varied nursing roles, and population needs.

Needs of a Nation's Families

Well-functioning societies need healthy people. So, a big question is how can the family units that make up a society be healthier? What do families need most? In what ways do the needs of individuals and families differ from those of society? What can nurses do better? How do we set policy that encourages strong families? How do we provide the kinds of care that people really need? Family-focused care can address immediate care needs but it always asks about broader family concerns for now and in the future. Nurses who *think family* remember that factors that influence illness and health transcend solitary settings and single points in time.

As technologies change and information increases, real needs must be in the forefront of care. Affordability and access to health care services are important, but so are answers to questions about health equity and fair and just service distribution. For example, difficult decisions about who gets what care are important. What are the most efficient, effective, and affordable ways to manage the health of a nation's families? If families are society's building blocks, then shouldn't they be the focus of nurses' attention?

A wide cast of health care professionals is needed to fulfill society's needs. Nurses will need to address the challenges that best fit within their scope of practice. Are there traditional practices that need to be questioned? What should stay the same and what must change? What creative ideas can family nurses bring to practice? Attending to family units and global perspectives both require some new practice models. How can nurses use family-focused nursing as an avenue of change? What can nurses do to transform nursing practice so that it better meets society's needs?

Individual and Family Health Care Needs

Individuals and family units need clear information, adequate supports, and abilities to self-manage health and illness at home. Consumers must be able to navigate through health care systems. Some reorganization of care delivery is needed so individuals and family units can have more active roles in their care (U.S. Department of Health and Human Services, 2011). Health care systems are discussed as if they existed but little about care delivery is systematic. Families are rarely informed about what health care services to access. What is needed? How do people decide when and where to go? How do they choose among the public health department, a nearby clinic, or a medical practice? When should you visit urgent care or an emergency department? Care consumers do not always have good information about what steps to take.

Effective care delivery is not a motto, buzzword, or a mission statement. Effective care provides what people want, the means to solve real problems and answer their questions. Satisfaction levels are likely to be low if needs are ignored. Some people might even think that this is a form of disrespect. We speak of being partners in care. A partner is an associate, teammate, or collaborator. Partners have voices in decisions and make choices. Families need voices in the care they receive and need to be at the table where decisions are made (Box 3.6).

Needed Changes in Acute and Inpatient Care

The Institute for Healthcare Improvement has provided leadership to improve inpatient stays and hospital experiences (Box 3.7). Rather than being treated paternalistically, as in the past, families should be considered an essential part of the care team. Nurses who *think family* do that. Respectful partnerships equip people to participate in their care. They are encouraged

BOX 3-6

Changes for Meeting Individual and Family Health Care Needs

ORGANIZATION PERSPECTIVE	PATIENT/FAMILY PERSPECTIVE
Choices and decisions need to be made by the persons most affected.	Consumers have choices and rights.
Safety is a concern inside the care setting, but a critical need for those at home.	Individuals and family members need full disclosure and clear explanation about what is occurring in care settings.
Family members are not obstacles in the way of efficient care delivery, but important caregivers with responsibilities to the individual receiving care.	Family members need to be informed about diagnosis, care needs, ways to best support unique individuals, and how to care for themselves.
Patient and family satisfaction and outcomes are likely to be improved when they are empowered by nurses and other health care professionals.	Individual and family members need information about care to be given, decisions that need to be made, problems that might be encountered, and ways to access needed supports and resources.
Family members are not just people to treat politely or view as optional to meeting care needs, but they are necessary and the true caregivers.	Individuals and family members want to be involved, know what is expected, and be prepared to meet the required needs in their households.

BOX 3-7

Criteria for Excellent Acute Care Delivery

The Institute of Medicine (2001) recommends redesign of health care systems and aims for improvement in six areas:

- Safety
- Effectiveness
- Patient-centeredness
- Timeliness
- Efficiency
- Equity

Care is respectful and responsive to individual needs, preferences, and values; it includes listening, effective communication, and family presence.

to ask questions so that all aspects of the care delivery are understood. Box 3.8 suggests steps nurses can use to gather information and use that evidence in nursing practice.

Nursing Care That Individuals Want and Need

What do people want when they enter health care settings? Research indicates that consumers do not make rational choices based upon high-quality and low-priced care (Lubalin & Harris-Kohetin, 1999). The weight given to quality-of-care information about health care services chosen does not indicate how quality-of-care information is used (Faber, Bosch, Wollersheim, Leatherman, & Grol, 2009). We lack strong evidence about the kinds of care most wanted.

BOX 3-8

Ideas for Moving Forward in Evidence-Based Practice

1. Define and clearly articulate the information needed to answer specific questions.
2. Identify and choose appropriate sources of information relevant to the question.
3. Develop and use clear and effective search strategies using predetermined terms.
4. Locate and retrieve all information that appears relevant to your question.
5. Evaluate the usefulness of the information retrieved.
6. Organize and analyze the information pertinent to your specific question.
7. Determine if any important facts relevant to the question asked are still missing (e.g., economics, legal information, social aspects, policy).
8. Synthesize the findings in ways that best answer the question asked.
9. Determine the strength of the evidence used to answer the question asked.
10. Decide whether evidence identified is strong enough to alter practice or if more information is needed.

Persons seeking care find that good manners, kind treatment, friendliness, genuineness, confidence, and passion of the nurses are important. Some of the best employees are identified as persons who know their strengths and use them to make contributions. Responses to an injection can be perceived differently. Those who receive injections from excellent nurses might report feeling less pain. Differences between the two groups can result from the way nurses set the stage before giving the injections. They might say something like "This might hurt, but I will try to be gentle." A show of empathy and compassion for the pain of the experience can cause nurses to be higher on a likability scale. Personal skills such as showing self-confidence, using etiquette, giving compliments, or using humor can help them seem approachable and encourage conversation. The best nurses get more compliments than complaints. Nurses who enjoy their work and create personal and positive experiences for those in their care might be viewed as more trustworthy. Nurses often have different beliefs and values than care recipients, but care experiences are transformed by use of nursing presence.

Delivering Excellent Nursing Care

Excellent care is more than hospitality. W. Edwards Deming (2000) is widely known for his work in quality measurement. He said that, if you cannot measure it, you cannot improve it. He also said that even though care delivery is important, most people want an experience that meets their unique needs. They want information they can use. Nurses who listen to individuals and family members, provide human touch, and show empathy are valued by most.

Being in a strange bed, sitting alone in the emergency department, waiting to learn of surgery outcomes, hearing unfamiliar medical jargon, and dealing with technical procedures and clinical care systems can be stressful. Nurses who *think family* offer care that puts people at ease, addresses fears, and answers questions. Dr. Marilyn Friedman was one of the first nurses to pay careful attention to the need for completing family assessments; her textbooks have been used by thousands of nursing students since the 1980s (Box 3.9).

Having Meaningful Conversations

Nursing students and some nurses may fear having certain conversations with individuals. They worry about saying the wrong thing or not knowing all the answers. Sometimes talking with strangers and the uncertainty of what to discuss can be uncomfortable and they avoid situations by busying themselves with tasks. But those diversionary tasks are

---

BOX 3-9

Family Tree

Marilyn M. Friedman, PhD (United States)

Marilyn M. Friedman is professor emerita from the California State University School of Nursing in Los Angeles, California. She is recognized as the author of the first family nursing textbook. In the late 1970s, while teaching community health nursing to students, she recognized the lack of adequate teaching materials about family care. She envisioned having a book to use in teaching nursing students that would conceptually define family nursing practice. She developed a family assessment framework that has been used by countless thousands of nurses as they have studied family and community health. She used the sociological literature available at the time to create an assessment tool that could be used to measure a family's structural-functional dimensions. Dr. Friedman has made an important contribution to nursing as she identified that family nursing is distinct and different from ideas of nursing care for individuals. She has helped us realize the importance of family as the unit of care, differentiate potential risks and needs of various types of families, understand the developmental stages of families, and consider behaviors of a well family. Her early work enabled nurses to use theory as they considered the health care needs of families and stressed the importance of completing a comprehensive family assessment. In 1981, the first edition of *Family Nursing: Theory and Assessment* was published. Over the years the book was revised several times (1986, 1992, 1998), and in 2003, the final version of *Family Nursing: Research, Theory, and Practice* was published. In 2005, at the Seventh International Family Nursing Conference in Victoria, British Columbia, Canada, Dr. Friedman was awarded the Distinguished Contribution to Family Nursing Award for her important contributions to the field of family nursing.

---

sometimes read as rudeness, disinterest, or not caring. For example, what does it mean if the nurse has a furrowed brow when telling a person he has "bad veins?"

What is a meaningful conversation? It is not measured by length but by the quality of the interaction. Maybe it demonstrates empathy. Perhaps it is about sharing what will happen in a particular experience. What questions do families have as they wait for a surgical outcome? If someone said it was an invasive surgery, what does that mean? Nurses might see some medical procedures as mundane, but the family waiting might recall hearing about air bubbles that could kill you, "blowing out" veins, or "bleeding out." These ideas produce anxiety.

Speaking about death can be an awkward situation and too often these conversations never occur. Yet it is an experience that all humans will face. When is the right time to speak of death? Medical providers might be hesitant or sidestep the topic. Facing the end of life is not a single or simple thing. It is shared with others. It can be a conversation that happens over time. It might not occur until very late in treatment of stage 4 cancer, maybe only weeks or even days before death is inevitable. What opportunities might be lost through this delay?

How do nurses gain expertise in conversing about uncomfortable things? How does one learn the best ways to approach difficult subjects? Nursing students need skills and experience to be at ease. Sometimes it can be easier to talk with strangers than with those who are closest. The best conversations are dialogues, involving give and take. The nurse might say something like "When you think about what is happening, what is of most concern?" When nurses *think family*, they realize dialogue means listening. Nurses are not required to have "the answer" or give advice. Being an active listener is important. Active listeners ask questions that encourage others to tell their story—it is not your story!

Family Content in Nursing Education

Ideas about nursing education are continually evolving but are based in the biomedical model that guides medical diagnosis and illness treatment in the Western world. This focus is on problems, issues that are "not normal." Nurses learn to do health histories, physical examination techniques, and observation, and use laboratory findings to treat and manage illness. They are taught to view people across the life span and holistically, including family and other related factors (e.g., culture, emotions, spirituality, environment).

Yet nurses are not always well prepared to work with family units (e.g., involve them in decision making, support caregiver needs, include them in care) in care settings (Institute of Medicine, 2001) because their education is focused on episodic illness needs. They know they are to address wellness, health promotion, and disease prevention, but do not always know how. Nurses know that coordinated care is needed, but they are not always well prepared to ensure that what is needed at home is addressed in the acute care setting. Nurses who *think family* learn to organize care to anticipate unique needs that might occur in different settings.

Preparation to Address Family Health Needs

To address family and societal health, nurses need to learn more about integrated care. Integrated care is more than cures and treatments. It includes family health history, genetics, current concerns, availability of support, adequacy of resources, personal goals, individual values, community, and environments. It involves consultations with interprofessional caregivers and use of conventional medicine and complementary therapy providers. Integrated care uses an array of cost-effective therapeutic services and processes.

Changing the approach to nursing care requires changes in what is learned and how that knowledge is applied in practice. Perhaps concepts of wellness, the power of the brain, and mind-body relationships need more attention. Letting go of tradition, changing ideas previously learned, and incorporating new knowledge may not be easy. How can nurses be leaders in delivery of new care forms? Will nurses lead or will they follow? Dr. Marilyn McCubbin is an example of a leader; her work has helped nurses around the world understand the problem of stress for individuals and families (Box 3.10).

BOX 3-10

Family Tree

Marilyn McCubbin, PhD (United States)

Dr. Marilyn McCubbin served as the former faculty director at the University of Wisconsin–Madison School of Nursing and as the director of the Nursing Center for Research on Health Disparities at the University of Hawaii at Manoa. Along with her husband, she developed the Resiliency Model of Family Stress, Adjustment and Adaptation. Her research and scholarship advanced knowledge of family responses in health and illness and provided important directions to health professionals who worked to improve family care. Her research underscores the importance of strengthening individual and family resiliency as a mechanism for improving family adaptation. Dr. McCubbin's work was instrumental in changing the ways in which we understand and conduct research about families with chronic illness. Her important work has moved the focus from family dysfunction and pathology to family resiliency and adaptation. Her work has been translated into German and Icelandic and contributed to our understanding about families from Germany, Korea, Japan, Iceland, Thailand, Taiwan, and the United States. In 1996, Dr. McCubbin was selected as a Fellow in the American Academy of Nursing in recognition of her significant nursing leadership in the United States. She has also received an award from the Family Health Research Section of the Midwest Nursing Research Society and, in 2007, was awarded for her distinguished contribution to family nursing research at the Eighth International Family Nursing Conference in Thailand.

To *think family*, nurses need to include family responses to health and illness, have greater communication expertise, and be more familiar with family dynamics, health policy, and ways to do family interventions. Becoming a family nurse requires exposure to the lived experiences and concerns of those receiving care. It also involves the ability to perceive things from a different point of view.

Varied clinical experiences that allow nursing students to see broad life experiences of individuals and their families are needed (Benner, Sutphen, Leonard, & Day, 2009). These exposures can provide greater insights about larger life experiences. That means reaching beyond personal knowing and experience and investigating the other—those different from you. What does health or illness mean personally? Do personal views differ from those of other family members? Is the family prepared to handle needs related to an illness, injury, or disability? Clinical situations suggest questions about ways to *think family*.

Shifting the Focus to Family

Learning to *think family* requires some new care orientations and philosophies. How can societal care and efficient, cost-effective, high-quality, and safe individual care be delivered? What is the best way to meet needs? How can nursing practice be transformed so that it meets the unique care needs of particular individuals and families?

Shifting focus from individual to family care will not occur without some battles. Most health care experiences involve only the individual. Some family members may accompany the person to the visit or sit in waiting areas, but they are neither addressed nor included in the care delivery. Unlike in some countries, home care in the United States is mainly for people with disabilities, those unable to travel, and those who are dying with hospice care. Most nurses never learn about household experiences because they never see individuals in their home settings. For example, hospitalized individuals in Malawi are dependent upon family members to bring food from home daily. Their overcrowded hospitals are just not prepared to provide for this basic need. Thus, family remains a constant in each individual's life and nurses see them and identify their important caring roles.

Learning to *think family* is a process. Intentionally focusing one's mind on family as a critical aspect of individual care might seem tedious at first. Family-focused nursing care has expectations whether family is present or not. Think about yourself; although your family is not always physically present, your family is still with you. Human connections occur in minds and hearts. Family-focused care is more than just comfort care, it includes intentional nursing involvement to satisfy unique needs presented.

Approaches to Family Care

Being a family nurse cannot be prescriptive. All will not look or act the same. A definition of a family nurse is one who identifies and attends to family as the unit of care in a breadth of care situations. Classroom, peer, and clinical experiences help one practice and gain understandings about the variety and breadth of family experience. Box 3.11 identifies different forms of nursing care, family-friendly care, and family-focused care. Box 3.12 differentiates individual and family care approaches.

Inadequate preparation for thinking family is a roadblock to providing family-focused care. Being a family nurse means investing time and examining personal assumptions and biases, incorporating evidence about complex family lives into practice, and honing skills for working with family units living in diverse community settings.

BOX 3-11
Diverse Forms of Family Care

	TRADITIONAL NURSING CARE	FAMILY-FRIENDLY CARE	FAMILY-FOCUSED CARE

Primary focus	Individuals:
	   Acute or presenting needs
	   Cure or "fixing" the problem
	   Treatments
	   Procedures
		Aesthetics:
		   Sitting rooms
		   Open visiting hours
		   Private spaces
		   Comfort measures
			Family as care unit:
			   Intentionally included
			   Inclusion
			   Holistic measures
			   Support
			   Empowerment

Nursing role	Expert	Consultant	Collaborator or partner
Individual's role	Care seeker	Care recipient	Care recipient
Family role	Not involved in care	Care recipient	Care participant

BOX 3-12
Comparison of Individual and Family Care Focus

AREA	INDIVIDUAL CARE FOCUS	FAMILY CARE FOCUS
Care settings	Traditional approaches in diverse health care settings (e.g., acute care, ambulatory care, mental health, nursing home, rehabilitation)	Care needs in traditional and other care settings (e.g., hospice, public health, community) Family household Aware of importance of family roles in care
Assumptions	Diagnose and treat Individuals make decisions and family might be involved Individuals act alone and self-management is tied to individual Meet needs of solitary persons	Complex interrelated care needs include family members and household perspectives Individuals include family, and household members are part of self-management Individuals are never isolated from others and needs of multiple interdependent persons must be met
Solutions to concerns	Educate and counsel single persons Interventions target single individuals	Assess needs and capacities of multiple members for needs linked with education and counseling Interventions target needs of multiple family members and household concerns

Practical Application of Family Content

Knowledge about families is useful when it can be artfully applied to situations in ways that meets care recipients' needs. Nurses who *think family* act responsively and deliberately to address diverse needs during clinical care situations. That approach requires prior thought and preplanning to select purposeful actions that satisfy distinct needs. Skillfully applying what has been learned in deliberate ways to satisfy family unit's needs is the backbone of family nursing. Using deliberate actions implies that the nurse performs as follows:

- Exerts conscious efforts to reflect on assessed and voiced concerns.
- Enters into interactions with individuals about family unit concerns that provide answers to questions and information or support for identified problems.
- Collaborates with the family unit to identify solutions.
- Assists family units with finding needed resources.
- Evaluates care outcomes.

Thinking family is not just a cognitive experience, it is an attitude that nurses develop and use. Family nurses know that families have similar needs, but express them in unique ways. For example, the initial loss of vision in a 48-year-old woman with type 1 diabetes may result in uncertainty and fear about the future. However, if the nurse doesn't understand the concerns of family household members, ideas about what is needed are vague. Asking questions will clarify those needs: Does she have a job and will the vision loss affect her economic security? Is she the only driver in the family? What safety risks need to be considered? Is she the caregiver for others? What adaptations need to be made in her lifestyle? In what ways does she need assistance and who will help her? How will she spend her time if she cannot see? Is she responsible for cooking and cleaning? How will she manage daily activities without her vision? As the answers are forthcoming, it is likely that additional questions will arise. What will this vision loss mean to other family members? What are their questions and needs? Thinking family recognizes that every diagnosis not only raises questions for the individual, but also for the family unit. Thinking family encourages potential vulnerabilities of the individual and family unit to be disclosed (Fig. 3.2).

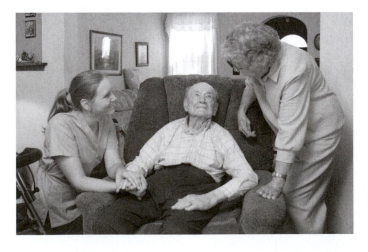

FIGURE 3-2 Nurse uses deliberate actions to collaborate with a family.

We tend to connect with what we know and have previously experienced. What do you know about yourself?

- Do you acknowledge the way things are or the way you want them to be?
- What is it like for you to be vulnerable?
- How do you experience others when they are vulnerable?

Learning new things sometimes means earlier ideas have to be unlearned or modified and that is not easy. Are you aware of things that you might need to unlearn as you consider thinking family? For example, does your behavior change in different situations (e.g., in an elevator, waiting in line, sitting in a waiting room, being with friends)? When we are in familiar situations, we know how to speak, where to look, and how to behave. In America, it is customary to walk to the right and let persons pass on the left. Did someone teach this to us? Or did we learn through observation? Notice how awkward it seems when someone tries to pass you on the right side. Yet, persons in other cultures might find our ways unnatural. Learning to forfeit what seems natural to learn new approaches takes time and effort.

Gaining Confidence

How is the confidence to interact with individuals and family units gained? Research used a pre- and post-test design to examine the self-efficacy of nursing students in a family nursing clinical practicum as they learned about family practice, home visiting, and collaborative practice (Ford-Gilboe, Laschinger, Laforet-Fliesser, Ward-Griffin, & Foran, 1997). Self-efficacy is the term used to explain perceptions about abilities to be successful in specific situations (Bandura, 1971). Perceptions of success are often remembered observations made over time. Those with high self-efficacy are likely to believe they perform well and often see difficult tasks as things to be mastered not things to avoid. Students took the pre-tests at the beginning of the school year and then again at 4 and 8 months later. It was only after the second post-test that their self-efficacy was noted to demonstrate significant difference. This study found that performing family nursing skills in a clinical setting was an essential source for gaining self-efficacy. Another study completed with nursing students in a community setting yielded similar results (Laschinger, McWilliam, & Weston, 1999). So, learning and practicing skills in clinical settings can enhance self-confidence and perhaps skill use.

Thinking Family

The idea of thinking family is not new to this textbook. In 1997, a paper published by Clarissa Green described that concept as a primary building block for nursing care. She explained that this idea involved "understanding and appreciating the interactive complexity of family life from a systems perspective" (p 231). She suggested that a critical focus of nursing practice should be aimed at helping families develop skills and confidence in managing illness experiences and adjusting to challenges.

Students had previously completed a course in basic family dynamics. One assignment involved topics in a fictitious case (e.g., divorce, substance abuse, a caregiving crisis, an unexpected serious illness, loss associated with death, financial vulnerability). A second major assignment involved the student development of a fictional family to answer the question: "What is this family's experience with difficulty?" Students found these topics challenging because they did not have much personal experience with conditions in family lives. The cases caused students to focus on three things: (a) factors contributing to or shaping the situation and related pertinent history, (b) family behaviors exhibited, and (c) what happens over time as the family members cope with difficulties. Students worked in small groups to consider what would constitute effective discharge planning, ways family health policies influence caregiving capacity, tools family members need to provide adequate care, and ways problems affect family roles, decision making, and health practices. Students were engaged with the ideas, but also evaluated their own thinking. The cases challenged the students and caused emotional responses and some personal discomfort. Students learned about strengths in troubled families and found that even big problems can get resolved without long-term harm to family members. Students were frustrated when they realized that they were ill-equipped to make their families do anything; it was family members and their unique circumstances that guided outcomes. Activities such as these are frustrating at times, but learning from them can help one gain the ability to *think family*.

Putting Family Knowledge into Actions

Critical thinking, decision making, problem solving, and effective communication are essential skills to master to be an effective family nurse. Varied laboratory and clinical experiences provide great opportunities to focus on the reading, writing, listening, talking, and reflecting needed to actively learn these skills. Simulated laboratory experiences can incorporate thinking family into case scenarios and provide time for shared learning experiences during debriefing.

In those experiences, the nurse begins to learn about family care. What does the family want to achieve? What things are needed? Even small changes in the right direction can provide a sense of accomplishment. You might not focus on personal concerns but rather on the immediate family need. For example, how will I answer questions about turning off the ventilator and allowing their father to die? Small things count. Listening, being present, and showing genuine care can make it easier to have difficult conversations once a trusting relationship is formed. Most people know that easy answers to hard questions do not exist.

Spending time doing critical analysis of family nursing and how it fits with nursing practice enhances practice (Hartwick, 1998). Sharing personal stories among peers can affirm that other families with different experiences can have similar responses. Nurses find other useful ways to handle problem situations and collaborate with family members by hearing what their colleagues have done. Nurses who *think family* are in touch with emotions and notice ways they respond to others.

Objective and Subjective Aspects of Nursing Practice

Nursing care is objective because it uses scientific evidence, skills, knowledge, formal policies, and standard procedures to guide care implementation. This objective work relates to the science of nursing. However, in the performance of care, the practice of nursing is also subjective and an art. For example, consider two nurses who perform the same procedure with a hospitalized person. Both nurses carefully follow the same steps of the procedure and demonstrate knowledge, skills, and competency. In reviewing the outcomes, one might find that satisfaction does not rest in nurses' competency skills. Responses to the treatment might relate to the nurse's attitude or behaviors. A business-like nurse might be seen as less helpful and receive a lower satisfaction score than the outgoing nurse who engages in conversation and appears genuinely interested. *Thinking family* has both objective and subjective aspects in care delivery. See the case study about a family facing many dilemmas when trying to understand health care (Box 3.13).

Work with families requires emotional balance or what some might call emotional intelligence. One needs to show concern, but not demonstrate extremes. Family nurses are not without emotion. They respectfully show empathy and compassion, but remain logical and competent. Nurses are bound to have times when intense emotions are triggered. Also, people show emotions differently. Critically reflecting on laboratory simulation or clinical experiences

---

BOX 3-13

Family Circle

Larry Hopsen had an excellent job until the recession hit. After a year of fear and frustration as he looked for work, he found a job. On his first day, he attended an orientation program and received information about health insurance options. He was told to return the paperwork by the end of the week. He took the papers home and gave them to his wife. She asked, "What do you want me to do with this?" He replied, "We have to choose a plan." The Hopsens are in their early 30s and have two children. David, their 2-year-old, was born with a form of spina bifida called meningocele. Sandra has just turned 4 and appears healthy. Larry had asthma as a child, but it was well controlled until they moved into this new apartment, which seems to have mold. The Hopsens think that they might want another child. Mrs. Hopsen experienced gestational diabetes with Sandra. Many Americans do not understand their health insurance plans. They do not know how to choose a plan. If you were to counsel the Hopsen family, what would you suggest they consider? Consumers need two skills to understand health plans. One is the ability to read and understand the choices. The second need is numeracy, or the ability to reason with numbers and use mathematical concepts. Here are some questions to consider:

Traditional approach:

1. What can you afford? What are the monthly, quarterly, or annual payments?
2. How much is the co-pay? Are there any deductibles?
3. Are you or is anyone in your family being treated for any illnesses?

Family-focused approach:

1. What is the best value for your family? Tell me about potential problems in your family that might lead to health concerns.
2. Do you have any questions about the meanings of terms like co-insurance, annual benefit limit, out-of-pocket limit, drug tier, or allowed amount?
3. Is anyone in your family taking any specialty drugs? Do you know how much they cost?

It is a good idea to focus on wellness and health. Let us review the health care plans together and see what each family member needs.

---

allows nurses to safely discuss responses to care situations. Reflection about things that happened in clinical environments can help one examine alternative ways to approach care.

Interacting with Families

Family members can be intimidating. The following situation illustrates this point. A co-worker came to the nurses' station and asked if she could be reassigned to a different patient as she was quite disturbed by the way the patient's wife acted. It seems she had a notebook and every time the nurse entered the room, she wrote something down. The nurse complained, "She makes me nervous, I think she is trying to build a case against me for a lawsuit." The nurse manager went to speak with the wife and inquired: "I see that you are writing things down in a book. . . ." The wife readily answered: "I am trying to keep a record of things, so I will remember them later. People come and go all day and each one tells me things. My memory is not as good as it used to be. Things happen one after another all day and it gets confusing. I am afraid I will forget, so I just write it down. Besides, it gives me something to do."

Boredom and confusion that come from sitting all day in a hospital room seemed good reasons to keep a written record. She was not trying to catch anyone doing something wrong, but merely passing time and ensuring that she could recall things later. A brief conversation easily clarified things. The other nurse was informed about reasons for writing. Later that day, the first nurse reported that she had spoken with the woman and discovered that they shared a common interest in quilting. Finding ways to relieve anxieties and get better acquainted with family members is a good way to correct false perceptions.

Working with Difficult Situations

Some situations can be difficult. For example, one might seem to be an intruder when entering a space that a family seems to claim as theirs. Maintaining privacy is not easy in an acute care setting. As nurses and others attend to clinical care needs, they often disrupt conversations. Nurses who *think family* learn ways to enter a family's private space. For example, concerns about genetics and related diseases can be troubling for families. Dr. Marcia VanRiper has long engaged in research with families with Down syndrome and has demonstrated many ways nurses can work with these families (Box 3.14). They manage some common problems, such as setting boundaries, forming relationships, and finding things to talk about and learn to effectively ask tough questions.

Wondering what you will talk about with a family can be troubling, but recognizing the family's strengths and competence can help (Wright & Leahey, 2013). For instance, the nurse might say: "Today, when the doctor explained the surgical procedure to your wife, I noticed that you listened carefully and asked several good questions." This positive remark might be followed with something like: "I was just wondering if all of your questions were answered or if there is something else you would like to know." Entering a conversation in this manner can seem welcoming and easy conversation can follow. Sometimes it is useful to be silent and just listen, then commend actions or behavior and ask for further details. Routine use of immediate and delayed affirmative responses can engage family members in useful conversations.

Using Narrative Approaches

A narrative approach can encourage family members to tell stories linked with everyday concerns and suffering; it is a valuable way for nurses to learn ways to take actions (Chesla, 2005). Conversation and stories can put family members at ease. It is good to have a few general questions that you can use in speaking with any family member, such as, what is most troubling to you about this situation? What can I do today to put you most at ease?

BOX 3-14

Evidence-Based Family Nursing Practice

Marcia Van Riper, RN, PhD (United States)

Dr. Van Riper is currently a Professor at University of North Carolina at Chapel Hill, with a joint appointment in the School of Nursing and the Carolina Center for Genome Sciences. Dr. Van Riper teaches genetics courses. The main focus of Dr. Van Riper's research has been the family experience of being tested for or living with a genetic condition. She has conducted numerous studies with national and international colleagues concerning families of children with Down syndrome. Dr. Van Riper completed a Mentored Research Scientist Career Development Award where she examined how families define and manage the ethical issues that emerge during four types of genetic testing: maternal serum screening for Down syndrome, carrier testing for cystic fibrosis (CF), *BRCA1* and *BRCA2* testing for families at high risk for breast cancer, and mutation analysis for Huntington disease. As part of this work, she engaged in a 3-year intensive, supervised career development/training plan that included (a) formal coursework in genetics, bioethics, and qualitative methods, and (b) interdisciplinary experiences, such as clinic and laboratory rotations, case rounds, journal clubs, and workshops. She recently completed a study about feeding issues in children with Down syndrome. Other work includes pilot studies on how minority families make sense of and use the results of genetic testing. Dr. Van Riper has been active in ISONG and served as the first president of the International Association for Family Nursing.

What do you think is the biggest problem your family needs to solve? Who is having the greatest difficulty? Family members will tell their stories if invited. Family insights offer the best guidance for nursing intervention. Meaningful conversations with family members create a therapeutic context for healing changes. Stories can help nurses gather information, organize it, make sense of it, and use it to plan nursing actions or interventions.

Chapter Summary

Nurses need to understand the ways health and illness are defined and regarded by the larger society. Not everyone sees these conditions in the same ways. Families are the building blocks of a society. Some health care services may not be what the family needs most Nurses have a social contract. this encourages them to think about what society needs and apply this understanding to the nation's families. The family household has great sway in determining individuals' needs and resources. Much about health and illness is learned first from family and then influenced by larger societal forces. Individuals stay healthy or get sick in the presence of family members. Nurses who *think family* can take the reins in modifying clinical practice so that it better addresses family and societal needs. These nurses are keenly aware of the complex factors that influence health and illness.

Providing family care does not always come naturally. Practicing skills in class, in clinical situations, and with peers can be useful for determining the best ways to provide family-focused nursing care. This chapter introduces many topics that will be explored more deeply later in this book.

REFERENCES

American Association of Colleges of Nursing. (2011). *The essentials of master's education for advanced nursing practice.* Washington, DC: Author.

American Nurses Association. (2010). Nursing's Social Policy Statement. Silver Spring, MD: Author.

Bailey, B., Conway, J., Zipper, L., & Watson, J. (2011). Achieving an exceptional patient and family experience of inpatient hospital care. IHI Innovation Series white paper. Cambridge, MA: Institute for Healthcare Improvement. Retrieved March 3, 2012 from www.IHI.org

Bandura, A. (1971). *Social learning theory.* New York: General Learning Press.

Behringer, B., & Friedell, G. H. (2006). Appalachia: Where place matters in health. *Preventing Chronic Disease, 3*(4), A113.

Benner, P., Sutphen, M., Leonard, V., & Day, D. (2009). *Educating nurses: A call for radical transformation.* San Francisco: Jossey-Bass.

Cai, L., Lubitz, J., Flegal, K. M., & Pamuk, E. R. (2010). The predicted effects of chronic obesity in middle age on Medicare costs and mortality. *Medical Care, 48*(6), 510–517.

Cawley, J., & Meyerhoefer, C. (2010). The medical costs of obesity: An instrumental variables approach. National Bureau of Economic Research, Working Paper No. 16467. Retrieved February 2, 2012 from http://www.nber.org/papers/w16467

Centers for Disease Control and Prevention. (2011). Adult obesity. Overweight and obesity. Retrieved February 1, 2012 from http://www.cdc.gov/obesity/data/adult.html

Chesla, C. A. (2005). Highlights from the 7th International Family Nursing Conference. Plenary Address: Nursing science and chronic illness: Articulating suffering and possibility in family life. *Journal of Family Nursing, 11*(4), 371–387.

Cummins, S., Curtis, S., Diez-Roux, A. V., & Macintyre, S. (2007). Understanding and representing "place" in health research: A relational approach. *Social Science & Medicine, 65*(9), 1825–1838.

Deming, W. E. (2000). *Out of the crisis.* Cambridge: MIT Press.

Dubos, R. (1987). *Mirage of health.* New Brunswick, NJ: Rutgers University Press.

Faber, M., Bosch, M., Wollersheim, H., Leatherman, S., & Grol, R. (2009). Public reporting in health care: How do consumers use quality-of-care information? Systematic review. *Medical Care, 47*(1), 1–8.

Finkelstein, E. A., Trogdon, J. G., Cohen, J. W., & Dietz, W. (2009). Annual medical spending attributable to obesity: Payer- and service-specific estimates. *Health Affairs, 28,* w822–831.

Ford-Gilboe, M., Laschinger, H. S., Laforet-Fliesser, Y., Ward-Griffin, C., & Foran, S. (1997). The effect of a clinical practicum on undergraduate nursing students' self-efficacy for community-based family nursing practice. *Journal of Nursing Education, 36*(5), 212–219.

Gerteis, M., Edgman-Levitan, S., Daley, J., & Delbanco, T. L. (Eds.). (2002). *Through the patient's eyes: Understanding and promoting patient-centered care.* San Francisco: Jossey-Bass.

Green, C. P. (1997). Teaching students how to "*think family.*" *Journal of Family Nursing, 3,* 230–246.

Haas, S. A., Schaefer, D. R., & Kornienko, O. (2010). Health and structure of adolescent social networks. *Journal of Health and Social Behavior, 51*(4), 424–439.

Hartwick, G. (1998). A critical pedagogy for family nursing. *Journal of Nursing Education, 37*(2), 80–84.

Hogan, C., Lunney, J., Gabel, J., & Lynn, J. (2001). Medicare beneficiaries' costs of care in the last year of life. *Health Affairs, 20*(4), 188–195.

Illich, I. (1975). *Medical nemesis: The expropriation of health.* London: Marian Boyars.

Institute of Medicine. (2001). *Crossing the quality chasm: A new health system for the 21st century.* Washington, DC: National Academy Press.

Jennings, B., Ryndes, T., D'Onofrio, C., & Baily, M. A. (2010). Access to hospice care: Expanding boundaries, overcoming barriers. In D. E. Meier, S. L. Isaacs, & R. G. Hughes (Eds.), *Palliative care: Transforming the care of serious illness.* San Francisco: Jossey-Bass.

Laschinger, H. S., McWilliam, C. L., & Weston, W. (1999).The effects of family nursing and family medicine clinical rotations on nursing and medical students' self-efficacy for health promotion counseling. *Journal of Nursing Education, 38*(8), 347–356.

Lubalin, J. S., & Harris-Kojetin, L. (1999). What do consumers want and need to know in making health care choices? *Medical Care Research & Review, 56*(suppl. 1), 67–102.

National Organization of Nurse Practitioner Faculties National Panel for NP Practice Doctorate Competencies (2006). Practice doctorate nurse practitioner entry-level competencies. Retrieved from http://www.nonpf.com/associations/10789/files/DNP%20NP%20competenciesApril2006.pdf

Organization for Economic Cooperation and Development (OECD). (2011). OECD health at 2011. Retrieved on January 12, 2012 from http://www.oecd.org/document/30/0,3746,en_2649_37407_12968734_1_1_1_37407,00.html

Reinhart, W. E. (2006). The pricing of U.S. hospital services: Chaos behind a veil of secrecy. *Health Affairs, 25*(1), 57–69.

Renne, K. S. (1974). Measurement of social health in a general population survey. *Social Science Research, 3*(1), 25–44.

Royal College of Physicians and Surgeons of Canada (2011). Addressing societal health needs. Retrieved January 12, 2012 from http://www.royalcollege.ca/shared/documents/fmec/societal_health_needs.pdf

Scitovsky, A. A. (2005). "The high cost of dying": What do the data show? *Millbank Quarterly, 83*(4), 825–841.

Song, L. (2011). Social capital and psychological stress. *Journal of Health and Social Behavior, 52*(4), 478–492.

Umberson, D., & Montez, J. K. (2010). Social relationships and health: A flashpoint for health policy. *Journal of Health and Social Behavior, 51*(1), S54–S66.

U.S. Department of Veterans Affairs. (2014). National center for PTSD. Retrieved August 20, 2014 from http://www.ptsd.va.gov

U.S. Department of Health and Human Services. (2011). National strategy for quality improvement in health care. Washington, DC: DHHS. Retrieved March 3, 2012 from http://www.healthcare.gov/law/resources/reports/quality03212011a.html

Wang, C. Y., McPherson, K., Marsh, T., Gortmaker, S., & Brown, M. (2011). Health and economic burdens of the projected obesity trends in the USA and the UK. *Lancet, 378,* 815–831.

Woolf, S. H., & Laudan, A. (Eds.). (2013). *U.S. health in international perspective: Shorter lives, poorer health.* Washington, DC: The National Academies Press.

World Health Organization (1947). The constitution of the World Health Organization. *WHO Chronicle 1*, 6–24.

World Health Organization. (2012). Social determinants of health. Retrieved January 12, 2012 from http://www.who.int/social_determinants/en/

Wright, L., & Leahey, M. (2013). *Nurses and families: A guide to family assessment and intervention* (6th ed.). Philadelphia: F. A. Davis.

Zhang, B., Wright, A. A., Huskamp, H. A., Nilsson, M. E., Maciejewski, M. L., Earle, C. C., . . . Prigerson, H. G. (2009). Health care costs in the last week of life. *Archives of Internal Medicine, 169*(5), 480–488.

CHAPTER 4

Communication With and About Families

Sandra Eggenberger • Sonja Meiers • Sharon A. Denham

CHAPTER OBJECTIVES

1. Discuss forms of communication aimed at assessment, care delivery, and health education.
2. Describe use of the individual-nurse-family relationship in communication.
3. Explain nurses' roles in communication to meet health and illness needs.
4. Identify nursing actions in addressing literacy, health literacy, and information needs during acute and chronic care situations.
5. Identify various communication models to guide interactions with individuals, families, communities, and populations.
6. Apply ideas for communication with diverse groups.

CHAPTER CONCEPTS

- Asking questions
- Building trust
- Communication
- Communication barriers
- Communication breakdowns
- Communication theory
- Exchange and resource theory
- Family systems theory
- Feedback
- Individual-nurse-family relationship
- Life course theory
- Literacy
- Low health literacy
- Managing conflict
- Motivational interviewing
- Privacy and confidentiality
- Role theory
- Social learning theory
- Symbolic interactionism
- Trust

Introduction

Communication is central to the human experience. Skillful communication is essential for nurses to interact with those receiving health and illness care and make sure appropriate care is provided, health is promoted, and comfort given (Hagerty & Patusky, 2003; Peplau, 1997). Nurses communicate with patients, families, and other health professionals to form relationships, convey information, clarify perceptions, and manage distress. Students often have more opportunities to learn about individual communication but less experience communicating with or about families. Family, as the primary social structure unit, needs to communicate with nurses who are capable and confident in their communication skills. Most individuals accessing health care settings experience a sense of power imbalance. They are unfamiliar with the setting or systems, unclear about health care roles, and may not understand medical terms. Care seekers often assume dependent roles, while health professionals adopt a more powerful position. In this interaction individuals and families may feel uncomfortable and vulnerable. They may not know what is expected or how to respond. Even though family members are often physically present, clear and thorough communication with them is often absent. This chapter describes some basics of effective communication and ways nurses can use them to guide individual and family unit interactions.

Providing Effective Communication

Effective communication needs to be a high priority in nursing practice. Nurses who use effective communication create satisfying care environments. Communication is a transactional process. It is how people create, share, and regulate meanings of complex experiences in relationships (Dance, 1967; Segrin & Flora, 2011; Travelbee, 1966). Communication is the transmission of messages from person to person through processes such as writing, speaking, texting, teaching, e-mail, and body language. We are always communicating! Communication requires a transmitter and a recipient. Messages focus on what is intended to be said but often include a relationship message such as how the message is sent, how it influences the relationship and interaction (Watzlawick, Beavin, & Jackson, 1967). Was the intended message conveyed? Effective communication happens when questions are asked, information is given and understood, and comfort is provided. Nurses who *think family* aim for effective communication with members of the family and the family unit.

Reflect on how you communicate? Like most people, learning some basic skills can improve the way you communicate. Quality communication requires more than just knowing how to speak. It is being cognizant of how your messages are sent and, more importantly, received by the recipient. To analyze your communication skills you need to examine responses of the recipient, reflect on how the message was received and the response, and listen to critiques from others. Effective communication takes practice and conscious effort to improve. Dr. Lorraine Wright has played a key role in promoting awareness of family-focused nursing care and continues her important work worldwide (Box 4.1).

BOX 4-1

Family Tree

Lorraine M. Wright, PhD, RN (Canada)

Lorraine M. Wright, PhD, RN, a native of Canada, is an international lecturer and consultant. She has a strong background in family therapy that she has used in thinking about the ways communication assessment should occur with family members. Her early work about human problems, suffering, and the family dynamics when illness occurs greatly influenced her future work. She collaborated with Dr. Janice Bell in the development of the Illness Beliefs Model. Dr. Wright and Dr. Maureen Leahey developed the Calgary Family Assessment and Intervention Models. She was the director for the Family Nursing Unit at the University of Calgary for 20 years. The sixth edition of the textbook entitled *Nurses and Families: A Guide to Family Assessment and Intervention* (2013) provides excellent guidance for the best approaches to meeting the needs of multiple family members. In addition to

BOX 4-1

Family Tree—cont'd

this work, she also developed the Trinity Model and, in 2005, published a book entitled *Spirituality, Suffering, and Illness: Ideas for Healing.* Dr. Wright has widely published many scholarly papers, written many book chapters, and produced educational films and DVDs that demonstrate nursing assessment methods. Her personal Web site <http://www.lorrainewright.com/index.htm> provides much information about her work and some direct contact information. You can visit her blog page, The Wright Perspective, on the Web site, where she shares some personal stories. Dr. Wright has greatly influenced family nursing practice and has paved the way for many students and nurses to grow in their knowledge and communication practices with families. Although now retired, she travels regularly and continues to share her highly respected family work world wide.

Privacy and Confidentiality

Privacy and confidentiality are often addressed separately from communication, but they are essential to building the trust that is needed when providing nursing care. Individuals and families have private information they do not want to share with everyone and they have to know that their information will be protected by nurses. Privacy about health is central to ethical practice and the development of trust relationships (American Nurses Association, 2001). We live in an age in which nothing seems private, and with the increasing use of electronic medical records and communication, individuals and families want to be certain that their privacy is always maintained. What does it mean to keep things private and confidential?

In 2003, the Privacy Rule was added to the 1996 Health Insurance Portability and Accountability Act (HIPAA) to regulate the use and disclosure of protected health information, which is any information held by the person seeking care that concerns health status, provision of health care, or payment of health care linked to an individual—essentially, any part of an individual's medical record or payment history. However, the law allows health professionals to use judgment and experience to decide if uses and disclosures are in a person's best interests. The idea of best interests is often used with underage children, but it also applies to adults. Best interests are also linked with mental health conditions, physical disabilities, comatose states, and persons unable to understand or speak. It is not easy to make judgments about what is in someone else's best interest. It is challenging for outsiders to decide who has the right to know and what information can be shared. Today's families are complicated and past social mores do not fit as well with current family configurations. So, determining with whom information can be shared can be difficult. Yet, nurses must be able to consider the family's needs and concerns when communicating.

Agencies can establish rules for ways in which they verify relationships (Health and Human Services, 2008), but this practice is not mandated. Individuals can always give permission for information to be shared or discussed with friends, family, and others. If a person states that he is a family member, friend, or involved in the patient's care, then HIPAA (1996) does not require proof. Nurses need to be aware of what the HIPAA does and does not regulate. Based on professional judgment, information can be shared by any method when others need to know or are involved in care. HIPAA does not forbid family members staying past visiting hours even when a room is shared. Calling out names is not an infringement of law and neither is posting a name at the patient's bedside, as these incidental events cannot be directly tied to medical information. Some states interpret regulations differently and this might determine who can be viewed as a family member (e.g., domestic partners). Yet, the nurse must consider the individual and family member's wishes and needs.

Rights to Information

Individuals and families need information that is clear and understandable so they know what to do, when to do it, and how to do it, and are aware of choices available to them. They need to understand the benefits, risks, and alternatives of care and procedures before they consent to them. They also need to know that they have a right to request other medical opinions, refuse treatments, or choose alternative practitioners or health care facilities. And family members need to know that they have rights as well. (Aspeling & Van Wyk, 2008; Bell, 2011)

Challenges can occur when someone the individual considers family is not legally recognized and health care providers need to discern who has the right to make decisions. Who can decide? Sociocultural influences, end-of-life situations, and decision making can create challenging situations at times. Occasionally a person's condition may warrant a nurse sharing health information without direct permission from a family member (Zerwekh, 2006). It is useful to have the person receiving care select a spokesperson for sharing family communication and most providers have the individual sign a document defining who they can share information with, if time permits. Nurses who *think family* know that rules for family communication must be fluid, be respectful, and consider privacy and confidentiality while developing relationships. Breach of confidential and private health information in our technological world is addressed by position statements of the ANA (2006). Health system personnel and regulatory systems need to thoughtfully cooperate as standards, policies, and laws to protect patient privacy and the confidentiality of health records and personal information change.

Communication and Nursing Practice

The social contract between nurses and society identifies needs for practice that support the attainment of positive health outcomes (ANA Social Policy Statement, 2010). Nurses need to use best practices as information is gathered and shared with families, messages are clearly transmitted, and collaborative relationships established. Nurses are connectors to broad forms of health care information that serve families and nursing practice with families (Box 4.2). Nursing care requires nurses who develop relationships with individuals and families through a focus on communication. Communication with and about families has potential to develop relationships that promote health and ease their suffering (Aspeling & van Wyk, 2008).

Nurses who *think family* collect information about socially linked persons during assessment. They learn about needs, resources, and supports useful in care coordination. If a nurse fails to collect family information during the initial assessment and health history, then essential information that can influence care can be missed. Clear nurse-to-family

---

BOX 4-2

Developing the Individual-Nurse-Family Relationship

The individual-nurse-family interaction uses several primary areas of communication to accomplish important goals Meleis, 2012; (Schuster & Nykolyn, 2010):

- Exchange sound information between nurse and family.
- Ensure accuracy in delivering and interpreting of information messages.
- Share patient and family information with diverse health care providers.
- Transfer responsibility to and from the family during the care episode.

communication conveys authentic care that shows acceptance and support. Nurses who *think family* use each contact to enhance health outcomes, guard safety, educate, and support. Family-focused communication not only addresses individual needs but also involves the family unit in appropriate ways.

Cultural groups have traditions, customs, values, norms, and behaviors that influence contexts for communication (Box 4.3). Terms, dialects, and health literacy issues influence communication. For example, a nursing student may try to initiate a caring relationship through a teaching project about women's health with a young Somali woman who is a practicing Muslim. Conversation might be difficult if the Somali woman is uncomfortable with the nursing student. An older Somali woman observing tells the student, "Please cover your breasts more fully if you will be working with my community; it is disrespectful to be showing so much." The nursing student might think she can dress however she likes, but cultural respect for the values of others is an essential aspect of meaningful communication.

Nurse-Family Communication Perspectives

Health and illness situations and environments present complex challenges that can make therapeutic relationships difficult. Families bring unique life experiences and needs to care situations but nurses see situations through lenses of expert knowledge and professional experiences. These divergent views affect the sender and receiver of all messages (Box 4.4). Differing perspectives create ambiguities, and misinterpretations can hamper effective relationships. For example, parents of a young child with depression may believe that the child simply needs to act different and be stronger. They might not recognize the importance

---

BOX 4-3

Communication and Culturally Sensitive Actions

Culturally sensitive nursing actions pay attention to the answers to such questions as:

- Who in the family has the greatest influence on member health?
- What are the family expectations?
- Where do ideas about health and illness get attended to in daily life?
- When do family members seek health care services?
- How do decisions get made in this family?

BOX 4-4

Communication Needs of Families

In a health or illness care situation, families need:

- Consistently shared honest information
- Cooperative and collaborative partnership built upon rapport
- Recognition of individual and family perspectives
- Autonomy that honors and recognizes individual and family needs
- Purposeful interactions in an environment where information is not withheld and trust and inclusion are fostered

Source: Rollnick, S., Miller, W. R., & Butler, C. C. (2008). *Motivational interviewing in health care: Helping patients change behavior.* New York: Guilford Press.

of scheduled follow-up counselor appointments or the important differences a medication can make. On the other hand, the nurse might view their lack of follow-through as non-adherent behaviors and ineffectual parent care. Ineffective communication could mean missed opportunities for beneficial changes.

Medical language is easily misunderstood. For example, a person may be told that a newly prescribed medication will help with fluid retention. They may assume this means that the medicine will help them hold their fluids better and become concerned when they experience frequent urination. Suppose a nurse fails to clearly inform a person that a further diagnostic procedure needs to be scheduled after a clinic visit. The patient might think that the time is scheduled and assume that the procedure is not needed if she is not called. Individuals may be given guidelines for dietary changes to improve obesity, yet family members may not have the same understandings. Involvement of family members in these situations could prevent mistaken understandings. Nurses can use therapeutic relationships to address the humanity and uniqueness of family units, motivate them in positive ways, and value their strengths in making needed changes (Rollnick, Miller, & Butler, 2008; Wright & Leahey, 2013).

Individual-Nurse-Family Communications

Communication is the way individuals, family members, and nurses come to know and understand each other in the context of the family health experience (Meiers & Tomlinson, 2003). Clear communication can assist persons seeking care and help the family unit achieve wellness and maximize potential health outcomes. Nurses understand that individuals are part of a whole and cannot be separated from their family. Thus, every individual met in a practice setting should cause the nurse to *think family*. Even absent family members are still present in the mind and life of the individual seeking care. Individuals have valued relationships beyond the immediate situation and these ties have strong implications for care management and caregiving. Families need not only to be treated in respectful ways but also to be included as part of the care team.

Thinking Family to Communicate

Nurses who *think family* regard family as full partners in decision making about treatment options. Nurses' roles entail clear communication to achieve the following:

- Deliver family-focused care rather than only individual-focused care.
- Act as a health teacher, coach, and counselor to meet individual and family needs.
- Use strengths-based perspectives when planning care and nursing actions.
- Address the various ecological dimensions pertinent to a health or illness situation.
- Assist families to prevent illness, maintain wellness, manage disease, promote health, and restore health to household members.
- Improve care outcomes.
- Act as an advocate for the person seeking care and the family unit.
- Increase satisfaction with health and illness care situations.

Caring relationships are often time limited but changes in health care delivery models could help nurses to advocate for care that is continuous and coordinated.

Nurses often face complex care situations and may have different opinions from administrators, supervisors, peers, and an array of health care providers. However, those seeking care most often turn to nurses when help is needed and when that occurs. Nurses who *think family* must effectively advocate for the best care options for the individual and families. That responsibility requires the ability to effectively communicate with all persons involved to ensure the best outcomes (Fig. 4.1).

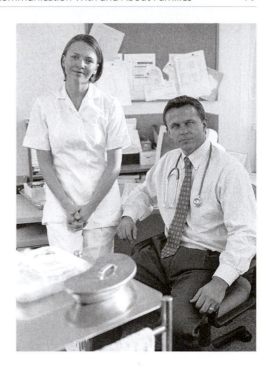

FIGURE 4-1 Families benefit when physicians and nurses collaborate.

Using the Individual-Nurse-Family Relationships to Communicate

Family-focused care implies that nurses are sensitive to even unspoken individual and family unit needs. Student nurses may be uncertain as they learn ways to provide competent and safe care, but family nurses can learn to use the individual-nurse-family relationship to encourage care seekers to share concerns, describe needs, and ask questions. Nurses don't always have the answers or solutions but they listen and collaborate to find answers and solve problems.

Meaningful communication is built on trust, respect, and professional concern. Therefore, family nurses must maintain appropriate boundaries, abstain from inappropriately disclosing personal information, and choose to behave ethically. Developing individual-nurse-family relationships can mean shifting away from some traditional practices, for example, viewing the individual and family as experts about their personal lives and moving more care from the acute care setting to the home. Even though nurses will always play crucial roles in providing care, they will increasingly become facilitators for care that extends beyond the present and no longer involves them directly but rather shifts the responsibility for health and illness care to families (Quinnet et al 2012).

Nurses who *think family* know that families need to be well prepared to give proper and adequate care at home. Nurses who value individual-nurse-family relationships see themselves as "in between"—they are often the potential links between "what is" and "what can be." Nurses offer support and teach families how to define a critical event and when an emergency room visit is unnecessary, how to stay healthy, and how to manage their disease. To do that, nurses need to be aware of potential health outcomes and financial constraints associated with treatments and actions and be able to provide expert information, clear instructions, caring support, and proper referrals.

Communication: A Basic Tool for Exchanging Information

Connectedness is a basic need and part of the human condition. A sender, receiver, message, and the nature of the relationship are all involved (Barnlund, 2008). Figure 4.2 suggests

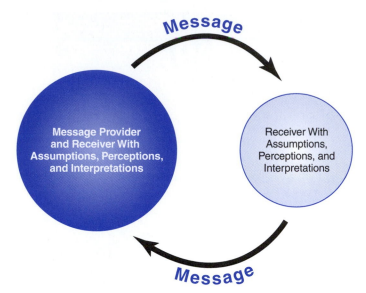

FIGURE 4-2 Traditional person-to-person communication models.

aspects in usual person-to-person communication. Nurse communication is rarely a single person-to-person interaction. Communication uses verbal and nonverbal behaviors as messages are sent, received, and interpreted (Arnold & Boggs, 2010). Verbal elements include the spoken, electronic, or written word, while nonverbal communication refers to the voice tone, body motions, facial expressions, eye motions, hand gestures, and body positions (Schuster & Nykolyn, 2010).

Communication occurs constantly. Although some communication is intended, it is not always deliberate or purposeful. Miscommunication occurs when communication is not clear and meanings may not be grasped. In health care, the transfer of accurate information is critical. Failure to listen, interpret appropriately, or understand can lead to medical errors, safety risks, and untoward outcomes. It can also cause unnecessary suffering and increased uncertainty (Spath, 2000). In addition, unintended messages interfere with relationship building and can result in dissatisfaction with the care and less than optimal outcomes.

When communicating, perceptions, assumptions, and interpretations are critical. For example, a nurse enters a hospital room to complete caregiving tasks. Family members use this situation to ask questions. The nurse might view the questions as interruptions to the individual's care delivery. On the other hand, family members might assume that nurse presence signals availability to answer questions. If the nurse fails to respectfully acknowledge questions, the response might be viewed as rude and cause negative family behavioral responses. People become defensive when they think that they are perceived as unimportant or bothersome. A nurse's negative relational stance can create future tensions and ineffective communication (Tapp, 2000). Box 4.5 identifies a number of strategies to improve communication.

Families need information about the best ways to care for their members. For example, the admitting nurse in a health care system documents the health history of an elderly gentleman with heart failure and notes his usual medications and daily activities. If the family is present, it is optimal to also obtain other information that may influence his care. For example, the family might describe his episodes of shortness of breath when climbing stairs or doing simple activities or discuss that he may not always take his medications as prescribed. Their information can be an important factor in evaluating his acute episode. If the individual is unable to effectively communicate, that resource is even more important.

BOX 4-5

Facilitating Individual-Nurse-Family Communication Strategies

A number of verbal and nonverbal actions can be taken to facilitate the effectiveness of communication. Consider the following:

Introduce self and role to initiate interaction:
"My name is Angela May. I am the registered nurse who will be caring for William today. Can you tell me who you are?"

Eye contact:
Be culturally sensitive to what is appropriate use with individuals and families:
"Tell me how your family was caring for your father in the home (make eye contact with each family member)."

Attention to family:
Be aware of who is accompanying the individual seeking care, note if no one is present, observe interactions and ways of communicating with one another: "Would you like to include your wife in your next clinic visit so we can review your medications?"

Create an environment that includes family:
"Would you like to help me walk with your wife down the hallway?"

Acknowledge illness experience:
"This illness must be a difficult time for your family."

Speak with a tone of authenticity and curiosity about family perception:
"I can see how stressful this illness is for your family. What can I most do for you and your family at this time?"

Make or schedule time to focus on family without tasks:
"Would it be acceptable to you if we asked your family to come to the next clinic visit so we can discuss your x-ray results and next steps?"

Use touch when it seems appropriate:
Recognize cultural and personal differences in this regard.

Express empathy for family struggle, distress, and suffering:
"Coping with these many care needs can be difficult; what needs does your family still have in giving you the support that you need?"

Purposefully involve family members in care:
"Come to the head of the bed and I will explain the purposes of these machines."

Use nonverbal communication such as hand gestures to suggest the inclusion of family members:
"Please come in the room while I ask your husband some questions. Your name is . . . ? Would that be okay with you (addressing husband)?"

When you speak with other nurses and health care professionals during bedside report, introduce and include family members.

Communication Breakdowns

Despite the importance of communication, breakdowns happen when nurses and the health care team face multiple competing demands or fail to fully convey or receive information (Callery & Milnes, 2012; Curtis, Tzannes, & Rudge, 2011; Ellington, Reblin, Clayton, Berry, & Mooney, 2012; Jones, Woodhouse, & Rowe, 2007). Ineffective communication results from faulty assumptions of senders and receivers. For example, a nurse appears hurried as an elderly woman is discharged after surgery. The family senses this and does not ask what an elevated body temperature means even though they are told to monitor it at home. The nurse did not explain the term "elevated temperature," when to check it or how to keep track of it, when it should be reported, or who gets the report. The nurse mistakenly assumes that everyone knows what an elevated temperature is and when to re-port it. Suppose the family mistakenly heard "a temperature is expected" and fails to report an elevated temperature of more than 48 hours. The woman appears in the emergency room because "she is getting worse not better." She is readmitted and diagnosed with sepsis. Ineffective communication too often results in poor outcomes, costly hospital readmissions, and dissatisfaction.

Even though nurses are busy and often working in stressful situations, they should always strive to avoid failed communication because it can create unnecessary risks such as accidents, errors, unsafe environments, poorer quality care outcomes, and decreased satisfaction (Schuster & Nykolyn, 2010). A landmark report by the Institute of Medicine (2001) estimated that 44,000 to 98,000 people die annually from medical errors and that communication breakdowns are the cause for about 70% of these errors. A report titled Crossing the Quality Chasm emphasized the need to establish effective communication and collaborative relationships to positively influence care delivery that results in therapeutic outcomes (IOM, 2001). Health care teams need to communicate effectively for a variety of reasons (Box 4.6).

Barriers to Family-Focused Communication

Health care systems are complex and not always systematic; weaving one's way through a web of services and practitioners can be baffling. For example, various levels of nurses and numerous roles of various medical professionals and specialists exist in practice. These dis-tinctions can be confusing to those working in health care but even more so to care seekers.

Several factors in health care such as the system, literacy, stress, and time make effective communication even more difficult. Barriers to communication can exist from the individ-ual, system, nurse, or family perspective (Table 4.1). Barriers signal the need to find alter-native approaches to developing family-focused communication.

System Barriers

The stress of an unknown environment with its many technologies and strangers creates uncertainty, and dealing with unfamiliar physical settings, lack of privacy, need to contin-ually interact with unfamiliar persons, strange smells, and noise contribute to increase anx-iety. Trying to develop interpersonal relationships while managing technical communication within computer-mediated communication systems are concerns for care providers and care recipients (Hrarbe, 2005). While electronic medical devices, medical records, health information technologies (HIT), computerized medical databases, the Internet, telehealth, and social media might be viewed as beneficial, they can also contribute barriers to com-fortable and effective communication for some people.

BOX 4-6

Health Care Teams' Use of Communication Skills

Growing evidence over the past two decades suggests that collaborative health care teams with excellent communication skills do the following:

- Produce quality outcomes in complex situations that reduce mortality rates in intensive care units (Knaus, Draper, Wagner, & Zimmerman, 1986).
- Reduce lengths of hospital stays and readmissions (Cowan et al., 2006).
- Improve chronic disease management (Bourbonniere & Evans, 2002).

TABLE 4-1	Barriers to Family-Focused Communication
Individual	Poor written, document, and oral literacy Low health literacy Individual emotional, cognitive, or sensory factors
System	Busy, unfamiliar environment Technology-rich environment Potential for unintentional breach of privacy/confidentiality
Nurse	Inaccurate assumptions Style of hostility and overtones of power Emotional stance (anger, aloof, distracted, irritated) Cultural biases, prejudices
Family	Negative attitudes Discomfort with family communication skills Negative past experiences with nurses or the health care system Emotional stance (anger, distracted, irritated, fear, uncertainty, anxiety, distrust) Lack of hope, uncertainty, need for information, lack of proximity to the patient

Nurse Barriers

Inaccurate assumptions about people and situations are barriers. Suppose a nurse assumes that adult children do not want to be involved in the care of their father who suffers from Huntington's disease. They seldom visit in the long-term care facility. This absence causes the nurse to assume that the family doesn't care and that they are uninterested in their father's care. The nurse has been heard saying negative things about them to a coworker. This nurse doesn't know about the family's complicated personal lives that make visiting hard. She is not aware that two of them are showing early signs of Huntington's disease and are fearful about their futures. Erroneous beliefs and bias produce communication barriers.

Nurses might assume that the recipients fully understands the information they provided and that the recipients will "do as told." Research has shown that nurses often use verbal and nonverbal strategies with an overtone of hostility, exclude the family from care, or maintain distance and a position of power over the family (Abraham & Moretz, 2012; Chesla, 1996; Nelms & Eggenberger, 2010; Soderstrom, Benzein, & Saveman, 2003). Nurses can seem aloof, irritated, angry, or distracted, and fail to respond in ways valued by individuals and family members. This negative communication can increase suffering, vulnerability, and uncertainty, all of which can lead to mistrust of the nurse (Eggenberger & Nelms, 2007). Nurses often admit they lack sufficient personal experience with some forms of communication, but projecting that attitude can produce ineffective individual-nurse-family communication (Soderstrom et al., 2003). Nurses who *think family* always strive to be conscious of their responses to others.

Family Barriers

Similar to nurses, with the stress of an illness or complex health care system, family members may also project emotions, anger, distractions, or irritation at nurses. Nursing students and even experienced nurses can be intimidated by these behaviors but must avoid responding negatively to them by retreating, avoiding the family, or blaming them. For instance, a nurse upset by a family might say to a peer, "The Smith family is so demanding." Rather than resolving the misunderstandings, nurses might blame the person or family and those perceptions may alter the way other team members relate to the families. On the other hand, some family members can use approaches that are frustrating and confrontational. The family nurse strives to understand the family's perception, experience, and responses in developing ways to partner with and connect with families.

Care seekers and families see communication as important to clinical care (Curtis & White, 2008). Nurse interaction may be the single most important aspect of care from the family perspective (Levine & Zuckerman, 2000). Families use this transactional process to create, share, and regulate meaning for their world (Dance, 1967; Gubrium & Holstein, 1993; Seagrin & Flora, 2011). Emotional state, worry, and other factors affect family experiences and perceptions. While some families freely express their concerns, others are silent, so the nurse who cares for the family from a perspective of understanding works to improve communication and nurse-family interaction.

When one family member is ill, other members also have needs. Needs for realistic hope, answers to questions, desire to be included, knowledge that optimum care is received, and current information about changes in condition are family concerns (Benzein, Hagberg, & Saveman, 2008; Eggenberger & Nelms, 2007; Meiers & Tomlinson, 2003). When a loved one is ill, family members often want to be near and included (Vandall-Walker & Clark, 2011). Inability to be near the ill family member increases anxiety and distress in some families as they may sense a family obligation or responsibility to be nearby when a member is ill. Communication that excludes the family or policies that deter their needs to be present and fulfill their family role can result in mistrust and anger. Box 4.7 provides information about Dr. Maureen Leahey, an expert clinician and leader in changing the ways nurses communicate with individuals and families.

Written Communications

Written communication can influence relationships. The way that care or a family response is documented can alter perceptions of the family when read by another health care provider. Objective information, rather than subjective information of opinions, can help prevent assumptions that may influence care.

BOX 4-7

Family Tree

Maureen Leahey, PhD, RN (Canada)

Dr. Leahey is an expert clinician, an author of many published journal articles and books, educator, and consultant. She is a graduate of Cornell University–New York Hospital School of Nursing and the University of Calgary. She has been an Adjunct Professor in both the Faculty of Nursing and Faculty of Medicine at the University of Calgary. She managed the outpatient mental health programs in Calgary and directed the Family Therapy Training Program. She is a member of the Canadian Nurses Association and a registered psychologist. She is also a clinical member, Approved Supervisor, and a long-standing Fellow with the American Association for Marriage and Family Therapy. Since the 1980s, she has been in the forefront of implementation of mental health programs in the Health Region. Dr. Leahey has collabored with Dr. Lorraine Wright and together they developed the Calgary Family Assessment and Intervention Models. Further, she and Dr. Wright have worked together in the writing of six editions of the family textbook *Nurses and Families: A Guide to Family Assessment and Intervention* (2013). This textbook is widely used by international audiences. She also worked with Dr. Wright on the series of eight videos in the How To Family Nursing series. She is a member of the International Family Nurses Association.

Care instructions for individuals and families must be clearly written. Written information is best when it supplements and is not a substitute for a verbal explanation. Clearly written information at the appropriate reading level ensuring the recipient's ability to read, level of reading, language, and culture are needed. Avoid using technical medical terminology. Poor instructions can have negative outcomes. For example, a child returns home after same-day surgery, but the family may not fully understand the written instructions about what to do if nausea and vomiting occur. Should they call the doctor if the child gags or spits up a small amount of vomitus or did the instructions mean vomiting that persists for 24 hours?

Written information must be effectively shared and communicated among health care team members to support safe and quality clinical decisions (Burns, 2011; Curtis et al., 2011; Dufault et al., 2010). Nurses regularly review medical orders and depend upon accurate written communication. It is essential that documentation describing observations, treatments, and other nursing actions is accurate. Nursing documentation is a legal record of the care provided. Be aware when creating written instructions that smart technologies sometimes correct spelling and if the wrong words are inserted, the information could be incorrect. Avoid using street language, slang, or symbols used in texting messages in any professional communication such as in nursing notes.

Literacy

Accuracy often depends upon the literacy skills of the care recipient. Literacy is the ability to use printed and written information to function in society, achieve one's goals, and develop one's knowledge and potential (White & McCloskey, 2003). In the United States, one in three young adults have dropped out of high school. The United States is the only country among 30 Organization for Economic Cooperation and Development (OECD) free-market countries where the current generation is less well educated than the previous one (National Commission on Adult Literacy, 2008). Persons with low literacy might be unable to understand some oral language, and to use printed materials successfully the writing must be at an understandable level. Not everyone will admit to not being able to read so it may be difficult to determine if illiteracy exists. Sometimes using pictures or videos rather than describing procedures will be more effective. One can be literate in one language, but illiterate in another. Functionally illiterate persons often develop ways to manage their daily life without reading.

Low Health Literacy

Health literacy refers to the ability to read, understand, and act on health information. In 2003, the first-ever National Assessment of Adult Health Literacy was conducted. Only 12% of those surveyed were found to be proficient, 53% were at the intermediate level, 21% were at the basic level, and 14% were below basic (National Assessment of Adult Literacy, 2003). Adults in the basic or below basic health literacy category are less likely to access health information from written sources than adults with higher literacy levels. Those with lower literacy get health information from television and radio. Without adequate health literacy, millions have trouble with common tasks (e.g., reading prescription labels, adhering to an immunization schedule). Even high school and college graduates can have low health literacy. Improving health literacy is a goal of Healthy People 2020 (U.S. Department of Health and Human Services [USDHHS], 2010a) and the National Action Plan to Improve Health Literacy (USDHHS, 2010b). Health literacy skills can be learned through Internet courses.

Low health literacy is related to poor health outcomes and poor quality of care (Berkman et al., 2004). Forms of health literacy include document literacy, a measure to understand information in forms, schedules, charts, graphs, and other information. Quantitative literacy refers to the use of numbers found in written materials. People need quantitative literacy to follow recipes, calculate tips, and tally costs. These skills are also needed for medication dosage and prescribed medicines. For example, 20% to 30% of medication prescriptions are never filled and about 50% of medications prescribed for chronic diseases are not taken as prescribed (Haynes, Ackloo, Sahota, McDonald, & Yao, 2008). Health literacy skills are needed to follow medication instructions, prepare for diagnostic examinations, understand health insurance plans, identify benefits or risks of medical treatments, calculate nutritional content, understand written test results, and complete a patient history form. Nurses who *think family* avoid using unnecessary medical jargon and complex general language. The best results for learners occur when information is grounded in experience. Listening to questions and observing behaviors when sharing information are helpful (Roter, 2011). Using dialogue or conversation to convey specific information is needed. Individualizing verbal instructions encourages optimal outcomes. See Box 4.8 to review a case study that provides an opportunity to reflect on the ways nurses can communicate with individuals and their family members.

BOX 4-8

Family Circle

The Natchez family includes a son, Juan (44 years old), and daughter, Maria (54 years old). They have been caring for their widowed father, Carlos (84 years old), who has chronic obstructive pulmonary disease (COPD). Carlos has been living with Juan and his wife, who have adult children and a grandchild. Maria lives nearby and helps much. She also works full time as a grocery clerk. Carlos is hospitalized with pneumonia and deteriorating COPD. A nurse conducts a brief family interview. The nurse says, "This must be a difficult time for you." She begins to acknowledge the family's experience. The nurse says, "Tell me more about the ways you have been helping your father." She is seeking information and providing the opportunity to find the strengths and challenges in the family. The nurse asks: "What are you the most worried about at this time?" This question allows a chance to uncover areas of concern. The nurse who takes this family-focused approach does not have assumptions about the family that might be barriers to communication. The nurse intentionally creates a context that supports making meaning of events and experiences with nurse-family and family member interactions.

During an individual-nurse-family interaction on the following day, the nurse asks the family to share their story about the illness: "When did your father's lung problems begin? Can you tell me about the time of diagnosis and how his treatment and condition have changed with time?" The nurse sits at the bedside with the family and listens attentively to their responses. She asks Juan and Maria about their work, family, and life responsibilities and explores ways they meet caregiving demands. This family communication recognizes the demands, needs for resources, and challenges of illness. The nurse carefully listens to the family story and notes the individual differences that exist in the family members. She begins to identify potential areas of concern for care and follow-up.

Carlos is discharged with plans for visits from the home care nursing services. The nurse prepares written materials and reviews them with the family. The hospital and home care nurse speak about the family. The hospital nurse introduces the home care nurse to the family. They had previously discussed a living will, but decisions have not yet been made. Carlos wanted to talk further with his family before completing the papers. The hospital nurse shares with the home care nurse concerns about whether Carlos and the family fully understand the discharge instructions, the chronic nature of his illness, and living will documentation.

In your next clinical rotation, try using the strategic methods applied in this case to improve personal communication. Discuss and compare your experiences with others.

- What are your nursing concerns for this family?
- What things would you communicate about with this family?
- What things would you say?
- How would you interact with different individuals and the family as a whole?

Theoretical Perspectives of Communication

Communication with one family can be different from that required by other families because families are unique. Given the many barriers to communication, it is important to have skills and experience that facilitate communication in some very varied situations. Theories provide road maps to identify needs from different points of view and suggest useful nursing actions. This section introduces several useful theories that nurses can use to communicate and plan, deliver, and evaluate nursing care.

Family Systems Theory

Nursing students usually learn about family systems theory, of which is derived from biological sciences where a system is defined as a set of interrelated elements (von Bertalanffy, 1975). This theory views family as an open dynamic system with a past, present, and future. Family members are interdependent and influence one another. Verbal and nonverbal communication occurs within the family and between them and the outside world. Thinking through this theory recognizes that illness in one family member affects the family unit and suggests that feedback loops are used to maintain equilibrium in the family system. For example, to understand the effects of a disease on the family unit, a nurse might say: "Tell me about the ways this cancer diagnosis and need for treatment has been experienced by your family." Family systems can help explain the varied ways multiple family members interact with health care systems and communicate with those outside the family unit. Nurses can support the well-being of families by considering family communication with various members (Fig. 4.3). When new situations occur, nurses can ask: How has your family communicated to solve problems in the past? Who, in the family, may have the most difficult time making the needed changes? Family systems thinking can help guide communication during troubled times.

Attachment Theory

Attachment occurs in infants through innate tendencies like following the parent visually and clinging to the mother. Infants attach to those who are the source of nourishment and protection (Bowlby, 1958). Attachment is relevant throughout life as persons continue to nurture, protect, and support one another. Death, divorce, lost abilities, geographical relocation, and

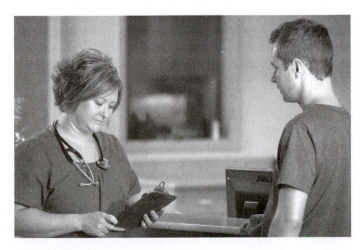

FIGURE 4-3 Communication with and about families is central to practice.

even hospital admission are examples of separation that can cause grief and emotional pain. Attachment is an essential human need; when separation occurs, nurses can help by providing the time and space for members to interact, offering to hear emotional stories to help individuals know they are cared for, and allowing family members to fulfill their need to protect. Nurses can facilitate connecting conversations during times of uncertainty and vulnerability.

Social Learning Theory

Social learning theory (Bandura, 1977) unites psychology and behavior by focusing on the performance of a learned behavior through reinforcement. Modeling is a central element of social learning theory. For instance, children learn health and illness behaviors from their parents and other family members (Denham, 2003). Individuals learn about consequences and rewards for different forms of communication as they observe others. For example, in one family, frequent cell phone conversations throughout the day may be normal and welcome; others may see them as invasive or unnecessary. Nurses who *think family* are sensitive to what is defined as "normal" by a family. Nurses can use communication to model behaviors that provide mutual rewards to individuals and family members. For example, a mother worried about her 10-year-old daughter's obesity might describe her television habits after school. Yet, she might not perceive possible connections between the two. Nurses can use social learning perspectives to discuss pertinent ideas: Can you describe your family meals? Do you eat together every day? What kinds of physical activities does your family enjoy together? Open-ended questions can lead to discussion of current behaviors. Questions can help the nurse identify family health routines that need change or ones to strengthen (Denham, 2003). Helping family members identify valued behaviors suggests ways to modify or try new things in a supportive way without placing members on the defensive.

Life Course Theory

The family life course theory is a developmental approach that emphasizes specific expected and unexpected transitions that occur as a family changes over time (Carter & McGoldrick, 1999). For example, it is expected that children generally go to school and eventually leave home. But an unforeseen illness or death is not expected and can create unanticipated stressors. Life events affect both individual and family development (Meleis, 2010). Changes in family make-up cause altered member interactions (Duvall, 1977). Nursing actions can support family members when they are stressed by transitions or changes in a member's health. For instance, an elderly grandmother suffers from some memory loss and the safety of living alone is in question. A nurse might suggest a family meeting to discuss and anticipate possible outcomes of decisions.

Role Theory

People play many roles in their personal lives. Role theory explains purposes of different interactions. Roles can be prescribed behaviors used to construct a valued life or maintain integrity during troubled times. Roles help members maximize their use of household resources and identify ways members care for one another (Yu-Nu, Yea-Ing Lotus, Min-Chi, & Pei-Shan, 2011). Parent, child, caregiver, wage earner, organizer, disciplinarian, nurturer, encourager, decision maker, and protector are just some of the common roles seen in family units. Some roles tend to be gender or culturally oriented. In the United States and even worldwide, ideas about gender roles are changing. Roles often signify what it means to be part of a particular family and are tied to identity; they might suggest ways family work is done. Some family roles evolve, but some stay the same. For example, keeper of the family finances might be viewed as a lifetime role. However, that member's death or changing responsibilities means someone else will have to do it. Role changes can be temporary, as during an extended acute illness, during which other family members need to do tasks that the hospitalized person normally does. Role theory can be used to help families communicate about expectations associated with any role changes that occur because of a member's hospitalization.

Discussion about roles might occur formally or informally. Suppose a home care nurse notices a mother's conflict as she cares for her terminally father. The nurse can say, "It must be hard to make choices about being here for your father and attending your son's school events." Indirect questions can lead to conversations and perhaps disclosure about conflicts. The nurse might note, "Others have told me about the difficulties experienced as they try to balance personal needs and the demands of caring for a dying person. How is this for you?" Normalizing a tough emotional battle can steer the conversation to roles and forms of support needed. The nurse might ask: "Would you like me to tell you about some community resources for respite care?" Therapeutic conversation can assist the nurse to identify areas where information, teaching, counseling, or coaching are needed.

Exchange and Resource Theory

Exchange and resource theories focus on ways relationships develop and how resources are distributed or used. Exchange theory describes the flow of information among family members and those outside the family unit (McDonald, 1981; Vangelisti, 2004). Resource theory describes the flow of resources and decisions that affects member relationships inside the family. The ways things are shared influences development and use of social networks. Exchange and resource theory can suggest new ways to access resources and supports during times of illness. Well-connected families often have a great deal of social capital to manage stressful situations (Looman & Lindeke, 2005). Social capital refers to the networks of family, friends, neighbors, and associates that can be called upon.

Nurses aware of exchange and resource theory note the importance of information exchanges and resources available within a unique family. Identifying resource gaps suggests ways for nurses to act. Nurses can use what they learn to assist families to make decisions, solve problems, and access resources. If a family experiences a traumatic event or a life-threatening surgery, social networks are important. A social media Internet site (e.g., Caring Bridge, Care Pages, Facebook) is a way to remain connected with peers, neighbors, church friends, or others. Online networks are available to receive notes of support when the ill person or family unit is ready for them.

Symbolic Interactionism

Symbolic interactionists assert that people act toward things and other people based on their meanings (Blumer, 1969). People interpret their world based upon prior experiences and use this information to solve problems and create meanings (Buber, 1970; LaRossa & Reitzes, 1993; Mead, 1956/1934). Families maintain or transform their identities as their personal world evolves and new experiences occur. People construct and share stories that become the reality of family experience. For example, parents of a 6-month-old child who has had several cardiac surgeries and never left the intensive care unit are planning for her imminent death because no further treatment is possible. The infant is dressed in infant clothing and her mother is rocking her as she is dying. A nurse comes into the room and says, "Oh, I'm so sorry this is happening." The mother says, "There is no room for pity here. For the first time in her life, she has no tubes. She has real clothing on. And, I am rocking her like a normal child. We are so thankful to have had her, even for this short time." In contrast, a nurse with a different reality says, "This must be difficult for you, but you are comforting your child." The mother responds: "It is sad for us to lose her so soon, but this is the first chance that I have had to be her mother." The nurse's words trigger different responses and conversations. Recognition of the experience and commendation of positive actions can help the mother clarify an experience's symbolic meanings.

Relationship-Focused Communication

Humans are innately social beings who need relationships to ease pain and suffering, effectively cope with stress, learn from life experiences, and maintain or regain health (Travelbee, 1966). Nursing is an interpersonal process between humans in complex environments filled with other beings (Paterson & Zderad, 1976; Travelbee, 1966). Relationships between nurses and care recipients are part of nursing care's foundation and the context in which nursing practice occurs (Bell, 2011; Fawcett, 1995; Hagerty & Patusky, 2003; Peplau, 1991). In the past, these ideas have largely centered on communication with single care recipients rather than a family unit.

Relationship-based care places the needs and priorities of individuals and families as central elements in nursing care (Koloroutis, 2004). Family-focused communication occurs through caring relationships with the individual and family unit. Communicating compassion can create healing relationships that improve health outcomes, satisfaction with care, and nurse satisfaction (Chesla, 2010; Koloroutis, 2004; Matire & Schulz, 2007). Approaches such as active listening are used to understand others' experiences. Intentional caring approaches have potential to produce quality outcomes and increase satisfaction. Relationship-based care that uses clear communication can create effective interactions with the family unit that can positively influence the health of all (Meiers & Tomlinson, 2003; Nelms & Eggenberger, 2010; Weihs, Fisher, & Baird, 2002; Wright & Bell, 2010). Nurses who *think family* recognize the importance and power of communication among family members, between the nurse and family, and with other health care professionals. Nurses who fail to include family members in decisions about a critically ill family member's treatment can amplify the family's suffering (Eggenberger & Nelms, 2007; Meiers & Tomlinson, 2003).

Evidence indicates that the use of psychoeducational and relationship-focused family interventions during illness can be more effective than medical care (Chesla, 2010; Hartmann, Bazner, Wild, Eisler, & Herzog, 2010). Medical care often treats symptoms of the problem, but often does not fully address behavioral and family implications. Psychoeducational interventions are used to educate about specifics restraints of an illness and explain ways to manage. This form of communication aims to help families develop needed skills, resolve conflicts, aid decision making, facilitate goal setting, and support problem solving (Chesla, 2010; Eggenberger, Meiers, Krumwiede, Bliesmer, & Earle, 2011; Heru, 2013; Weihs et al., 2002). Nurses who *think family* intentionally include the family unit in conversations about management of daily routines, medical treatments, and prevention of potential complications.

Building Trust

Trust develops through sincere and honest sharing of pertinent personal information in thoughtful ways. Trust has different levels and evolves over time. The foundation of trust is mutual intention, and reciprocity, expectations, and relationships affect abilities to communicate and levels of satisfaction (Lynn-McHale & Deatrick, 2000). Intentional relationships consider what needs to be accomplished and involve cooperation to identify the best ways to reach goals. Some conversations begin with sharing personal experiences or information relevant to a current situation. A nurse might say, "I see that your mother has breast cancer. I know how you feel because my mother had breast cancer, too." Nurses can tell too much of their personal stories and misuse valuable time. Our stories are important, but they should not be the focus in the care of others. Another nurse might say: "It sure has been hot lately, have you been keeping cool?" or "How about those Yankees, do you think they are going to win?" These remarks lead the nurse to spend valuable time talking about irrelevant things. Nurses who *think family* use all working time to intentionally communicate. In an acute care setting, nurses are often in and out of rooms many times during a single shift. Add up those minutes and ask yourself:

- Who in the family do I need to communicate with?
- What topics should I discuss today as I complete tasks?
- Where is the best place to have a private conversation?
- What is the best time to bring up topics that need to be discussed?
- How do I best use my time to develop trusting relationships during this shift?
- How do I make sure that the most important needs of each person are met?

Trust relies on the competence and willingness of someone to protect, rather than harm, persons one cares about (Cody, 2013). Trust, respect, and mutuality are essential to relationships (Tarlier, 2004; Cody, 2013). Treating others as worthy equals, accepting, engaging, and attempting to understand is respectful (Cody, 2013). When persons are met, ask: "What is the most important thing that I can do for you today?" Nurses can't do everything, but they can usually do one important thing for each person given care. Box 4.9 identifies several useful factors to help differentiate between actions that build trust versus mistrust.

BOX 4-9

Trust Versus Mistrust in a Therapeutic Relationship

TRUST	MISTRUST
Use direct communication to solve problems and reinforce strengths	Talk about problem with many others without including the persons directly involved
Be generous with saying "thank you" and give credit to everyone; find ways to commend others	Take credit yourself or expect others to lavish credit on you
Only make promises you can keep	Fail to follow-through on promises made
Be direct in all forms of communication, and if you have uncertainties, then share then openly	Do not say exactly what you mean; keep people guessing about what you will do next
Be approachable and willing to engage in open conversation	Be unavailable, leave without answering questions, and do not give clear answers
Be timely in your responses	Do not answer clearly and blame things on others, authority, or some outside force
Admit when you are wrong and own up to your mistakes	Always take the position that you are right and others are wrong
Allow others to ask questions, express their concerns, and express their frustrations	Assume you know all the answers, fail to listen to the needs of others, and talk only about yourself
Acknowledge uncertainty	Fail to disclose the unknowns

Asking Questions

Asking questions is a tool to gather information and understand the main issues confronting persons or family member (Rollnick et al., 2008). Specific information can be learned by questions such as: Where do you hurt? Has your mother been taking her medications?

How long has it been since you, as a family, ate a meal all together? Broader information can be learned by asking more open questions: In what ways can I be most helpful to your family today? What is most worrying your family about this current situation? Open-ended questions allow room for responses. Closed questions often get only single-word answers. The nature of the open question is that it clearly demonstrates that the nurse does not "know it all." When open-ended questions are coupled with appropriate nonverbal behaviors (e.g., eye contact, attentive listening, a nonjudgmental context), individuals and families can safely explore their challenges and pose solutions (Rosengren, 2009).

Listening

Learning to listen authentically is a key to healthy communication and ensures that others have been heard and understand you. Think about the "who, what, where, when, and how" that needs to happen during communication. Listening is an opportunity to not just learn information, but also to connect. Listening checks for accuracy and relays information that can be valued, believed, and viewed as important (Rollnick et al., 2008). Sometimes people appear to listen, but they are just waiting for a time to take charge and get their points across. When professionals take time to listen, individuals often think that the time spent with them is longer. Listening is a window to see things through others' eyes and better understand their experience. It demonstrates curious attitudes and a way to "live-out" relationship-based care. Good listening habits enable nurses to:

- Use wording that will be understood correctly.
- Share personal feelings about comments that were heard.
- Ask questions that help clarify experiences.
- Use silence when necessary to allow others time to collect thoughts.
- Summarize what is heard through reflective statements.

Listening enables nurses to see things differently and hear silences that share meanings. Listening is the milieu for collaborative partnerships and solving real problems.

Informing

Informing is the exchange of information that may be new or different. Information should be offered, not imposed. It involves giving facts, not opinions. It is a give-and-take experience. Informing includes giving feedback to further clarify and direct communication (Box 4.10). For example, after teaching a person with a cardiac condition, the nurse might say, "After all this information, I am not sure what you are thinking. Perhaps it has created more questions or stress. Would you like to share with me anything that is not yet clear?"

Giving Feedback

Nurses need to be culturally sensitive as they respond to things learned. For example, the nurse observes a family member who begins to cry and she's not sure why. Feedback might involve saying something like "Your feelings are very strong; do you want to talk about what is going on?" Persons who sit silently, avoid eye contact, fail to respond to questions, or leave the room during conversations are likely to be disengaged or be signaling some form of conflict. Nurses who *think family* realize cues and gently confront future trouble spots at the appropriate time. Unanswered questions, lack of attention to detail, and misunderstandings can send unintended messages (Box 4.10). Lack of timely feedback can inhibit positive care outcomes or satisfaction.

Complex Communication in Family-Focused Care

Acute and chronic illness may cause suffering and distress that interrupts the family's usual communication patterns and overwhelms their coping abilities. Kind and respectful interactions can create a calm healing environment, decrease anxiety and depressive symptoms, and improve satisfaction with care (Curtis, Patrick, Caldwell, Greenlee, & Collier, 1999). Nurses shepherd those unfamiliar with medical management of disease and illness through a chaotic maze.

Nursing Actions

Nurses use many skills to understand the family's experience. Many issues come to the forefront when families face health and illness challenges. These concerns upset the comfortable routines of daily life. Nurses are not privy to private family interactions, but must quickly gain insights into key aspects of their lives. Even spending small amounts of time with families or using purposeful conversation while conducting task-oriented care can help identify needs and concerns (Nelms & Eggenberger, 2010). Describing what others can expect from you as a nurse is a good way to start. People need to know what to expect, how long they will wait, what will happen, and how they will be involved. Competence in nursing is greater than the ability to perform tasks (Eggenberger & Reagan, 2010); it is about being able to do expected things while simultaneously engaging in relationship-building practices (Benner, 1983; Brown & Hartrick Doane, 2008). Effective communicators recognize that time during a work shift might go very fast, but for those in distress seconds can seem like days.

Taking Part in Challenging Conversations

The presence of a nurse often invites questions about medical matters such as wounds, indigestion, pain, constipation, impotence, menstrual irregularities, fears of memory loss, or organ donation in situations in which they may not normally come up. Managing these conversations effectively requires an awareness of the sacred trust granted through a caring relationship. Nurses can use this sacred trust to communicate about difficult

---

BOX 4-10

Communicating with Individuals and Families

- Find out if the information is wanted before you give it.
- Ask permission before sharing information, particularly if you are uncertain whether they want it.
- Describe information within the context of other clients. For example, "In my work with other families managing diabetes, I have found. . . ."
- Give people the space to disagree, agree, and ask questions.
- Provide options that might be workable.

Source: Rosengren, D. B. (2009). *Building motivational interviewing skills: A practitioner workbook.* New York: Guilford Press.

topics in ways that are supportive and preserve dignity. While nurses are familiar with having difficult conversations at work, such topics may be unnerving in the community. Nurses are often seen as health professionals in the community not just when they are "on the clock." Professionalism means nurses always respond respectfully within their scope of practice.

Managing Conflict

Persons usually have some prior personal or shared health agency experiences. If a family faces an end-of-life situation in which the wishes of the dying member have not been previously discussed, family members might need nurses' help to communicate with one another in constructive ways (Wiegand, 2006). Nurses can help family members discuss their feelings and differences with one another. Family members can worry, become angry, and get frustrated as they cope with various health care providers. Nurses must not side with persons, but listen, remain objective and help family members communicate. Nurses should first reflect upon their own behavior. Sometimes personal behaviors create defensive barriers and create awkward and uncomfortable situations (Box 4.11). Some people have volatile personalities and families may have a history of communication difficulties, which may be heightened by illness. In some cultures, people speak louder and are sharper. An ability to disagree, compromise, and not blame others is a healthy communication approach. Nurses must not side with persons, but remain objective. Whether an acute illness requires hospitalization or a chronic illness demands care transitions for home, communication is critical if quality outcomes are to be realized.

Caregivers

The illness burden, health maintenance, chronic disease management, palliative care needs, and other things linked with family care can create great stress on caregivers. This burden has been linked to depression (Clark & Diamond, 2010), stress (Matire & Schulz, 2007), and other adverse psychological and physical health effects (Clark & Diamond, 2010; Sherwood, Given, Given, & Von Eye, 2005). Complex caregiving roles are common to many families, particularly today when parents are living longer and more people work outside the home. Nurses need to be aware of caregiver burden. Astute family nurses acknowledge multiple struggles families might be facing. Healing conversations about caregiver need might seem uncomfortable at first, but many will appreciate your

---

BOX 4-11

Reflections About Personal Actions

Here are some examples of personal behaviors to consider about yourself as you communicate with others:

- Is your tone of voice and body language welcoming?
- Are you sharp or sarcastic in your responses?
- Do you intimidate others by the ways you approach them or things you say?
- Are you sensitive to individual preferences and needs?
- Do you appear impatient or hurried?

concern. Families might have other family concerns, but the current difficulty can be the one that overwhelms their coping abilities. Families might be dealing with such issues as grandparents raising grandchildren, the imprisonment of an adult child, a recently lost job, care of a son with schizophrenia, lack of health care insurance, or other life difficulties. These often unspoken pressures can be part of the caregiver burden faced by families as they manage a new dilemma.

Developing Relationship-Based Care

Relationship-based care built upon effective communication assists individuals and family members to better manage stress and the uncertainties of illness (Koloroutis, 2004). If a family is comfortable communicating with the nurse, members are more likely to eagerly request information to manage care associated with an illness (Benzein et al., 2008). All too often, nurses busily enter hospital rooms thinking about the tasks to be completed without acknowledging the family member. The following script demonstrates the nurse's role in such an interaction:

> *Good afternoon. My name is Janet Jones. I am the nurse caring for Mr. Hazelton today. Would you mind sharing with me your name and relationship to Mr. Hazelton? Have you thought of how you would most like to be involved in your [state family member's relationship] care today? How could I help you do that?*

Failure to ask questions about family's wishes or ways members are involved in caregiving activities can lead to false assumptions. Family is a critical part of coordinated care.

Variations in Types of Communication

Care delivery in different clinical and community settings calls for different forms of communication. In a stressful critical care situation, the focus might be to assist a family member in managing caregiving ambiguity, encourage them to be physically present, and assume a protection role (Tomlinson, Swiggum, & Harbaugh, 1999). In contrast, the mother is concerned that her young daughter is gaining too much weight and fears she is at risk for developing type 2 diabetes. In this instance, the nurse's focus might be on health teaching about preparation of nutritious meals and increased physical activity. Situations require very different care forms and communications. Table 4.2 identifies a variety of communication elements nurses can consider as they *think family* and provide care. Who is the target of the communication? Will the communication occur with individuals separately or with the family unit? For instance, if the nurse is caring for a comatose person, then family members are the best informants. If the person is a 45-year-old woman with multiple sclerosis being cared for at home, communication about mobility strategies might be targeted at her and caregiver needs simultaneously.

Consider the context of the message and the timing of its delivery. Is the message to be communicated at a highly stressful time and in an unfamiliar setting? If so, how do these factors influence ways the message might be received? Receipt of the message will be influenced by typical communication patterns. For example, if usual communication is initiated with the family matriarch, but the nurse delivers the message to a child first, the matriarch could resist the message. Perceptions of communication to convey information can affect its acceptance.

TABLE 4-2	Important Communication Elements in Family-Focused Care	

ELEMENTS OF COMMUNICATION	DESCRIPTION	FAMILY-FOCUSED ASSESSMENT CONSIDERATIONS
Communicators	Originators of the message (facts, thoughts, feelings)	Individual-family-nurse communicate to meet needs of individuals and families
Context	Physical, temporal, social, biological, psychological, cultural, spiritual, and professional	Consider context of health care setting for family conversations that may increase stress, fear, and vulnerability What is family's perception of the context?
Critical thought process	Cognitive deliberations to assess best strategy, select communication strategy, create and deliver message, and then evaluate effect and response Facilitate common meaning	Attend to and evaluate individual and family in the communication strategy Recognize unique meanings may exist among family members Identify shared family meanings
Message	Factors, thoughts, or feelings Content and relational element Verbal behavior Nonverbal behavior	Consider "fit" with family's typical communication patterns Recognize differences in family members perception and interpretation Consider verbal and nonverbal behavior of family members Consider relational elements of family members
Method	Face to face Technology	Consider whether to share information with designated person or family as a whole Family as a unit or family member Family face to face or via technology
Assign meaning	Communicators assign meaning to message based on personal experiences	Consider "fit" of message with family goals and family health Consider individual differences of family members in assigning meanings
Effects	Intentional and unintentional effects of the communication	What does the message imply for family actions? What is the effect on individual family members that will impact the family unit?
Feedback	Response to message	Is it necessary to receive feedback from all family members to determine if message was heard?
Communication risk factors	Communication risk factors such as physical, psychological, physiological, and semantic risk factors	Consider risk factors; family unit conflicts; prior experiences; usual family communication patterns Consider family culture, faith beliefs, traditions for particular approach to communication Observe nonverbal cues Think about members' various interpretations of the messages Recognize language and literacy barriers.

TABLE 4-2	*Important Communication Elements in Family-Focused Care —cont'd*	
ELEMENTS OF COMMUNICATION	**DESCRIPTION**	**FAMILY-FOCUSED ASSESSMENT CONSIDERATIONS**
Person-safety communication strategies	Purposeful communication strategies used to overcome risk factors when interacting	Individual-nurse-family communication to assess, plan, implement family care Engage family members in reducing safety risks
Transformation	An outcome of communication process with change as a result of communication	A family change in the health experience supports health of individual members and family unit Move toward individual well-being and family health

Source: Adapted from Schuster, P. M., & Nykolyn, L. (2010). *Communication for nurses: How to prevent harmful events and promote patient safety.* Philadelphia: F. A. Davis.

Sharing Messages With Families

Messages can be shared with a family decision maker or the family as a whole in a face-to-face method or using some form of technology. Regardless of the method, persons tend to receive messages based on whether things fit with family life goals, beliefs, values, and usual routines. For example, a family is managing the home care of a 7-month-old medically fragile child. They want to attend a family reunion and bring their child to "meet the family" for the first time. On the morning of the reunion, the home care nurse notices that the child has spiked a fever of 102°F. This common experience is usually managed with antipyretics. On this day, the message brings tears to the parents' eyes because it means a significant change in plans. In this case, the child cannot be introduced to the larger family. The family will need to manage the fever, but also cope with the sadness of loss linked with missing the important family event.

Nurses that *think family* can be sensitive to situations in which the response received is not the one expected. If a message is about daily decision making, such as in medication administration, perhaps the schedule and information about side effects needs to be given to only those directly involved. However, if the message is about end-of-life decisions, perhaps multiple family members and even a close family friend might need to be involved. Consider a 43-year-old woman who lives alone and is scheduled for knee surgery; the nurse must identify who will assist her at discharge and what supports will be available for the 10 days when her activity will be limited, driving prohibited, and on-going physical therapy needed. Discussion about who caregivers will be might involve extended family, neighbors, and friends. Making sure these temporary caregivers know physical limitations, medication regimens, and other care particulars will be different from a single caregiver responsibility. Message delivery can also be challenging with families in which other conflicts already exist, as in the following situations:

- The son says he is homosexual and the parents do not acknowledge his partner's rights to make decisions.
- Messages were delivered to the woman seeking care but the family's culture teaches that the man in the family is the decision maker.
- Instructions for a low-sodium diet need to be given to an 80-year-old Hispanic woman who does not speak English.
- A person's medical condition quickly deteriorates to life-support decisions.
- Parents are faced with the birth of a child with a severe disability.
- A colleague administers an incorrect medication to someone allergic to it.

When such events occur, nurses might need time to debrief and acknowledge personal feelings and experiences. Acknowledgment of personal loss, emotions, and distress can support nurses' healthy coping. Debriefing includes information sharing and event processing that reflects on the event actions, outcome, and experience (Dreifuerst, 2009; Hanna & Romana, 2007). Nurses use debriefing to reflect "on action" and "in-action" (Tanner, 2006) and find resolutions that build personal confidence in difficult situations.

Motivational Interviewing

Motivational interviewing (MI) is a communication form that originated from addictions recovery and behaviorism (Rollnick et al., 2008). It has been adapted for use in a variety of situations in which counselors assist persons in changing health behaviors; for example, smoking cessation, weight loss, physical activity, nutrition enhancement, hypertension, cardiovascular disease, diabetes, and psychosis are situations in which MI may be beneficial. Communication aims to strengthen family's knowledge and support positive behavior changes (Rollnick et al., 2008). Nurses can use MI to motivate or encourage changes by identifying beneficial reasons to make changes. MI focuses on the development of a cooperative and collaborative partnership (Box 4.12). Individuals identify their resources for change, try new behaviors, and celebrate successes as changes are made.

MI guides rather than directs. Nurses act as a coaches or tutors. Nurses are viewed as resources and suggest what is possible and offer alternative ideas or directions for behavior changes. Three core communication skills particularly helpful in guiding behavior change are asking, informing, and listening. The nurse asks the individual specifically to identify the desired change. Active listening allows individuals to explore concerns, fears, and ambivalence that might prevent change. With this knowledge, the nurse informs the person about treatment choices, research evidence related to the problem, and some actions others have found effective to manage the problem. At the close of the session, the nurse assists the individual in identifying specific behavioral goals and ways successes can be evaluated. At a follow-up session, the nurse checks to see how the client is doing with those goals and coaches about any needed revisions. When the client is the family, MI can be adapted through the use of modeling as suggested by social learning theory (Bandura, 1977). The family can set goals, identify barriers, plan ways to deal with barriers, identify potential solutions, and evaluate outcomes of the actions taken. Table 4.3 presents the similarities between the techniques of family interviewing and motivational interviewing strategies identifying facilitating and constraining family beliefs (Wright & Bell, 2010).

BOX 4-12

Principles of Motivational Interviewing

Four distinct principles can be used by nurses in motivational interviewing (Dreifuerst, 2009; Rollnick et al., 2008):

1. Nurses must resist the reflex to "right" the individual's behavior by "telling" them what to think or what they need to change. Instead nurses' role is to assist individuals to voice personal desires to change.
2. Nurses seek to understand individual interests, concerns, and motivations for making a behavior change; this knowledge helps them to deal with the ambivalence often experienced toward change.
3. Nurses recognize the importance of listening with empathetic interest as motivations are shared.
4. Nurses inform by exploring ways in which a difference in one's health can be made.

TABLE 4-3	*Family Interviewing and Motivational Interviewing Techniques*
FAMILY INTERVIEWING TECHNIQUES	**MOTIVATIONAL INTERVIEWING STRATEGIES**
Generate hypotheses prior to interview	Draw out ideas and solutions from the client
Comfortable interview setting	Comfortable interview setting
As many members as possible present	Client only
Family-nurse relationship of reciprocity, nonhierarchical, respect for unique expertise and strengths	Collaboration/partnership with client
Therapeutic conversations	Reflective listening
Manners and respectful	Focus on behaviors
Family genogram (and ecomap)	_____
Therapeutic questions	Open-ended questions
Commendations	Affirmations
Engagement	Resist the righting reflex
Assessment	Understand your client's motivation
Intervention	Listen to your client/change talk
Termination	Engage your client/summarize needed information

Source: Meiers & Jenson (2011) based on Wright & Leahy (2013) and Rollnick, Miller, & Butler (2008).

Creating Therapeutic Conversations

Purposeful conversations invite family members to join, ask questions about areas of concern, and offer involvement with potential to be therapeutic, healing, and affirming (Wright & Leahey, 2013). Commending family strengths is a communication strategy that helps family members develop their strengths and reduce distress (Wright & Leahey, 2013). Asking key questions about the family's concerns, challenges, and expectations provides useful information for the nurse to identify ways to involve the family (Wright & Leahey, 2013). As families share their personal stories, nurses better understand what is needed, and trusting relationships are made (Lynn-McHale & Deatrick, 2001; Wright & Leahey, 2013). More information about topics in this section is found in Chapter 8.

Eliciting the Family Story

Families perceive a need to share their stories and be heard whenever uncertainty is faced (Henriksson & Andershed, 2007; Henriksson, Benzein, Ternestedt, & Andershed, 2011). These conversations require clear communication and a partnership with the individual seeking care and family. Hearing the family story acknowledges needs and struggles and it takes time, but knowing that story might save time later and even avoid medical errors or other problems. Box 4.13 identifies the importance of using evidence-based nursing interventions when hearing the family story and helping members alter their routines.

Interventive Questioning

Interventive questions are used intentionally to collect information that can help nurses better understand situations. Linear and circular questioning techniques are skills used to assist the family in making meaningful changes. Linear questions may provide information while

> **BOX 4-13**
>
> **Evidence-Based Family Nursing Practice**
>
> Strong evidence has shown links between smoking and lung cancer, yet people continue to smoke. Research has demonstrated links between individual behavior changes and the relational processes with their family members. Evidence shows that having a supportive partner increases smoking cessation. Social environments also influence individual behaviors. A qualitative study was conducted with 16 families, in which 13 had lung cancer and 3 had serious lung diseases and the individual with the disease smoked. Study participants were concerned about continuing smoking and wanted the ill person to stop. The family members who continued to smoke were concerned about ill members and altered some smoking behaviors in response. Love and concern for the other were factors in behavioral changes. Many thought the smoking decisions were individual ones. Smoking can be a long-standing relationship dimension between family members, and many members continued to see that preserving the relationship was important and they modified their smoking behaviors. When the relationship with one another is the priority, then adaptive smoking behaviors can serve both parties well. Other individuals in this study thought that it was their responsibility to influence the decisions about smoking cessation for those around them. In this situation, family members were willing to risk the relationship for the short term if they could enable the long-term gain of protecting well family members from lung cancer. This pattern was not successful in positively influencing smoking cessation and created tensions at a vulnerable time. Nurses are in a unique position to help individuals and families with smoking cessation. Many excellent evidence-based programs exist, but these might be more effective if relationships and interactions are considered. Unfortunately, family dynamics (e.g., communication, family processes) are not often regarded when smoking cessation is needed. When family members of the person with lung cancer or other lung diseases smoke, then including them in the plans for actions could be important. Effective interventions with family members might also be useful with other kinds of health or illness concerns.
>
> _____
>
> Source: Robinson, C. A., Bottotoff, J. L., & Torchalla, I. (2011). Exploring family relationships: Directions for smoking cessation. In E. K. Svavarsdottir and H. Jonsdottir (Eds.), *Family nursing in action* (pp 137–159). Reykjavik, Iceland: University of Iceland Press.

the circular questions suggest possibilities for new understandings about relationships and meanings (Wright & Leahey, 2013). Linear questions are used to explore family meaning or perceptions about a health experience. A nurse often uses linear questions as new information about an illness or health concern is collected. For example, a family brings a young child with shortness of breath to the emergency department. The nurse may ask a family member linear questions such as: When did your daughter's symptoms start? What do you think might have caused them? Is this the first time this has happened? Circular questions are used to determine the family's understandings, understand the relationships, and examine beliefs and thinking processes (Wright & Leahey, 2013). Circular questions linked to this episodic situation might be: What is your greatest fear about your daughter's condition? Who in your family has the most difficulty handling stressful situations? How does her older sister respond when this distressful breathing occurs? Has your family made any changes since she was diagnosed with asthma? Both forms of questioning are useful and enable the nurse to gain insights into the family's response to this illness situation.

Chapter Summary

Communication is a vital element of family-focused nursing practice. Individuals and family units can face highly stressful times with enormous barriers and great challenges when managing health alterations. Family nurses need skills and experience to share clear messages in trusting environments. A variety of communication strategies can ensure the safety of an ill family member, ease the distress experienced by uncertainties, and increase the comfort of those seeking care. Intentional communication strategies aimed at building and enhancing trusted relationships are important. Relationship-based care includes authentic interactions that recognize the importance of the family unit. Reflection about what has or has not been adequately communicated can help nurses to gain confidence and become more proficient. This chapter has provided information about many skills (e.g., listening, asking, informing, giving feedback, motivational interviewing) to use in building strong individual and family unit relationships.

REFERENCES

Abraham, M., & Moretz, J. G. (2012). Implementing patient- and family-centered care: Part I—understanding the challenges. *Pediatric Nursing, 38*(1), 44–47.

American Nurses Association. (2001). *Code of ethics for nurse with interpretative statements.* Washington, DC: Nursebooks.org.

American Nurses Association (2006). *Position statement on privacy and confidentiality.* Washington, DC: Nursebooks.org.

American Nurses Association (2010). *Nursing's social policy statement: The essence of the profession.* Washington, DC: Nursebooks.org.

Anderson, H., & Goolishan, H. (1988). Human systems as linguistic systems: Preliminary and evolving ideals about the implications for clinical theory. *Family Process, 27,* 371–393.

Arnold, E. C., & Boggs, K. U. (2010). *Interpersonal relationships: Professional communication skills for nurses* (6th ed.). Philadelphia: W. B. Saunders.

Aspeling, H. E., & van Wyk, N. (2008). Factors associated with adherence to antiretroviral therapy for the treatment of HIV-infected women attending an urban care facility. *International Journal of Nursing Practice, 14*(1), 3–10.

Bandura, A. (1977). *Social learning theory.* New York: General Learning Press.

Barnlund, D. C. (2008). A transactional model of communication. In. C. D. Mortensen (Ed.), *Communication theory* (2nd ed., pp 47–57). New Brunswick, NJ: Transaction.

Bell, J. M. (2011). Relationships: The heart of the matter in family nursing. Journal of Family Nursing, 17(1), 3-10, doi:10.1177/1074840711398464

Bengston, V. L., Acock, A. C., Allen, K. R., Dilworth-Anderson, P., % Klein, D. M. (1993). *Sourcebook of family theory & research.* Thousand Oaks, CA: Sage Publications.

Benner, P. (1983). Uncovering the knowledge embedded in clinical practice. *Image, 15*(2), 36–41.

Bennett, C. L., Ferriera, M. R., Davis, T. C., et al. (1998). Relation between literacy, race, and stage of presentation among low-income patients with prostate cancer. *Journal of Clinical Oncology, 16,* 3101–3104.

Benzein, E. G., Hagberg, M., & Saveman, B. I. (2008). "Being appropriately unusual": A challenge for nurses in health-promoting conversations with families. *Nursing Inquiry, 15*(2), 106–115.

Berkman, N. D., DeWalt, D. A., Pignone, M. P., Sheridan, S. L., Lohr, K. N., Lux L., . . . Bonito, A. J. (2004). *Literacy and health outcomes* (AHRQ Publication No. 04-E007-2). Washington, DC: Agency for Healthcare Research and Quality.

Blumer, H. (1969). *Symbolic interactionism: Perspective and method.* Englewood Cliffs, NJ: Prentice Hall.

Bourbonnier, M., & Evans, L. K. (2002). Advanced practice nursing in the care of frail older adults. *Journal of the American Geriatric Society, 50,* 2062–2076.

Bowlby, J. (1958). The child's tie to his mother. *International Journal of Psycho-analysis, 39,* 1–23.

Brown, H., & Hartrick Doane, G. (2008). From filling a bucket to lighting a fire: Aligning nursing education and nursing practice. In L. Young & B. Patterson (Eds.), *Teaching nursing: Developing a student-centered learning environment* (pp 97–118). Philadelphia: Lippincott Williams & Wilkins.

Buber, M. (1970). *I and thou.* New York: Scribner.

Burns, K. (2011). Nurse-physician rounds: A collaborative approach to improving communication, efficiencies, and perception of care. *Medsurg Nursing, 20*(4), 194–199.

Callery, P., & Milnes, L. (2012). Communication between nurses, children and their parents in asthma review consultations. *Journal of Clinical Nursing, 21*(11/12), 1641–1650.

Carter, B., & McGoldrick, M (1999). *The expanded family life cycle: Individual, family and social perspectives* (3rd ed.). Boston: Allyn & Bacon.

Chesla, C. (1996). Reconciling technologic and family care in critical care nursing. *Image:Journal of Nursing Scholarship, 28*(3), 199–203.

Chesla, C. (2010). Do family interventions improve health? *Journal of Family Nursing, 16*(4), 355–377. doi:10.1177/1074840710383145

Clark, M. C., & Diamond, P. M. (2010). Depression in family caregivers of elders: A theoretical model of caregiver burden, sociotropy, and autonomy. *Research in Nursing and Health, 33,* 20–34.

Cody, W. K. (Ed.). (2013). *Philosophical and theoretical perspectives for advanced nursing practice* (5th ed.). Burlington, MA: Jones & Bartlett Learning.

Cowan, M. J., Shapiro, M., Hays, R. D., Afifi, A., Vazirani, S., Ward, C. R., & Ettner, S. L. (2006). The effective of multidisciplinary hospitalist/physician and advanced practice nurse collaboration on hospital costs. *Journal of Nursing Administration, 36*(2), 79–85.

Curtis, J. R., Patrick, D. L., Caldwell, E., Greenlee, H., & Collier, A. C. (1999). The quality of patient-doctor communication about end-of-life care: A study of patients with advanced AIDS and their primary care clinicians. *AIDS, 13,* 1123–1131.

Curtis, J. R., & White, D. B. (2008). Practical guidelines for evidence-based ICU family conferences. *Chest, 134*(4), 835–843.

Curtis, K., Tzannes A., & Rudge T. (2011). How to talk to doctors—a guide for effective communication. *International Nursing Review*, 58(1), 13–20. Retrieved from http://dx.doi.org/10.1111/j.1466-7657.2010.00847.x

Dance, F. E. X. (1967). *Human communication theory.* New York: Holt.

Denham, S. A. (2003). *Family health: A framework for nursing.* (2003). Philadelphia: F. A. Davis.

Denham, S. A., & Looman, W. (2010). Families with chronic illness. In J. R. Kaakinen, V. Gedaly-Duff, D. P. Coehlo, & S. M. Harmon Hanson (Eds.), *Family health care nursing: Theory, practice and research* (4th ed.). Philadelphia: F. A. Davis.

Doane, G. A. H. (2002). Beyond behavioral skills to human-involved processes: Relational nursing practice and interpretive pedagogy. *Journal of Nursing Education, 41,* 400–404.

Dreifuerst, K. T. (2009). The essentials of debriefing in simulation learning: A concept analysis. *Nursing Education Perspectives, 30*(2), 109–114.

Dufault, M., Duquette, C. E., Ehmann, K., Hehl, R., Lavin, M., Martin, V., . . . & Willey, C. (2010). Translating an evidence-based protocol for nurse-to-nurse shift handoffs. *Worldviews on Evidence-Based Nursing, 7*(2), 59–75.

Duvall, E. M. (1977). *Marriage and family development* (5th ed.). Philadelphia: Lippincott.

Eggenberger, S. K., & Nelms, T. P. (2007). Being family: The family experience when an adult member is hospitalized with a critical illness. *Journal of Clinical Nursing, 16*(9), 1618–1628.

Eggenberger, S. K., & Regan, M. (2010). Expanding simulation to teach family nursing. *Journal of Nursing Education, 49*(10), 550–558.

Eggenberger, S. K., Meiers, S. J., Krumwiede, N. K., Bliesmer, M., & Earle, P. (2011). Reintegration in families in the context of chronic illness: A family health promotion model. *Journal of Nursing and Healthcare of Chronic Illness, 3,* 283–292. doi:10.111j1752-9824.2011.01101.x

Ellington, L., Reblin, M., Clayton, M., Berry, P., & Mooney, K. (2012). Hospice nurse communication with patients with cancer and their family caregivers. *Journal of Palliative Medicine, 15*(3), 262–268.

Fawcett, J. (2005). *Contemporary nursing knowledge.* Philadelphia: F. A. Davis.

Gubrium, J. F., & Holstein, J. A. (1993). Phenomenology, ethnomethodology and family discourse. In P. G. Boss, W. J. Doherty, W. R. LaRossa, W. R. Schumm, & S. K. Steinmetz (Eds.), *Sourcebook of family theories and methods: A contextual approach* (pp 651–672). New York: Plenum Press.

Hagerty, B. M., & Patusky, K. L. (2003). Reconceptualizing the nurse-patient relationship. *Journal of Nursing Scholarship, 35*(2), 145–150.

Hanna, D. R., & Romana, M. (August 2007). Debriefing after a crisis: What's the best way to resolve moral distress? Don't suffer in silence. *Nursing Management,* 39–47.

Hartmann, M., Bazner, E., Wild, B., Eisler, I., & Herzog, W. (2010). Effects of interventions involving the family in the treatment of adult patients with chronic physical disease: A meta-analysis. *Psychotherapy and Psychosomatics, 79*(3), 136–148.

Haynes, R. B., Ackloo, E., Sahota, N., McDonald, H. P., & Yao, X. (2008). Interventions for enhancing medication adherence. *Cochrane Database System Review,* CD000011.

Health and Human Services. (2008). Health information privacy. Retrieved July 31, 2012 from http://www.hhs.gov/ocr/privacy/hipaa/faq/disclosures_to_friends_and_family/534.html

Henriksson, A., & Andershed, B. (2007). A support group programme for relatives during the late palliative phase. *International Journal of Palliative Nursing, 13*(4), 175–183.

Henriksson, A., Benzein, E., Ternestedt, B., & Andershed, B. (2011). Meeting needs of family members with life-threatening illness: A support group program during ongoing palliative care. *Palliative and Supportive Care, 9,* 263–271.

Heru, A. M. (2013). *Working with families in medical settings: A multidisciplinary guide for psychiatrists and other health professionals.* New York: Routledge.

Hrabe, D. P. (2005). Peplau in cyberspace: An analysis of Peplau's interpersonal relations theory and computer-mediated communication. *Issues in Mental Health Nursing, 26*(4), 397–414.

Institute of Medicine. (1999). To err is human: Building a safer health system. A report of the Committee on Quality of Health Care in American. National Academy Press.

Institute of Medicine. (2001). Crossing the quality chasm: A new health system for the 21st century. Washington, DC: Committee on the Quality Health Care in America, National Academy of Science, National Academy Press.

Jones, L., Woodhouse, D., & Rowe, J. (2007). Effective nurse parent communication: A study of parents' perceptions in the NICU environment. *Patient Education & Counseling, 69*(1–3), 206–212.

Kendall-Tacket, K. A. (1993). *Postpartum depression: A comprehensive approach for nurses.* Newbury Park: Sage.

Knaus, W. A., Draper, E. A., Wagner, D. P., & Zimmerman, J. E. (1986). An evaluation of outcome from intensive care in major medical centers. *Annals of Internal Medicine, 104,* 410–418.

Koloroutis, M. (Ed.). (2004). *Relationship-based care: A model for transforming practice.* Minneapolis: Creative Health Management.

LaRossa, R., & Reitzes, D. C. (1993). Symbolic interactionism and family studies. In P. G. Boss, W. J. Doherty, W. R. LaRossa, W. R. Schumm, & S. K. Steinmetz (Eds.), *Sourcebook of family theories and methods: A contextual approach* (pp 135–166). New York: Plenum Press.

Levine, C., & Zuckerman, C. (2000). Hands on/hands off: Why health care professionals depend on families but keep them at arm's length. *Journal of Law, Medicine & Ethics, 28,* 5–18.

Looman, W. S., & Lindeke, L. I. (2005). Health and social context: Social capital's utility as a construct for nursing and health promotion. *Journal of Pediatric Health Care 19*(2), 90–94.

Lynn-McHale, D. J., & Deatrick, J. A. (2000). Trust between family and health care provider. *Journal of Family Nursing, 6*(3), 210–230.

Machnowski, G. P. (1997, Fall). Correlation seen between communication skills and malpractice risk. *Details in Professional Liability, 11*(3), 1.

Mason, P., & Butler, C. C. (2010). *Health behavior change.* Toronto: Elsevier.

Matire, L. M., & Schulz, R. (2007). Involving family in psychosocial interventions for chronic illness. *Current Directions in Psychological Science, 16*(2), 90–94.

Mayberry, L. S., Kripalani, S., Roghman, R. L., & Osborn, C. Y. (2011). Bridging the digital divide in diabetes; Family support and implications for health literacy. *Diabetes Technology Therapeutics, 13*(10), 1005–1012.

McDonald, G. W. (1981). Structural exchange and marital interaction. *Journal of Marriage and Family, 43*(4), 825–839.

Mead, G. H. (1956). *On social psychology: Selected papers* (Anselm Straus, Ed.). Chicago: University of Chicago Press (originally published in 1934).

Meiers, S. J. (2002). *Family-nurse co-construction of meaning: Caring in the family health experience* (Doctoral dissertation). Dissertation Abstracts. Minneapolis: University of Minnesota. Retrieved from UMI Order AAI3041946.

Meiers, S. J., & Jenson, C. (2011). *Family interviewing and motivational interviewing: Comparisons and contrasts*. Unpublished manuscript. Rochester, MN: Winona State University, Department of Nursing.

Meiers, S., & Tomlinson, P. (2003). Family-nurse co-construction of meaning: A central phenomenon of family caring. *Scandinavian Journal of Caring Sciences, 17*(2), 193–201.

Meleis, A. I. (2012). *Theoretical nursing: Development and progress* (5th ed.). Philadelphia: Wolters Kluwer Health.

Meleis, A. I. (Ed.). (2010). *Transitions theory: Middle range and situation specific theories in nursing research and practice*. New York: Springer.

National Assessment of Adult Literacy (2003). Institute of Education Sciences, National Center for Education Statistics, U.S. Department of Education. Retrieved from http://nces.ed.gov/NAAL/kf_demographics.asp

National Commission on Adult Literacy. (2008). *Reach higher, America: Overcoming crisis in the U.S. workforce*. New York: Council for Advancement of Adult Literacy.

Nelms, T. P., & Eggenberger, S. K. (2010). Essence of the family critical illness experience and family meetings. *Journal of Family Nursing, 16*(4), 462–486.

Paterson, J. G., & Zderad, L. T. (1976). *Humanistic nursing*. New York: John Wiley.

Peplau, H. E. (1991). *Interpersonal relations in nursing: A conceptual frame of references for psychodynamic nursing*. New York: Springer. (Original work published in 1952.)

Peplau, H. E. (1997). Peplau's theory of interpersonal relations. *Nursing Science Quarterly, 10*(4), 162–167.

Quinn, J. R., Schmitt, M. H., Baggs, J. G., Norton, S. A., Dombeck, M. T., & Seller, C. R. (2012). Family members' informal roles in end-of-life decision making in adult intensive care units. *American Journal of Critical Care, 21*(1), 43–51.

Robinson, C. A., Bottotoff, J. L., & Torchalla, I. (2011). Exploring family relationships: Directions for smoking cessation. In E. K. Svavarsdottir and H. Jonsdottir (Eds.), *Family nursing in action* (pp 137–159). Reykjavik, Iceland: University of Iceland Press.

Rollnick, S., Miller, W. R., & Butler, C. C. (2008). *Motivational interviewing in health care: Helping patients change behavior*. New York: Guilford Press.

Rosengren, D. B. (2009). *Building motivational interviewing skills: A practitioner workbook*. New York: Guilford Press.

Roter, D. L. (2011). Oral literacy demand of health care communication: Challenges and solutions. *Nursing Outlook, 69*, 79–84.

Rubin, R. (1984). *Maternal identity and the maternal experience*. New York: Springer.

Sarkar, U., Karter, A. J, Lieu, J. Y., Adler, N. E., Nguyen, R., Lopez, A., . . . Nykolyn, L. (2010). *Communication for nurses: How to prevent harmful events and promote patient safety*. Philadelphia: F. A. Davis.

Schuster, P. M., & Nykolyn, L. (2010). *Communication for nurses: How to prevent harmful events and promote patient safety*. Philadelphia: F. A. Davis.

Segrin, C., & Flora, J. (2011). *Family communication* (2nd ed.). New York: Taylor & Francis.

Sherwood, P. R., Given, C. W., Given, B. A., & Von Eye, A. (2005). Caregiver burden and depressive symptoms: Analysis of common outcomes in caregivers of elderly patients. *Journal of Aging and Health, 17*, 125–147.

Soderstrom, I., Benzein, E., & Saveman, B. (2003). Nurses' experiences of interactions with family members in intensive care unit. *Scandinavian Journal of Caring Sciences 17*, 185–192.

Sorenson, D. L. S. (1990). Uncertainty in pregnancy. *Clinical Issues in Perinatal Women's Health Nursing, 3*(1), 289–296.

Spath, P. (2000). Reducing errors through work system improvements. In P. Spath (Ed.), *Error reduction in health care* (pp 199–234). San Francisco: Jossey-Bass.

Spinda, B. (1997, Fall). What prompts a patient to sue? *Details in Professional Liability, 11*(3), 2.

Tanner, C. A. (2006). Thinking like a nurse: A research-based model of clinical judgment in nursing. *Journal of Nursing Education, 45*(6), 204–211.

Tapp, D. M. (2000). The ethics of relational stance in family nursing: Resisting the view of 'Nurse as Expert.' Journal of Family Nursing, 6(1), 69.

Tarlier, D. (2004). Beyond caring: The moral and ethical bases of responsive nurse-patient relationships. *Nursing Philosophy, 5,* 230–241.

Tomlinson, P. S., Swiggum, P., & Harbaugh, B. (1999). Identification of nurse-family intervention sites to decrease health-related boundary ambiguity in PICU. *Issues in Comprehensive Pediatric Nursing, 22*(1), 27–47.

Travelbee, J. (1966). *Interpersonal aspects of nursing.* Philadelphia: F. A. Davis.

U.S. Department of Health and Human Services (USDHHS) (2010a). Healthy people 2020. Retrieved from http://www.healthypeopole.gov/2020/

U.S. Department of Health and Human Services (USDHHS) (2010b). National action plan to improve health literacy. Retrieved from http://www.health.gov/communcation/HLActionPlan/

Vandall-Walker, V., & Clark, A. M. (2011). It starts with access! A grounded theory of family members working to get through critical illness. *Journal of Family Nursing, 17*(2), 148–181.

Vangelisti, A. L. (Ed.). (2004). *Handbook of family communication.* Mahwah, NJ: Lawrence Erlbaum Assoc.

von Bertalanffy, L. (1975). Perspectives on General Systems Theory. In E. Taschdjian (Ed.), *Scientific-philosophical studies.* New York: George Braziller.

Walsh, F. (Ed.). *Normal family processes* (3rd ed.) (pp 424–459). New York: Guilford Press.

Watzlawick, P., Beavin, J. H., & Jackson, D. D. (1967). *Pragmatics of human communication.* New York: Norton.

Weihs, K., Fisher, L., & Baird, M. (2002). Families, health and behavior: A section of the Commissioned Report by the Committee on Health and Behavior: Research, Practice and Policy. *Families, Systems and Health, 20*(1), 7–46.

Weiss, B. D., Mays, M. Z., Martz, W., Castro, K. M., DeWalt, D. A., Pignone, M. P., . . . Hale, F. A. (2005). Quick assessment of literacy in primary care: The newest vital sign. *Annals of Family Medicine, 3*(6), 514–522. doi:10.1370/afmm.405

White, S., and McCloskey, M. (2003). Framework for the 2003 National Assessment of Adult Literacy (NCES 2005-531). Washington, DC: U.S. Department of Education, National Center for Education Statistics. Retrieved from http://nces.ed.gov/naal/fr_definition.asp - top

Wiegand, D. L. M (2006). Withdrawal of life-sustaining therapy after sudden, unexpected life-threatening illness or injury: Interactions between patients' families, health care providers, and the healthcare system. *American Journal of Critical Care, 15*(2), 178–187.

Williams, M. V., Baker, D. W., Parker, R. M., & Nurss, J. R. (1998). Relationships of functional health literacy to patients' knowledge of their chronic disease. A study of patients with hypertension and diabetes. *Archives of Internal Medicine, 158,* 166–172.

Wright, L. M., & Bell, J. M. (2010). *Beliefs and illness: A model of healing.* Calgary, Alberta, Canada: 4th Floor Press.

Wright, L. M., & Leahy, M. (2013). *Nurses and families: A guide to family assessment and intervention* (6th ed). Philadelphia: F. A. Davis.

Yu-Nu, W., Yea-Ing Lotus, S., Min-Chi, C., & Pei-Shan, Y. (2011). Reconciling work and family caregiving among adult-child family caregivers of older people with dementia: Effects on role strain and depressive symptoms. *Journal of Advanced Nursing, 67*(4), 829–840. doi:10.1111/j.1365-2648.2010.05505.x

Zerwekh, J. V. (2006). *Nursing care at the end of life: Palliative care for patients and families.* Philadelphia: F. A. Davis.

CHAPTER 5

Family Assessment

Sonja J. Meiers • Norma K. Krumwiede • Sharon A. Denham
• Sue Ellen Bell

CHAPTER OBJECTIVES

1. Differentiate between individual, family, and community assessment.
2. Discuss assessment that includes the predictive and protective factors influencing the health and illness of individuals, families, communities, and populations.
3. Explain ways that genograms, ecograms, and ecomaps can be used to assess family from an ecological point of view.
4. Describe ways that computer-based geographical information systems can be used to understand family, community, and population health needs.
5. Recognize ways that genetics and genomics influence health, disease prevention, treatments, screening, and outcomes.

CHAPTER CONCEPTS

- Assessment
- Clinical nursing judgments
- Ecomap
- Family pedigree
- Family unit assessment
- Genetics
- Genogram
- Geographical information systems
- Individual assessment
- Nursing process
- Social capital
- Spiritual assessment

Introduction

Regardless of the type of care setting, the best nursing care occurs when nurses *think family*. Although several nursing theorists have discussed the roles of families in health and illness care (Neuman & Fawcett, 2011), many nurses still view the family as the "context of care." Family members might be included in some discussions when they are present, but this is seldom planned or noted in personal health records. Family-focused nursing recognizes that the accuracy and breadth of assessment data are improved by purposely including family. Thinking family could increase awareness of the breadth of possible causative factors for symptoms (Tanner, 2006). This chapter introduces ways to intentionally *think family* during assessments, especially about aspects of life pertinent to those living in the family household and within the community. Health and illness outcomes can be improved when predictive factors (those factors that cause risk or benefit to health) and protective factors (those factors that provide a buffer to illness, injury, or disability) are simultaneously considered. This chapter reviews critical aspects of assessments and describes ways to include family units.

Nursing Process

Nurses use the nursing process, a modified version of the scientific method that is holistic and personalized to assess individual needs in planning care (American Nurses Association, 2012). Nursing process includes assessment, diagnosis, care planning, implementation of the planned care, and evaluation. This chapter focuses on assessment. Use of an ecological framework aids understandings about the individuals, families, household, neighborhood, and community links with health and illness (Bronfenbrenner, 1979). A holistic assessment can suggest multiple risk determinants and related nursing actions.

Assessments

Assessments are tools for gathering holistic information to guide nursing actions that support health promotion, disease prevention, illness management, restorative outcomes, and well-being. Assessment is the first step in nursing care and can be used to identify nursing diagnoses (Jensen, 2011; Lunney, 2009) and in planning nursing actions. It is the way nurses come to know the needs of others. Similar assessment processes are used in all forms of care settings.

Individual Assessments

Assessment identifies problems and leads to a medical diagnosis or nursing diagnosis. Assessments are initially conducted when persons enter a health care encounter and completed during care delivery and before discharge to another setting. In fast-paced health care systems, nursing assessments mainly focus on individuals' physiological status, health histories, and limited social information. The assessment would include the individual's presenting problem, history of illness events, symptoms, current medications, and other pertinent clinical information. This baseline information can help health care practitioners identify facts about the presenting condition.

In care directed by medical model thinking, nurses can provide dependent and independent nursing functions (Fig. 5.1). Dependent nursing functions are actions that directly respond to medical orders given by a physician or other professional provider. These actions guide many treatments nurses provide. Independent nursing functions are actions within the scope of nursing practice and do not require a physician's order. Independent nursing functions can be used in response to individual needs (Snyder & Lindquist, 2009).

Family Unit Assessments

Most assessments consider little about the family unit. A family unit assessment is a systematic process used to collect family household information that is baseline knowledge about resources, strengths, and risks aligned with individual care needs. Family unit assessments identify individual, family, household, and community components. The family household provides important information about their usual lives such as the ways members function independently, as a unit, and with social networks. Family structure assessment aids in identifying family health routines that can be threats or supports for the person needing care or suggest potential risk factors for illness. Hospice programs have long collected and used this type of information in the care of dying persons and their family units.

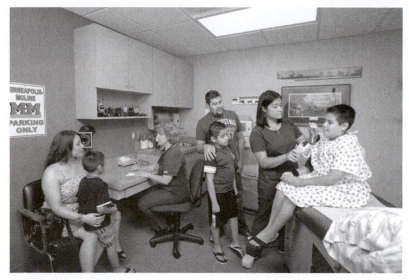

FIGURE 5-1 Family assessment includes independent and dependent functions.

Clinical Nursing Judgments

Clinical nursing judgments involve observation, reasoning, analysis, synthesis, and critical thinking. In a review of about 200 studies on clinical judgment, Tanner (2006) identified that clinical nursing judgments are:

- Influenced by what nurses bring to situations
- Linked with knowing individuals and their responses
- Influenced by the context of the situation and culture of the nursing unit
- Influenced by the nurses' reasoning skills

Tanner found that reflections about actions taken can improve clinical reasoning. Making appropriate clinical judgments is grounded in what is known. If the nurse has assessed only biophysical data, then few tools for holistic clinical nursing judgments might be available. Nurses who *think family* want a fully equipped clinical nursing judgment toolbox ready to employ.

Moving from an Individual to a Family Assessment

Nurses who *think family* know that individual assessment, which focuses on the presenting symptoms or complaints, is only the beginning and collecting a family assessment offers a much better insight into health patterns and risks for both the individual and family. Suppose you are admitting a 54-year-old gentleman who complains of upper back pain. What kinds of information do you need to discover during the assessment process (Box 5.1)?

Completing the Physical Assessment

As nurses complete health assessments, they gather objective data that will help formulate a plan of care:

- Screen for general well-being
- Develop a baseline for comparison with future assessments

BOX 5-1
Components of an Individual Health History

COMPONENT	DETAILED ASSESSMENT	EXAMPLE OF DATA COLLECTED
Biographical data	Name, contact information, birth date, age, marital/partnered status, religion, nationality, emergency contact, language, health care providers.	Mr. M. is a 54-year-old, single, Somalian, practicing Muslim, whose emergency contact is his sister. He does not have a regular physician. He speaks English.
Current physical and emotional complaints	Questions are asked to determine the type of symptom, the duration and severity of the symptom, and how the symptom is affecting daily life.	If upper back pain is the symptom, the nurse would ask how long Mr. M. has been experiencing pain; whether the pain is dull or sharp; what activities Mr. M. is not able to do because of the symptoms; and on a scale of 0–10, with 0 being no pain and 10 being the worst possible pain, what number Mr. M. would assign to the pain.
Past medical history and health habits	The individual presenting for assessment usually completes a form asking if there have been any health problems in the past; the list of possible health problems is typically organized according to body systems and includes surgeries, injuries, hospitalizations, allergies, immunizations, medications; health habits such as smoking, exercise, diet, and drug use are also included.	Mr. M.'s health history includes a past work-related back injury, allergy to aspirin, and a history of hypercholesterolemia and hypertension. He is minimally physically active in his role as a small grocery store owner. He does not smoke tobacco or drink alcohol.
Past and current ability to perform activities of daily living (ADLs)	The individual may respond to questions about whether the current back pain is limiting his daily activity, either on a paper/electronic form or in response to verbal questions asked by the nurse.	Mr. M. states that he is not able to lift boxes and stock shelves in his grocery store because of his back pain. He also has pain while getting into and out of his automobile.
Available support systems, coping and patterns, perceived stressors	The individual responds to questions about who is present to support him in his daily activities given the pain he is experiencing, how he typically copes with pain and discomfort, and if there are any additional life stressors with which he is dealing.	Mr. M. states that his father, who is 80, is helping him at the grocery store. Mr. M. typically manages back pain by taking acetaminophen and using a heating pad to the area. He is having trouble maintaining his grocery store, which is his source of income, and this is stressful to him. He feels supported by his faith community at the local mosque.

BOX 5-1

Components of an Individual Health History—cont'd

COMPONENT	DETAILED ASSESSMENT	EXAMPLE OF DATA COLLECTED
Socioeconomic factors	The individual responds to written or verbal questions about income level, education level, occupation status, and housing status.	Mr. M. is a small business owner, with a high school education, who lives with his elderly parents in an apartment. The family has a combined annual income of about $45,000.
Spiritual and cultural practices, preferences, and concerns	The individual responds to written or verbal questions about religion and/or spirituality, culture, and related practices, preferences, and concerns.	Mr. M. practices the daily Islamic prayer rituals and celebrates Muslim holidays. He does not eat pork or pork products in adherence to Islamic dietary laws.
Family patterns of illness	The individual responds to written or verbal questions about family history of major physical or mental illnesses or illnesses related to the presenting health issue. Alternatively, a family medical pedigree may also be created by the individual.	Mr. M. does not have a history of rheumatoid arthritis in his family. His parents both have hypertension, high triglycerides, and high cholesterol.
Other assessments (health risk appraisal; dental, nutritional, developmental, vision, and hearing screening; immunizations; tuberculosis screening; and fall risk assessment)	These assessments are appropriately used based upon the age of the person.	Mr. M. is screened for tuberculosis based on his history of having spent time in a refugee camp as part of his immigration experience and an immunization history to determine his immunity status.

- Validation of the complaints that bring an individual to seek health care
- Monitoring for changes in the current health problem

This assessment can be a comprehensive assessment or a focused assessment if it is being done in episodic care to address a specific symptom or problem. It is within the nurse's purview to expand assessment so that multiple factors that influence individual health or illness are also included.

A complete physical assessment identifies normal and abnormal findings and relates them to the health history for a complete picture. The assessment includes vital signs, general appearance, health habits, past medical and illness-related history, social connectedness, and education level; combined with results of diagnostic tests, this information helps identify possible nursing diagnoses (Goolsby & Grubbs, 2011). The way the nurse communicates during this assessment can set the tone for the relationship. Assessment findings are analyzed and synthesized to formulate opinions or clinical nursing judgments about the best courses of action to take. Components of a physical examination from individual and family perspectives are included in Box 5.2.

Since the beginning of professional nursing, the goal has been to assess individuals within the environment and pay attention to the healing potential of the family (Nightingale, 1859 and 1946). Nightingale believed nurses should attend to spiritual needs and return individuals to the caring families where they would best be healed. Professional nursing has always included the family as a healing instrument; perhaps this is the true meaning of holistic care. For example, Mr. M. lives with his elderly parents who have similar cardiovascular risk markers. Mr. M. needs to make some nutritional modifications as a result of his recent myocardial infarction. As the nurse caring for him, you realize the importance of dietary routines. What kinds of assessment data will you need to make effective clinical

BOX 5-2
Components of the Physical Examination

PHYSICAL EXAMINATION COMPONENT	INDIVIDUAL COMPONENT DESCRIPTION	FAMILY COMPONENT DESCRIPTION
Vital signs	Measure the individual's respirations, pulse, temperature, blood pressure, and assess for pain.	Obtain a genogram; collect information on the type and amount of family resources.
General appearance	Collect information about the individual's physical presence, psychological presence, and signs and symptoms of distress.	Observe the family's physical and psychological presence and signs and symptoms of distress to actual or perceived threats.
Health habits	Elicit information about the individual's lifestyle that can affect health.	Ask about the health practices and health maintenance activities of the family.
Past medical and health related events	Collect information on the individual's health status and health-related events from birth.	Complete the family health history and pedigree; collect information on the health-related events the family has faced in the past and ascertain how the family dealt with them.
Social connectedness	Collect the social history, determine interpersonal relationships, and create an individual ecomap.	Obtain a family level ecomap, collect the family social history, and identify interpersonal relationships.
Education	Determine the individual's ability to read and write and level of health understanding.	Determine the health literacy of the family and tailor questions and teaching to this level.

nursing judgments and a collaborate with him in a plan for home? Family members who live in a shared household share resources, dietary routines, and habits. When nurses *think family*, it is important to understand that the family household is the place where health and illness are produced.

Gathering Information From Family Members

Family members often possess valuable information about care needs. For instance, a young man is in the clinic because of intense suffering due to migraine headaches. An individual assessment might just focus on the presentation, duration, intensity, frequency, and exacerbation of symptoms. The young man describes the pain as excruciating and limiting his ability to work. He is primarily seeking medicine or treatment for pain relief. A nurse who thinks family understands the importance of the family household and so initiates a conversation about his family. She discovers that he is married. The nurse knows that his wife might likely have some additional knowledge about the illness trajectory. Even though his wife is not present in the clinic, the nurse wants to include her in their conversation.

The nurse asks, "If your wife were here with you today, what do you think she might say about your symptoms?" He responds, "Well, she would really like me to tell you about the difficulty I have staying awake during the day. Even when doing simple activities I get tired." He adds, "She has been asking me if missing sleep could cause the migraines." The nurse then asks more specific questions about the sleep loss. His answers could lead to some additional testing. Without that additional information, the sleep disorder would have been missed and the course of treatment less effective.

Taking a family-focused approach can occur even if family members are absent. Use of circular questioning along with linear questioning during assessments can draw out important information about family members that can assist nurses in making appropriate clinical nursing judgments (Wright & Leahy, 2009). Circular and linear types of questioning were described in Chapter 4. Use of the question, "What do you think your family [family member] would say about . . ." is a valuable open-ended question that naturally takes a family-focused perspective. Using this question during assessments can elicit important information that challenges potential assumptions.

Challenges in Completing Assessments

The importance of information that family members can share during delivery of individual care may not always be valued. But nurses who *think family* know that health determinants in one's household, neighborhood, and larger community often have relevance to the presenting symptoms. Exploring them can help the nurse identify critical factors about ways the individual and family unit have been managing a presenting condition or even why the condition occurred. Family nurses use sincere and concerned language and nonverbal cues while completing the assessment. It can be a challenge during an assessment to listen carefully, ask curious and related questions, and accurately document observations in the health record but the information obtained can have a profound effect on outcomes.

Evaluating Nursing Outcomes

Assessment is ongoing and used to later evaluate nursing care outcomes. For instance, the Jones family is greatly stressed because their 14-year-old son Alex with type 1 diabetes consistently has high blood sugar levels and is unsuccessful in meeting the target hemoglobin

A_{1c} of 6.5 to 7.5. At the time of diagnosis, when he was 11 years old, his parents attended classes with him and discussed the need for family change with a diabetes educator and dietitian. The family has tried to make appropriate modifications to their lifestyle, but has not fully adopted all needed changes. Alex has always been a gamer and spent many solitary hours playing. As he has gotten older, he has taken to closing himself in his room alone for hours every day with the video games. He seems withdrawn and not interested in interacting in real life with friends, but says he has many friends online. His parents encourage him to be more physically active, but he refuses. His sedentary lifestyle and frequent high-carbohydrate snacks of highly processed foods are likely part of the reason for the uncontrolled blood glucose levels.

Earlier assessments and education had only addressed ways to modify Alex's diet, explained insulin use, and discussed medical management. The early assessments had treated the diabetes as if it was his problem and not a family matter. Family health routines were ignored and goals to address the family unit's dietary and lifestyle behaviors were not included in the plans. Target blood sugar readings were not discussed and no one was keeping track of things on a regular basis. Alex was partially responsible for the high readings, but what roles did his family have? How does his family unit factor into his diabetes management? What kinds of things need to be assessed? What is known about his school work, peer group influences, and reasons for socially withdrawing? Depression is sometimes linked with diabetes. Could this be a concern? A thorough assessment of family household factors could provide broader ideas about goals to set and strategies to plan. A plan that only considers Alex and ignores his family household, peer group, and other social factors might be ineffective in making needed changes. An assessment that clarifies relationships among things like his high carbohydrate intake, metabolism, school schedules, grades, peer associations, levels of sadness, and physical activity is important. Nurses who *think family* realize those connections. An evaluation that only gives a verdict of failure is not likely to encourage meaningful change. Contributing factors leading to repeated high blood sugar levels and an inability to reach a target hemoglobin A_{1c} can be altered with family support.

Completing a Family Assessment

Nurses who *think family* can discover relationships among individuals, family units, and the community that can influence care and outcomes. Using an ecological model such as the Family Health Model (Denham, 2003) can be a good guideline for providing those assessments and make it easier to identify family factors. The household is where health is produced and also where illness, disability, and crisis occur. Family unit assessments can include elements about the individual, family, and community (Box 5.3).

Using a single assessment form for everything does help with regulation compliance for accreditations or reimbursement. But use of single standardized forms can miss the mark by not focusing on specific problems. A better approach might be devising instruments that go beyond the general assessment and using targeted approaches along with addressing the supporting roles family members or family health routines play. This type of assessment allows for goal setting, formulating strategic plans for reaching goals, and identifying threats as well as strengths.

It is possible to view the family and the individual simultaneously as the foreground context for any health experience; this approach is important in family-focused care (Denham, 2003). Foreground context implies that individuals and families are essential,

BOX 5-3

Comparing Individual, Family, and Community Assessments

CARE CONCERN	INDIVIDUAL ASSESSMENT COMPONENT	FAMILY ASSESSMENT COMPONENT	COMMUNITY ASSESSMENT COMPONENT
Child abuse of a 2-year-old boy	Physical and psychological symptoms	Parental knowledge of growth and development	Availability of quality, affordable child care
Obesity in an elderly woman	Physical and psychological symptoms	Understanding of nutritional and activity requirements within the family	Availability of nutritious food and areas for safe exercise in the community
Sleep disturbance in a middle-aged man	Physical and psychological symptoms	Family stress level	Ambient noise or ongoing, sudden noises in community
Eating disorder of an adolescent girl	Physical and psychological symptoms	Recent losses in family or relocation stress	Peer pressure or bullying in the school setting

not optional! The entire family can be the target for care. Family assessment acknowl-edges the uniqueness of each family's needs and priorities (Wright & Leahy, 2009), even when individuals are respected and treated as the important care seekers. Family assess-ments identify specific concerns that need attention and can use a strengths-based or support-enhancing approach during data collection, one that discovers strengths for health promotion or behavior changes (Haggman-Laitila, Tanninen, & Pietila, 2010). Regardless of whether a needs- or strength-based perspective is used, an intentional systems-focused assessment approach that includes individual, family, and community is part of a family unit plan (Denham, 2003).

Interactions of multiple household members influence one another in ways that can sup-port or sabotage wellness or disease management (Denham, Manoogian, & Schuster, 2007; Manoogian, Harter, & Denham, 2010). When nurses *think family*, they consider the im-portant family roles and individual responsibilities that can influence outcomes and develop skills for completing assessments useful for family care (Bell, 2003).

Family Assessment Strategies

Family assessment requires perceptual skills or abilities to clearly observe, conceptual skills or the ability to think, and executive skills or the ability to follow through (Bell, 2003). Six things are needed as the nurse completes a comprehensive family assessment:

1. A systematic method for data collection and recording of the data
2. Excellent communication and observation skills
3. Careful analysis of the information collected from the individual and family members
4. Critical thinking skills to determine which areas of care most need attention

5. Sensitivity to what is valued by the individual and family
6. Imagination that allows one to identify ways to use nursing actions creatively to provide family-focused coordinated care

Nurses who *think family* also know that four areas give a family perspective to individual situations and provide cues about things to notice and assess:

1. Nonverbal behavior (e.g., affect, silence, eye contact, hesitancy to respond)
2. Verbal behaviors (e.g., who speaks, voice tones, content of dialogue, questions)
3. Interpersonal behaviors (e.g., individual behaviors, types of interactions with others, visitors)
4. Environment (e.g., household location, work, dependent relationships)

A systematic family assessment requires awareness of the verbal and nonverbal communication of those interviewed and observed. This means paying attention to who is and is not speaking. While collecting data, observe the ways family members interact with the individual seeking care and with one another. Does one person talk for another? Does one person never speak? What do these things mean for this family? Respectful attention given to the individual and the family unit needs during these encounters builds trust. A template for a brief family-focused assessment charts how family type, functions, and processes come together (Table 5.1).

TABLE 5-1	*Brief Family-Focused Assessment*
ELEMENT:	**NOTES:**
Individual demographic data	
Family demographic data	
Illness or health promotion concern of the individual	
Illness or health promotion concern of the family	
Family structure and developmental information	Complete genogram
Family routines disrupted by illness	
Family health promotion activities	
Family economic status	
Family cultural status	
Family connections to the larger community	Complete ecomap
Usual ways family manages an illness, injury, or developmental transition	
How is this illness or health promotion activity influencing usual management of activities of daily living?	
How do you, as a person, typically communicate, solve problems, and make decisions about health and illness? What things help? What things create barriers?	
How do you, as a family, typically communicate, solve problems, and make decisions about health and illness? What things help? What things create barriers?	
Who or what in your community do you believe could be helpful to you in managing this health/illness challenge?	
How can we, as health care professionals, best help your healing, as a person?	
How can we, as health care professionals, best help your healing, as a family?	

Case Study: The Cox-Halverson Family

Meet Randy Cox and Sheila Halverson, both 38 years old, the family being discussed throughout the rest of this chapter (Fehl, 2012). Some information is based on a real family that agreed to share some of their story, but some facts and names have been altered to protect their identity. This family provides a way to learn how conceptual ideas apply to family experiences.

Assessment of Family Types

Family types are somewhat different from in the past. Individuals in a single household may be extremely different from one another. Multiracial families are more common as a result of increasing globalization, immigration, ethnic diversity in a geographical region, economic shifts, and changing social values. Family forms are increasingly diverse and a growing number of gay, lesbian, bisexual, and transgender (GLBT) people live openly as family units. Nurses in clinical practice are likely to meet transgender and gender-nonconforming people and their families as they seek medical care and some face discrimination in doctor's offices, emergency departments, mental health clinics, and drug treatment programs and by emergency medical transporters (Grant, Mottet, & Tanis, 2011). Health and illness concerns of GLBT families are important. For instance, the Injustice at Every Turn study noted that only 43% of transgendered people maintained most of their family bonds, and 57% experienced significant family rejection (Grant et al., 2011). This study also found that 19% of the participants reported being refused medical care and 50% of transgendered persons had to teach their medical providers about care needs. Transgendered or gender-nonconforming people might have little or no contact with their family of origin and may have experienced an alarming amount of harassment, physical assault, sexual violence, and discrimination in their lifetime. Nurses who *think family* realize that their practice role calls for them to be tolerant and caring regardless of the family type.

Randy Cox and Sheila Halverson are a blended family. Randy and Sheila started dating about 2 years ago and their relationship became serious rather quickly. Both had previously been in unsuccessful long-term relationships and decided not to marry, but to live together. They each brought children to the relationship, seven of them (Table 5.2). Randy has five children, four biological children from his previous marriage and Brendan who was adopted as an infant when he married his mother. Randy has had contact with his daughter Jess throughout her life, but not custody. She recently moved to the area trying to make a new life. She stayed with her father and Sheila for about 6 months, but has found a job and an apartment. She still has frequent contact with them.

Randy receives a monthly Social Security disability payment based on the debilitating effects of his rheumatoid arthritis and he receives 40 hours a week of assistive services to help with his activities of daily living (ADL). He took Dilaudid and Oxycontin on a daily basis for pain control before therapeutic surgeries and for the first time in years he is not taking prescription pain medications. He has recovered well from his surgeries, but still struggles with knee pain due to years of walking with an impaired gait. The pain is mostly manageable, but flairs often enough to effect his ADL. Randy has been a smoker since the age of 14, but quit after his surgeries with the help of electronic cigarettes. He has struggled to remain smoke free and still uses them and smokes cigars several times each week. At 6 ft tall and 200 lb, he has no other significant health concerns.

Sheila has two children. Amanda, Sheila's daughter from a teenage relationship, was adopted by Sheila's parents and had little contact with her until the last 4 years. Initially the relationship was very strained, but it has grown stronger over time. If you use the Family Health Model (Denham, 2003) to understand the family from an ecological perspective,

TABLE 5-2	Cox-Halverson Children		
RANDY'S CHILDREN	**CONCERNS**	**SHEILA'S CHILDREN**	**CONCERNS**
Bailey, female, age 11 years, in 6th grade	Mostly healthy, average weight and height, has shown some signs of asthma lately	Amanda, female, age 19 years	Born from teen relationship; adopted by Sheila's parents; currently living with Randy and Sheila along with her two daughters
Liam, male, age 12 years, in 7th grade	Attention deficit-hyperactivity disorder (ADHD) and anxiety; takes medication; social difficulties; in special education; conflicts with Alex	Travis, male, age 14 years, in 8th grade	ADHD and oppositional defiant disorder (ODD); takes medication daily (took Abilify and made remarkable progress but had symptoms of tardive dyskinesia and drug was discontinued); serious social and education difficulties
Alex, male, age 14 years, in 8th grade	ODD without ADHD; no medications; attends school for behavioral disorders; 90th percentile for weight relative to height; conflicts with Liam	Sasha, female, age 2 years, biracial (Amanda's daughter)	Quiet child, does not interact much with others, has temper tantrums and screams when she does not get what she wants
Brendan, male, age 16 years, in 11th grade	Adopted, but does not know this; well adjusted; works part time	Autumn, female, age 5 months, healthy at this time (Amanda's daughter)	Cries often and Amanda becomes very frustrated; Bailey takes care of her much of the time when she is available
Jess, female, age 19 years, has a General Educational Development (GED) diploma	Born from a short teen relationship; little contact over the years; lived with them for about 6 months and now has contact	_____	_____

you would consider more than the family type and number of children (Box 5.4). The family lives in a three-bedroom, two-bath home in a rural community. They have two cars available for transportation. Currently Randy, Sheila, Alex, Travis, Liam, Amanda, and her two daughters live in the home. Amanda was having difficulties and they encouraged her to move in with them, making their home a bit cramped. At the age of 16, Amanda had Sasha,

BOX 5-4

Implications of Family Type

Consider the information provided about the Cox-Halverson family and their blended family living situation. Take some time to consider the various factors associated with the family members described in the family type section. Think about what daily life for this family might be like. What are the implications of these known factors on members' health and illness?

Answer these questions:

1. List risk factors you see for this family based upon what you know about family type.
2. List the strengths you see in this family based upon family type.
3. Given the risks and strengths identified through the family type assessment data available, what one or two things would be a priority for Randy's care needs if you were a nurse talking with him during a physician visit?
4. Now *think family* and identify two or three other things that the nurse might discuss with Randy that could be important for his family's wellness or illness prevention or management.
5. Using an ecological model to think about this family, what other questions do you have about the family's context (i.e., interacting factors linked with family, neighborhood, and larger social environments)? List three areas you might want to further assess.

her first daughter, but she has no contact with Sasha's father. Amanda realized she was pregnant again soon after she moved to live with Randy and Sheila and her second daughter, Autumn, is now 5 months old.

Sheila Halverson is overweight and has hypothyroidism, polycystic ovaries, and anxiety. At 5 ft 9 in. tall and approximately 260 lb, she has an increased risk for an array of weight-related conditions. She gained much weight while her hypothyroidism was undiagnosed. At the age of 15 she had an induced abortion. She then, at the age of 16, gave birth to a daughter who her father and stepmother adopted as a toddler. Later, at 22 years, she gave birth to a son who she has raised primarily as a single parent. She takes Levothyroxine and oral contraceptives daily. Sheila smokes 5 to 10 cigarettes per day and struggles to find time to make exercise a daily part of her routine.

Neither Randy nor Sheila identifies as religious, but Randy attends church sometimes with the children and extended family. Some of the children occasionally attend youth activities at the church. Although they do not identify themselves as religious, they define themselves as spiritual. Sheila explains this as feelings of respect for others, contributing to society, and striving to be a good person. Randy and Sheila, both raised on the East Coast, have little knowledge of their family heritage. Although at first Randy and Sheila thought it unlikely that they would ever marry, they decided to blend their family in a more formal way and just recently married.

Learning this background information through an assessment helps one know more about this family. Nurses who *think family* and use an ecological perspective can determine the factors and traits linked with the family household that have potential implications for the health or illness of the person. Things like culture, religion, ethnicity, and personal values all have implications for health and need to be assessed. One cannot fully understand the struggles multiple household members face by merely noting that this is a blended family. If a genogram and ecomap (described later in this chapter) are completed, even more could be understood about family risks and household needs. Family stories can also help nurses see individuals as whole people and identify nursing actions that can support care needs.

Assessment of Family Function

Most nursing assessments miss information about things like caregivers, family resources, social networks, and ways family work is accomplished. At minimum, the projected setting where the person will go after discharge is usually recorded and the caregiver for a dependent individual will be noted. The word *caregiver* often refers to a person caring for those seen as dependent but fails to consider caregiving when persons are more able or independent. In families, members give different forms of care to each other. For example, someone does the grocery shopping and food preparation; these tasks are linked with nutrition and diet and are relevant to many illnesses. That person would be the caregiver if dietary changes are needed. Although this person contributes to an individual's care, they are likely overlooked as a caregiver in the traditional sense.

Family functioning has to do with things like member tasks and roles. In well-functioning families, members' needs are met and the family unit promotes well-being for individuals. Nurses who *think family* know that all members may not function at optimal levels and some households fail to provide adequate support and resources for members. Although families share some needs, these needs are often prioritized and accomplished in distinct ways. Family members assume different roles for the work of caring and nurturing with or without the presence of illness (Meiers, Eggenberger, Krumwiede, Bliesmer, & Earle, 2009). Assessments provide bits of relevant information. For instance, nurses caring for a medically fragile newborn or a disabled veteran living in a rural community need to know about the family's abilities to provide needed care. Systematic assessment considers five functional roles:

1. Who organizes things in the family and makes certain needed supplies or resources are available for members?
2. How do family members communicate with one another in sharing family work, making decisions, or planning care and how do they maintain connections with primary health care providers?
3. What roles do members take in parenting, disciplining, and nurturing needed by various members?
4. Who are the financial "bread-winners" who assure things like an adequate salary, family income, and health benefits are available to meet members' needs?
5. Who are the family's social coordinators, who maintain connections between the family unit, social networks, and larger community to meet various forms of support needs?

When roles are optimally fulfilled, the family's caring work can be completed with maximized outcomes met and minimized stress or confusion (Box 5.5).

Functionally the Cox-Halverson family faces significant challenges. Sheila is the chief financial provider for the family. She contributes the major portion of the family income and is the financial manager who pays the bills and handles the money. She was recently promoted to a program coordinator at an adult foster home. This has been a financial benefit, but it means a greater time commitment, more responsibility, and additional stress. Randy and Sheila are supporting four children and two grandchildren, a difficult task for even the most financially stable couple. They live in a home that is not ideal, have regular transportation issues due to an unreliable vehicle, and have few prospects for improvement in the future.

Sheila is responsible for much of the family's health management. She arranges medical appointments for household members and usually accompanies them. She ensures that medications are taken as scheduled and prescription reorders are processed. It was under Sheila's urging that Randy was able to decide to have the hip surgeries done. Randy's

BOX 5-5

Implications of Family Functions

As you review the five functional roles in families, think about what you know about the Cox-Halverson family from the family type and family function session. Then answer these questions:

1. Who organizes what is needed in this family?
2. How effective is communication among members of this family and their health care providers?
3. Who plays what roles when it comes to parenting, discipline, and nurturing in this family?
4. Who are the "bread-winners" in this family and what conflicts do they have?
5. How well are members in this family connected to one another? Are they linked with other social networks? How effective are their connections to the larger community in obtaining the supports that are needed?
6. Given the risks and strengths identified through the family type and functional assessment data available, what one or two things would be a priority linked with Randy's care needs if you were a nurse talking with him during a physician visit?
7. Now based upon the family type and functional assessment data available, *think family* and identify two or three other things that the nurse might discuss with Randy that could be important for his family's wellness or illness prevention or management.
8. Using an ecological model to think about this family, what other questions do you have about the family's context (i.e., interacting factors linked with family, neighborhood, and larger social environments)? List three areas you might want to further assess.

disabilities limit his physical activities, but the surgery outcomes are enabling him to be more active with his family. He loves to cook, but does not embrace healthful cooking methods. This is a concern for Sheila as she battles with weight. Randy enjoys video games and plays with the older boys. Sheila has never had a little girl before and has enjoyed the experience of spending time with Bailey doing "girly" things. Although these parents love their children, they have many problems.

The family supported Randy as he took the necessary, yet somewhat frightening, steps to have the two hip surgeries. The family now has questions about how to move forward. Randy is an experienced mechanic. He doubts that he can physically return to that job and lacks skills to begin a career with less physical demands. He would love to make a substantial financial contribution to his family, but there are concerns about him returning to work before he is ready or to a position that is too physically demanding. Returning to work also means they will lose his Social Security benefits. They also face the dilemma that if he is unable to maintain employment because of physical disability, he might have difficulty regaining these benefits. This loss could put the family at significant financial risk.

Assessment of Family Processes

Family processes are the actions or activities members use as they interact and accomplish family tasks. Family processes include daily household activities, promote member health, parent children, instill rituals and routines, make transitions or accommodate changes, manage conflict, solve problems, make decisions, demonstrate affection, and satisfy individual needs (Walsh, 2003). A family managing a chronic illness such as Alzheimer's disease needs to identify goals, plan family work, and manage daily caregiving tasks. As the affected individual's cognition declines, the individual needs to find new ways of including the member in valued traditions. The Family Health Model (Denham, 2003) identified seven core processes that can be used to assess family's health and illness needs systematically and plan interventions: caregiving, cathexis, celebration, change, communication, connectedness, and coordination. These core functions are useful ways to work collaboratively with family units and are fully described in Chapter 14 of this text.

Think about the ways your family managed the last illness of one of your family members. What family processes came into play? How did your family members communicate needs? Were roles or communications different? Was decision making altered? How did your family negotiate and coordinate various tasks? Who invested the most emotional energy or physical energy in caring for the ill member? How did family members support change as healing occurred? How did your family celebrate the healing? Did the ill member facilitate or hinder usual family work? For instance, did a young child learn to comfort the parent? How was connectedness fostered? What steps were taken to coordinate efforts? The next time you complete an assessment, consider what usual family life is like for the family and the disarray potentially experienced with this member's condition.

When a member tries to change his or her lifestyle to self-manage a chronic condition or focus on wellness, others can support or sabotage behaviors. Perceived threats to the routine, possibly related to loss of control or power, can be emotional and cause feelings of grief, loss, anger, or frustration. Nurses who *think family* understand that perceived threats can have a dramatic effect on family members. Members do not always discuss their concerns in ways that create positive change. When members are cooperative, they will respect one another, provide support, and negotiate differences. However, not all people live in ideal families! Nurses who *think family* use their communication and assessment skills to learn what families need most.

When power is shared, communication is apt to be more direct, honest, and affirming. Families with shared power are more likely to be flexible, adaptable, willing to admit mistakes, and comfortable trying new things. But not all families are caring or deeply concerned for other members. Some are self-interested, inattentive to others' needs, and controlling. When family power is unbalanced, members might experience anxieties, depression, distrust, distress, or dissatisfaction. These concerns might not be identified if the assessment focuses only on physiological symptoms. Pause and reflect. How would you handle a situation when family members demonstrate power imbalances? What would you say? How might you facilitate the conversation so that the most powerful person begins to relate to the others from an equal or relational position (Knudson-Martin, 2013).

The Cox-Halversons have many challenges with their blended household and multiple members (Box 5.6). Those living in the household have changed over 2 years. Randy previously shared custody of the four children with Mandy, his ex-wife. She moved away after losing her job, giving Randy full custody of the four children. About a year ago, Mandy moved back into the area and now has custody of Brendan and Bailey and they visit the home every other weekend. Randy and Mandy try to be amicable and flexible with the visitation schedule. Sheila has full custody of Travis, her son who has never met his biological father. The father does not provide any financial support. Sheila and Mandy get along, but Mandy sometimes speaks negatively about Sheila to Brendan and Bailey. Despite what might seem like chaos, Randy, Sheila, the children, and the dogs manage their busy household with strengths that mostly complement one another.

Sheila and Randy make most decisions collaboratively, talk openly with one another about concerns, and can usually weigh options and come to decisions together. Children are sometimes included in conversations and are listened to when it is relevant. Several of the children have conflicts with one another. When Randy needed the hip replacement surgery, they needed to discuss how the children would be cared for during that time. They

> **BOX 5-6**
>
> **Implications of Family Processes**
>
> The Cox-Halverson family has a total of nine children for whom they share some responsibility. In turn, they have complications of others who are also involved somewhat with parenting tasks. The children, although connected in some ways to one another, also have connections to other extended family members that differ from one another. Although daily life may not always involve all of these people, at times the family does have to manage these social connections. Sometimes these connections are supportive, but at other times they are stressful.
>
> As a family nurse consider what you know about the Cox-Halverson family's type, functions, and process. Now think about the Randy's discharge home and his needs in the next 3 to 4 weeks as he recuperates after his surgery. As a nurse who *thinks family*, how might you answer the following questions?
>
> 1. What is the support that Randy will likely need at the time of his discharge?
> 2. Identify three or four particular accommodations that the family might need to make for Randy's homecoming.
> 3. List two or three problems the family nurse might anticipate in family care based on what is known from the assessment data that should be considered when doing discharge planning.
> 4. If you could ask three questions to gain more information you consider essential to satisfy these needs, what they would be?
> 5. Identify three social networks or community supports that would be useful to this family. Explain what they are and the usefulness of their inclusion.

considered delaying his surgery and making various arrangements for the children. In the end, they decided that it was best to just make the situation work. A similar problem-solving approach was used when Jess and Amanda needed to move into the home within a month of each other. Ten people were living under one roof and Randy was still actively recovering from his surgeries; it was a stressful time. Randy's extended family provided emotional support and his mother, stepfather, and brother were available to help occasionally when needed. Sheila's mother lives out of state and is neither supportive nor reliable; no other extended family are available. Amanda just became employed by the same company where Sheila works and is at the top of the waiting list for subsidized housing. She recently passed her driving test. Amanda is still in contact with Autumn's father, Aaron, who is 17 years old and still in high school. She is looking forward to moving in with him and her children and being more self-sufficient. Randy and Sheila have mixed feelings about her moving and are concerned about her parenting abilities and immaturity. They anticipate continuing to help her after she moves.

Nurses can use assessments to identify steps for Randy and Sheila to improve their member and family health. For example, the family would benefit if Sheila quit smoking. Second-hand smoke exposure is bad for the children's health; it increases risks for asthma, upper respiratory infections, and ear infections. In households where parents smoke, risks for children smoking increase. Cigarettes are expensive and the family could also benefit from the financial savings. Several family members have emotional and behavioral concerns. Some counseling or behavioral training could assist children and parents, but resources to pay for such help and accessibility to services are limited. Randy could benefit from a referral to a vocational rehabilitation program as it is often most effective to keep persons with rheumatoid arthritis active and the family is likely to benefit from his being more fully employed.

Moving From Family to Community Assessment

Nurses who *think family* acknowledge that the true primary care environment for individuals is the family household and the community where the family lives. Nurses who realize their role is to increase the family's capacity to support individual members think differently about the consequences and adequacy of community supports. Nurses who *think family* recognize their central role is to prepare those receiving care to self-manage their conditions to their fullest capacity independently. An ecological perspective incorporates different nursing actions than those derived through the more narrow thinking of the medical model. It means nurses assess the household environments, neighborhoods, and communities where families live in relation to risks, threats, benefits, and supports aligned with health or illness concerns.

Most nurses have had some exposure to community health or public health nursing and may have experience in community assessment using a technique known as a windshield survey, when a nurse may assess risks, supports, and other barriers to well-being or health that might be present in the neighborhood or larger community by driving, walking, or riding public transportation within the neighborhood. However, nurses who *think family* can also use a family ecomap to identify community threats or supports; these are described later in this chapter. This tool can be used to anticipate concerns and resources needed in a care transition.

Household Location in Community

Just as individuals and families are unique, so are communities. Understanding the risks and benefits of a particular household or community is similar to thinking about an individual. For instance, it is useful to know whether an elderly woman in an ethnic community is willing to assist a new single parenting mother. A single parent may need the support of a community of people if she is from a culture outside the mainstream. Although it is impossible for nurses to learn everything about multiple persons met during a day's work, learning to elicit and hear stories about family households and community neighborhoods provides information for care.

Nurses who *think family* conduct assessments that identify individual connections with family and the community. The Family Health Model suggests family-focused care is aligned with ways individuals are situated within households nested in neighborhoods, communities, and the larger society (Denham, 2003). This perspective encourages questions about what needs to be known about where people live, work, learn, play, and pray. Persons are usually seen in a health care setting outside their home environment, so some important environmental influences are overlooked. The following are three scenarios faced by home care nurses conducting the initial posthospital discharge visit; none of this information was noted on the original referral for care:

1. Trash piled high and cluttering the entire living room from groceries consumed by an obese caregiver living on a couch while the elderly gentleman needing nursing care was confined to a bed in the same room
2. A blind elderly man with type 2 diabetes and open sores requiring treatment and daily dressing changes living alone in a home without running water
3. A semiparalyzed 27-year-old wheelchair-bound woman living alone with her pet in a house littered with dog urine and excrement from when the dog could not get outside

These findings were not expected and in each case they called for immediate problem-solving actions by the home care nurse at the clinical visit. When nurses *think family*, the assessment includes information linked with household and community.

Coordinated family care relies upon collection of information that provides an accurate picture of the actual living conditions. Dr. Duhamel and many others are working in

Canada and other nations to advance family-focused nursing care (Box 5.7). Assessing household information including neighborhood safety, access to necessary resources, availability of transportation, and distances to medical care provides a baseline for determining appropriate nursing actions. An ecological model encourages the family nurse to learn if the family household poses risks or offers supports for individuals and family units (Fig. 5.2). Remember, families are greatly influenced by the ways their lives connect with pets, friends, social networks, and many other things in the community where they live.

Family Links With Community

Assessing community factors that predict and protect individual and family health requires innovative thinking about how families are linked within communities and openness to new models of care and technologies. Dr. Janice Bell has global recognition for her work with families and has inspired many to look at nursing differently (Box 5.8). Suppose a family wants to vacation at a mountain retreat where they have gone for years, but they are concerned that the mother's compromised mobility from multiple sclerosis will make it impossible. The nurse might help the family explore solutions for the transportation problems such as renting a motorized wheelchair from a durable equipment company or facts about a van with a platform lift for raising and lowering a wheelchair because she knows the valued shared time together and memory-making for the family are important. Comprehensive assessment not only examines physiological, psychosocial, and emotional needs, but also identifies whether resources are available or threats need to be addressed.

Interrelationships of larger community factors predict individual and population health (U.S. Department of Health and Human Services, 2010), and family health is often tied to the economic and environmental factors of the family's community. We need a community-based framework to help identify ways to decrease health disparities and promote healthy lifestyles from a family perspective. Two such frameworks are Healthy People 2020 and the one used by the Red Cross Nurse (RCN) in a disaster.

BOX 5-7

Family Tree

Fabie Duhamel, PhD (Canada)

Dr. Fabie Duhamel, PhD, is a professor at the Faculty of Nursing in the University of Montreal, Quebec, Canada. She received her doctorate from the University of Calgary, Ontario, Canada. In 2010 Dr. Duhamel and colleagues founded the Center for Excellence in Family Nursing, a partnership between the Faculty of Nursing and several Montreal health institutions. The center's mission is to promote and sustain advancement of the family systems nursing knowledge through education, research, and clinical practice for graduate nurses. The center provides a unique opportunity for exchanging knowledge among practitioners, researchers, and academicians.

Dr. Duhamel's scholarship demonstrates a commitment to research focused on family interventions and the implementation of family systems nursing in practice. Her research activities focus on family systems nursing, chronic illness, and knowledge exchange. Dr. Duhamel has numerous family nursing publications in English and French. She has developed a tool, called the Family Genograph, to assist nurses in using genograms and ecomaps in family assessment.

Dr. Duhamel has received funding from the Canadian Institutes of Health Research to bring together family systems nursing colleagues from six countries (Canada, Iceland, Japan, Sweden, Thailand, United States) to create an international collaborative effort focused on knowledge transfer of family nursing to practice settings. She is a member of the International Family Nursing Association and is currently serving on the Board of Directors.

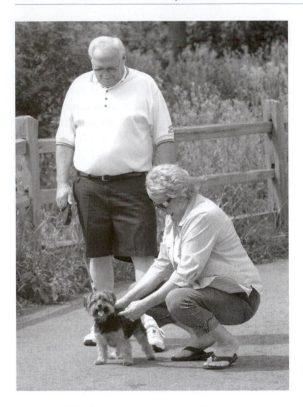

FIGURE 5-2 Ecological model encourages the nurse to assess the family environment.

BOX 5-8

Family Tree

Janice Bell, PhD (Canada)

Janice M. Bell, PhD, is a nurse educator and registered psychologist who has focused her career on building capacity in nurses and others to care for families with competence, confidence, and compassion. Dr. Bell provides global leadership in family health with a focus on family system nursing. Dr. Bell served as a member of the faculty team of the Family Nursing Unit, University of Calgary (1986–2002), and as the Director of the Family Nursing Unit, University of Calgary (2002–2007). This unique faculty practice unit was built upon an innovative educational model that provided extensive opportunities for faculty and student scholarship.

Dr. Bell and her Canadian colleagues have taught the Calgary Family Assessment and Intervention Model to thousands of practicing health care professionals, graduate students, and academics in Canada, United States, Japan, Thailand, Hong Kong, Singapore, Iceland, Finland, Sweden, Switzerland, Brazil, Portugal, and Poland. Dr. Bell has focused on Family Systems Nursing as a way to guide nursing practice through which nurses form relationships with persons and enter into therapeutic conversations with families. She co-developed the Illness Beliefs Model and focuses her scholarship on illness suffering, family healing, therapeutic conversations, family interventions in health care, and research. Dr. Bell is widely published and greatly respected throughout the world for her work with family nursing.

Dr. Bell is the founding editor of the *Journal of Family Nursing*. This journal, first published in 1995, is now a leading reference for work linked with extending understandings of the family experience during health and illness and improving care to families. Dr. Bell was instrumental in the planning and hosting of seven international family nursing conferences (1988–2009). She is a founding member of the International Family Nursing Association and is on the Board of Directors.

Dr. Bell is highly respected and internationally known for her commitment to discovering and translating knowledge that informs practice. She currently offers workshops and consultation about practice knowledge with families to an international community of nurses and other health care professionals.

Healthy People 2020 identifies 26 Leading Health Indicators (LHIs) organized into 12 topical areas. They include access to health care; clinical preventive services; environmental quality; injury and violence; maternal, infant, and child health; mental health; nutrition, physical activity, and obesity; oral health; reproductive and sexual health; social determinants; substance abuse; and tobacco use. The LHIs are guides for national health assessments and interventions; they provide guidelines and benchmarks to measure progress or outcomes. LHIs extend across the life span to address social and physical environments, multisector policies, individual behaviors, health services, and biological or genetic factors that influence the ability of individuals and communities to be healthy. The LHIs apply to health at the individual, family, and community levels and provide focus for assessment when the family enters a disaster shelter.

In disaster nursing, the RCN uses an initial intake and assessment form to collect data about families that include immediate and long-term shelter needs, mental health concerns, and planning for the future. Family members who require assessment beyond the immediate concerns about nutrition and shelter are seen by the shelter RCN for a more in-depth assessment. The Red Cross Shelter intake process connects shelter clients with their broader families through local and nationalized disaster disposition databases. When the intake assessment is completed, the result is a conclusion about what the family will continue to need for the duration of the shelter stay and upon reentry into the community of origin. A similar assessment could offer systematic ways to collect a breadth of information for care management relevant to a usual community where families live even when disaster is not at hand.

A Family Health Record

A family health record could go a long way to ensure continuity of care once the individual moves out of the health care setting and back into the home. A multitude of issues can negatively influence outcomes if not addressed. For example, if the person needs to see a medical specialist for a referral, is transportation available after he is at home? Do special arrangements need to be made? Is there someone to transport the person if he can't do this independently? Does the family believe follow-up care is important and will they see that it occurs? Does the person have a smartphone and is he willing to receive reminders about care management? Is the family willing to spend their money on resources for this visit (e.g., gasoline costs, meals out, co-pays for a medical visit)? In the past, this type of follow-up belonged to social workers. However, nurses who *think family* can intentionally discuss these relevant family issues to help streamline care from an acute setting or primary care to home and community, possibly preventing hospital readmissions because the families are prepared for self- or family-management. Box 5.9 suggests that family research occurring in Finland needs to expand and faculty in schools of nursing are helping students learn about ways to include families in nursing care.

Thinking family provides ways to view the interdependent care needs of multiple family members simultaneously. For instance, a single family health record could note several things:

- The decline in musculoskeletal function of one of its members
- Family responses to falls related to a hypoglycemic incident in that member
- Physical therapist notes about member's declining abilities to navigate uneven surfaces
- Family's response to these events
- Abilities hindered because of barriers and lack of resources in the community

Electronic medical records may or may not be the answer, as they remain largely untested. But some form of an ongoing plan for some chronic conditions that identifies goals, strategies, supports, and outcomes linked with family unit needs and individual

---

BOX 5-9

Evidence-Based Family Nursing

Family Nursing Interventions in Finland: Benefits for Families

Nursing interventions are actions taken to support and help individuals and families promote personal health, care for self and each other, and die gracefully. The researchers in Finland have determined more research about effective nursing actions is needed in Finland. Family nursing aims to strengthen family resources and resolve problems in all stages of life, and many families are open to these ideas. However, in the Finnish culture, adult persons tend to be viewed as unique individuals living within a family rather than as members of families. When illness occurs, family members show concern and often need support themselves. Interventions that have been shown to be useful for Finnish families include meeting with and obtaining supportive care from nurses. However, family members are not well incorporated into assisting with care for their ill family member. Work in research and practice is only beginning in this nation and much still needs to be studied and better understood. Dr. Paivi Åstedt-Kurki and her colleagues at the University of Tampere, Finland, are leading the way in developing family nursing curricula at the graduate level that assist nurses in incorporating the family in care for the individual ill family member.

Source: Åstedt-Kurki, P., & Kaunonen, M. (2011). Family nursing interventions in Finland: Benefits for families. In E. K. Svavarsdottir & H. Jonsdottir (Eds.), *Family nursing in action* (pp 115–129). Reykjavik, Iceland: University of Iceland Press.

---

conditions could be instrumental in improving outcomes. Emerging models must include family unit and household information if coordinated care linked with individual and family health is ever to be fully achieved (Calman, Hauser, Lurio, Wu, & Pichardo, 2012).

Tools to Guide Assessment

Many types of survey tools are available that could be used to guide assessments and collect pertinent data about families units, individuals within families, and families within communities. Some of these tools include genograms (McGoldrick, Gerson, & Shellenberger, 1999) and ecomaps (Hartman, 1995). In addition, geographical information systems (GIS) capture, store, analyze, and display referenced information about specific environmental concerns that are geographically and ecologically pertinent to families (Choi, Afzal, & Sattler, 2006). GIS can be used to identify health risks based upon geographical locations. Tying GIS with social determinants of health, demographic information, and epidemiological data could provide new ways to consider risks for family units. Personal and family health records that take genetics, genomics, and social determinants into account are other tools for assessment.

Using a Family Genogram

A genogram is a visual representation of the family's membership and health history. A genogram is an effective way to represent visually multiple generations, areas of support, and other information for decision making. Genograms enhance nursing family assessment (McGoldrick & Gerson, 1985). They can be constructed to reveal facts about many different elements. For instance, family type(s), roles, relationships between the family members, demographics, age, developmental level, gender, number of members, employment status, immediate health problems of individual family members, trends of health problems, and genetic illnesses of the family over time can all be depicted. Genograms efficiently organize a breadth of family information to present a useful family picture visually.

Detailed illness information can be added to the genogram to create a family pedigree depicting transmission of such features as genetic conditions, familial conditions, and psychosocial patterns, such as chemical dependency and suicide. A family pedigree refers to family groups or line of ancestors; this is useful to identify the passing of genetic traits or conditions. A genogram can be useful for early diagnosis, identification of risk factors for particular conditions, and suggestions for prevention. The genogram is arranged by generation, with three generations considered a minimum data set (Kaakinen, Gedaly-Duff, Coehlo, & Hanson, 2010). Figure 5.3 provides some information about the various symbols that can be used to create a family genogram. It is also possible to show the strength of relationships on a genogram (Fig. 5.4). Think back to the Cox-Halverson family; the complicated blended family membership can be clarified with a genogram (Fig. 5.5). Nurses can construct a genogram by eliciting health and demographic information about the individual and family (first, second, and third generations).

Using a Family Ecomap

An ecomap is a different structural form that can be used to visualize the various activities and relationships of the family with the larger ecological environment. To draw the ecomap, the genogram is first placed in the center and then the connections among persons within the family and the entities outside the family are drawn. Entities are drawn as circles surrounding the family genogram. Examples of surrounding environment

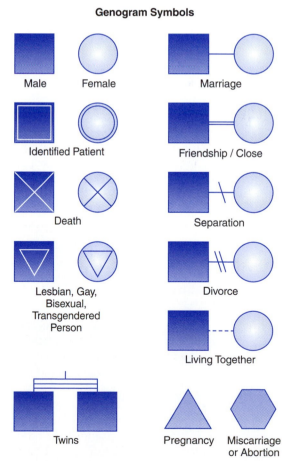

Genogram Symbols

Male   Female   Marriage

Identified Patient   Friendship / Close

Death   Separation

Lesbian, Gay, Bisexual, Transgendered Person   Divorce

Living Together

Twins   Pregnancy   Miscarriage or Abortion

FIGURE 5-3 Genogram symbols.

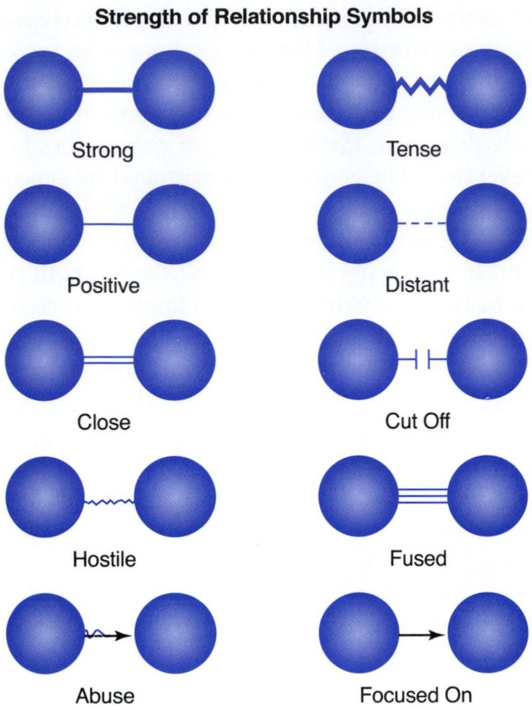

Strength of Relationship Symbols

Strong

Tense

Positive

Distant

Close

Cut Off

Hostile

Fused

Abuse

Focused On

FIGURE 5-4 Strength of relationship symbols.

Cox-Halverson Genogram

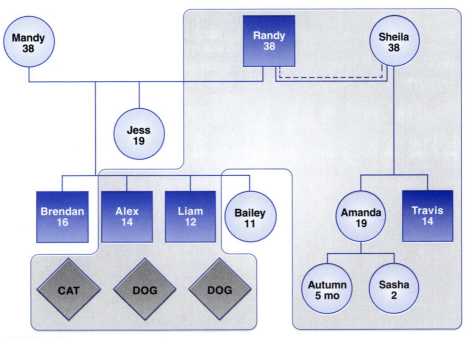

FIGURE 5-5 Cox-Halverson genogram.

entities are extended family, school, work, health care institutions, social services, recreation, and friends (Wright & Leahy, 2009). Recall the Cox-Halverson family and consider the multiple interactions members might have with their larger community and related systems (Fig. 5.6). Even more complexity can be added to the ecomap by making specific connections between each genogram member and persons or entities in the larger environment.

Geographical Information Systems

Geographical information system (GIS) databases are powerful epidemiological tools that can be used to highlight geospatial patterns of concern that occur in residential living environments (Bloch, 2012). The GIS is a way for health professionals to use electronic means and expand the traditional windshield survey. This type of assessment shows the interconnected nature of individuals and community health (Berkman & Glass, 2000). Understanding the distribution or lack of physical program resources within communities assists nurses

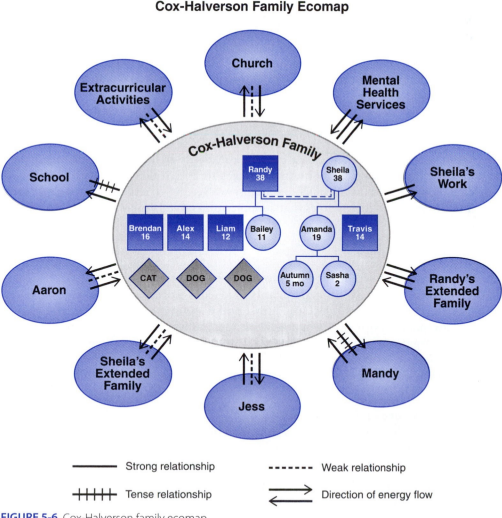

FIGURE 5-6 Cox-Halverson family ecomap.

to plan community-located nursing actions with implications for and potential to change health or lifestyle behaviors.

GIS software can be used to identify social determinants of health locally, regionally, and nationally. For instance, geographical locations of spatial attributes can be entered into a map of the area. Each map point has a latitude and longitude identity, similar to Google maps or any type of global positioning system (GPS). Additional data might be added for analysis, such as race, immigration status, and primary care clinics. Nurses can search the map based on different attributes to look for patterns of concern, track improvement or decline in health disparities, or illustrate family or community resources available that may help with health promotion, disease prevention, or management of illness. GIS also gives information about physical, program, and potential social capital resources available to persons or families in the geographical area.

Geographical distribution of morbidity and mortality patterns can be geospatially analyzed by policy makers and health care systems to determine service needs of a region, state, or country. GIS databases can be used to examine trends in health behaviors and lifestyle that can identify community assets that support health, such as healthy diet and physical activity (Gebel, Bauman, Sugiyama, & Owens, 2011). Public health nurses have used epidemiological statistics and methods for decades to plan population-level interventions and are now using GIS databases to design these interventions (Caley, 2004). Community partnerships have created Web sites that can be used to fine-tune action plans that support healthy communities. An example of an interactive map to support healthy living has been designed by Healthy Living Rochester. Their Web site map can be accessed to identify community resources that can help support a family that wants to become more physically active.

Nurses who use GIS databases as part of routine community assessments can attend to many factors that support or deter healthy behaviors for individuals and families. Many of the GIS databases and map systems contain tutorials or learning modules so that those using the sites can readily access data useful for evidence-based decision making. Nurses can work with community persons and agencies to design GIS databases that support health and contribute to family and community well-being. These can be used to assume active and futuristic advocacy roles that support vulnerable families.

Genetic Assessments

Genetics is the study of the transmission of inherited traits from one generation to another among similar or related organisms. Genes are used to transport traits or characteristics through family descendants, and genetics is concerned with the traits passed from one ancestor to the next generation. Genomics is the study of all genes of a particular organism; the human genome is made up of approximately 35,000 genes (Cutting, 2005). Genomics includes the ways genes interact within persons and with their environment. Nurses need to be concerned about four areas of genomics (Scanlon & Fibison, 1995):

- Basic knowledge of genetic terms
- Ability to understand genetic terms such as chromosomal variations
- Ability to explain genetic inheritance
- Ability to apply knowledge of genetics and genomics in nursing practice

Nurses' roles in the genomic era include individual and family genetic counseling, clinical care, health education, policy development and analysis, advocacy, and research (Table 5.3).

TABLE 5-3	*Societal Concerns Linked With Genetics*
SOCIETAL CONCERNS	**QUESTIONS RAISED**
Fairness in the use of genetic information	Who should have access to personal genetic information? How will it be used?
Privacy and confidentiality	Who owns and controls genetic information?
Psychological impact and stigmatization	How does personal genetic information affect an individual and society's perceptions of that individual? How does genomic information affect members of minority communities?
Reproductive issues	Do health care personnel properly counsel parents about the risks and limitations of genetic technology? How reliable and useful is fetal genetic testing? What are the larger societal issues raised by new reproductive technologies?
Clinical issues	How will genetic tests be evaluated and regulated for accuracy, reliability, and utility? How do educators prepare health care professionals for the new genetics? How do nurses prepare the public to make informed choices? How does a society balance current scientific limitations and social risk with long-term benefits?
Uncertainties	Should testing be performed when no treatment is available? Should parents have the right to have their minor children tested for adult-onset diseases? Are genetic tests reliable and interpretable by the medical community?
Conceptual and philosophical implications	Do people's genes make them behave in a particular way? Can people always control their behavior? What is considered acceptable diversity? Where is the line between medical treatment and enhancement?
Health and environmental issues	Are genetically modified foods and other products safe for humans and the environment? How will these technologies affect developing nations' dependence on the West?
Commercialization of products	Who owns genes and other pieces of DNA? Will patenting DNA sequences limit their accessibility and development into useful products?

* Adapted from U.S. Department of Energy Human Genome Project. Ethical, legal, and social issues. (2011). Retrieved from http://www.ornl.gov/sci/techresources/Human_Genome/elsi/elsi.shtml

Genomic influences and risk factors are important to the health of individuals, families, and communities. In 1996, the National Coalition of Health Professionals Education in Genetics (NCHPEG) was formed to develop core competencies related to genetics for all health care professionals (National Human Genome Research Institute, 2012). An important basic element in genetic competency is the ability to draft a three-generation genetic history for an individual and family (American Medical Association, 2012). Such a genetic history can reveal health risks that deserve attention and tracking to enhance preventive care. For example, the death of a biological first-degree relative at a young age from a heart attack indicates potential risk for other family members. In this instance, identification of high blood pressure in another family member at a young age would be a concern. Many leading causes of death have genetic aspects including heart disease, cancer, cerebrovascular diseases, chronic lower respiratory diseases, diabetes, pneumonia, Alzheimer's disease, and kidney disease. Knowledge about genetic predispositions can be useful in assisting persons to understand family risks and make informed lifestyle choices.

Genetic Linkages

Genetic linkages considered during family-focused assessments can identify many diseases. Family members are often unaware of conditions their ancestors have experienced and are not able to track patterns of disease transmission. Nurses who *think family* assess for incidences of all diseases and disorders known to have been diagnosed in the family, speak to the family about their health history, assist them to reduce risks, obtain health information, and speak with their doctors about high-risk concerns (Kaphingst et al., 2012).

It is important to include the age at onset of the diseases and disorders. For instance, family clusters of breast, ovarian, colon, and endometrial cancer might indicate possible hereditary cancer syndromes. Medical disorders such as heart disease before age 40 to 50, dementia before age 60, hearing loss before age 50 to 60, venous thromboembolism before age 50, three or more pregnancy losses, several family members with the same condition, or multisystem and bilateral occurrences may indicate genetic disorders (Goolsby & Grubbs, 2011).

A report by the Consensus Panel (2009) has noted that nurses need to be able to incorporate genetic and genomic information into practice and be aware of personal attitudes, beliefs and values. They need to be aware of many things including those such as:

- The genetic and genomic basis of health or illness linked with care needs.
- Ways to obtain a three generation family health history.
- Newborns at risk for morbidity or mortality resulting from genetic metabolism errors.
- Couples at risk for having a child with a genetic disorder.
- Persons with questions about genetics and genomics.
- Persons at risk based on assessment data that might benefit from more information or a referral.

Genetic Patterns

Genetic patterns of inheritance are important not only for individuals and families, but also communities. Some autosomal recessive disorders are more commonly seen among certain racial/ethnic groups. Examples include Tay-Sachs disease in Ashkenazi Jews, cystic fibrosis and hemochromatosis in Caucasians, sickle cell anemia in black Americans, and beta-thalassemia in persons of Mediterranean origin, such as Greeks and Italians (Vallance & Ford, 2003). Amish people also exhibit some rare diseases (e.g., Troyer syndrome, Amish lethal microcephaly) unique to their community due to small founding groups and generations of close marriages. Most Amish people can trace their roots back to a few hundred German-Swiss settlers who came to the United States in the 18th century. It is important for closely related communities to know their genetic histories. It is possible for both parents to be carriers of a genetic disorder without any outward expression of the autosomal recessive disease. If one parent is a carrier, there is a 25% chance of the child having the condition. If both parents are carriers, there is a 50% chance of the child having the condition. In such cases, genetic counseling is helpful for expectant parents or those contemplating pregnancy to determine the risks of having affected children. Family nurses are attuned to these genetic risks and spend time doing assessments, health counseling, and education relevant to unique risks.

Spiritual and Religious Assessments

Spirituality is not a topic always closely associated with health, illness, or health care in the United States as it is sometimes thought to be unscientific because of the lack of evidence needed to validate it for use in modern health care practices (Chidarikire, 2012; Swinton & Pattison, 2010). However, spirituality and religion are topics that often arise, especially in palliative care, hospice, and at the end of life. Some people use faith and beliefs as a coping resource and these beliefs often originate from and are informed by family culture and traditions. Many who do not ascribe to any formal religious tradition may practice a form of spirituality that deepens meaningful connection with and beyond the self. Consider the Cox-Halverson family. They identified with spirituality more than religious practices and had personal ways to define the experience. Spirituality can be described as a search for purpose and meaning in life, whereas religion is the formal framework used by many to channel the spiritual journey (Power, 2006).

Nurses are sometimes unsure about how to approach assessment of religion, faith, or spirituality (Cook, 2012). Nurses who do assess spiritual care beliefs and listen to illness stories and personal concerns do this with no great predictability (Mamier, 2011). Nurses most likely to engage in spiritual care practices are those who perceive spiritual issues occur frequently in the setting, are spiritual themselves, do not work in pediatrics, and have received education about spiritual care (Mamier, 2011).

Evidence abounds that spiritual beliefs, practices, and experiences are relevant to nursing practice. A systematic review of the literature found spiritual outcome measures and 85 tools that are used in research about spirituality (Selman, Harding, Gysels, Speck, & Higginson, 2011). Spiritual well-being can be assessed with questions that are not specifically related to religion (Table 5.4). Areas to cover in a spiritual assessment include views of a higher power, sources of strength and hope, and religious practices (Carson, 1989). Within a single family, the nurse is likely to find differences of opinion, beliefs, and practices. If appropriate, discussion with the individual seeking care or other family members can provide additional information. Family beliefs and values about spiritual and religious practices can be elicited through a therapeutic family interview (see Chapter 4). Preferences for a clergy visit, orientation to places that can be used for prayer and meditation, or the placement of religious items at the bedside can offer clues about individual practices.

Social Capital Assessment

The completion of a family ecomap can help you gain an understanding about family links to others and with the surrounding community. These links can be both positive or negative influences on the family unit and its members. Social capital is the term given to the positive, health-promoting resources that provide beneficial supports to persons and families; it refers to human networks, social norms, and relationships that create mutual benefits (Carpiano & Hystad, 2011). Social capital viewed from a neighborhood perspective is an accessible network of community resources that potentially facilitate well-being and health. Social capital includes the actual or potential material, informational, and affective resources that persons and families have access to within family and friendship networks. Social capital is typically a benefit to individuals, families, and communities and positively affects health. However, loosely established neighborhood relationships can negatively

TABLE 5-4	*Things to Consider in a Spiritual Assessment*				
SPIRITUAL IDEAS TO ASSESS	**NOT AT ALL**	**A LITTLE**	**SOMEWHAT**	**QUITE A BIT**	**VERY MUCH**
I feel peaceful.					
I have a reason for living.					
My life has been productive.					
I have trouble feeling peace of mind.					
I feel a sense of purpose in my life.					
I am able to reach down deep in myself for comfort.					
I feel a sense of harmony within myself.					
My life lacks meaning and purpose.					
I find comfort in my faith and spiritual beliefs.					
I find strength in my faith or spiritual beliefs.					
My illness has strengthened my faith or spiritual beliefs.					
I know that whatever happens with my illness, things will be okay.					

Source: Bradle, J. M., Salsman, J. M., Debb, S. M., Arnold, B. J., & Cella, D. (2011). Spiritual well-being as a component of health-related quality of life: The Functional Assessment of Chronic Illness Therapy-Spiritual Well-Being Scale (FACIT-Sp). *Religions, 2,* 77–94.

influence attitudes, constrain opportunities, and create actions that are detrimental to individual and family health and safety (Carpiano, 2008).

Social capital includes supports and abilities to access needed resources, receive information, and maintain social order (Carpiano, 2008). When the terms *social capital* and *social support* are compared, common ideas such as social networks, social engagement, sense of belonging, and reciprocity are identified (Kritsotakis & Gamarnikow, 2004). For example, a study of female primary caregivers of children demonstrated that women with social support from their neighbors have less parenting strain and master the parenting role (Carpiano & Kimbro, 2012). Conversely, youth gangs provide social support and social cohesion, but have negative effects because such social capital also promotes a culture of violence. Having people in one's life willing to do favors increases mental health for urban and rural dwellers (Carpiano & Hystad, 2011). Persons with wide social networks might possess more social capital to manage immediate challenges related to health and illness. Nurses who *think family* assess social capital to identify availability of supports and gaps to fill.

In 2001, Robert Putnam published a highly acclaimed book titled *Bowling Alone*. In his book, he described how more people are taking up bowling as a form of recreation, but they are doing it alone as opposed to joining organized leagues. He described the ways contemporary middle-class Americans have focused on work, material consumption, and leisure with less interest in civic engagement or collective activities than in the past. Over the past few decades, there has been less engagement in things like social organizations, church attendance, family dinners, having friends over, and voting. Decreased social connectedness may limit opportunities to build social capital and negatively influence private and public lives. Persons with high neighborhood social participation, more favorable neighborhood perceptions, and high general trust and those who live in lower income households are more likely to have strong core neighborhood ties (Moore et al., 2011). Researchers of a large international study on social capital in 50 countries discovered that higher levels of education were directly related to health and life satisfaction and that these people were less dependent on social capital (Elgar et al., 2011). More educated persons are likely to have spatial ties that reach beyond the local area. Those with higher incomes are inclined to have greater access to resources outside their neighborhood and fewer ties to their neighborhood. However, this can be detrimental if instrumental support is needed for caregiving. Wealthier more educated persons will likely hire help. But those with greater social capital may have family and volunteer resources available.

Chapter Summary

Nurses who *think family* always consider the family unit strengths and threats as they do an assessment. Although a number of components of a family assessment have been presented, perhaps no single model or framework is all-inclusive or the only correct one. This chapter has reviewed differences among individual, family, and community assessments. Predictive and protective factors such as family type, family function, and family processes that influence health of individuals, families, and communities are described. Genograms, ecomaps, and other tools can be used to describe the structure of families and the connections between members and larger communities. GIS are introduced as resources for community assessment. Ideas about genetics and genomics, spiritual assessment, and social capital are also identified as factors to consider in the assessment process. Some challenges in communicating and documenting family-focused assessments are discussed. More exploration and further development and refinement around the best ways to document family-related assessment data and better ways to tie to the community are still needed.

REFERENCES

American Medical Association. (2012). Family medical history. Retrieved from http://www.ama-assn .org/ama/pub/physician-resources/medical-science/genetics- molecular-medicine/family-history.page

American Nurses Association. (2012). The nursing process. Retrieved from http://nursingworld.org/ EspeciallyForYou/StudentNurses/Thenursingprocess.aspx

Åstedt-Kurki, P., & Kaunonen, M. (2011). Family nursing interventions in Finland: Benefits for families. In E. K. Svavarsdottir & H. Jonsdottir (Eds.), *Family nursing in action* (pp. 115–129). Reykjavik, Iceland: University of Iceland Press.

Bell, J. M. (2003). Clinical scholarship in family nursing. *Journal of Family Nursing, 9*(2),127–129.

Berkman, L., & Glass, T. (2000). Social integration, social networks, social support and health. In L. Berkman & I. Kawachi (Eds.), *Social epidemiology*. London: Oxford.

Bloch, J. R. (2012). Using geographic information systems to explore disparities in preterm birth rates among foreign-born and U.S.-born black mothers. *Journal of Obstetric Gynecologic and Neonatal Nursing, 40*, 544–554. doi:10.111/j1552-6909.2011.01273.x

Bradle, J. M., Salsman, J. M., Debb, S. M., Arnold, B. J., & Cella, D. (2011). Spiritual well-being as a component of health-related quality of life: The Functional Assessment of Chronic Illness Therapy-Spiritual Well-Being Scale (FACIT-Sp). *Religions, 2*, 77–94.

Bronfenbrenner, U. (1979). *The ecology of human development: Experiments by nature and design.* Cambridge, MA: Harvard University Press.

Bronfenbrenner, U. (1997). Ecology of the family as a context for human development: Research perspectives. In J. L. Paul, M. Churton, H. Rosselli-Kostoryz, W. C. Morse, K. Marfo, C. Lavely, & D. Thomas (Eds.), *Foundations of special education* (pp. 49–83). Pacific Grove, CA: Brooks/Cole.

Caley, L. M. (2004). Using geographic information systems to design population-based interventions. *Public Health Nursing, 21*(6), 547–554.

Calman, N., Hauser, D., Lurio, J., Wu, W. Y., & Pichardo, M. (2012). Strengthening public health and primary care collaboration through electronic health records. *American Journal of Public Health, 102*, e13–e 18. doi:10.2105/AJPH.2012.301000

Carpiano, R. M. (2008). Actual or potential neighborhood resources and access to them: Testing hypotheses of social capital for the health of female caregivers. *Social Science and Medicine, 67*(4), 568–582.

Carpiano, R. M., & Hystad, P. W. (2011). "Sense of community belonging" in health surveys: What social capital is it measuring? *Health and Place, 17*, 606–617.

Carpiano, R. M., & Kimbro, R. T. (2012). Neighborhood social capital, parenting strain, and personal mastery among female primary caregivers of children. *Journal of Health and Social Behavior, 53*(2), 232–247.

Carson, V. B. (1989). *Spiritual dimensions of nursing practice.* Philadelphia: W. B. Saunders.

Chidarikire, S. (2012). Spirituality: The neglected dimension of holistic mental health care. *Advances in Mental Health, 10*(3), 298–302.

Choi, M., Afzal, B., & Sattler, B. (2006). Geographic information systems: A new tool for environmental health assessments. *Public Health Nursing, 23*(5), 381–391.

Consensus Panel. (2009). Essentials of genetic and genomic nursing: Competencies, curricula guidelines, and outcome indicators (2nd ed.). Silver Springs, MD: American Nurses Association. ISBN-13: 978-1-55810-263-7

Cook, C. (2012). Pathway to accommodate individuals' spiritual needs. *Nursing Management 19*(2), 33–37.

Cutting, G. R. (2005). Modifier genetics: Cystic fibrosis. *Annual Review of Genomics and Human Genetics, 6*, 237–260. doi:10.1146/annurev.genom.6080604.162254

Denham, S. A. (2003). *Family health: A framework for nursing.* Philadelphia: F. A. Davis.

Denham, S. A., Manoogian, M., & Schuster, L. (2007). Managing family support and dietary routines: Type 2 diabetes in rural Appalachian families. *Families, Systems, & Health, 25*(1), 36–52.

Elgar, F. J., Davis, C. G., Wohl, M. J., Trites, S. J., Zelenski, J. M., & Martin, M. S. (2011). Social capital, health and life satisfaction in 50 countries. *Health and Place, 17*, 1044–1053.

Fehl, W. M. (2012). Cox-Halverson family assessment data. Unpublished raw data.

Gebel, K., Bauman, A. E., Sugiyama, T., & Owen, N. (2011). Mismatch between perceived and objectively assessed neighborhood walkability attributes: Prospective relationships with walking and weight gain. *Health & Place, 17*, 519–524. doi:10.1016/j.healthplace.2010.12.008

Goolsby, M. J., & Grubbs, L. (2011). *Advanced assessment: Interpreting findings and formulating differential diagnoses.* Philadelphia: F. A. Davis.

Grant, J. M., Mottet, L. A., & Tanis, J. (2011). Injustice at every turn: A report of the national transgender discrimination survey. Executive summary. Washington, DC: National Center for Transgender Equality. Retrieved from http://www.thetaskforce.org/downloads/reports/reports/ntds_summary.pdf

Haggman-Laitila, A., Tanninen, H. M., & Pietila, A. M. (2010). Effectiveness of resource-enhancing family-oriented intervention. *Journal of Clinical Nursing, 19*, 2500–2510. doi:10.1111/j.1365-2702.2010.03288.x

Hartman, A. (1995). Diagrammatic assessment of family relationships. *Families in Society, 76*, 111–122.

Jensen, S. (2011). *Nursing health assessment: A best practice approach.* Philadelphia: Wolters Kluwer Health/Lippincott Williams & Wilkins.

Kaakinen, J. R., Gedaly-Duff, V., Coehlo, D. P., & Hanson, S. M. H., (2010). *Family health care nursing: Theory, practice, and research* (4th ed.). Philadelphia: F. A. Davis.

Kaphingst, K. A., Goodman, M., Pandya, C., Garg, P., Stafford, J., & Lachance, C. (2012). Individual perceptions, preference, and participation: Factors affecting frequency of communication about family health history with family members and doctors in a medically underserved population. *Individual Education and Counseling, 88*(2), 291–297. doi:10.1016/j.pec.2011.11.013

Knudson-Martin, C. (2013). Why power matters: Creating a foundation of mutual support in couple relationships. *Family Process, 52*(1), 5–18.

Kritsotakis, G., & Gamarnikow, E. (2004). What is social capital and how does it relate to health? *International Journal of Nursing Studies, 41*, 43–50.

Lunney, M. (2009). *Critical thinking to achieve positive health outcomes: Nursing case studies and analysis.* Boston: Wiley-Blackwell.

Mamier, I. (2011). *Nurses' spiritual care practices: Assessment type, frequency, and correlates.* Ann Arbor, MI: ProQuest, UMI Dissertation Publishing.

Manoogian, M. M., Harter, L. M., & Denham, S. A. (2010). The storied nature of health legacies in the familial experience of type 2 diabetes. *Journal of Family Communication, 10*, 1–17.

McGoldrick, M., & Gerson, R. (1985). *Genograms in family assessment.* New York: W. W. Norton.

McGoldrick, M., Gerson, R., & Shellenberger, S. (1999). *Genograms: Assessment and intervention* (2nd ed.). New York: W. W. Norton.

Meiers, S., Eggenberger, S., Krumwiede, N., Bliesmer, M., & Earle, P. (2009). Enduring acts of balance: Rural families creating health. In H. Lee (Ed.), *Conceptual basis for rural nursing* (3rd ed.). New York: Springer.

Moore, S., Bockenholt, U., Daniel, M., Frohlich., K., Kestens, Y., & Richard, L. (2011). Social capital and core network ties: A validation study of individual-level social capital measures and their association with extra-and intra-neighborhood ties, and self-rated health. *Health and Place, 17*(2), 536–544.

NANDA International. (2012). *Nursing diagnoses: Definitions and classifications 2012–2014.* Boston: Wiley-Blackwell.

National Human Genome Research Institute. (2012). Specific genetic disorders. Retrieved from http://www.genome.gov/10001204

Neuman, B., & Fawcett, J. (Eds.). (2011). *The Neuman systems model* (5th ed.). Upper Saddle River, NJ: Pearson.

Nightingale, F. (1859 and 1946). *Notes on nursing.* Philadelphia: J. B. Lippincott.

Power, J. (2006). Spiritual assessment: Developing an assessment tool. *Nursing Older People, 18*(2), 16–18.

Putnam, R. D. (2001). *Bowling alone: The collapse and revival of American community.* New York: Simon & Schuster.

Riner, M. E., Cunningham, C., & Johnson, A. (2004). Public health education and practice using geographic information system technology. *Public Health Nursing, 21*(1), 57–65.

Roy, S. C. (2009). *The Roy adaptation model* (3rd ed.). Upper Saddle River, NJ: Prentice-Hall.

Scanlon, C., & Fibison, W. (1995). *Managing genetic information: Implications for nurses.* Washington, DC: American Nurses Publishing.

Selman, L., Harding, R., Gysels, M., Speck, P., & Higginson, I. J. (2011). The measurement of spirituality in palliative care and the content of tools validated cross-culturally: A systematic review. *Journal of Pain and Symptom Management, 41*(4), 728–753.

Snyder, M., & Lindquist, R. (2009). *Complementary and alternative therapies in nursing* (6th ed.). New York: Springer.

Swinton, J., & Pattison, S. (2010). Moving beyond clarity: Towards a thin, vague, and useful understanding of spirituality in nursing care. *Nursing Philosophy, 11*, 226–237.

Tanner, C. A. (2006). Thinking like a nurse: A research-based model of clinical judgment in nursing. *Journal of Nursing Education, 45*(6), 204–211.

U.S. Department of Health and Human Services. (2010, November). Office of Disease Prevention and Health Promotion. Healthy People 2020, ODPHP Publication No. B0132 www.healthypeople.gov

Vallance, H., & Ford, J. (2003). Carrier testing for autosomal-recessive disorders. *Critical Reviews in Clinical Laboratory Sciences, 40*(4), 473–497. doi:1040-8363/03

Walsh, F. (2003). *Normal family processes.* New York/London: Guilford Press.

Wright, L., & Leahy, M. (2009). The Calgary Family Assessment Model. In L. Wright, & J. Leahy (Eds.), *Nurses and families: A guide to family assessment and intervention* (pp. 47–142). Philadelphia: F. A. Davis.

CHAPTER 6

Cultural and Diversity Aspects of Health and Illness Care Needs

Hans-Peter de Ruiter • Jennifer M. Demma • Marianne Kriegl • Joachim Schulze

CHAPTER OBJECTIVES

1. Describe ways cultural diversity influences views of health and illness.
2. Discuss ways that using a family lens redefines ideas about culture and diversity.
3. Explain ways nurses need to tailor care, communication, and nursing actions with diverse cultural groups.
4. Discuss relationships between culture and communication.

CHAPTER CONCEPTS

- Communication barriers
- Cultural ambiguity
- Cultural competency
- Cultural desire
- Cultural humility
- Cultural knowledge
- Cultural nuances
- Culturally sensitive care
- Culture
- Diversity
- Literacy
- Low health literacy
- Routines
- Stereotypes
- Time management

Introduction

Family nurses are aware of cultural differences and use culturally sensitive ways as they meet and care for individuals and families. *Thinking family* suggests thoughtful consideration of the breadth of ways that cultural diversity factors into health and illness. Families differ in the ways they live their daily lives. Ideas about wellness and disease or birth and death are often linked with family traditions and routines. Family culture influences the ways children are socialized about health and illness. Nurses should examine personal bias, prejudice, and assumptions about race, social class, ethnicity, age, and sexuality to understand their worldview before they can effectively care for others whose views differ. This chapter invites you to look through a family lens as culturally competent and sensitive nursing actions are examined. Nurses working with family units recognize that diversity occurs within families and not just between families. Giving culturally sensitive care requires curious, thoughtful, and intentional nurses. This chapter explores culture from family unit, family household, and community perspectives.

Cultural Distinctiveness

The United States is a nation of family immigrants and ancestors from all over the world (Fig. 6.1). Cultures have blended over time so that many are different from their origins. As the nation was settled, early immigrants often lived near others who shared similar race, traditions, ideas, beliefs, values, rituals, ethnicity, and religion. Large groups of Europeans came and settled in the lands of the indigenous people, and slave traders followed, bringing Africans. Immigrants have come in waves, settled the land, managed their differences, and created a place called America, a land where being an American was based more on shared values than on ethnicity. Initial settlements were along the coastlines and then they moved inland. Today's immigrants are from many places, including Mexico, India, Somalia, China, the Philippines, Cuba, and the Dominican Republic. Some immigrant populations settle in distinct locations. For instance, the largest numbers of Somali immigrants have settled in Minneapolis, Minnesota, and Columbus, Ohio. Some are not constrained to a particular geographical region, but are dispersed throughout the country. The United States has been called a melting pot, but perhaps it is really more like a stew. In the United States, even after many generations some remnants of original cultural traits remain, but more importantly, Americans share many blended factors that unify them as a people. Families often retain some traditions from earlier lifestyles even when they no longer know their origin.

Early settlers came for many reasons and still do. Early settlers forged frontiers, farmed land, and labored in factories. Today, many live in cities, work in service industries, and have sedentary jobs. Family relocation often means extended family is remote and supports they might bring are lacking. Families may have fewer children and face the challenge of caring for ill persons or aging parents. Families share similarities, but also vary widely in the ways members give and receive care.

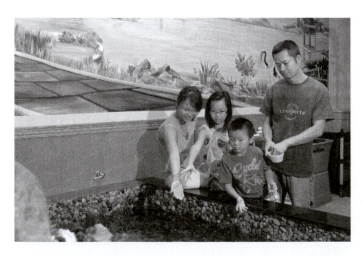

FIGURE 6-1 Culturally distinct family.

Defining Culture

Culture refers to the behaviors and beliefs that characterize a particular group of people, society, or nation. The idea of culture comes from anthropology. It is somewhat intangible, vague, and elusive and involves symbols, customs, social interactions, forms of dress, speech, and occupations. Culture flavors opinions or viewpoints and influences the ways in which behavior is interpreted. Cultural groups value different artifacts, material goods, and behaviors. Culture has nuances; it can be diverse even within the same group.

Cultural Nuances

Culture displays a breadth of ideas and attitudes about what is acceptable or prized (e.g., sexual orientations, race, gender, national origins, aging, youth). This diversity must be considered. Popular culture influences what is currently in vogue or style (e.g., fashion trends, films, music, books, slang), but may have generational differences. The world is a smaller place than it once was; there are few isolated pockets, and access is now universal. Videos and YouTube create bridges for people sharing ideas rapidly and in new ways. A viral video could mean the whole world is dancing Gangnam style. Cultural distinctiveness implies one has ideas or beliefs different from the mainstream (Box 6.1). All people have culture derived from familial ancestors, residence, and their expectations and values. Diversity occurs within a single culture and all from a particular culture are not the same.

Using a Family Lens to Understand Cultural Diversity

A family lens is needed to assess unique cultural perspectives of those seeking care for health and illness. A family lens can help dissolve preconceived ideas. Using this lens means striving to see things as they are, not making textbook knowledge fit. Even a culturally distinct family can have members who differ. Cultures can clash when birth, illness, or death occur. Cultural variation can be noted with prevention, wellness, chronic disease management, or rehabilitative practices. Diversity implies the many forms in which culture can be expressed. Consider this example:

You are working in a birthing unit in a hospital. You are assigned to Ms. D., a woman who gave birth to her second baby just 12 hours ago. At the start of the shift, you observed Ms. D. breastfeeding, smiling as she looked at the baby, stroking his head, and talking to him. He appeared to be feeding well and she appeared content. Several hours have passed. You notice Ms. D. is still in bed and has not interacted with her son except for breastfeeding. A man is in the room and is asleep on a cot in the corner. Another woman in the room is sitting on blankets on the floor and holds the newborn. Other than feeding, she performs all the baby's care. You suggest to Ms. D. that she walk around the hallway for physical activity. Ms. D. says she is tired and her family wants her to rest.

BOX 6-1

Levels of Culture

Tylor (1909) spoke of culture as having three different levels:

- Cultural traditions that distinguish a particular society (e.g., Chinese, French, German, Dutch)
- Subculture with shared traits in a different society (e.g., food traditions, language, traditions)
- Cultural universals (e.g., grammatical rules, sexual division of work, rules for sexual behaviors, ideas for raising children, kinship, good or bad behaviors, leadership roles, art, jokes, games)

In this example, cultural identifiers were purposely left out of the story. Imagine how you might respond and interact to this situation based on specific cultural identifiers:

- Scenario A: Ms. D is an 18-year-old single Caucasian, American, Catholic student from a rural Midwestern town; the man in the room is 19 years old, father of the baby, involved and supportive; the woman is Ms. D's 16-year-old half-sister.
- Scenario B: Ms. D is a 36-year-old married, Hmong, Buddhist, stay-at-home mother and lives in a suburban West Coast city; the man is her 62-year-old father; and the woman in the room is her 58-year-old mother. Both recently arrived from Laos to help Ms. D take care of her children, and they have not seen her in 5 years.
- Scenario C: Ms. D is 28 years old; the child's father is a Mexican American, agnostic lawyer who lives in an urban East Coast city; the man in the room is her 68-year-old father; and the woman is her 32-year-old Canadian, Caucasian life partner.

Situations challenge norms, traditions, and values we hold. What different ideas do these situations suggest? What biases or assumptions flavor your thinking? Take a few minutes to read about the work of Drs. Benzein and Saveman, family-focused nurses from Sweden who are leading the way in helping students and other nurses learn about the importance of involving families in the care of individuals (Box 6.2).

How nurses respond creates barriers or facilitates effective relationships. For example, in scenario B, how would you interpret the situation if you had learned that Southeast

---

BOX 6-2

Family Tree

Eva Benzein, RN, PhD (Sweden)

Britt-Inger Saveman, RN, PhD (Sweden)

Britt-Inger Saveman, RNT, PhD, is a professor at the Department of Nursing, Umeå University, in Umeå, Sweden. Eva Benzein, RNT, PhD, is a professor at the School of Health and Caring Sciences, Linnaeus University (formerly Kalmar University), in Kalmar, Sweden. These leaders have provided sustained, visionary leadership in establishing family-focused nursing in Sweden. In 2005, their efforts were recognized with an Innovative Contribution to Family Nursing Award from the *Journal of Family Nursing.* In 2012, Dr. Saveman received an honorary doctorate from the University of Tampere in Finland for her contributions to family nursing and health science. Dr. Benzein was awarded a multimillion dollar award from the Kamprad Family Foundation to establish a palliative care center in Småland with an emphasis on family-focused care. Their family nursing interest was influenced by Dr. Lorraine Wright and the work of the Family Nursing Unit at the University of Calgary. These two leaders, in 2002, translated *Beliefs: The Heart of Healing in Families and Illness,* a textbook by Wright, Watson, and Bell (1996) into Swedish. In 2004, they established the Family-Focused Nursing Unit (Omvardnadsmottagning foer familjer) at Kalmar University where therapeutic conversations were offered to families using a research process. They call these interventions "health promoting conversations." In 2002, they organized the First Nordic Conference on family-focused nursing at Kalmar University with family nursing scholars from Denmark, Finland, Iceland, Norway, and Sweden. In 2006, they hosted the Second Nordic Conference, followed by a third conference in 2010. They have studied Swedish nurses' attitudes about the importance of involving families in care. They developed and revised an instrument called Families' Importance in Nursing Care—Nurses' Attitudes (FINC-NA) used by family nursing researchers. Their publications focus on the family illness experience and offering family interventions. Their research is now examining the efficacy of family nursing interventions and translating this knowledge to practice settings. In 2012, Benzein, Saveman, and Hagberg published *Meeting With Families in Health and Community Care.* Published in Swedish, this book describes the Family Health Conversation Model.

Asian families traditionally care for newborns and women are encouraged to rest often for 30 to 40 days? What nursing actions would you take? If you were to assume what you learned was true without doing an assessment, could you overlook uncontrolled pain or depression? Suppose she does not believe like her parents, and wants to be more involved? Assumptions about a culture based on stereotyped behaviors instead of critical thinking lead to incompetent cultural practices. Families need their unique family stories and needs associated with health, illness, and usual lifestyles to be understood. Families met in care settings are often ill at ease with unfamiliar situations. Many have uncertainties about the foreign world of health care and do not know what to expect. Nurses also have uncertainties about what individuals need and families expect. Bridges to meet needs must be built.

Culturally Sensitive Care

The only culture that can be truly known is one's own, and self-knowledge is the starting point of understanding. Culturally sensitive care begins with understanding one's personal biases and assumptions. One does not gain cultural sensitivity through learning about beliefs and customs of particular people, but through listening and learning about their needs and preferences (Simon & Kodish, 2005). A deep sense of sincere curiosity and a spirit of inquiry are needed. Rather than being judgmental and letting prejudice color attitudes, find a place of neutrality that negates reliance on stereotypes and generalizations. Try these steps:

1. Know yourself as the key starting point.
2. Identify personal biases about culture and families.
3. Find neutrality instead of judgment.
4. Use curiosity and interest as tools to understand culture and family.

Knowing the cultural context of a family can change the way relationships are created. Education emphasizes culture, but some learning only reinforces assumptions and stereotypes. Generalizations are not helpful for learning about specific family needs. Although some things are true for some families, there are differences. Nurses who *think family* approach each individual and family unit without preformed ideas. Learning to be culturally sensitive is likely a career process, learned over time, as nurses gain knowledge, skills, and experience.

Providing Culturally Sensitive Care

Nurses often provide care and meet people in unpredictable settings. For example, if giving care in a family household, members interrupt, phones ring, visitors arrive, children cry, and dogs bark. In acute care, call lights signal needs, transporters arrive, staff members interrupt, and emergencies occur. Delivery of culturally sensitive care happens in the midst of everyday work. One doesn't decide to do it; instead, it catches you by surprise. Here is an example:

> When I came to the hospital, I felt lost. It was hard if not impossible to understand what was going on and why. At home, when I feel sick, I like to eat white bread toast with marmalade, but that was not available. I tried to explain my history to the nurse, but she seemed rushed and asked me several times to "get to the point." At home I relax by calling people, I was not allowed to use my cell phone. I was hoping that a few of my family members could stay with me, but I was told that hospital policy restricted visiting to one person.—Hermann, age 86 years

This situation is not uncommon. Care is frequently delivered based on what is most convenient for the health care institution or care providers.

Consider how the nurse could have handled the encounter differently:

• How did the nurse sound to this gentleman when telling him he could not have marmalade?

Were other choices offered?

- When he was told that he could not use his cell phone, could this have been handled in a more sensitive way?
- Could the nurse use personal experiences of being in a strange place with loss of control about personal choices to increase empathy with this man's situation?

Cultural Differentiation

When speaking of cultural differentiation, race and ethnicity immediately come to mind, but other factors are equally important, such as age, country of origin, education, gender identity, social class, family of origin, employment, language, religion, and relationship status. Even within families, cultures can differ. For instance, a sibling with a professional degree working in a high-income career will have a different culture than one who may have adopted a drug-using behavior. Nurses need to see their uniqueness. Cultural traditions exist around many things. Foods eaten during celebration or illness vary. Forms of dress have special meanings. Some traditional remedies in the treatment of illness or disease may be used. Faith healers or shamanistic healers may be called. In some places, goods or services are bartered for health services. Complementary and alternative modalities may be viewed as means of healing. Beliefs about evil spirits or the "evil eye" or customs of prayers, talismans, colors, jewelry, or other adornment may be needed to keep bad things from happening.

Gender Rules

Some cultures have social, legal, and religious rules about the roles and rights of women and men. Taboos might be related to men and women being alone in a room together, shaking hands, or making eye contact. Wrongful or improper behaviors are easily interpreted as offensive. Inquiring about expectations if things are unclear is always a good way to begin. Cultural ideals can be misunderstood by the nurse or those seeking care. Thus, it is always good to clarify if expectations are not clear. Inappropriate actions can be serious roadblocks to building therapeutic individual-nurse-family relationships. Nurses who *think family* know that satisfaction is often related to ways things are perceived. It is impossible to know everyone's preference and so inquiry is a good way to begin.

Seeking Health Services

Culture can influence where, when, and how individuals seek health care. Families socialize their members about health and illness (Denham, 2003). Some families are more apt to seek medical care for every problem but others delay and come only after a disease has greatly progressed. For example, cancer death rates are decreasing overall throughout the United States, but immigrant minorities continue to have much higher incidence and mortality rates (Gany, Herrera, Avallone, & Changrani, 2006). What might be the reasons for this delay in seeking care? Could the reasons be tied to culture in some way? Research about health-seeking behaviors of minority groups related to cancer found that cultural, linguistic, and system barriers accounted for much misinformation (Gany et al., 2006). Tailored community-based approaches for culturally distinct groups are recommended.

Stereotypical Images

Personal biases and assumptions can cloud perspectives and responses. Stereotypes are oversimplified ideas about traits observed, imagined, or attributed to a specific group. They are the views that one group holds about another. A positive stereotype might be something like black men are great athletes. A negative stereotype is the assumption that women are terrible drivers. These things might be true in some cases but not all the time. Both ideas are as likely to be false as true. Stereotypes, once formed, are not easy to dispel. The important thing is that nurses recognize when their thoughts are biased.

For instance, a Native American from a large reservation was admitted to an urban hospital for an organ transplant, and 12 family members accompanied him. One of the family members, the patient's uncle, was considered a healer. At admission, the intake nurse was fascinated by the family support, beliefs about traditional healing, and different life views expressed. She shared her enthusiasm with her peers. The nurses agreed that this was going to be a good experience for all and an opportunity to be exposed to a rich ancient culture. After a few days the novelty wore off. Nurses were frustrated that the family was present. A healing ritual using tobacco was performed. A smoke alarm went off and caused some chaos. The family members ate the food in the patient's refrigerator and slept in the unit family room. Before long, this family had earned the label of difficult and unmanageable. Hospital administration and patient relations were called to resolve what was identified as a big problem.

What went wrong? Part of the problem was rooted in biases of the admitting nurse and her colleagues. They held views of Native Americans based on their own cultural ideas. Nurses viewed their welcoming attitude to the Native Americans as being culturally sensitive. However, the nurses' views were actually based on stereotypes. It is more difficult to identify positive stereotypes than negative ones because we tend to see positive feelings held about others as good and not problematic (Box 6.3).

Cultural Ambiguity

We tend to see our culture as the norm and are often unaware of it until we meet differences. A term used to describe this behavior is ethnocentric. It implies that when we become aware of worldviews or cultural ideas, we tend to see them through our personal experience and think our way is best. We do not notice our personal traits unless someone points them out and notes the differences. If you are an American, you might notice that people call things by different names. For example, it is "soda" in New York, "pop" in Kentucky,

---

BOX 6-3

Identifying Positive Stereotypes

Often when stereotypes are considered, we tend to identify negative traits. Take some time to think about what might be positive stereotypes associated with culture.

1. Identify some positive ideas about different cultural groups. For example:
   - Japanese people are . . . ?
   - Young people are . . . ?
   - Persons in the military are . . . ?
   - Caucasians are . . . ?
   - Gay men are . . . ?
   - Old people are . . . ?
2. How did you come to have these ideas? What has informed your thoughts?

What could be the result of having these positive biases or stereotypes in everyday care in a hospital or other health care setting?

and "Coke" in Texas. In Wisconsin, you might drink from a "bubbler," whereas in neighboring Minnesota, you drink from a "water fountain." Naming products, foods, or activities is tied to regional cultures.

Some nursing students have difficulty defining their culture. Think about popular culture. In the 1950s, American culture might have been described with words like "baseball, Chevrolet, and apple pie." In the 1990s, it was football, blue jeans, hamburgers and fries, and Mickey Mouse. Today, we might refer to technologies like smart phones, tablets, apps, and YouTube. Americans may differ on what defines their culture, but ideas like independent, patriotic, convenience, and freedom of choice may be common themes. Cultural icons and heros tell of generational differences. American college graduates in the year 2013 will recall Princess Diana, Oprah, Madonna, Britney Spears, Michael Jordan, Barney, the Power Rangers, and the Spice Girls as childhood influences. They will also recall the bombing of the twin towers, Iraq and Afghanistan, and hurricane Katrina. Whereas, 1970 college graduates recall Muhammed Ali, Evil Knievel, Jackie Onassis, Elvis Presley, Martin Luther King Jr., Marilyn Monroe, the Beatles, and Willie Mays. Memories would include *Sputnik*, President Kennedy's death, and Vietnam. Culture can be described by what is popular at a particular time. Popular with whom? Cultural ideas can be ambiguous, vague, and even debatable.

Using Culture in the Care of Families

Cultural differences are most obvious when we meet situations in which the dominant culture is in stark contrast to our own. We can be intrigued by differences that are far off but appalled when we are directly confronted with them—similar to the nurses caring for the Native American family. One becomes culturally sensitive as one experiences differences. One sometimes needs to be a bit of a risk taker to try something unfamiliar and uncomfortable. Suppose you were a Thanksgiving guest with friends, a time previously celebrated only with your family. And what if the foods served were none of those traditionally served at Thanksgiving? Can you recall a holiday or event with a family other than yours? What differences did you notice? How did you react? Was it comfortable? What did you learn about yourself or your family as a result? Even when we share times with those similar to us we can still find differences. Although families differ, they are also alike as they connect with one another, support, give identity, and supply needed resources.

Curiosity allows one to risk new situations. Cultural sensitivity is less about understanding cultural traits and more about being open to the needs of unique individuals and families. Cultural knowledge is useful but false perceptions are barriers. Reliance on ambiguous ideas is insufficient. We live in a time when growing numbers of interracial, mixed ethnicities, and those with big religious differences unite and become family. Consider a nuclear family with an American mother born and raised in Japan in a military family. The father is a native from a small farming community in Peru. Their two children were born in Germany where their parents were studying. They now live in Canada. How would you regard this family? What is their culture? The children are exposed to multiple cultures. How will they think about culture? It is challenging to be culturally sensitive and relationships can be complicated. Cultural knowledge needs to be accompanied by listening, asking relevant questions, and being sensitive to unique needs (Box 6.4).

Cultural Competence in the Delivery of Family Nursing Care

What do you talk about while you are delivering care? Do you ask about beliefs, traditions, values, taboos, and practices? Cultural knowledge that identifies traits is not enough;

> ## BOX 6-4
> ### Thinking About Cultural Ambiguity
>
> Take some time to consider your family and others you know. It is easy to form opinions quickly without giving thought to the multiple factors that might be involved. It is easy to have a bias, prejudice, or opinion based upon face value without understanding full explanations. Think about the ways you might answer these questions about your family. Are there some things about which others in a health care setting could have misunderstandings?
>
> 1. With what culture does your family identify?
> 2. Do you have more than a single culture linked with your family? If so, what does this mean to you?
> 3. What are some "cultural family facts" about the culture(s) with which your family identifies? In what ways is your family similar to or different from others of that culture?
> 4. What influenced your family to decide which cultural ideas to adopt, value, and celebrate?
>
> When you meet individuals and families from a particular race, ethnicity, same sex and other diverse relationships, or religion, it is important to recall that stereotypical viewpoints are unlikely to describe their uniqueness.

knowledge about unique needs must also occur. Meanings and values of legacies, traditions, rituals, and routines are just as important as their accompanying behaviors. Nurses can address cultural needs using these five constructs: cultural awareness, humility, knowledge, skill, and desire (Campinha-Bacote, 2002).

Cultural Awareness

Cultural awareness begins with self-examination, which is an in-depth exploration of one's culture and ethnicity. Discovering one's roots or ancestry can provide a breadth of understanding not previously realized. For example, Mary, a nurse of West African descent, works in a long-term care facility in a suburban area of Chicago. She notices that many elderly persons get infrequent visits from their children. She finds it hard to understand. In West Africa no one is admitted to a long-term care facility. Mary catches herself being critical of the families because in her culture families have the responsibility to care for the elders. Questions to consider in cultural awareness are as follows:

- Why am I reacting so critically to this situation?
- What makes it hard for me to accept this family the way they are?
- What is making me so uncomfortable with this individual or family?
- Do I truly understand what this individual or family wants or needs?
- What do I need to learn about this culture so that I can better meet individual and family care needs?

Everyone has some bias. Offering culturally sensitive care must start with awareness (Box 6.5). Take time to discuss these ideas with others.

Cultural Humility

Humility implies meekness, a term not often used. It means being unassuming, modest, and not presumptuous. Nurses who *think family* recognize power imbalances between care providers and those receiving care. It is not unusual for nurses to be critical when others act in ways not well understood. A home care nurse might get frustrated with members of

---

BOX 6-5

Examination of Cultural Identity

These questions are designed to help find your cultural identity as you examine your past and present. Carefully consider each question and decide the best ways to get answers. You may need to talk with immediate or extended family members, complete some genealogical research, look at old family artifacts, or do some personal soul-searching in this quest. You might want to create a journal and keep track of what you find so that you can reflect on it, add to it, and share it with others. You will examine your personal identity and answer this question: Who am I?

1. Discover your racial and ethnic heritage. What are your family origins? Trace your family back as far as you can and explore maternal and paternal sides of your family. How are they alike? How are they different? Where did they live? What did they do? How have family members changed or stayed the same over the years? Can you find old pictures that you can view and compare with your present family?

2. Consider your personal culture in relationship to your racial and ethnic heritage. What do people say about these ethnic or racial groups? How does popular media depict these groups? What does published literature report about these groups? What do you think about them?

3. Identify how your personal cultural beliefs and identity fit with your heritage. In what ways do you see your life as similar to or different from these ancestral groups? What are your personal values and beliefs? Do these values and beliefs have origins rooted in your family history? Are your religious beliefs or faith similar to that of family members from the past? What traditions, celebrations, or ways of life are legacies of the past? What items do you have in your family home that have been handed down over several generations? Do you know the stories that accompany these items?

4. Identify your popular culture perspectives. Think about the present time: What things do you value in your present life? Is this linked with the past in any way? What beliefs or personal philosophy do you hold? How do you identify yourself in your everyday life? What material things in your current home or life do you deeply value? Might these be things you would want to pass to future generations?

---

an Orthodox Jewish family. Relying on their traditions of eating Kosher foods, they have conflicts about the foods the sick individual should eat and when they should be eaten. Their family member is on dialysis and has dietary constraints that conflict with Rabbinic Law of the Torah. The nurse might prefer to ignore the conflict. Unfamiliarity with Judaism and a Kosher diet create uncertainty. How should this situation be approached? Their arguing is loud and it makes the nurse uncomfortable. Yet, the family needs nutritional information and a dietary plan. What would you do in this situation? Remember, thinking family implies collaboration with the family and assisting them to form a workable solution.

Cultural Knowledge

Education about culture must be aligned with clinical actions. Cultural knowledge includes the following:

- Various cultural worldviews or varying points of view
- Unique beliefs about wellness, disease, and healing
- Areas of particular risk to a given group or population
- Biophysiological or genetic variations

Standards to define culturally and linguistically appropriate services exist (Office of Minority Health, 2007). Box 6.6 identifies standards to assist in providing culturally sensitive care. For example, preferences of Korean women after giving birth may differ from others. Telling her to drink ice water or cold fluids might cause conflict if she holds beliefs that a new mother should not drink cold things. A family of Muslim faith might want to be near their dying member as death approaches, but not show excessive expressions of grief when the death occurs. It is often the custom to bury the person quickly and burial practices might be unfamiliar to the nurse. Cultural knowledge is not enough if the woman is a third-generation American-Korean woman or if the deceased has accepted different faith beliefs. Nurses who *think family* use their cultural knowledge to ask questions about needs in a particular situation.

BOX 6-6

National Standards on Culturally and Linguistically Appropriate Services

These standards are primarily intended for health care organizations, but they are useful for nurses who aim to provide culturally sensitive nursing care. These standards recommend that all health care organizations do the following things:

- Ensure that staff provides care that is effective, understandable, and respectful in ways compatible to health beliefs and preferred language.
- Employ staff that is representative of the demographic characteristics of the area.
- Provide continuing education in culturally and linguistically appropriate service delivery.
- Provide language assistance at no cost to the consumer at all points of contact and during all hours of operation.
- Provide individuals with oral and written notices about their rights to receive language assistance services in their preferred language.
- Ensure the competence of language assistance to persons with limited English proficiency by providing interpreters and bilingual staff; family should not be used to provide interpretive services (except on request of the individual receiving care).
- Ensure that written patient materials and signage are in the language of commonly encountered groups.
- Employ a strategic plan that outlines clear goals, policies, operational plans, and management accountability to provide culturally and linguistically appropriate services.
- Conduct initial and ongoing assessments of activities that integrate cultural and linguistic measures into internal audits, performance improvement programs, patient satisfaction assessments, and outcome-based evaluations.
- Ensure that data about race, ethnicity, and spoken and written language are documented in the health record, integrated into the organization's information systems, and periodically updated.
- Maintain a current demographic, cultural, and epidemiological profile of the community to use for planning and implementing services that meet the cultural needs of the service area.
- Develop community partnerships using formal and informal mechanisms to design and implement culturally appropriate activities.
- Ensure that conflict and grievance resolution processes are culturally and linguistically sensitive and able to identify, prevent, and resolve cross-cultural conflicts or complaints by care consumers.
- Make information about successful innovations for implementing culturally and language appropriate standards available to the public.

Source: Adapted from the Office of Minority Health. (2007). National Standards on Culturally and Linguistically Appropriate Services (CLAS). Department of Health and Human Services. Retrieved May 11, 2012 from http://minorityhealth.hhs.gov/templates/browse.aspx?lvl=2&lvlID=15

Cultural Skills

Nurses use cultural skills to collect and use culturally relevant information about a person's health history and presenting problem. Abilities to conduct individual and family assessments in culturally sensitive ways are needed. This is typically not learned solely in the classroom but in practice areas. For instance, a nurse might be unsure whether shaking hands with the community or religious leaders visiting a hospitalized individual or family is appropriate. Is it permissible to shake hands with a Buddhist monk? An Ashkenazi rabbi? An Amish bishop or a Native American traditional healer? The best approach for learning cultural skills is to become familiar with some general ideas about the culture of persons with whom you are interacting. However, it is appropriate to ask those involved what they prefer. In everyday practice, these actions get skipped if the nurse is uncomfortable or finds the situation awkward. Cultural skills are mastered by making a commitment to learn through experience; this learning is a lifelong experience. Learning can occur even when events turn out differently than anticipated.

Cultural Desire

Culturally competent nurses do not gain skills automatically; they take conscious efforts and have a desire to understand what people need. Cultural desire arises when the benefits of culturally sensitive nursing care are understood. Cultural desire fosters tolerance for differences, compassion, authenticity, humility, openness, availability, and flexibility. It is a commitment to quality care. It is usual to have some discomfort or conflicted emotions when communicating with persons who see the world differently. Cultural desire puts aside personal unease to address real care needs. Campinha-Bacote (2002) challenges nurses to be sure they have ASKED the right questions:

A(wareness): Are you aware of biases? Did you notice the reflection in your voice that might have sounded as if you were disgusted?

S(kill): Do you possess the experience needed to listen to multiple family members' stories when completing an assessment?

K(nowledge): Do you understand the particular perspectives of this family?

E(ncounters): Do you know how to interact with families from this cultural group?

D(esire): Do you want to learn more effective ways for working with families from different nations?

Cultural desire actively seeks ways to increase cultural understandings. Culturally congruent care is consistently doing what is needed by those receiving care.

Using Cultural Knowledge in Practice

Textbooks offer general information about demographics, family structures, and health practices of some cultural groups. General cultural information, however, does not describe the unique qualities of diverse people. For example, the terms Caucasian, African American, and Hispanic are often used. What mental pictures do you see? Stereotypical assumptions without checking are misleading. Reflect on how learning more details changes the way you visualize each family. How does what you think influence your desire to give care? In what ways do your beliefs alter what you think about the family unit and their household lives?

Several years ago, a nurse colleague shared that a nurse manager came into the nurses' station irritated. The nurse manager said, "Who has the patient in room 204? She needs to get down there and ask all of those visitors to leave." The person hospitalized, a

Caucasian woman in her early 20s, had surgery earlier in the day and was in her bed resting. When the nurse went into the room, three black male visitors were present. The nurse manager had not spoken to them but had some assumptions about race. Rather than inquire and talk with the visitors, she insisted that someone else deal with the situation. Her communication and personal bias had little to do with hospital rules that allowed two visitors. We seldom recognize our own bias. Consider the following scenario.

Mrs. Johnson, a 72-year-old woman, was admitted to the hospital after she broke her hip. Her daughter found her 6 hours after she had fallen. She was brought to the emergency room at a nearby hospital and went directly into surgery for a hip replacement. Her family is waiting. Now add the following information: replace the first sentence with the following:

- "Mrs. Johnson, a 72-year-old Caucasian woman who struggled with alcohol abuse most of her life."
- "Mrs. Johnson, a 72-year-old Japanese American woman who worked as a researcher at a major research university."
- "Mrs. Johnson, a 72-year-old Native American woman."
- "Mrs. Johnson, a 72-year-old African American mother of 5 children and grandmother of 18 who lived in a small Midwestern town all her life."

How do these details influence the ways you might consider individual and family care?

An Increasingly Diverse World

Improved transportation and communication allow for racial and ethnic cultural diversity to grow not only in North America but across the world. Health disparities disproportionately affect certain racial and ethnic groups. Qualities such as race, ethnicity, language barriers, socioeconomic status, and perceptions of discrimination affect access to quality health care.

Family Households

The 2010 U.S. Census reported that household factors in families continue to change (Table 6.1). Family units influence members' ideas. Growing up in one family household type can cause you to have a biased perspective about the right type of family unit and might cause personal conflict and less tolerance for other family types. Ideas about family forms may conflict with those the nurse values the most. Abilities to be tolerant or open to various family types can affect communication. Nurses must be cautious to not let personal beliefs interfere in professional practice. Nurses do not have to agree with others' beliefs or practices, but all persons seeking care still need to be treated in respectful ways.

Aging Populations

Aging has already been discussed as a trending concern for the future. It is a factor that might be responded to in cultural ways. In some cultures, elders are greatly honored and a central part of all family decision making, even when pertaining to younger generations' decisions. In other cultures individual autonomy is valued and elders have a more limited role in decisions. Some cultures value productivity and elders who are not contributing to the family's welfare may not be involved in decision making. However, regardless of ways a culture treats aging, not all families act the same. In the United States, for several generations, greater focus has been on youth than on elderly people.

TABLE 6-1	Differences in Family Households Between 2000 and 2010	
HOUSEHOLD TYPE	**2000**	**2010**
Husband-wife households	51.7%	48.4%
Female household, no spouse	12.2%	13.1%
Male household, no spouse	4.2%	5.0%
Male householder, living alone	11.2%	11.9%
Female householder, living alone	14.6%	14.8%
Unmarried couples	5.2%	6.6%
Opposite-sex partners	4.6%	5.9%
Same-sex partners	0.6%	0.8%
Average household size	2.59 persons	2.58 persons
Average family size	3.14 persons	3.14 persons

Source: 2010 U.S. Census.

The U.S. Census statistics suggest that the population of Americans aged 65 or older will reach 70 million by 2030 (Box 6.7). More elderly people will live alone as they age. Societal institutions, such as education, housing, retirement, taxation, Social Security, and churches, are likely to be influenced by these population shifts. Since the 1980s, the sandwich generation has been described as people who care for children and aging parents. This will continue but those caring for their very old parents (in their 80s and 90s) will likely be in their 60s and 70s. Caregiving will fall to a smaller number of adult children often living distant from their parents. Many will be working full time as retirement age gets extended. Availability of long-term care may be limited and expensive, putting it out of reach for many. Well elders and those with chronic illnesses will be independent but need support. Acute care will be brief with caregivers having greater responsibility. How do you think increases in the elderly population will influence culture? How might this affect nursing practice?

Stereotypical ideas that elderly people are dependent and frail are contradicted by the majority of older people with good health and active lives. Over the next decade, aging persons will likely need more help with activities of daily living. Fewer family members will be available to give care. Those living independently in rural places may have limited resources. What kinds of care will families need at home? Some will reside in care facilities, but not everyone. In what ways will a well older population influence society (e.g., civic, workforce, volunteer)? How might an aging population with great health costs tax family and national resources?

BOX 6-7

Aging in America

During the 20th century, while the number of persons under 65 has tripled, the number of those 65 years and older has increased 11-fold (U.S. Census, 2010). In 1900, those age 65 years and older accounted for only 1 in every 25 Americans; by 1994 this ratio was 1 in 8, and it is expected to increase to 1 in 5 by 2050. As the "baby boomers" age between years 2010 and 2030, each year will show a 2.8% annual increase in the number of elderly persons. Those 85 and older are the most rapidly growing elderly group.

How will care needs be provided by fewer health professionals? Nurses need knowledge about elderly populations, geriatric care, family care, and support needs.

Religion, Faith, and Spirituality

Factors such as birth, death, and illness often create an awareness of the spiritual aspects of our existence. Many believe the spirit gives meaning and purpose. Spiritual well-being, faith, and religion are often linked with health and disease. Spiritual well-being is an inner state that influences and may even govern the way one fulfills their needs, goals, and life aspirations (Carson, 1989). Figure 6.2 depicts complex relationships that occur around spirituality.

Variations in Beliefs

Religion, faith, and medicine share a history in which they were once dispensed by the same person, such as a witch doctor or shaman. Although faith can be separate from religion, the two are often entangled. Religion might imply the regularity of church attendance, prayer, devout adherence to religious practices, or the comfort it brings to believers. Religion can be orthodox with strict practices, a practice of daily rituals, or an anchor in times of trouble and need. Religion and faith are often linked and deeply tied to values. Although practices are shared by some families, others have big differences. Views include fundamental believers from the Bible Belt (a region in the south and south-central part of the United States) along with those with traditional Protestant, Catholic, Jewish, Mormon, Jehovah's Witnesses, Quaker, Amish, or other types of beliefs. Others hold one of the other world

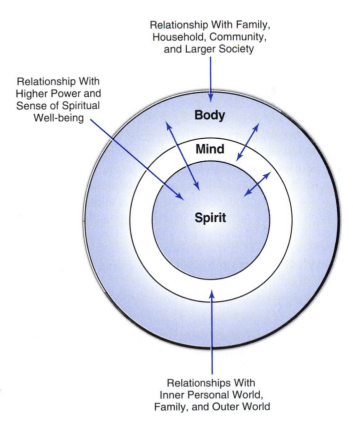

FIGURE 6-2 Relationships of body, mind, and spirit.

religions as sacred, such as Muslim, Hinduism, Buddhism, Islam, and Taoism. Others may be agnostic, atheist, pagan, wiccan, or scientologists, or may even be Gypsies or Roma. Religions often have practices linked with health, illness, and healing and influence personal lives, family lifestyles, and daily routines. When fear and uncertainty occur, religion and faith are comforts, provide peace, and give hope.

Nursing Practice to Meet Spiritual Care Needs

Nurses meet persons with different beliefs. Empirical evidence from thousands of studies documents relationships among religiousness, spirituality, faith, and health (Koenig, King, & Carson, 2012). Some strongly value their faith; others do not believe. Within a single family, religious practices may differ. Nurses who *think family* respect the beliefs of others. Culturally competent nurses are curious, respectful, and tolerant, and allow time and space for spiritual beliefs and rituals. In family-focused care, spirituality and faith should be part of assessments and be considered with nursing actions or interventions (Tanyi, 2006). For example, some may have alternative or complementary therapies tied with belief systems.

Gender Orientations

Additionally, sexuality and gender orientations can create cultural distinctions not shared by the mainstream. In 1973, the American Psychiatric Association eliminated homosexuality from its list of disorders. Families with gay, lesbian, bisexual, or transgender members (referred to as GLBT) have unique problems when it comes to health care. Who has the right to make important health care decisions? Gay and lesbian couples are often treated differently than their heterosexual couple counterparts in decision-making autonomy. Consider this situation:

Patricia and Dorothy are in their early 70s and have lived together as partners for the last 40 years. Before retirement Patricia was an English college professor at a small liberal arts college, and Dorothy was a nurse manager on a medical/surgical unit. Even though most people in their community know they live together, only their closest friends know of their committed relationship. Many of Patricia and Dorothy's family members also are not aware of the nature of their relationship. A few days ago Dorothy was admitted to a neurological unit with a severe stroke. She is out of the critical phase, but her motor abilities on the left side of her body are severely impaired and she is aphasic. Patricia has spent many hours at the bedside, but now two of Dorothy's siblings who live out of state have arrived and started to make decisions regarding Dorothy's future. Patricia has different ideas about the situation, but finds it hard to speak up as the siblings consider her merely a roommate.

As a nurse caring for Dorothy, what actions would you take? Do you have responsibilities as a family advocate? What do your state laws dictate about rights of cohabiting partners in health care decision making? Laws and rights are changing. Nurses can find a situation such as this awkward and might try to avoid the room or discussion. Box 6.8 provides information to consider in caring for GLBT individuals or families.

Transgender Individuals

Caring for a transgendered person might seem a challenge to cultural sensitivities. A transgendered person is one born with certain sexual organs but believes his or her true gender is the opposite. Gender dysphoria is not the same as sexual orientation or being a transsexual or transvestite. Although sexual orientation speaks to a physical or emotional attraction to another person (e.g., straight, gay, bisexual, lesbian), gender dysphoria has to do with a personal sense of knowing you are of a different sex. Chaz Bono is perhaps the

> **BOX 6-8**
>
> **Caring for Gay, Lesbian, Bisexual, and Transgender (GLBT) Persons and Families**
>
> Nurses often do not have experience giving care or working with GLBT persons or their families. Here are some things to consider in developing a caring and culturally sensitive relationship:
>
> - People who are identified as GLBT should be treated as unique individuals rather than seeing them as a certain type of person.
> - Some clients might express being GLBT to you as a professional/confidante, but might not yet have discussed this with their family. Respecting confidentiality is thus an important obligation to maintain.
> - Therapies such as "conversion therapy" have been shown to be highly ineffective and even harmful.
> - Identify who the patient has chosen as primary contacts and respect the patient's wishes.
> - Nurses should ensure that the rights of GLBT patients are incorporated in hospital policies, standards, and guidelines (e.g., visiting policies).
> - Nurses have a professional responsibility to take action when they witness discriminatory behavior toward GLBT persons or any other patients.
> - A patient's race, gender, or sexual orientation should never be grounds for refusing care or giving a lesser standard of care.

best known transgendered person. New questions about gender identity arise with the case of Army Pfc. Bradley Manning, the man who tested complex questions about espionage, journalism, and treason by leaking classified documents. He has been sentenced to 35 years in a male prison, but wants to be known as Chelsea Manning. Courts have decided that not providing hormone therapy to inmates is cruel and unusual treatment, but this decision has not been tested by the military. What bias or assumptions about transgendered persons do you hold? What does being culturally sensitive in this situation imply? What needs does a family with a transgendered member have?

Intersex Individuals

Other sexual differences are also found. Intersex people, those with disorders of sexual development or sexual anatomy, can cause great consternation to physicians and parents. Gender usually gets labeled at birth. The first question people ask is: Was it a boy or girl? Biological variations or ambiguous genitalia are not always clearly visible at birth. The need to distinguish gender has led to morally questionable decisions and troubling surgical procedures. Cultural implications of gender orientation raise questions of fear, shame, secrecy, bullying, and other troubles for families. Nurses meet individuals and families that are coping with the uncertainty and stress of these types of obscure situations. Families need nurses who can offer safe, respectful, and sensitive responses during these emotionally painful times.

The Power of Family Stories for Learning About Cultural Needs

Every family has stories, noteworthy descriptions of what is valued. Some stories are told repeatedly at family gatherings or at special times. Stories are powerful tools for understanding responses to health, illness, caregiving, and hardships. Nurses meet people at times of crisis or stress, when relationships and resources are strained. Stories can help nurses learn the ways problems get solved, decisions made, family work divided or shared, and traditional life patterns maintained. Stories provide insights into family roles and behaviors. Nurses who *think family* value family stories as a way to learn and collaborate in decision making and planning care.

When families are in a highly stressful situation, they often refer to past situations or experiences. For example, they might preface things with words such as "my aunt said . . .," "my cousin told me . . .," or "when my father went to the hospital. . . ." Initially, this information might not seem pertinent. Yet, it can offer insights into the ways families assist their members. If a family member talks about when her daughter experienced uncontrollable pain and nothing could be done about it, this might indicate fears about current treatment. A grandmother reflecting about how she delivered her baby can convey information about culture or values. Stories might refer to media where members get advice.

As people share their stories, pay close attention to body language. When do people stop talking or withdraw? Are there topics that change the dynamics of the conversation? Do people change the topic when sensitive things are discussed? Note these things and, if appropriate, ask for clarification. For example, you might say something like "I noticed that the tone of the conversation changed when the diagnosis was brought up; does this mean something special?" Silence might occur. It might be tempting to think it is the nurse's responsibility to break this silence. However, allowing silence can be an important form of communication. The family's culture might allow more time for quiet, or it might be full of vigorous and loud member interactions. Nurses can be curious and inquire about stories to clarify understanding:

- How have you handled similar situations in the past?
- Tell me about some of your family strengths.
- What roles do family members have in giving care to the ill person?
- What would be most helpful, in your view?

Information obtained, the findings, can be turned into a customized plan of care and include the following:

- Accommodations (e.g., location, type, adequacy of family household)
- Use of culturally sensitive assessment tools (e.g., pain scale)
- Identification of those to involve in decision making

Building Trust

Trust is an essential factor when it comes to nursing care. It takes time to get to know someone and build a foundation for competently delivering needed care. Consider this case:

A former high school principal was admitted to a home care program after a stroke. The family anxiously awaits the intake nurse's arrival. Family members have questions about special aids they think will help (e.g., bars in the bathroom, an alarm system, hospital bed). His daughter has questions about prescribed medications and worries about side effects. His wife, a legal immigrant from Taiwan, has concerns about the social effects of his aphasia. When the nurse arrives, she has pages of paperwork to complete and another visit to complete. Some questions are about insurance and whether he meets payment criteria. The nurse has multiple assessments to complete. She starts on the forms immediately and often looks at her watch when family speaks. The nurse has trouble understanding his wife and directs most questions to the daughter who questions her mother and repeats responses. The nurse completes the assessments and leaves. After the nurse is gone, family members realize that none of their questions were answered. As the nurse drives away, she reflects on what happened and thinks, "They are a nice family; this was a successful intake visit."

Think about that situation. Does the family think the visit went well? Did the nurse focus on tasks or family's needs? What might have been done differently to better satisfy this family's needs? Were there any cultural barriers? Each family situation offers opportunities and choices to build trust. What things might this nurse have done differently?

Good communication requires intentional verbal and nonverbal presence. Developing trust should be a priority before getting "right to the point" of the care delivery. Quickly creating a safe place for families where they can share their stories takes a nurse with strong family communication skills. Showing empathy with the suffering and needs of others can help build trust. As nurses, most have had the experience of losing someone or something we love and can use this experience to help sense what it is like to be in the shoes of others facing loss. Quickly creating a safe place for families where they can share their stories takes a nurse with strong family communication skills (Box 6.9).

Managing Time

The first step in making a trust connection is taking time to be present with families. Nurses always have a plethora of tasks and responsibilities. With many demands on highly valued time, it might seem overwhelming to think about talking with families. You might be tempted to classify this activity as nonessential. Trust is an important building block for highly valued relationships. Taking time to listen is an important way to break through barriers and minimize future caregiving challenges. Thoughtful sharing can provide insight and awareness of needs. When you hurry or are unable to spend time, tell those getting care when you will return. Be sure to keep your word and return as promised.

Small Talk or High-Level Assessment

Talking with others in meaningful ways does not come easily to everyone. Nurses are often unaware of topics they avoid or things they ignore. Nurses often spend time engaged in

---

BOX 6-9

Evidence-Based Family Nursing Practice

Cross-cultural measurement of family phenomena can be especially challenging when the desire is to consider illness or health-related phenomena. Families are social groups with different subjective experiences that can be best understood using an ecological framework or theory. If we are to exchange ideas among people from different nations or ethnicities, then understandings about culture and language must be considered. These things can be especially different based upon whether the culture is individualistic or collectivist. Individualistic implies that ties are loose and everyone is expected to care for oneself and their family. Collectivism implies people are integrated into cohesive groups that have a sense of duty, responsibility, and interdependence upon one another. Key considerations for research and practice are selection of the instrument or assessment tool, determination of the goal of evaluation, translation of the survey instrument, and the cross-cultural equivalence of measures. Five dimensions of cross-cultural equivalence should be considered: content, semantics, technical, criterion, and conceptual. Families assess their own environment and describe it based upon their experience. Nurses must first be aware of their personal cultural experience before they can become more fully aware of the family's culture. It is important to guard against thinking that individual members of a group can be predicted by group characteristics. The general characteristics of a group of people should not be applied automatically to a particular family.

Source: Looman, W. (2011). Cross-cultural considerations for measurement in family nursing. In E. K. Svavrsdottir & H. Jonsdottir (Eds.), *Family nursing in action*. Reykjavik, Iceland: University of Iceland Press.

what might be called "small talk," which is easy chatter that occurs when giving care. High-level assessment implies thoughtful interactions around meaningful and pertinent topics relevant to present or potential needs. This approach implies asking the difficult questions and having conversations about things that might be less comfortable. Consider two different scenarios involving families are met in a hospice setting:

> Ben, a newly graduated nurse, is admitting a patient to the hospice program. Multiple family members are present. Ben enters the room and while standing says, "I have some assessment information to collect from you." Ben proceeds with the survey. He thinks some questions are awkward, such as: Do you have any sexual concerns? Have you been emotionally or physically abused? Do you have any religious beliefs that might affect your care? He asks the questions, quickly writes down the answers, and goes to the next question. He is uncomfortable, fidgets with his pen, and shifts from one leg to another. He completes the form. As he walks away he thinks: "I am glad that is over, I have so many important things yet to get done."

In the next room Sarah, a nurse with 8 years of experience, is admitting a hospice patient. Rather than having the form in front of her, she introduces herself, sits down and speaks to the gentleman being admitted and his family. She involves them all. They explain how hard it is to see these latest changes. Sarah nods her head and says, "This must be very painful. . . . How has it changed the ways you relate to one another?" They openly discuss how the disease has changed their lives and physical intimacy. She turns to other family members and asks, "What are your biggest concerns right now?" Patiently, Sarah nods her head as she listens to the things they share. During the conversation, Sarah takes a few notes on her pad. Sarah then says, "I want to give you some time to get settled. I will be back in about 10 minutes to complete the intake assessment form." Sarah goes to the nursing station and documents some things she observed and learned. She looks at her watch to be sure to return in 10 minutes to complete the assessment.

In our rapidly paced society taking time to listen might seem like a luxury, but is it? Think about these two different approaches. If this was your family, which nurse would you rather have? Whenever we meet new people, expect some barriers. A first step is always wise use of our time. Every interaction is an opportunity to add information and gather facts. Rather than merely acting based upon our own assumptions or needs, we can use time and tasks to build trust, develop relationships, and satisfy needs of those needing care (de Ruiter & Demma, 2011). High-level assessment can help avoid misunderstandings and future frustrations.

Cultural assessment is ongoing as more information is needed over time. A basic question like "How are you doing?" is not intended as small talk, but as a way to gather useful information about care needs. Use of open-ended questions is a useful way to obtain information about culturally unique needs:

- What kinds of things would assist you to be more comfortable while you are here?
- What questions do you have about plans for your care?
- When you go home, what uncertainties do have in managing care?
- The doctor has suggested a special diet for you. How will this fit with the way you usually eat at home?

Inquiry about family needs for care at home is a good conversation starter. Open-ended questions can help you learn about culturally distinct needs and lead to teaching moments. High-level assessment often feels like an ongoing conversation, not just questions. See Box 6.10 to identify a situation where you can begin putting your knowledge about culture to work.

BOX 6-10
Family Circle

Martin, a 17-year-old male patient with terminal leukemia, was recently admitted to a pediatric oncology unit for care. He has lived in a large extended family household with his mother, grandmother, aunt, and three cousins for the last 10 years. Martin's grandmother came to the United States from Cuba when her daughters were young teens. Martin's mother, a single parent, is juggling two full-time jobs to make ends meet. She is often stressed about the troubling situations faced as she tries to meet financial costs and care for her terminally ill son. Martin's grandmother gains strength from her religion and is active at her church. She has taken her grandchildren to church with her and instilled strong moral values. Most days she is busy taking care of her grandchildren while her daughters work. Martin has a 16-year-old girlfriend, Josephine. She has an unstable home life and little contact with her family. She often stays with friends. Josephine has been Martin's main support over the last few months. During the current admission Martin's family has not been able to stay at the hospital very much. Martin's girlfriend has stayed overnight at his home on several occasions with his mother's consent, but his grandmother does not approve. His girlfriend is spending a great deal of time at the hospital and wants to stay at night. One of the nurses said that she needs a note from her parents giving her permission to stay. She says that she has no contact with her parents. As a nurse caring for Martin, consider two different perspectives you might take. How might you respond differently if you approached their care from a traditional perspective or one that is family focused? In the following list of questions, identify some ways you might respond using each perspective:

1. As a nurse, what might you say to Martin's girlfriend?
2. As a nurse, what kinds of things will you say to Martin?
3. As a nurse, what things will you discuss with Martin's mother on her next visit? With his grandmother?
4. In what ways might religion be a factor in this family situation?
5. What cultural concerns will you address?
6. How will you identify and plan for the pressing concerns this family is likely facing?

Transcultural Nursing Assessment Tool

The Transcultural Assessment Model is a basic assessment tool that includes six areas that reflect ways people demonstrate culturally distinct patterns of identifiable behaviors (Giger & Davidhizar, 1991, 2002). Be cautious and observe for variations within a single culture. Age, gender, religion, and other features can create these variances (Box 6.11). This model encourages individual participation in assessment so the complexities of family life can be learned.

Culture and Communication Barriers

Cultural differences can create troublesome barriers to effective communication. To the extent possible, nurses need to be creative and maintain maximum flexibility to best satisfy care needs. Nurses, as advocates, can help create or adapt systems in ways that better address cultural needs. Routinization occurs when nurses' institutional tasks become routine (Chambliss, 1996). Some tasks are done on a routine basis and it can be difficult to see how others perceive these actions. Suppose that while resuscitating a patient nurses were also viewing television in the room. Nurses may be comfortable with resuscitation, but the family is not and could perceive this action as indifference. Care must be taken to avoid doing things in a robotic fashion. Before changes can be made, needs must be recognized.

BOX 6-11

Assessment of Culturally Distinct Behaviors

The following six areas reflect ways people demonstrate culturally distinct patterns of identifiable behaviors:

1. Communication: Verbal and nonverbal differences in communication can lead to misunderstandings and miscommunication that creates riffs between the nurse and person(s) receiving care. For instance, eye contact is a behavior with different cultural meanings.
2. Space: Closeness and distance of personal space differ, as do body movements, touching, and closeness or distance.
3. Social organization: Those from different cultures may have different rules linked with their dominant culture (e.g., respect, member roles, inheritance, gender, age expectations).
4. Time: Values concerning time may be different in relation to valuing the past and its traditions, importance of the present, and regard for the future.
5. Environmental control: Environment describes where one lives, but also the dynamic systems and processes that influence health or illness (e.g., health practices, religious beliefs, rituals, taboos).
6. Biological variation: Consider similarities and differences in body structure, skin coloring, hair texture, physical traits, genetic characteristics, and nutritional preferences.

Source: Giger, J. N., & Davidhizar, R. E. (1991). *Transcultural nursing: Assessment and intervention*. St. Louis: Mosby.

Culture, Literacy, and Low Health Literacy

Do not confuse literacy with health literacy. Literacy is the ability to read and use numbers. Health literacy is defined as the capacity to obtain, process, and understand basic health information and access services needed to make health decisions (U.S. Department of Health and Human Services, 2014). Even well-educated persons can have low health literacy. Thus, all information shared must satisfy the needs of those seeking care. If individuals have low language proficiency, whatever the reason, nurses need to use assistive tools or devices to effectively communicate. Brochures, written documents, or quick verbal directions can be inadequate ways to transfer information. Low health literacy can mean appointment cards or medication labels are not understood. Failure to comprehend can lead to devastating, unwanted, and detrimental outcomes. Families need to be able to follow prescribed treatment safely, know how to prevent risks and complications, and be able to describe needs for follow-up care.

Assessments must include literacy and health literacy. It is a disservice to assume persons are literate or illiterate because they are from a certain cultural background. When language differences occur, nurses must be responsive. Dealing with multiple health professionals, services, systems, and treatments is a hurdle for those who read at a sixth-grade level or below. Thinking family is a good starting point when previously successful care strategies (e.g., ways medications are taken at home) are explored for planning to meet current care needs.

Culture and Privacy, Confidentiality, and Ethics

Some issues around privacy and confidentiality were discussed in Chapter 4. Using a cultural lens to address family concerns can result in unpredictable issues related to what is private, confidential, or ethical. Some may be uncomfortable speaking about diagnosis with others. Topics like mental illness and sexual behaviors are often accompanied by cultural values.

When medically prescribed treatments are not valued in cultural terms, culture can support or thwart adherence. What is private and what can be shared? Questions about who owns or has rights to information can vary depending upon cultural ideas. With which family members can information be shared? What is considered confidential may be interpreted differently based upon cultural beliefs. Nurses who *think family* are sensitive to cultural nuances that influence ways in which families view information, actions, and relationships. Nurses can be in delicate positions when deciding the who, what, when, and how in sharing information. Although these are concerns for all families, it can be even more challenging when cultural barriers exist.

Ethical dilemmas about ways to have trusting relationships with persons calling themselves family can arise. When persons receiving care can clearly state what they want and control the flow of information, things are relatively easy. However, when persons cannot speak for themselves, knowing how to communicate information appropriately and who to speak with can be misunderstood. Persons might not want some information disclosed. Absolute answers to solve ethical dilemmas are not available. Using ethical principles and applying them to culturally sensitive family-focused care can help. Sometimes decisions must be made quickly or under duress. Maintaining confidentiality is always important and being culturally sensitive can help prevent behaviors or actions that might be interpreted incorrectly. During initial assessments gather and document information about who is privy to personal information, but also who to include in decision making and planning. Asking questions to access needed information can prevent facing dilemmas later. Of course, laws, guidelines, regulations, and policies must be followed.

Chapter Summary

The cultural complexity of society continues to grow. Nurses will be giving care to people and families with varied cultural beliefs, values, and practices. The provision of culturally sensitive care must not be taken lightly. Although cultural knowledge is important, sensitivity to unique needs within cultures and family units must be considered. Nurses can learn about cultures as they meet families with curiosity and inquiry. Culturally sensitive nurses have examined their personal biases and assumptions around varied topics that address cultural diversity. Employment of excellent communication skills that address areas of distinct needs will help nurses develop effective relationships with those in their care.

REFERENCES

Anderson, G. F., & Hussey, P. S. (2000). Population aging: A comparison among industrialized countries. *Health Affairs, 12,* 191–203.

Campinha-Bacote, J. (2002). The process of cultural competence in the delivery of healthcare services: A model of care. *Journal of Transcultural Nursing, 13*(3), 181–184.

Carson, V. B. (1989). *Spiritual dimensions of nursing practice.* Philadelphia: W. B. Saunders.

Chambliss, D. (1996). *Beyond caring: Hospitals, nurses, and the social organization of ethics.* Chicago: University of Chicago Press.

Denham, S. A. (2003). *Family health: A framework for nursing.* Philadelphia: F. A. Davis.

De Ruiter, H. P., & Demma, J. (2011). Nursing: The skill and art of being in a society of multitasking. *Creative Nursing, 17*(1), 25–29.

Gany, F. M., Herrera, A. P., Avallone, M., & Changrani, J. (2006). Attitudes, knowledge, and health-seeking behaviors of five immigrant minority communities in the prevention and screening of cancer: A focus group approach. *Ethnicity & Health, 11*(1), 19–39.

Giger, J. N., & Davidhizar, R. E. (1991). *Transcultural nursing: Assessment and intervention*. St. Louis: Mosby.

Giger, J. N., & Davidhizar, R. (2002). The Giger and Davidhizar Transcultural Assessment Model. *Journal of Transcultural Nursing, 13*, 185–188. doi:10.1177/10459602013003004

Koenig, H. G., King, D. E., & Carson, V. B. (2012). *Handbook of religion and health* (2nd ed.). New York: Oxford University Press.

Looman, W. (2011). Cross-cultural considerations for measurement in family nursing. In E. K. Svavrsdottir & H. Jonsdottir (Eds.), *Family nursing in action*. Reykjavik, Iceland: University of Iceland Press.

Oe, M. (2006). Problems and implications of Japan's aging society for future urban developments. Policy and Governance Working Paper Series No. 89. Retrieved June 11, 2012 from http://coe21-policy.sfc.keio.ac.jp/ja/wp/WP89.pdf

Office of Minority Health. (2007). National Standards on Culturally and Linguistically Appropriate Services (CLAS). Department of Health and Human Services. Retrieved May 11, 2012 from http://minorityhealth.hhs.gov/templates/browse.aspx?lvl=2&lvlID=15

Simon, C. M., & Kodish, E. (2005). "Step into my zapatos, Doc": Understanding and reducing communication disparities in the multicultural informed consent setting. *Perspectives in Biology and Medicine, 48*(1), 123–138.

Tanyi, R. A. (2006). Spirituality and family nursing: Spiritual assessment and interventions for families. *Journal of Advanced Nursing, 53*(3), 287–294.

Tylor, E. (1909). *Anthropology: An introduction to the study of man and civilization*. New York: D. Appleton.

U. S. Department of Health and Human Services. (2014). Healthy people 2020 topics and objectives: Health communication and health information technology. Retrieved September 3, 2014 from http://healthypeople.gov/2020/topicsobjectives2020/overview.aspx?topicid=18

CHAPTER 7

Using Family Theory to Guide Nursing Practice

Sonja J. Meiers

Introduction

Family theories, whether family science, family therapy, or family nursing theories, are useful in guiding nurses' ideas about *thinking family* and practicing innovative family-focused care. Family theories help nurses move beyond what they know from personal experiences of their own families. Personal family experiences are powerful influences on perceptions, biases, and assumptions about family. Family theories can help nurses expand thinking and provide templates for more holistic assessment. In addition, use of family theories can encourage nurses to consider broader possibilities for family-focused nursing actions than are known from their personal family lives.

This chapter presents examples of how theoretical perspectives can be used to guide family-focused thinking and actions. Core elements of family science and family therapy theories are described and differentiated from family nursing theories. Finally this chapter demonstrates how existing family science, family therapy, and family nursing theories and models can guide family-focused nursing actions when considering the realms of family coping, development, interaction, and integrity.

Family Theories: What They Are and How They Help

The family, as a system, socially constructs its reality (Reiss, 1987). When families initially form and then later add members, they seldom fully plan the future or see future challenges. Risks and threats to the family system happen when unintended events occur in families. Life happens. Life events influence choices and decisions. Families evolve and develop boundaries that are open to influences from the outside, closed to such influences, or flexible (Olson & Gorall, 2003). This fluctuation can depend upon the situation, but also on family roles, goals, and purposes. Family boundaries also differ and may change over time. Attention needs to be given to boundaries. Behaviors such as touching, hugging, and personal distance signal some information about these boundaries. A family might be predominately opened or closed, but stress can cause the family to take a contrary position until the stressor is decreased or suffering is lessened. For instance, a family may appear open to others, but this openness might be due to one member with an especially extroverted personality. If this person becomes critically ill, more introverted family members might be less welcoming. Nurses' understandings about family systems have grown over time. An early family nursing theory contributed by Marilyn Friedman drew upon ideas of structural-functional systems and family development theories (Friedman, 1981). Friedman suggested that family is an open system that interacts with a variety of societal institutions (e.g., health care, education, religion). Her family assessment ideas are widely taught in nursing classes across the world.

Family Science

Family scientists and family nursing professionals base their ideas and recommendations for family care on observations of family life and member interactions. These theories are mainly concerned with the ways that families function, develop, and interact with environments. Nurses are mostly concerned with what occurs around families' health and illness experiences. Family theories developed by family scientists, when used by nurses, are generally viewed as borrowed theories. Nurses use family science theories to understand complex family member interactions and the varied dynamics that influence health and illness (McEwin & Wills, 2011). Family science has enhanced discovery of approaches to family nursing care. Social science theories largely focus on the form or structure of families (e.g., nuclear, single parent, cohabiting), ways members interact to accomplish needed functions (e.g., parenting, socialization, economics), and developmental tasks (e.g., young versus middle age or older families). Those ideas are often only loosely relevant to nursing practice. For example, a nurse assesses a family's type and finds that it is a cohabiting family. This helps the nurse know who to include in parenting tasks if the mother is acutely ill. However, theories about family type and evidence about effectiveness of the cohabiting parents may not be especially useful at the time of a critical illness or to direct care.

The family satisfies certain core societal functions such as in the nurture and protection of children or the provision of stable economics. Another core function of families is fostering societal survival by producing new members to replace dying members and socializing these new members to eventually enacting adult roles. Families also transmit shared norms and values from one generation to the next. To meet these functional needs, families are structured in ways that use differentiated roles such as parent, child, economic provider, and home organizer.

Think about your own family. What roles does each person serve? What happens if a member does not fulfill an expected role? Think about a crisis or acute situation, when surgery or an intensive care stay in the hospital is required. What happens within the family? Who is filling usual roles? How might families differ in needs? Suppose a mother caring for an autistic child is unexpectedly hospitalized as a result of an automobile accident. What stressors might she and her family have? Can an individual crisis become a family crisis? Family science theories can be used to consider the complexity of what needs to be assessed and can guide nursing actions in organized and purposeful ways.

Family Therapy

Family therapy aims to understand relationships and interactions within family groups rather than merely considering needs of single individuals. Nurses need some knowledge from what is known about family therapy even though they are not involved in psychotherapy. Nurses need to know how to sensitively collaborate within the family to meet family expectations. Family therapy usually involves several family meetings and is focused on resolving problems within the family. Family-focused nursing differs from this type of intense family therapy. Nurses with family therapy backgrounds use family therapy theories to contribute knowledge for family-focused nursing (Wright & Leahy, 2013). Yet, family therapy theories cannot always adequately guide nursing actions when it comes to health and illness.

Usefulness of Family Nursing Theories and Models

Using family nursing theories to guide nursing actions begins with careful assessment of situations involving those seeking care. Nurses who work with families recognize the interdependence of families with other social units and larger communities. Nurses who *think family* assess family needs and capacities for supporting health and illness. Family nursing theories provide perspectives for planning, implementing, and evaluating care (Box 7.1).

Theories are like road maps; they suggest paths of action or directions to a desired destination. A mapped destination can be compared to a desired goal or outcome. Assessment data provide specific information about things to consider in choosing destinations and directions. Assessment continues along the path to the destination and ensures that the

---

BOX 7-1

Usefulness of Family Theories

Family theories can suggest ways nurses can:

- Empathize with and interpret family members' strengths and limitations.
- Comprehend the family and community context that influences needs and outcomes.
- Collaborate or partner with family units throughout the health or illness experience.

Family nursing practice, like most other aspects of nursing practice, requires the nurse to have a cadre of strategies in the nursing practice toolkit:

- Scientific or evidence-based knowledge
- Experience with various methods of communicating
- Skills for interacting in culturally sensitive ways
- Theoretical ideas for forming and directing nursing practice
- Artful ways to partner with individuals and family members whenever and wherever nursing care is provided

target point is reached in an efficient and timely way. Theories equip nurses with particular mind-sets that can help them think about their actions in coherent ways. Along the path to meeting goals, nurses make meaningful discoveries about family fears, uncertainties, and strengths that can be used in work with families (Meiers & Tomlinson, 2003).

Planned strategies for reaching goals need to be analyzed to see which strategies best fit with the family. For instance, if you were taking a trip, you might consider the type and size of luggage, what things to take along, best ways to travel, and how much money will be needed. Planning for family care uses the same process. Moving from a novice nurse to an experienced one takes time and effort (Benner, 1982). Beginning nurses learn basic tasks through direct instruction. As they become experts within the clinical context, they develop an intuitive grasp of clinical nursing practice. Family-focused nursing can seem incredibly challenging to the novice, but becomes less daunting with experience. Theory can guide family-focused practice, redirect courses of action when needed, and help nurses use nurse-family relationships to clarify ideas and employ the best actions in timely ways.

Family Nursing Theories and Models

Family nursing science addresses broad ideas to help nurses understand how families influence and are influenced by illness experiences and the ways members support others, increase healing, and decrease suffering (Wright & Bell, 2009). Family nursing theories can enhance understanding about the family process to promote well-being and health and manage ways illness events affect families. Five family nursing theories or models that guide nursing actions are presented in the following section. Each theory provides a unique framework or way to think about family-focused nursing practice. Family nurses can use theories and models to guide partnerships with families.

Calgary Family Intervention Model

Wright and Leahey (2013) developed the Calgary Family Assessment Model (CFAM) and the companion model, the Calgary Family Intervention Model (CFIM). These models have led the way for family nursing practice worldwide by helping nurses identify family strengths, resources, and actions to take in situations of health and illness. The CFAM suggests that illness situations have concerns primarily focused on a particular member, but the situation is best evaluated when related problems are linked within the larger family context. The CFAM guides the nurse to assess family developmental stages, structure, and function to gain the relevant information for guiding nursing actions. The CFIM is strength based and resiliency based with the goal of supporting optimal family functioning. CFIM-guided nursing actions promote, improve, or sustain family functioning in the cognitive, affective, and functional domains associated with family life (Box 7.2). Nursing actions are tailored to family needs and an area of family functioning is identified for action. The CFIM can guide actions across a range of health promotion and illness situations.

Family Health System Model

The Family Health System Model (FHS) considers family health and informally guides family nursing practice (Anderson & Tomlinson, 1992). This model assumes that family health is systemic, process based, and includes individual and family unit interactions. The health of the individual affects the whole family. Changes in health demand or imply needed changes in member roles, household resource demands, or alterations in daily

---

BOX 7-2

Using the Calgary Family Intervention Model (CFIM)

Several nursing actions may be guided by the CFIM:

- Commending family and individual strengths
- Offering information and opinions
- Validating or normalizing responses
- Encouraging the telling of illness narratives
- Drawing forth family support
- Encouraging family members to be caregivers and offering caregiver support
- Encouraging respite
- Devising rituals

Source: Wright, L., & Leahy, M. (2013). *Nurses and families: A guide to family assessment and intervention* (6th ed.). Philadelphia: F. A. Davis.

---

activities. These changes influence the individual and the family simultaneously. The FHS proposes that family health and illness events include biopsychosocial aspects along with contextual systems. The goal is to achieve optimal responses in five realms and assessment in these realms can inform nursing actions (Box 7.3).

This model also suggests that it is impossible to separate family health into truly independent realms because they interact and are deeply intertwined. Nurses can use these realms to guide thinking and clinical practice in integrated ways. Individual family members and the family unit are viewed as a whole. This approach to nursing practice uses a comprehensive family assessment to address health and illness concerns (Anderson, 2000). For example, the nurse using the FHS would plan nursing actions that simultaneously consider the developmental task of becoming a new parent, of learning to interact with health care providers of a medically fragile child, the concurrent stress of family financial concerns, and the value of maintaining family privacy. The family-focused nurse is alert to the delicate intertwining and stressful nature of this situation.

Family Management Style Framework

The Family Management Style Framework (FMSF) is based upon ideas about the family's response to childhood chronic illness (Knafl & Deatrick, 1990). This model has been

---

BOX 7-3

Aspects of the Family Health Systems (FHS) Model

The FHS model identifies five realms of the family health experience:

- Interactive processes such as relationships, communication, support, nurture, other roles
- Developmental processes such as family transitions, task completion, individual development
- Coping processes such as problem solving, resource use, handling of stress and crisis
- Integrity processes such as values, beliefs, identity, rituals, and spirituality
- Health processes such as health beliefs and behaviors, illness stressors, caretaking

Source: Anderson, K. A., & Tomlinson, P. S. (1992). The family health system as an emerging paradigmatic view for nursing. *Image: Journal of Nursing Scholarship, 24,* 57–63.

refined over the past two decades (Knafl & Deatrick, 2003, 2006) and has three major components—the definition of the situation, management behaviors, and perceived consequences. The Family Management Measure (FaMM) developed from this model measures ways families manage caring for a child with a chronic illness condition and how this care management fits into everyday family life (Knafl et al., 2009). Take time to review Box 7.4 as it provides additional information about Dr. Kathy Knafl, an important American family nurse leader. Box 7.5 describes more about Dr. Janet Deatrick, an expert working with children and their families. Family members are viewed as important persons who shape and manage children's chronic conditions and incorporate chronic illness management into family life. The three components of this model shape the ways family members manage efforts. Families managing childhood chronic diseases do so in five different styles: thriving, accommodating, enduring, struggling, and floundering. Nurses working with families with young children or teens can use this theory to identify factors that support or impede optimal care of the child and support family functioning as illness care is provided, recognizing that the care approaches needed by families will be diverse and culturally distinct. For instance, three different families with female 7-year-olds with leukemia are likely to approach care needs and manage situations differently.

Illness Beliefs Model

The Illness Beliefs Model (Wright & Bell, 2009) was developed as a clinical practice model to use in family care. The model is used to identify and enhance the therapeutic ways nurses help families who are suffering in their experience of serious illness. It is

---

BOX 7-4

Family Tree

Kathleen Knafl, PhD, FAAN (United States)

Kathleen Knafl, PhD, FAAN, a Professor and Associate Dean for Research and Frances Hill Fox Distinguished Professor at the University of North Carolina at Chapel Hill, is a renowned scholar. Dr. Knafl has developed a program of research focused on describing distinct patterns of family response to the challenges presented by childhood chronic conditions leading to descriptions of family management styles that can influence family outcomes. She has explored the interplay between the ways family members define disease conditions and manage family life in the context of a child's chronic condition. She is widely published and recognized as an expert in family and research methods.

Dr. Knafl serves as a consultant to universities and mentors other researchers. She sits on editorial boards for *Research in Nursing and Health*, *Nursing Outlook*, and the *Journal of Family Nursing* and serves as a consultant to the National Institutes of Health, universities, and researchers. She was intricately involved in the formation of the International Family Nursing Association (IFNA) and instrumental in organizing the first IFNA conference in Minneapolis, Minnesota, in June 2013 and continues to serve as a leader in this organization, among others.

In collaboration with her colleagues, Janet Deatrick, RN, PhD, FAAN, and Agatha Gallo, RN, PhD, FAAN, she worked to develop the Family Management Measure (FaMM) , a valid and reliable measure of how families manage a child's chronic condition that will foster the development of interventions that support the quality of life of families living with a chronic illness. Dr. Knafl has long believed that nurses and other health care professionals can play pivotal roles in helping families adapt to a child's chronic condition. She emphasizes that we must understand the different ways families manage a child's chronic conditions, relationships between family management styles, and child and family outcomes.

BOX 7-5

Family Tree

Janet Deatrick, PhD, RN, FAAN (United States)

Dr. Janet Deatrick, a Professor of Nursing at the University of Pennsylvania's School of Nursing in Philadelphia, Pennsylvania, has served as the Co-Director of the Center for Health Equity Research. Dr. Deatrick is an expert in advanced practice pediatric nursing and caring for children with chronic conditions such as cancer. In 1995, she received the Christian and Mary Lindback Award for Distinguished Teaching. In 1997 she was recognized for her contributions to nursing research and she won the Excellence in Nursing Research Award from the Society of Pediatric Nurses.

Her efforts to explain children's and family's involvement in health-related decisions and careful observations of family management of childhood illness provide invaluable information to clinicians. Her theory-based efforts provide direction for pediatric nursing and research. She is well respected for her methodological expertise in qualitative, mixed methods, and family research. Current research focuses on caregivers and adolescent and young adult survivors of childhood brain tumors living at home with their parents. This research extends family management into oncology populations and provides a family context to caregiving research.

She has been the Principal Investigator for a series of studies funded by the Oncology Nursing Society Foundation and National Institutes of Health/National Institute of Nursing Research (NIH/NINR) regarding caregiver and survivor perception of family management and quality of life. Results will be used to develop interventions to enhance caregiver's perceived competence and survivor's quality of life. Dr. Deatrick's research collaborations with Dr. Kathleen A. Knafl has helped to develop the Family Management Measure (FaMM). This measure systematically recognizes multidimensional family processes involved in disease management for children with serious health problems. Dr. Deatrick has supported the development, mission, and conferences of the International Family Nursing Association.

---

used to discover family core and value-laden beliefs that may constrain or facilitate health or healing. Constraining beliefs are those that are self-sabotaging to health and may be debilitating. For instance, a belief that one is completely responsible for care of an illness, accident, or injury can influence engagement of family caregivers. Similarly, in a family that feels suffering is deserved and to be endured, the family may not seek outside help in times of need. Once beliefs are identified, they can be discussed with family members and might direct ways to collaborate and solve problems. The Illness Beliefs Model can be used to create therapeutic conversations that uncover and challenge constraining beliefs. It can also be used to facilitate beliefs that lead to more healthful actions. The nurse carefully listens to what is said, observes nonverbal actions, and identifies with the family what is needed.

Family Health Model

The Family Health Model (FHM), described earlier in Chapter 2, is used throughout this textbook to demonstrate ways health and illness are intricately linked with individual, family, and community lives (Denham, 2003). This theory explains or predicts some ways ecological ideas can influence family health and illness and describes ways interdependent member interactions influence outcomes. The family household niche, a central aspect of the FHM, is where:

- Family health is potentially produced or threatened.
- Individuals are socialized about health and illness.
- Rituals and routine patterns with health potentials and threats are practiced.

The domains of the FHM, contextual, functional, and structural, provide ways to view how complex systems influence multimember households' responses to health and illness over time. The three domains suggest areas to assess; ways to identify, plan, and implement nursing actions; and methods for evaluating care outcomes. For example, the core processes—caregiving, cathexis, celebration, change, communication, connectedness, and coordination—are ways to *think family* and plan nursing actions. The core processes are explained in more depth in Chapter 14. Nurses who *think family* can use the FHM to address multiple household factors that come into play with health or illness. For example, Mr. Smith is a long-time employee of Amazon. He has received a promotion to manage an outlet store in a rural area. After only living in an urban area, he is uncertain what the move will mean for his family. The promotion means a large pay increase and an opportunity to move up in the company, but his wife has lupus and regularly sees a specialist in their current community. She has had flare-ups over the past few months and he is worried about her changing care providers. The move means finding a new specialist and the nearest one will be an hour drive. If he decides to move and his wife is admitted to the hospital where you work, the FHM can help you understand the family's multiple stressors and plan ways to best address care needs.

Major Realms of Family Science Important for Family-Focused Care

The realms of family coping, development, interactions, and integrity are areas that must be considered when *thinking family*. These realms are relevant to family nursing practice (Anderson & Tomlinson, 1992) and are common areas of consideration across family science, family therapy, and family nursing theories and models. Regardless of the theory or model chosen to guide assessment and to guide nursing actions, consideration of these realms can broaden family-focused nursing practice. Various approaches can be taken to family-focused care while considering these major realms.

Family Coping

Family losses are central to stressful events (Boss, 2003). Illness places great demands on individuals and family capacities as stressors pile up and vulnerability increases (Kaakinen, Coehlo, Steele, Tabacco, & Hanson, 2015). Material and emotional resources can be severely strained by the stress of illness experiences. Usual ways of managing may be ineffective when unexpected events occur or severe long-term illness is experienced. Even families that usually manage daily stressors well may be poorly equipped to handle crisis, illness consequences, or permanent disabilities. Daily family life presents many areas to balance and it can be challenging to manage normal health-promoting measures or other changes, especially when multiple crises are occurring simultaneously.

Nurses may observe only a small portion of a family's illness experience and may be oblivious to the extensive or long-term effects of illnesses that remain after the acute episode is over. Families are often ill prepared to cope with chronic conditions, accidents that cause lasting changes, or terminal diagnoses. Nurses often focus on the immediate tasks of care delivery, but may be blinded to the troubling effects a situation has on the family unit. It often seems easier to attend to technology and teach about medication use, for instance, than attend to coping challenges for families.

Paying attention to emotional, functional, social, or resource difficulties in family coping is different from the more familiar nursing tasks of providing acute care. Illness can have an aftermath that extends far beyond the present. Injuries, terminal illness, and birth anomalies are often unexpected and alter the family's future and sometimes the family's identity in irreversible and tragic ways. To understand and support family coping, it is helpful for the nurse to learn the following:

- Usual actions or responses to sudden unknown or difficult events
- The ways members have cared for one another in past troubling times
- Strategies they have used successfully to handle other difficult problems

How families manage stress provides insight into possible solutions for other troubling times. Stress can disturb the equilibrium or balance that most families try to achieve. Managing stress often requires problem-solving skills of multiple-member households. Stress is often viewed from past personal experiences and perceptions. Thus, persons from a single family can experience shared experiences differently. Unexpected events can create strains and demands for which families are ill prepared and have no previous experience.

Managing Family Stress

Family stress occurs when the family unit is challenged by an environment that overwhelms collective resources and threatens member well-being and health (Boss, 2003). Hill (1971), one of the original family stress researchers, proposed the ABCX model. In this theory, the "A" factor pertains to the stressor or the provoking event that places pressure for change on the family system. Illness is often a stressor. The "B" factor represents the strengths and resources of the system that enable the family to deal with stressors (e.g., financial, cognitive, social support needs). The "C" factor is the meaning or perception of the event for the family. The meaning a particular family gives an event influences their perceptions. Reactions are based on perceptions of what is or might occur rather than the reality of the event. The "X" factor is the outcome of the "ABC" process; the outcome can be viewed as low to high stress or a crisis. Family resources, the B factors, are critical because they influence the ways family members manage the stress factors (McCubbin, McCubbin, Thompson, & Futrell (1998). Individual and family problem-solving abilities, communication patterns, flexibility, cohesion, and boundary clarity are some of the resources that influence family stress management (Kaakinen et al., 2015).

Figure 7.1 depicts the way the ABCX theory might work in the following situation. A 23-year-old husband (A. H.) and father is diagnosed with an aggressive form of acute myelogenous leukemia (AML). Think about his hospitalization and isolation in a bone marrow unit away from his child and other family members (the A factor). The strengths and resources of supportive parents, his faith community, the joy of being a parent of a 1-year-old (C. H.), and a happy marriage to B. H. are positive B factors. However, the lack of full health insurance coverage and worries about high out-of-pocket costs are negative B factors. The AML diagnosis is a perceived threat to this short marriage, new parenting role, and future plans, dreams, and family goals (the C factors). The resulting X factor may be the high stress as a result of the perception of threat to the integrity of the family. In daily work, nurses frequently meet families coping with high stress X factors yet may not comprehend the meaning of the stress to the family.

McCubbin and Patterson (1983) further developed Hill's (1971) ABCX model by adding the notion that family stressor pileup occurs when unresolved aspects of an initial stressor accumulate. An accumulation of stressful events limits abilities to resolve one problem before another event occurs. Thus, family resources are depleted. An example might be a family with a child diagnosed with cystic fibrosis who experiences frequent critical exacerbations requiring repeated hospitalizations. At the same time, an older sibling is experiencing bullying in school. The mother loses her job, which is the only job that has the needed health insurance. Pileup is a frequent occurrence in families with aging or younger persons and

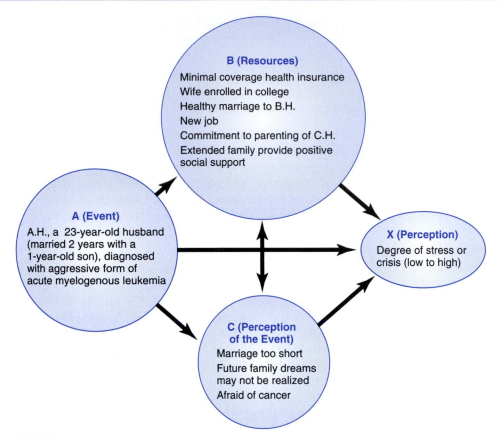

FIGURE 7-1 Family care based on Hill's ABC-X Model of Family Stress.
Adapted from Hill, R. (1971). *Families under stress.* Westport, CT: Greenwood Press (original work published 1949).

families with chronically ill family members. Technological advancements and innovative new therapies mean that today's families are living with uncertainties and tenuous situations of illness and it's not clearly visible unless a family assessment is done. Families that communicate easily with one another and have satisfactorily resolved problems in the past are likely to have a more effective toolkit for managing stress than others. Families with fragile communication or ongoing conflict might find resolving their coping difficulties hopeless.

Nursing Care to Enhance Family Coping

A goal for family-focused nursing is to assist persons and families in decreasing the stress linked with health and illness experiences and to help them find supports to enhance healing, manage care situations, and promote family health. The important topic of support is covered in Chapter 15. Identifying forms of family stress and coping during clinical experiences is important for providing family-focused nursing care (McCubbin et al., 1998b). Practical ways to solve problems and support networks are to mediate the negative stress effects and enhance well-being (Hupcey, 1999; Peterson & Bredow, 2004). Caregiving strategies, such as planning, monitoring, protecting, inquiring, vigilance, and balancing, assist family units in meeting life demands as they manage illness symptoms (Eggenberger, Krumwiede, Meiers, Bliesmer, & Earle, 2004). Family inquiry into the illness trajectory or treatment helps a family develop illness perspectives and actions that enable them to create a protective environment (Meiers, Eggenberger, Krumwiede, Bliesmer, & Earle, 2009).

Family-focused nurses encourage growth and support for family coping linked with illness by preparing families to use strategies that reduce stress. Health education, counseling, and coaching to support coping of specific families are tools family nurses use. For instance, teaching and informing parents of a medically fragile child to organize the medical care area in the child's bedroom can reduce the stress of finding things, reduce the illness reminders scattered through the house, and meet safety needs. Nursing care helps the family to have as normal a family life as possible.

Nurses can use research findings about strengths and resiliency to help families navigate through life transitions, crisis, and stress (McCubbin, McCubbin, Thompson, & Fromer, 1998a). Have you ever wondered why some people manage better than others? Have you met families that successfully manage problems and grow from stressful events while others deteriorate? Knowledge about a family's strengths and resiliency factors can help nurses establish relevant nursing actions to identify and support existing strengths. For example, A. H. gains joy and a high level of satisfaction from being with his 1-year-old child. Even though he is in protective isolation for treatment of AML, finding ways for him to remain connected could be health producing and stress reducing. Perhaps regular visual and audio connection (e.g., Skype, Face Time) through use of a computer, smartphone, or tablet would be helpful. Table 7.1 provides some other ideas for specific nursing actions to support A. H. and his family's coping using various perspectives from the five nursing models described earlier.

TABLE 7-1	*Nursing Actions to Support Family Coping Based on Family Models*	
FAMILY NURSING MODEL	**KEY MODEL CONCEPTS**	**POSSIBLE NURSING ACTIONS**
Calgary Family Intervention Model (Wright & Leahey, 2013)	Support the cognitive domain of family functioning.	• Provide literature to address uncertainties about care and community resources. • Commend family strengths: "Your family seems to work very well together to meet your challenges." • Identify specific questions of concern and collaborate to identify possible options for solutions.
Family Health System Model (FHS) (Anderson & Tomlinson, 1992)	Support five processes (i.e., interactive, developmental, coping, integrity, health).	• Help family members to understand why various members might be coping differently. • Arrange time for a family conference. • Identify ways spirituality or faith may play important roles in healing processes.
Family Management Style Framework (FMSF) (Knafl et al., 2009)	Identify important aspects of the family's definition of the situation, management of behaviors, and perceived consequences of the condition on family life.	• Guide the parents in conveying information about family member condition to siblings, friends, church members, and extended family. • Discuss perceptions of illness events.

Continued

TABLE 7-1	*Nursing Actions to Support Family Coping Based on Family Models—cont'd*	
FAMILY NURSING MODEL	**KEY MODEL CONCEPTS**	**POSSIBLE NURSING ACTIONS**
		• Affirm management behaviors. • Acknowledge fears and trauma caused by illness events throughout management of the chronic illness.
Family Health Model (Denham, 2003)	Address core processes (e.g., caregiving and cathexis).	• Provide information about specific pain management techniques and fatigue management strategies. • Listen to concerns of anticipatory grief. • Draw on the support of the church community for respite care so that couple time is preserved.
Illness Beliefs Model (Wright & Bell, 2009).	Foster conversations of affirmation and affection.	• Create a trusting, calm environment that invites open expression of family members' fears, anger, suffering and sadness, and beliefs about the illness experiences. • Commend family members for positive actions taken. • Invite questions and take time to carefully answer them.

Consider another situation. Suppose a small child is hospitalized after a severe insulin reaction that resulted in a seizure, broken teeth, and a skeletal injury from the fall that occurred during the seizure. His parents are extremely frightened as nothing like this has ever happened before. The nurse uses the Family Management Style Framework to assess coping and the plan of care (Knafl & Deatrick, 2003, 2006). What can the nurse do to identify the important aspects of the family's perceptions of the situation? Can the nurse guide the parents to diabetes-related care management information that can be conveyed to extended family, school teachers, and school friends? How can the nurse learn the family's typical management style? Think about one of the other family models previously discussed; what approaches might this model suggest? The Family Health Model (Denham, 2003) might encourage the nurse to use the structural domain and think about family health routines. The nurse might spend time doing health teaching specifically around diet or physical activity to prevent future insulin reactions. A family-focused nurse could affirm the family's positive behaviors and seek ways to build on family strengths.

Family Development

Family development is another area relevant to family-focused nursing practice. Nurses learn about various individual human developmental theories such as those of Maslow (1954), Piaget (1967), and Erickson (1950), but receive less education regarding family development theories (Table 7.2). Similar to individual development, family development describes stages or phases with associated tasks to be accomplished (Carter & McGoldrick, 1999; Duvall, 1977).

TABLE 7-2	Middle Class North American Family Life Cycle	
STAGE	**TASK OF STAGE**	**RELATIONAL STANCE OF THE NURSE**
1. Leaving home as single young adults	Accept emotional and financial responsibility for self.	Encourage independent decision making about health, lifestyle choices, intimate peer relationships, work and financial independence.
2. Joining of families through marriage: the new couple	Commit to new transitional family system.	Support the new couple in their process of constructing new family health routines.
3. Families with young children	Accept new members born or adopted into the family system.	Co-construct plans and action strategies with the family that promote healthy family lifestyles that meet unique child and family development needs.
4. Families with adolescents	Increase flexibility of family boundaries (e.g., children's growing independence, grandparent's increasing frailties).	Assist families in negotiating new family goals that integrate independence of adolescents. Counsel families on strategies for safe care of and resources for family elders.
5. Launching children and moving on	Accept the exits from and entries into the family system.	Encourage families to establish new forms of relationships from parent to adult to adult to adult as they consider various health and illness-related needs.
6. Families in later life	Accept and adapt to the shifting of generational roles.	Suggest creation of traditions and rituals that help families stay connected through shifting roles and identify ways these might be health or illness related.

Source: Adapted from Carter, B., & McGoldrick, M. (1999). *The expanded family life cycle: Individual, family and social perspectives* (3rd ed.). Boston: Allyn & Bacon.

Family Life Course

Family units and the members who compose them mature and develop over time through various developmental stages of family life (Bianchi & Casper, 2005). Developmental theories often leave gaps about such issues as launching family members at older ages into adulthood, when children leave home but return later with or without offspring, elders moving in with adult children, and the uncertain implications of aging family constellations living longer. In the past, individuals found life partners, had children, and lived together in a separate household until death. Marriage disruption, increased nonmarital cohabitation, out-of-wedlock childbirths, and multigenerational households alter the family landscape. Social mobility and migration create sometimes less than ideal geographical separations for many families. More research evidence is needed about these challenges to family development.

Family Life Course Theories consider that individuals transition from one stage of life to another (Bengston & Allen, 1993). This perspective involves the ideas of time, context, process, and other factors (Box 7.6). In Family Life Course Theory, early life events have implications for future life. Family life course is more about the evolutions families go through than fixed stages and expectations of those stages. These evolutions take in the total experience rather than a sequential ordering of age-linked events. Life course transitions can cause family conflict

---

BOX 7-6

Concepts in Life Course Theory

Life course theory principally involves the following ideas:

- Life changes are considered over a lifetime, not just at particular episodes.
- Lives are considered across a large series of cohorts rather than by a single family lineage.
- Lives are considered across life domains (e.g., work and family).
- Development is linked to personal characteristics, individual actions, cultural frames, and institutional structures.
- Lives are lived in the context of others (e.g., couples, families, cohorts).

Source: Mayer, K. U. (2009). New directions in life course research. *Annual Review of Sociology, 35,* 413–433. doi: 10.1146/annurev.soc.34.040507.134619

---

and disturbances. Think about your personal life course, which is likely briefer and different from that of your parents or grandparents. Variations among past state, current situation, and future hopes can affect responses to personal or family crisis. Talk to someone older and get a sense of how generational differences color the life course and help explain actions taken.

Families try to manage conflict and disturbances by decreasing chaos and disorganization. Family-focused nurses realize that life course transitions affect life management. Some families can adjust roles more easily than others. Think about the transition from being childless to being a parent. Once this change occurs and if the child tragically dies, the parent is unlikely to return to the same state of childlessness experienced before the birth. Many perspectives in this growing field still need to be explored, such as relationships of internal family dynamics and causal relationships, psychological processes, and social interactions. Social policies and preventive interventions need to consider what is experienced during these life course transitions (Mayer, 2009).

Uncertainty of the Life Course

Over time, families with children go through transitions. The empty nest might occur as children leave home and establish families in a different household. Some families have numerous life transitions at the same time (e.g., divorce, remarriage, parenting younger children, launching young adults, giving birth, caring for elder kinfolk). Families experience transitional points at disparate points in time. Many transitions do not fit neatly into past ideas of family development stages. Life events occur along a time trajectory linked with others in an extended family cohort across generations and time. How families change, operationalize daily lives, or structure their time to nurture and protect members is strongly influenced by the family's context and place in history (McCubbin et al., 1998b). Current experiences influence future behaviors. When nurses *think family*, they consider member placement and note life aspects that will influence care, well-being, and resources needed by those seeking care. A nurse's relational stance with those seeking care should acknowledge "not knowing" and curiosity about the family's developmental story (Wright & Leahey, 2013).

Goals to Enhance Family Development

In the developmental realm, family nurses aim to support individual and unit development throughout the life course (Table 7.3). A life course transitional approach can be useful. For instance, when caring for a family in which a 15-year-old son is learning to manage his diabetes independently, his father might be drawn away regularly to care for his 73-year-old paternal grandfather with dementia. The nurse can assist the family in

TABLE 7-3	*Nursing Actions That Support Family Development*

FAMILY NURSING MODEL	KEY CONCEPTS	NURSING ACTIONS
Calgary Family Intervention Model (Wright & Leahey, 2013)	Support behavioral functioning throughout developmental transitions.	• Ask, "What could your son do that would help you know how to help him manage his diabetes?" and "How long do you think you will be able to help your father manage living at home?" • Use questions to facilitate conversation and encourage the family to reflect upon possible impending changes from various member perspectives. • Make commendations as appropriate.
Family Health System Model (FHS) (Tomlinson, Peden-McAlpine, & Sherman, 2012)	Support five family processes (i.e., interactive, developmental, coping, integrity, health) as the members mature.	• Consider ways families interact as they mature and evolve over time. • Identify which of the five processes are most affected by the developmental changes within the family. • Identify which member processes require priority attention at any one time.
Family Management Style Framework (FMSF) (Knafl et al., 2009)	Consider the implications of the complexities of family life and parenting goals as needs of both teenager and an elderly grandfather are considered while son adjusts to care needs of a diabetes diagnosis.	• Invite the adult father to share his views of the grandfather with dementia and the extent to which those views focus on normality (e.g., life not challenged by needs of dementia) or dementia-related deficits (e.g., abilities, activities, and life compromised by dementia). • Follow up with a focus on the resources and abilities needed to assist the teenage son in maintaining normality in the face of managing diabetes (e.g., abilities to balance among activity, food, and insulin). • Compare, contrast, and commend for thriving in this difficult context.
Family Health Model (Denham, 2003)	Coordination processes	• Facilitate a conversation to discover the abiding family goals: "Within the next year, what do you hope to accomplish as a family?" and "What are your most significant health needs as a family?"

Continued

TABLE 7-3	*Nursing Actions That Support Family Development—cont'd*	
FAMILY NURSING MODEL	**KEY MODEL CONCEPTS**	**POSSIBLE NURSING ACTIONS**
		• Based upon the common family goals, discern from the family the abilities and skills they believe they will need to accomplish these goals. • Set goals and identify ways the family can work together as a team to accomplish them. • Talk together about ways to evaluate whether goals have been met.
Illness Beliefs Model (Wright & Bell, 2009).	Create a collaborative relationship and remove obstacles to change.	• Construct a family genogram and ecomap together that will reveal the illnesses across the generations. • Identify resources that can be drawn upon for support and information. • Ask the questions: "What is one characteristic that you most appreciate about [your father] [your son] [your grandfather]?" and follow up with "Who do you count on most for support these days?" • Remain curious about the answers. Focus the conversation to build on the family's strengths and ability to problem solve together.

negotiating practical family goals and help integrate independence for the teenage son while counseling the father on strategies for safe care and resources for the aging grandfather.

Developing families will likely inhabit a variety of households in various geographical locations over time and form unique attachments. Life events that occur in various places can influence individual life courses, which may or may not remarkably affect the family unit. As advocates, family nurses can be aware of the sociopolitical and economic environments of the communities where they are employed and seek ways to strengthen the context that influences family development (Denham, 2003). From this perspective, community-minded, family-focused nurses might advocate for after-school child care, anti-bullying policies, and contexts that support healthy eating and physical activity. An occupational health nurse can advocate for work safety policies that protect family members so that they can continue to economically provide for the family. Nurses who *think family* identify and address developmental concerns in the care they provide.

Family Interactions

Family interactions are dynamic, but at the same time have some consistency of pattern. Family interactions establish, build, and maintain relationships and are used to meet family goals and needs (Anderson & Tomlinson, 1992). Family interactions evolve over time and through life course transitions (Cowan & Cowan, 2003). These interactions include verbal and nonverbal communication, nurturance patterns, and expressions of intimacy (Anderson & Tomlinson, 1992). Family members provide mutual support when their interactions are satisfactory. The larger community provides supports and barriers for family units. Box 7.7 provides a case study for you to consider nurse partnerships with individuals and their families. Take some time to reflect about the best answers to the questions about a family-focused perspective.

Family Exosystems

The family household is the principal place where members interact in interdependent ways and interface with their many environments (Bubolz & Sontag, 1993; Denham, 2003). On a grand scale, one can imagine that family units are in some ways interdependent with all the world's people. For example, go through your closet and examine the labels on clothes. See where the items are produced and consider how you are intricately connected with persons the world over. Family units are continually influenced by many forces outside household boundaries. The word exosystem is used in ecological theory to describe the

---

BOX 7-7

Family Circle

Travis was born prematurely and discharged to go home at 4 months with his parents and 7-year-old twin siblings Brianna and Troy and a 4-year-old sister, Janie. Travis's primary health problems are bronchopulmonary dysplasia, oral aversion, pulmonary arterial hypertension, and right-sided cardiac failure. He is receiving home low-flow oxygen therapy by nasal cannula, furosemide (Lasix) and digoxin medication therapy, occupational therapy for the oral aversion, and feedings by percutaneous endoscope gastrostomy (PEG) tube. You are the home care nurse who provides direct care for the child overnight on weekends and during parent's workdays. Travis is now 6 months old. His parents work at a local factory. Some days they are on the same schedule and some days they have few overlapping hours. On some days Brianna and Troy are home for a portion of your shift. Janie is sometimes there when Mom or Dad is doing household tasks. You notice Janie is engaging in activities that do not seem safe for her age level (e.g., riding her tricycle on a country road, climbing the kitchen counter to retrieve a sharp knife, playing in the wading pool outside for long periods unattended). When Janie is near Travis, her speech is loud and it is difficult to calm Travis. Meanwhile, Travis is not gaining weight and is lagging in achieving developmental milestones. Mom and Dad are struggling with household bills and are considering filing for bankruptcy.

Questions from a traditional perspective:

1. What are the nursing problems you are managing for Travis?
2. What are the nursing actions you consider important to improve Travis's growth and development?
3. What are your goals for Travis's care?

Questions from a family-focused perspective:

1. What model or models of family-focused care do you believe could be helpful for Travis's family that would best support his growth and development?
2. What are your goals for this family's care from the different perspectives of the five family nursing models presented in this chapter?
3. What are the key concepts of concern regarding family coping, family development, family interaction, and family integrity for Travis's family?
4. List the proposed nursing actions you consider most important in the realms of family coping, family development, family interaction, and family integrity?

settings wherein a person may not actively participate but is still affected. For example, a parent's employer might alter the costs and services of health care insurance available to employees and families. These decisions greatly influence the members, but these members are not a part of the decisions made. Families interact with many social structures that affect their lives even when they are not noticed.

Family relationships affect members' health-seeking behaviors and family caregiving during illness. Individual personality, knowledge, motivation, and self-efficacy are some factors that can influence care behaviors. Some families faced with a stressful situation may disagree loudly and argue with great intensity when they disagree. These arguments may be usual communication patterns for a particular family, but upsetting to the nurse hearing the boisterous debate. Other families may be sullen, speak little, or seem overtly courteous and respectful of one another. Nurses observe outward behaviors, but these actions only reveal some parts of the family relationship. Observations might not always indicate how a family truly values its members or reveal how care is provided. Member roles influence individual actions. For instance, in an immigrant family from Sudan the mother expresses care for her family through traditional cooking and baking to retain memories of the country of origin. Family-focused nurses know that the behavioral patterns are tied to roles and values. The nurse does not usually aim to alter roles, but to understand and help family units use them beneficially in member care. For example, the family-focused nurse works with the mother in a Sudanese family to design a family-level intervention to improve nutrition that incorporates new information about low-fat cooking methods (Epstein, Ryan, Bishop, Miller, & Keitner, 2003).

Family Communication

Nurses need to know how family members communicate with one another. Communication is essential to relaying biomedical information and helping families with self-care or care management. Some messages are factual or intended to inform, but others are emotional. Family communication conveys beliefs and values linked with the past, present, and future. Language is used to share relevant information. Families have unique interpretative patterns developed over time that help members understand meanings. Nurses might not understand nonverbal family cues but can notice whether they seem congruent with what is said. Families often have their own language through which they privately share things. For example, Amish family members often live in the midst of an American or English community but hold very different ideas about appropriate behaviors. They interact with those outside their sect or community but hold unique ideas about electricity, automobiles, and technologies. They behave differently than those in the mainstream. Intentional minimal use of motorized vehicles, varying educational forms, and faith guide their lifestyles from birth to death. Family-focused nurses caring for the Amish will need to interact in some different ways. Listen to your emotional responses to families and recognize that there are likely reasons why a family is attentive, anxious, hostile, or withdrawn during care situations (Wright & Leahy, 2013).

Family Support

Families and communities frequently provide support to one another when a crisis occurs. For example, if a family has a member diagnosed with cancer, extended family, friends, and others might reach out and offer supports. A series of fund-raising events to raise money for medical costs might be organized. Where you live matters, and family and social resources may or may not be well met by agencies. When supports are lacking, those with inadequate resources can experience great despair. Amish families, for instance, do not usually have health care insurance and are largely self-employed. They depend upon one another for support. Family health is affected by whether members interact in health-producing or health-negating ways as they live and interact outside the view of nurses and other health care professionals (Denham, 2003). Through the individual-nurse-family relationship, supportive partnerships aimed at providing for individual and family needs can be formed.

Goals to Enhance Family Interaction

Family-focused nurses purposely *think family* and use intentional actions to assist individuals and family units to strengthen their capacities and face life transitions linked with health and illness. Nurses who *think family* set goals that support families in constructing life patterns that enhance health and manage illness. Nurses can use therapeutic conversations as they collaborate and co-evolve with the family during care experiences (Benzein & Saveman, 2008). Therapeutic conversations facilitate reciprocity, or mutual give and take, as nurses and families share opinions and values. This partnership focuses on the care responsibilities that best support identified family needs.

When nurses *think family* and caring actions are co-constructed, they are meaningful to the nurse, the individual needing care, and the family unit (Meiers & Tomlinson, 2003). Co-construction of meaning is central to caring in the family health experience; it is developed through caring interactions and partnerships. These interactions help the nurse to know the family and advocate for their identified needs using an existential and intentional perspective (Meiers & Brauer, 2008). This means the nurse respects the humanity of each person and recognizes they are self-determining and have free will (Gadow, 1989). The nurse in partnership practice with families seeks to understand the family's point of view of the world to inform nursing action. Family goals are set to reach mutually agreed upon outcomes. The family-focused nurse using this approach is, "someone you can share things with . . . who feels concern . . . , but doesn't put the pressure on you . . . so you just kind of relax and . . . know that there are other people close by that care ..." (Meiers, 2002, p. 60). Table 7.4 provides ideas for building therapeutic individual-family-nurse relationships.

TABLE 7-4	*Nursing Actions to Influence Family Health Beliefs Through Family Interactions*		
NURSING ACTION GOALS	**SUBCONCEPTS**	**RELATIONAL STANCE**	**SPECIFIC NURSING ACTIONS**
Recognize the power of co-constructed meanings.	Nurse-family interactions (verbal and nonverbal) implicitly influence interdependent and dependent future.	• Approach the nurse-family interaction as the major form of co-construction. • Nurse authenticity facilitates insight. • Caring actions hold potential for enhancing the family health experience.	Prepare the environment: Introduce yourself, offer the appropriate physical greeting (e.g., eye contact, handshake, smile).
Create a context for an ongoing collaborative relationship.	First impressions are long lasting.	Approach meetings with the goal of developing a therapeutic alliance.	Prepare for the session: • Outline goals for the interaction (e.g., I would like to discuss how I can be most helpful to you with choosing healthy eating approaches).

Continued

TABLE 7-4	Nursing Actions to Influence Family Health Beliefs Through Family Interactions—cont'd		
NURSING ACTION GOALS	**SUBCONCEPTS**	**RELATIONAL STANCE**	**SPECIFIC NURSING ACTIONS**
	Manners matter.		• Offer a plan for your time together (e.g., Today, I would like us to get to know each other; help me understand who is in your family and a bit about your family health background). • Offer ideas for the timeline for meetings (e.g., I will spend about 1 hour with you today and then an hour every 2 weeks). Ask the following questions: • Have you previously sought help as a family for healthy eating ideas? • What is the worst advice that you have been given by a provider about healthy eating? • What is the best advice you have been offered by a provider about healthy eating? Create the genogram (and ecomap, if appropriate): Ask the names, ages, occupations, & health concerns of family members. Follow questions in the instance of illness: • What is the one characteristic that best describes X? • What have you come to appreciate most about your XXX since this illness began? Follow with questions for health promoting actions: • Who do you count on the most for support these days? • Is there anyone else that you consider to be like "family"? • Are there any particular religious or spiritual or cultural beliefs that are helpful or not helpful to your or your family's health?

TABLE 7-4	Nursing Actions to Influence Family Health Beliefs Through Family Interactions—cont'd		
NURSING ACTION GOALS	**SUBCONCEPTS**	**RELATIONAL STANCE**	**SPECIFIC NURSING ACTIONS**
			End the session with the following: • Have you had a chance to tell your story? • Is this way of working a good fit for you?
Focus the therapeutic conversation.	Discover the family's perceptions and clarify the therapeutic work.	Adopt an attitude of constant vigilance against the idea that you have any degree of certainty about the family's perception.	• How are you hoping that we can be of most help to you? • What is causing you the biggest challenge these days? • What are you hoping we could talk about today? • If you could have just one question answered in our work today, what would it be?
Remove obstacles to change needed in the health care situation.	A family member who does not want to be present or is present under duress can be an obstacle.	Approach the situation with the courage to identify issues that are implicit and not within the realm of usual social conversation, things that might impede therapeutic conversation.	• Clearly address any nonverbal or verbal behavior that suggests there has been coercion to participate or signs of disinterest or resentment. • We cannot proceed as if this is a helping session because we need to talk about [the situation]. • What should we do about this? • Then proceed to co-construct a solution with which all can move forward.
	A family member who is dissatisfied can be an obstacle.	Acknowledge and talk about any strong emotions that seem to be present.	• I would be interested in knowing what is troubling you today. • Listen and try to understand the situation. • Acknowledge and clarify any misconceptions.
	Unclear expectations about the therapeutic conversation can be an obstacle.	Proceed from the perspective that the family's beliefs and expectations about the therapeutic process may be unclear.	Ask these questions if not already used: • What is the worst advice that you have been offered by a provider about healthy eating? • What is the best advice you have been offered by a provider about healthy eating?

Continued

TABLE 7-4	Nursing Actions to Influence Family Health Beliefs Through Family Interactions—cont'd		
NURSING ACTION GOALS	**SUBCONCEPTS**	**RELATIONAL STANCE**	**SPECIFIC NURSING ACTIONS**
	Previous negative experiences with health care providers can be an obstacle.	Seek to learn about the family's previous experiences within the health care system.	• Probe the idea that there has been a lack of fit between family and provider expectations. • Affirm the fact that the family is the expert about their experience. • Support the family's decision not to continue with care by a specific provider if the fit is not right for them.
	Simultaneous involvement with multiple health care providers can be an obstacle.	Honor family relationships with other health care providers.	How can I/we be helpful to you in a way that is different than other providers?
	Unrealistic or unknown expectations of the referring person about care or treatment can be obstacles.	Encourage family self-referral to give the family opportunity to clarify their perspective.	Ask the referring person to have the family speak directly with you to set the initial contact time and purpose.

Source: Meiers, S. J., & Tomlinson, P. S. (2003). Family-nurse co-construction of meaning: A central phenomenon of family caring. *Scandinavian Journal of Caring Sciences, 17(2),* 193–201.
Wright, L. M., & Bell, J. M. (2009). Creating a context for changing beliefs. In L. M. Wright & J. M. Bell (Eds.), *Beliefs and illness: A model of healing* (pp. 143–178). Calgary, Alberta, Canada: 4th Floor Press.

Family Integrity

The family integrity realm is the final area to explore. The term *integrity* refers to strength, solidarity, stability, and wholeness. Elements of family integrity are linked with family identity, values, boundaries, and health beliefs (Anderson & Tomlinson, 1992). Families create and maintain integrity through a variety of means and seek to retain it as they interact with larger societal systems (Box 7.8).

Family Boundaries

Family systems can be described along a cohesion continuum from disengaged, to engaged, to enmeshed or along an adaptability continuum from rigid to flexible (Olson, Russell, & Sprenkle, 1989). Things that complement family identity are beneficial but those that compete can create conflict and discord. For instance, family members can get caught between family and caregiving system boundaries. Families that might have been viewed as strong for years may be splintered, as responsibilities for care of an aged parent compete with needs to support children in school activities. Family disagreements can occur. A young

> **BOX 7-8**
>
> **Basic Family System Tenets**
>
> Family systems theorists propose the following basic tenets that are linked with integrity of these unique family systems:
>
> - A family system is a set of interrelationships of interdependent persons who mutually influence each other; what happens to one component influences all other components.
> - A family system has a hierarchy of components (e.g., subsystems, systems, suprasystems, exosystems).
> - Family systems are surrounded by permeable boundaries that interface with larger environments.
> - Family boundaries vary in permeability; some boundaries are open, others are closed, and some are more flexible.
> - Family systems take things in and have outputs that cross its boundaries.
> - Family systems use a variety of means to reach the goals to communicate with one another and manipulate information relevant to family identity.
> - Feedback loops regulate the family system, and information exchange occurs among system components, the system, and its multiple environments.
>
> Source: Whitchurch, G. G., & Constantine, L. L. (1993). In P. Boss, W. Doherty, R. LaRossa, W. R. Schumm, & S. K. Steinmetz (Eds.), *Sourcebook of family theories and methods: A contextual approach* (pp. 325–352). New York: Plenum.

teen insists she wants a visible tattoo because friends have gotten them. Parents do not want to allow the outside world to negatively influence their family ways. Nurses who *think family* consider family boundary issues in their practice. As nurses involve family dyads (e.g., parent-child, sibling-sibling, husband-wife), the goal is to create care approaches to respect existing system beliefs and practices and maintain integrity or wholeness of the family (Tomlinson, Peden-McAlpine, & Sherman, 2011).

Families create boundaries that determine "who is in" and "who is out," which describes who is or isn't included in the family circle of care and decision making. Family-focused nurses are attentive to the ways persons receiving care define family. Family boundaries are often renegotiated over time. This change is not always the result of conscious effort but might evolve from trial and error as attempts are made to reach valued goals. Family members may have boundaries with one another as well as with those outside the family. Siblings often set boundaries for one another. Nurses working with families need to be sensitive to what boundaries exist and what they mean. Who gets told the good or bad news in a health care situation is influenced by family boundaries.

Family Identity

Family identity involves common, mostly shared perceptions, goals, and values about who members are in relationship to others. Family identity influences unit behaviors, relationships with the external world, and internal interactions with each other. Wright and Leahy (2013) state "as a family thinketh, so it is." For instance, a family may see itself as "busy" and make choices based on current involvements. Families may demonstrate a range of behaviors that identify their commitment and loyalty to each other. A big brother may step in when children bully his younger brother.

The family's shared identity is linked to the family's history. For example, a Sudanese family may have a history as political refugees, and traumatic experiences and great loss may have occurred during that time. Even in a different environment, the family might find it difficult to trust those outside the immediate family. Outsiders include nurses and other health care providers. The nurse caring for such a family must invest time and gain their trust. Without trust, counsel may go unheeded.

Family values are connected to family identity and influence priorities. For instance, time given to physical activity in families differs. Some families value growth and change, and others resist it. Family identity plays roles in determining power structures and decision making. For instance, parental power can be used to control children or to strengthen their spirits and encourage personal choices. Family identity often guides choices of personal relationships. For example, if a family values getting regular physical activity, young adults are likely to choose physically active friends. Nurses who *think family* know when issues concerning family identity might need to be assessed and be included in a care plan. In some communities, the nurse might need to work with community elders to discern community-held beliefs about family identities and values.

Family Health Routines and Rituals

Family values can shape stories about health experiences and influence the behaviors, routines, and rituals of family health. Knowing about health beliefs helps family nurses better understand reasons for decisions and actions, especially when a new or ambiguous situation is faced (Antonovsky & Sourani, 1988; Reiss, 1987). Rolland (2003) identified some beliefs for nurses to inquire about:

- Causes of illness influenced by and outcomes of usual family life
- Meanings attached to symptoms linked with religion or culture
- Influences of prior generations
- Anticipated points of difficulty in managing an illness or promoting health

Family health beliefs influence health-seeking behaviors and family health routines. Health-related activities such as adhering to immunization schedules, going to the doctor, implementing dietary changes, and maintaining hygiene are influenced by family health beliefs (Denham, 2003). Health beliefs are influenced by the family's culture, values, education, and history, which are all linked to family integrity.

Family health routines are the usual daily activities (e.g., sleep, physical activity, diet) that promote or attend to health or illness care needs in daily life and are shaped by health beliefs and other family factors (Denham, 2003). Routines help families maintain member integrity and support the household production of health. Family health routines are shaped by values, attitudes, family influences, sociocultural mores, and faith. Rituals tied to traditions, celebration, and commemoration of special occasions can also influence some routines. Family-focused nurses recognize that they are temporary guests as they work with family health routines and honor family integrity (Denham, 2003; Tomlinson, Peden-McAlpine, & Sherman, 2011). More needs to be learned about the ways nursing interventions can make important differences for the health of individual members (Box 7.9).

Goals to Enhance Family Integrity

Family nurses consider family integrity in terms of family interactions, boundaries, identity, and routines. Nurses who *think family* know that care involves more than merely telling others what to do. Caring actions employ strategies that use trusting relationships to meet goals. Family-focused nurses avoid a "one size fits all" approach and communicate through specific messages for each family's needs and situations. For example, Todd, a 5-year-old boy, was lying on the sidewalk in front of the family's home after a hit-and-run motorcycle accident.

BOX 7-9

Evidence-Based Family Nursing

Global changes in health care are needed to reduce the costs of that care. Increased demands on nurses and other health professionals call for some changes in the health care systems. Short hospital stays and intense care needs, along with early discharge, call for shifts in the ways nursing is done. Family members need information, skills, and support to adequately provide quality coordinated care. A children's hospital in Iceland has been testing family interventions to identify and better respond to family needs. As new knowledge is identified and evidence of best practice becomes available, questions about how to translate this knowledge into clinical practice are often unanswered. The best ways to provide family nursing in a systematic way are a concern because there has been little evaluation of the effects of family nursing interventions on family relationships and family outcomes. A study investigated the effects of a short therapeutic conversation to see if it made differences in the ways families perceived support (Svavarsdóttir & Sigurdardottir, 2011). Thirty families of hospitalized children were randomly divided into a control group and an intervention group. All took part in a 15-minute or less therapeutic conversation. Those in the intervention group also participated in an average 25-minute family interview in which the nurse drew a genogram and an ecomap with help from the family. Therapeutic questions were used: What is the greatest challenge your family is facing? Who is suffering most? What one question do you need answered? Also, tailored questions about the specific child's condition were asked. After this interview those in the intervention group completed questionnaires while the child was still an inpatient (time 1). They then completed the surveys again on the fifth day after discharge (time 2). Those in the control group also completed surveys during the inpatient stay and again on the fifth day after discharge. Of those who started the study, 13 intervention and 11 control families completed all surveys. No significant difference was found on perceived family support between the experimental or control group at the beginning of the study or after the 15-minute therapeutic conversation. Those in the experimental or intervention group reported better family support after the 25-minute intervention than did the control group. Also, those in the intervention group experienced a significantly higher level of family and cognitive support after this intervention compared to before the intervention. Perceptions of family collaboration and problem-solving skills were the same in the intervention and control groups. Findings indicated that family intervention makes some differences, but more study about family practices that create efficient and valued outcomes is needed.

Source: Svavarsdóttir, E. K., & Sigurdardottir, A. O. (2011). Implementing family nursing in general pediatric nursing practice: The circularity between knowledge translation and clinical practice. In E. K. Svavarsdóttir & H. Jónsdóttir (Eds.), *Family nursing in action*. Reykjavik, Iceland: University of Iceland Press (pp. 161–184).

His father was working in the yard at the time of the accident. He called for emergency help. He accompanied the child to the emergency department. Todd was admitted to the pediatric intensive care unit (PICU). His mother was en route from an out-of-town business trip and could not be reached. Todd suffered multiple skeletal fractures and a possible spinal injury. In the opinion of the PICU diagnostic team, Todd needed a contrast MRI (magnetic resonance imaging) to determine the presence and extent of the spinal injury. However, because of the nature of the injury and the need for sedation, the MRI was considered a high-risk procedure. Todd had lost a considerable amount of blood and needed a blood transfusion. Dad was the sole decision maker and was having a difficult time deciding whether to have the MRI or blood transfusion done. Table 7.5 provides some suggestions for appropriate nursing actions that can support family integrity in this situation. The five family nursing models explained earlier in this chapter suggest various ways to consider family integrity and approach family care.

TABLE 7-5	Nursing Actions to Support Family Integrity Based on Family Models	
FAMILY NURSING MODEL	**KEY CONCEPTS**	**NURSING ACTIONS**
Calgary Family Intervention Model (Wright & Leahey, 2013)	Support the affective domain of family functioning.	Acknowledge the difficulty this must be causing the father and the threat posed by this injury to the family unit. State, "This must be difficult and frightening for you. How are you doing, especially without your wife here? Would you like to share what your thoughts were as this was happening? Is there someone I can call for you who could support you right now; a family member, friend or your clergy person?"
Family Health System Model (FHS) (Tomlinson, Peden-McAlpine, & Sherman, 2012)	Strengthen family boundaries, roles, values, meaning.	Assist the father in enacting his parenting role. For instance, state, "Your son may not be awake and or respond to you right now, but you can help him by sitting here at the bedside, touching his face, his arms, giving him a hug and kiss, and talking to him. He needs your strength and we are pretty sure he will sense your presence. If there are specific things you can do to help with his care, we invite you to do so if that is acceptable to you."
Family Management Style Framework (FMSF) (Knafl et al., 2009)	Not always applicable to a critical illness situation	During moments of critical care it might not seem obvious to address family management. In this case, the father might be inexperienced with some nurturing roles. However, as time goes by and both parents are available, strategies for care management will likely need to be identified.
Family Health Model (Denham, 2003)	Connected family processes, meanings of external environments, and family routines	Confirm parental roles and the uncertainty of the situation; show curiosity about normal family activities. For instance, state, "You are being strong for your son right now; this is important. What would your wife do if she were here? Would it be helpful for us to keep a few notes for her about what is happening so she can catch up when she arrives? What are you most concerned about her missing? Could we keep a journal for her and your son?"

TABLE 7-5	Nursing Actions to Support Family Integrity Based on Family Models—cont'd	
FAMILY NURSING MODEL	**KEY CONCEPTS**	**NURSING ACTIONS**
Illness Beliefs Model (Wright & Bell, 2009)	Intersection of family member beliefs, cultural values of those needing care and the health care providers linked with suffering	Strengthen facilitating beliefs and challenge constraining beliefs. Interpret what is happening physiologically and medically. Explain goals of medical care. Allow the father to share his feelings about the accident. See what questions about care need answers, clarify errors in understanding the situation.

Chapter Summary

Various theories can guide the delivery of family-focused nursing care. Theories provide perspectives and ways to think about approaching care. Family science and family therapy theories and models suggest ideas about how nursing actions can be aligned with care needs. Several family nursing theories have been identified as ways to think about different care approaches. Nurses who *think family* use theories to intentionally select nursing actions to meet family goals. Collaborative individual-nurse-family relationships are formed to plan actions that meet goals relevant to the health or illness need. In family-focused care, nurses give attention to family realms of concern (i.e., family coping, family development, family interaction, family integrity). These realms can be assessed and then plans of care determined. Nursing actions are intentional, respect the family experience, and address meaningful concerns from the family unit perspective.

REFERENCES

Anderson, K. (2000). The Family Health System approach to family systems nursing. *Journal of Family Nursing, 6*(2), 103–119.

Anderson, K. A., & Tomlinson, P. S. (1992). The family health system as an emerging paradigmatic view for nursing. *Image: Journal of Nursing Scholarship, 24,* 57–63.

Antonovsky, A., & Sourani, T. (1988). Family sense of coherence and family adaptation. *Journal of Marriage and the Family, 50,* 79–92.

Bengston, V. L., & Allen, K. R. (1993). The life course perspective applied to families over time. In P. Boss, W. J. Doherty, R. LaRossa, W. R. Schumm, & S. K. Steinmetz (Eds.), *Sourcebook of family theories and methods: A contextual approach* (pp. 469–499). New York: Plenum.

Benner, P. (1982). From novice to expert. *American Journal of Nursing, 82*(3), 402–407.

Benzein, E., & Saveman, B. (2008). Health-promoting conversations about hope and suffering with couples in palliative care. *International Journal of Palliative Nursing, 14,* 439–445.

Bianchi, S. M., & Casper, L. M. (2005). Explanations of family change: A family demographic perspective. In V. L. Bengston, A. C. Acock, K. R. Allen, P. Dilworth-Anderson, & D. M. Klein (Eds.), *Sourcebook of family theory and research* (pp. 93–103). Thousand Oaks, CA: Sage.

Boss, P. (2003). *Family stress management* (2nd ed.). Newbury Park: Sage.

Boss, P., Doherty, W., LaRossa, R., Schumm, W. R., & Steinmetz, S. K. (Eds.). (1993). *Sourcebook of family theories and methods: A contextual approach*. New York: Plenum.

Bubolz, M. M., & Sontag, M. S. (1993). Human ecology theory. In P. G. Boss, W. J. Doherty, R. LaRossa, W. R. Schumm, & S. K. Steinmetz (Eds.), *Sourcebook of family theories and methods: A contextual approach* (pp. 419–448). New York: Plenum.

Carter, B., & McGoldrick, M (1999). *The expanded family life cycle: Individual, family and social perspectives* (3rd ed.). Boston: Allyn & Bacon.

Cowan, P. A., & Cowan, C. P. (2003). Normative family transitions, normal processes and healthy child development. In F. Walsh (Ed.), *Normal family processes* (3rd ed., pp. 424–459). New York: Guilford Press.

Denham, S. A. (2003). *Family health: A framework for nursing*. Philadelphia: F. A. Davis.

Duvall, E. M. (1977). *Marriage and family development* (5th ed.). Philadelphia: Lippincott.

Eggenberger, S. K., Krumwiede, N. K., Meiers, S. J., Bliesmer, M., & Earle, P. (2004). Family caring strategies in neutropenia. *Clinical Journal of Oncology Nursing, 8*(6), 617–620.

Epstein, N. B, Ryan, C. E., Bishop, D. S., Miller, I. W., & Keitner, G. I. (2003). The McMaster Model: A view of healthy family functioning. In F. Walsh (Ed.), *Normal family processes* (3rd ed., pp. 581–607). New York: Guilford Press.

Erickson, E. H. (1950). *Childhood and society*. New York: Norton.

Friedman, M. M. (1981). *Family nursing: Theory and assessment*. New York: Appleton-Century-Crofts.

Gadow, S. (1989) An ethical case for patient self-determination. *Seminars in Oncology Nursing, 2*, 99–101.

Hill, R. (1971). *Families under stress*. Westport, CT: Greenwood Press. (Original work published 1949.)

Hupcey, J. (1999). Looking out for the patient and ourselves—the process of family integration into the ICU. *Journal of Clinical Nursing, 8*, 253–262.

Kaakinen, J. R., Coehlo, D. P., Steele, R., Tabacco, A., & Hanson, S. H. H. (2015). *Family health care nursing: Theory, practice, and research*. Philadelphia: F. A. Davis.

Knafl, K., & Deatrick, J. (1990). Family management behaviors: Concept synthesis. *Journal of Pediatric Nursing, 5*, 15–22.

Knafl, K., & Deatrick, J. (2003). Further refinement of the family management style framework. *Journal of Family Nursing, 9*, 232–256. doi:10.101177/1074840703255435

Knafl, K., & Deatrick, J. (2006). Family management style and the challenge of moving from conceptualization to measurement. *Journal of the Association of Pediatric Oncology, 23*, 12–18.

Knafl, K., Deatrick, J. A., Gallo, A., Dixon, J., Grey, M., Knafl, G., & O'Malley, J. (2009). Assessment of the psychometric properties of the Family Measurement Measure. *Journal of Pediatric Psychology, 36*(5), 494–505. doi:10.1093/jpepsy/jsp034

Maslow, A. (1954). *Motivation and personality*. New York: Harper.

Mayer, K. U. (2009). New directions in life course research. *Annual Review of Sociology, 35*, 413–433. doi:10.1146/annurev.soc.34.040507.134619

McCubbin, H. I., McCubbin, M., Thompson, E. A., & Fromer, J. E. (Eds.). (1998a). *Resiliency in ethnic minority families: Native and immigrant families* (Vol. 1). Thousand Oaks, CA: Sage.

McCubbin, H., McCubbin, M., Thompson, E., & Futrell, J. (Eds.). (1998b). *Stress, coping, and health in families: Sense of coherence and resiliency. Resiliency in families series* (Vol. 1). Thousand Oaks, CA: Sage.

McCubbin, H. I., & Patterson, J. M. (1983). The family stress process: The double ABCX model of adjustment and adaptation. In H. I. McCubbin, M. B. Sussman, & J. M. Patterson (Eds.), *Social stress and the family: Advanced and developments in family stress theory and research* (pp. 7–37). New York: Haworth.

McEwin, M., & Wills, E. M. (2011). *Theoretical basis for nursing*. Philadelphia: Lippincott Williams & Wilkins.

Meiers, S. J. (2002). *Family-nurse co-construction of meaning: Caring in the family health experience* (doctoral dissertation). Retrieved from UMI Order AAI3041946.

Meiers, S. J., & Brauer, D. J. (2008). Existential caring in the family health experience: A proposed conceptualization. *Scandinavian Journal of Caring Sciences, 22*, 110–117.

Meiers, S., Eggenberger, S., Krumwiede, N., Bliesmer, M., & Earle, P. (2009). Enduring acts of balance: Rural families creating health. In H. Lee (Ed.), *Conceptual basis for rural nursing* (3rd ed.). New York: Springer.

Meiers, S. J., & Tomlinson, P. S. (2003). Family-nurse co-construction of meaning: A central phenomenon of family caring. *Scandinavian Journal of Caring Sciences, 17*, 193–201.

Olson, D. H., & Gorall, D. M. (2003). Circumplex model of marital and family systems. In F. Walsh (Ed.), *Normal family processes* (3rd ed., pp. 514–547). New York: Guilford.

Olson, D. H., Russell, C. S., & Sprenkle, D. H. (Eds.). (1989). *Circumplex model: Systemic assessment and treatment of families*. New York: Haworth.

Peterson, S. J., & Bredow, T. S. (2004). *Middle range theories: Application to nursing research*. Philadelphia: Lippincott William & Wilkins.

Piaget, J. (1967). *Biology and knowledge*. Chicago: University Press.

Reiss, D. (1987). *The family's construction of reality*. Cambridge, MA: Harvard University Press.

Rolland, J. S. (2003). Mastering family challenges in serious illness and disability. In F. Walsh (Ed.), *Normal family processes* (3rd ed., pp. 460–489). New York: Guilford.

Svavarsdóttir, E. K., & Sigurdardottir, A. O. (2011). Implementing family nursing in general pediatric nursing practice: The circularity between knowledge translation and clinical practice. E. K. Svavarsdóttir & H. Jónsdóttir (Eds.), *Family nursing in action,* (pp. 161–184). Reykjavik, Iceland: University of Iceland Press.

Tomlinson, P. S., Peden-McAlpine, C., & Sherman, S. (2011). A family systems nursing intervention model for paediatric health crisis. *Journal of Advanced Nursing, 68*(3), 705–714. doi:10.1111/j.1365-2648.2011.05825.x

Whitchurch, G. G., & Constantine, L. L. (1993). In P. Boss, W. Doherty, R. LaRossa, W. R. Schumm, & S. K. Steinmetz (Eds.), *Sourcebook of family theories and methods: A contextual approach* (pp. 325–352). New York: Plenum.

Wright, L., & Bell, J. (2009). *Beliefs and illness: A model for healing*. Calgary, Alberta, Canada: 4th Floor Press.

Wright, L., & Leahy, M. (2013). *Nurses and families: A guide to family assessment and intervention* (6th ed.). Philadelphia: F. A. Davis.

CHAPTER 8

Developing a Family-Focused Nursing Practice

Kathryn Hoehn Anderson • Sharon A. Denham

CHAPTER OBJECTIVES

1. Describe the nature of the individual-nurse-family relationship and its importance in family nursing practice.
2. Describe the characteristics of a family practice model.
3. Discuss family nursing skills used to provide family nursing care.
4. Demonstrate use of a family nursing model and nursing actions to provide family nursing care.
5. Discuss family nursing approaches/models used in family nursing care practice.

CHAPTER CONCEPTS

- Circularity
- Clinical family nursing skills
- Family nursing practice
- Family unit perspective
- Hypothesizing
- Individual-nurse-family relationship
- Interventive questions
- Neutrality
- Practice model
- Selecting a family nursing model
- Therapeutic questioning

Introduction

About 35 years ago, the first edition of *Family-Focused Care* was published, and this thoughtful work crafted some early thinking around nursing actions and family interventions (Miller & Janosik, 1980). Since that time, the science around family-focused practice has grown. This chapter considers more current thinking about family practice and explains how this approach can be used in clinical work. By forging an individual-nurse-family relationship with every person receiving care, nurses can build collaborative partnerships with those seeking care. This chapter describes the development and use of an individual-nurse-family relationship, considers the importance of using practice models to guide clinical work with families, and discusses ideas about use of clinical skills in family nursing practice. It explains how to choose and apply a family nursing model when planning care for individual families and addresses the nature and development of the individual-nurse-family relationship with family nursing practice. It provides brief explanations of a few select family nursing models, describes several family nursing skills important to master, and provides a case example of family nursing care using the Family Health System model (Anderson, 2000). This chapter describes ways to effectively *think family* not just as a prelude to providing family nursing care, but throughout the caring endeavors.

Family-Focused Nursing Care

In family-focused care, nurses assume a mind-set that continually *thinks family* as they care for individuals and their families as a unit of care. Family nurses apply all their skills, using technical, mental, and emotional processes. Family theories, as presented in Chapter 7, can be used to guide clinical practice in the ways nurses give care with families, and take action. Nurses who desire to develop a family nursing practice need knowledge about families including dynamics, history, health patterns, lifestyles, and culture, member, and community connections.

Providing nursing care from a family unit perspective can be challenging and exciting. The family and nurse become true partners in care. Families have information and expertise about their concerns. Stories from their perspective tell of the stresses, difficulties, and worries experienced. They know what is and is not working. Nurses are in positions in which they can help families manage health and illness, developmental concerns, and transitions (Anderson, 2000). Family nursing can enhance awareness, meaning, and potentials of individuals and families (Hartrick, 1997). Family nursing is intentional collaboration and identifies the best ways to help families achieve their health goals. Family nursing looks beyond the individual and the present and includes family and potential future needs (Fig 8.1).

Family Nursing Practice

Nursing is a practice discipline, both an art and a science. The art of nursing is the therapeutic use of self in delivery of nursing care, and the science is based on research evidence. Nurses need to read and understand research findings and then use that information to help

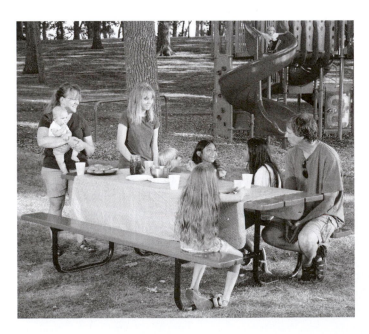

FIGURE 8-1 Family nursing looks beyond the individual and the present.

individuals and families promote health and manage illness. More still needs to be learned about the implications of intentional family inclusion in nursing actions (Anderson, 2000). Current knowledge is a foundation that clinicians, researchers, and scholars can build upon and use to develop even stronger evidence about what constitutes family nursing practice.

Family nursing practice addresses the needs of individuals and their families who seek health and illness care services. *Thinking family* includes learning how those seeking care and their family members relate to one another and what these relationships imply for care. Individuals are not just care recipients, but also partners in care with families who are part of the care experience. Nurses need to know how this happens and what it looks like in practice. These things can be demonstrated in clinical experiences, but also through active learning in the classroom.

Individual-Nurse-Family Relationships

When a family care approach is used, care is centered on the family unit and how to satisfy their health or illness needs (Anderson & Valentine, 1998). The concerns addressed are associated with the individual and who that person views as family. What individual and family perspectives need to be heard? People are social animals, often eager to engage others and be noticed. What happens when we get together with others? We often tell stories about what is happening in our life and find out what is happening in theirs. It happens everywhere—at work, with neighbors, with friends, and in families—people tell stories about their lives as they share their life experiences. During times of crisis, at critical life moments, in health or illness, people often want to tell about what happened and their responses.

Suppose you tempt fate and go out in a snowstorm against your better judgment. Two miles down the road on a steep rural incline you lose control and the car slides off the road and you sit alone in your car. You look around at the lonely desolate place, note the gas tank is half full and the outside temperature is 11 degrees. You put on your hazard lights but know they can't be seen until someone is dangerously nearby. You grab your cell phone and call someone who cares. Although this person is 30 miles away and not able to help you, the sound of her voice gives comfort and you tell the story of your dilemma. You are in a difficult situation, but here is someone who cares, will listen, and offers comfort. This helps! People usually show up willing to help. Strangers without names suggest tactics that might work, things to try, and ideas to solve the problem. Still fearful and uncertain, you trust their ideas may help get you out of a difficult or troubling situation.

In a way, nurses can be like these strangers, they are present to care in unusual and stressful situations. Individuals and their families enter unfamiliar health care settings filled with frightening things, faces, and rules. Often uncertainty about life and what is going on with a health condition is present. A nurse who cares shows up and is prepared to offer help. Though uncertain about the outcome, it is comforting not to be alone. Family nurses reach out to establish a caring connection to individuals and families. It is a relief to meet someone with ideas about things that might help and who is invested in acting in intentional ways to resolve the problem. The history of nursing tells of caring persons available during uncertain times, willing to listen, offer comfort, be present, and provide care.

A narrative or story of personal experience has new meanings, value, and potentials when it is heard and shared with others. Clearly, critical interventions must occur first, but even then care and support are important to care recipients and family units. Family nurses begin relationships by welcoming individuals and families into the relationship, establishing a caring connection leading to an individual-nursing-family relationship, and listening to the health or illness story that communicates individual and family needs and concerns.

Characteristics of the Individual-Nurse-Family Relationship

The individual-nurse-family relationship is a reflective one. This means that what is said or done is thoughtfully appraised from the perspective of others. It allows for acceptance of vulnerability and examines whether stressors might be physically based, relationship based, or from a prior experience, fears, or external determinants. Nurses establish thoughtful relationships with the individual and the family and notices that people often respond out of prior experiences and personal emotional pain. Although the current event might be in sharp contrast to previous ones, sometimes past events cause lingering impressions that cause present worry, fear, or other emotions. As nurses reflect on the situation at hand, they are careful to put aside biases and assumptions. Assessments help discover the obscure and gain a perspective of patterns and needs. Reflective practice requires checking personal reactions to situations and accepting differences without judgment. It acknowledges various points of view and gives authentic care that is sensitive to other's needs. The nurse evaluates various needs and whether a partnership to meet family unit goals is being successful. Reflective nurses know that troublesome situations are not always due to current circumstances, but may be responses to actions from other circumstances that need addressing from the family perspective.

Stop a minute. Think about what you read in the previous paragraph. How do you define reflective practice? How might reflection cause you to approach a practice situation differently? Do you think about needs and situations before planning care? What are you thinking about after care is given? Do you pause and consider what happened? How did your interaction help the family with healing and easing their suffering (Wright & Bell, 2009)? With helping them with what they are going through? What does the family want to improve in their situation? How might you have done things differently? Take time to reflect before and after care is provided (hypothesizing what is going on). Thus, you consider a variety of options. You might be thinking, "Oh, good, I am already doing just that!" But at other times you might be thinking "I need to learn more about how to *think family* in action or practice or how to react when others have differing values than mine." Self-reflection enhances nursing practice.

Actions of the Individual-Nurse-Family Relationship

Nursing actions can support individuals and their family members in many ways. Some nursing actions are aimed at immediate concerns, others are more relevant to the future. Family nurses focus on what the family determines are the priority concerns; the nurse adds expert input for family consideration. For example, a new mother is trying to decide whether to breastfeed her new infant. She may need to learn skills for making the process successful. Her husband and his mother might have an experience in which breastfeeding didn't work so well and may need information about the long-term health benefits for the child to be able to support the mother's wishes. When family members are included in the conversation, multiple needs can be addressed. Including family in discussions about breastfeeding could answer questions, explain benefits, and be more useful than just telling the mother that she should breastfeed without considering other family member support. The individual-nurse-family relationship uses a *think family* perspective including relevant scientific evidence and holistic care for the family unit based on their need priorities. Think about your family and ask yourself, if one of my family members were sick, how would I want to be treated as a family member? How would I want to be included? What would my family prefer? Take a few minutes to review Box 8.1 where you can learn about a family nurse leader from Finland who has been helping students learn about family care for many years.

Initiating the Individual-Nurse-Family Relationship

Individual-nurse-family relationships begin with introductions. Then take time to hear the family health story about their current situation. Communicate the purpose of the

---

BOX 8-1

Family Tree

Päivi Åstedt-Kurki, PhD, RN (Finland)

Päivi Åstedt-Kurki, PhD, RN, is a professor and chair of the discipline of Nursing Science in the School of Health Sciences, University of Tampere, Finland. A core societal belief held by the Finnish culture is that a patient and his family are the most important participants in health care. The need to advance science in this particular area of health care led to the establishment of Family Nursing Science at the University of Tampere. Dr. Åstedt-Kurki helped to develop a Family Nursing Science curriculum and has served as a supervisor of numerous doctoral dissertations in nursing science in which the topic is family nursing. She is a prolific researcher with over 200 data-based publications in Finnish and English that focus on family health, well-being, and family nursing interventions across the life span. Besides funded research and publications, Dr. Åstedt-Kurki and her colleagues co-developed two family nursing research instruments: Family Functioning, Health, and Social Support Instrument (FAFHES) and Parents' Perceptions of Care (PPC). In 1999, an International Family Nursing Congress, hosted by the University of Tampere, shared the development of Family Nursing Science in Finland. Dr. Åstedt-Kurki is a national leader and has twice been invited to serve as the chairperson of the Finnish Association of Caring Sciences. She is the Editor-in-Chief of the *Journal of Nursing Science* in Finland (2009–2010). In 2009 Dr. Åstedt-Kurki was honored with a Distinguished Contribution to Family Nursing Award from the *Journal of Family Nursing* for her outstanding and sustained leadership in family nursing leadership in Finland.

---

interaction and help the family share important information and understand the family view of the situation. The nurse can say "Tell me what brings you for care today." The story is a critical aspect of the initial meeting. The nurse gathers data from the health/illness story that can be included in the assessment data. It is the opportunity to learn important facts from the person's or family's point of view. You might be wondering how you encourage people to share their story in ways you can understand the family's view about how their illness came about and what needs they perceive. Also, you might wonder how you kindly interrupt someone when the story goes on too long or leads to other unconnected stories. Redirecting the story so that the most valuable information is gained in a timely way is a skill that is learned through practice and using your interviewing skills. Another way to start the interaction with the family is by asking "What brings you here today?" or "What led up to your admission today?" These open-ended questions easily lead to the telling of the health/illness story and get you started with your individual-nurse-family relationship and the nursing assessment. As you listen, ask for clarification if something is not clear, show that you are involved and interested. As you hear the story, you might want to write a few notes about points to discuss in more detail later.

The story might include facts about events leading up to the current care-seeking event or reasons why the situation is happening a certain way. Because of how busy nurses are, if the story interaction goes on too long and you must attend to other things, you can say to the family something like "I want to talk with you more about this, but I need to go and take care of some other important things related to your care (if possible state what this might be). But I will be back in about 10 minutes." Be sure to return as you stated. If something hinders you, check in and let them know you have not forgotten. Remember, waiting can be a stressful time that seems longer than it really is. These initial interactions set the stage for future ones. When you return, you might ask about pertinent stressors, greatest difficulties or related worries, what is and is not working, or the ways personal and family life is affected.

It is essential to determine what is most important to the individual and the family and what their concerns are. Communicate clearly in understandable ways. As the picture of the health/illness story emerges and meaningful interactions occur, trust is built and the groundwork for a relationship is established. As time permits, you can ask further questions about values and beliefs, developmental concerns, member roles, family communication, problem solving, conflict resolution, health practices, and routine family behaviors, continuing the process of assessing the family. Take time to consider alternative ways to assist. Avoid assumptions and be sure to get needed facts. The personalized story tells the nurse that this is not just an elderly woman with a broken hip who fell, but that this is a person, part of a unique family unit, who shares a household life in a particular neighborhood and community and is loved and cherished by her family. The families we care for are real people! They have interesting lives, distinct needs, caring friends, and social networks. This meaningful individual-nurse-family interaction is the foundation of family nursing practice.

Caring in the Individual-Nurse-Family Relationship

Traditional nursing education often approaches families as the "context of care"—such as including the parents in the care of a child patient. Family is often highlighted in obstetrical, hospice, or community clinical rotations. In a traditional mode, patients can be viewed as dependent and nurses as experts. *Thinking family* means that the family unit is the target of care and they are experts about their health and illness condition. Individuals are viewed are independent care-seeking agents who are part of a family. This unit point of view encourages families to participate in their own health achievement with a family nurse. Box 8.2 provides some information about the benefits to families of in-home intervention.

When the family unit is integral to individual needs and best interests, nurses do not just take control or give orders, they identify specific needs of multiple persons in a care situation based on what the family tells them. They unit use supportive therapeutic actions in ways that meet individual and family unit needs and address distinct needs in the best ways possible. Caring interventions are customized to diverse families.

Nurses who *think family* know the importance of family dynamics and the bidirectional influence family unit members have on one another (Anderson & Tomlinson, 1992). Family systems theory tells us that whatever happens to one person influences the family and whatever influences the family also influences persons who compose the family (Denham, 2003; von Bertalanffy, 1968). Family members have influence, roles, and meaning whether an individual is ill or wants to increase his wellness. In thinking family, nurses appreciate that individuals hold common family dynamics and experiences that are foundational to the family.

Nature of the Family Nurse Relationship

Family nursing is different from practice done by social workers or family therapists as discussed in Chapter 7. Family-focused nursing care includes several goals:

- Facilitating individual and family growth
- Enhancing individual and family knowledge and understanding
- Assisting individuals and family members in managing health symptoms
- Following evidence-based prescribed medical and nursing regimens
- Promoting and improving individual and family health
- Supporting behaviors to maintain and improve individual and family health

Sometimes how to work with families to achieve these goals are taught in a family nursing or community health course, but they are meant to be used in all aspects of providing care. Individual-nurse-family relationships are collaborative partnerships that can be used

BOX 8-2

Evidence-Based Practice in Family Nursing

Community Interventions for Families With Children

Attention deficit-hyperactivity disorder (ADHD), a condition that negatively affects children and families, is on the rise and affects about 4% to 7% of children worldwide. A nurse case management program intervention named Parents and Children Together (PACT) has been developed to focus on assessment and service delivery. A total of 87 families participated in this study. PACT focuses on family support, empowerment, and a strength-based perspective. The main aim of this form of nursing intervention is to focus on family support rather than disease management. The PACT intervention has four steps:

- Assessing strengths, resources, and risks to determine family level of need
- Setting goals and identifying type and level of services needed
- Providing direct service
- Ongoing monitoring

Nurse case managers (NCMs) received a month of intensive and specialized training focused around the common concerns experienced in families with a child who has ADHD. The intervention was family directed and the NCM was primarily a resource and facilitator. Families were not sure what to expect when they agreed to participate in the intervention and later said many of their perceptions were wrong, as were those of other health care providers. After working for an extended time with families (12 months), the NCM was observed to be like family because she understood the situations and believed the families. The PACT was a collaborative relationship designed to provide supportive services and not direct intensive care. Mothers of the children were highly satisfied with the intervention and thought the intervention was effective. A subset of the mothers ($N = 17$) reported that learning more about the neurobiology of the disorder and how problems were linked to executive function gave them more confidence in their parenting as they realized the behavior was not linked to poor parenting. Although providing a yearlong program in most situations is not feasible, several important things were learned. Families needed clear education about the physiology of the disease, the role executive function plays in child behavior, and parenting techniques for behavioral challenging behaviors. PACT is an example of a home visit nursing intervention, and study findings suggest that family education, ongoing assessment and monitoring, problem-solving skills, crisis intervention, and knowledge about community resources helped families be more successful in their daily management of this childhood disorder.

Source: Kendall, J., & Tabacco, A. (2011). Parents and children together: In-home intervention for families with children with attention-deficit/hyperactivity disorder. In E. K. Svarsdottir and H. Jonsdottir (Eds.), *Family nursing in action* (pp. 185–216). Reykjavik: University of Iceland Press.

---

to meet health and illness care needs of all ages in all forms of care settings. When nurses view the family as the expert on its life, they enter into respectful interactions knowing that the family is giving its best efforts (Anderson, 2000).

Caring interactions involve listening to the family, validating key concerns, noting expectations, and integrating family strengths and desires (Anderson, 2000). Nurses with this mind-set are open to the unexpected and alert to unusual or different family responses in meeting the primary concerns confronting the family (Kaakinen, Gedaly-Duff, Coehlo, & Hanson, 2014; Wright & Leahey, 2013) reflecting a nonjudgmental view of the family.

Family nurses create the context or atmosphere for therapeutic interactions to occur. Those seeking care are often unsure what to expect, so nurses take their clinical expertise into the family's world (Fig. 8.2). Nurses describe ways they can assist, explain environments or systems, address concerns, and clarify information not well understood. However, the family is always the expert when it comes to what is happening in their personal lives. Nurses learn about their needs directly from them.

A legendary family therapist, Virginia Satir (1967), said, "I believe the greatest gift I can conceive of having from anyone is to be seen, heard, understood and touched by them. The greatest gift I can give is to see, hear, understand and touch another person. When this is done, I feel contact has been made" (p. 31). Of course, Satir does not mean physically touching, but touching the heart through a caring tone and actions. These words are still true and hold wisdom for designing individual-nurse-family relationships. Nurses who *think family* respect the challenges being faced by the individual and family unit and assist those seeking care in recognizing their strengths and using them to solve problems.

Steps in Delivering Family Nursing Care

In family-focused nursing care, numerous skills are needed for competent care delivery. Although nurses who *think family* know that the individual and family are not separate, they also know that families do not always behave in unison. Some families are tragically fragmented by long histories of tragedies, misunderstandings, conflict, and selfishness. Thinking family does not imply that nurses need to solve family problems. Many issues require the skills of advanced practice nurses or therapists. Nurses need to direct their care toward specific concerns linked with health and illness at the generalist nurse skill level. When deep-seated emotional or social problems are identified, the family nurse advises the physician or other medical team member about them and they are often referred to another interprofessional health team member. Nurses who use sound nursing practices know the limits of their scope of practice, but they can act as connectors as they facilitate improved well-being of the family unit in areas requiring skill beyond their education. Thinking family includes some philosophical ideas about "doing for" and "being with." These ideas are fully discussed in Chapter 13.

In clinical nursing practice, family nurses consider ways family members' reciprocal relationships influence care outcomes. In collaboration with the family, intentional actions requiring numerous skills with families are used to set goals, plan care, find strategies that

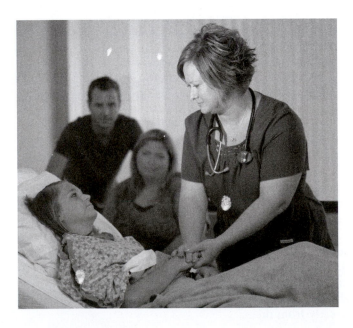

FIGURE 8-2 Nurses initiate the conversation and create the context for therapeutic interactions with the individual and family.

will work, and identify how successful outcomes can be measured. Family care approaches include neutrality, hypothesizing, and circularity (Wright & Leahey, 2013). Nurses also use interventive questions to discover what is most needed and facilitate problem solving.

Neutrality

A neutral view, not taking sides or making judgments, helps nurses be respectful of families' abilities and gain humility (Wright & Bell, 2009). Neutrality describes the nurse's attitude toward the family system that constrains them from taking sides or placing blame (Wright & Bell, 2009). The essence of neutrality is curiosity; this means that the nurse will entertain alternative points of view to more clearly understand a situation (Cecchin, 1987). You may not understand the multiple interpretations of a behavior, an event, a relationship, or interaction observed or experienced, but by taking a neutral stance you remain open to the many possibilities presented. Being neutral allows time to interpret conversations and events in ways different from your personal life experience. Neutrality implies that it is okay for families to act differently from the ways other mainstream families might respond. It implies that nurses do not need to decide how things get done. Family nurses foster openness and curiosity about the ways family members engage with and respond to health and illness problems. This attitude can help families consider ways to be open to other viewpoints also.

Hypothesizing

Hypothesizing is the use of propositions or hunches that suggest areas to explore, things that can help the nurse connect or attribute meanings to behaviors (Wright & Leahey, 2013). It keeps one open to the possibilities about what dynamics are at work in a situation. It can guide the use of questions or discussions, help the nurse weigh alternatives or optional actions, and explore potential strategies for problem solving. For example, you might wonder what happens if a family member is unsure how to act in a hypoglycemic event. Suppose the family member is afraid, freezes, and does nothing. Or suppose the family member knows something sweet should be given and has the person consume a big glass of orange juice and a candy bar. What might be the consequences of the family member's actions? Suppose the family knows exactly what to do, but the problem is something else. Can you see how hypothesizing helps you see needs from varied viewpoints? Being curious and considering possibilities is part of critical thinking.

Using questions to confirm a hypothesis can lead to thinking about life or illness differently. As the nurse works with a family member, she might ask: Suppose your husband gets weak, says his lips are tingling and he starts perspiring, what would you do? What do you think about when that happens to him? Or if the nurse wants to educate about nutrition, he might say: If you went shopping and had to buy items for three well-balanced meals for a day, what things would you buy? Use of hypothesizing questions can validate the nurse's ideas and guide their thinking and responses (Wright & Bell, 2009). A nonconfirming reply to a hypothesis can prepare the nurse to revise the teaching to be done as new information is included. A hypothesizing view opens the door for new possibilities and alternative explanations.

Circularity

Circularity refers to reciprocal influences that occur as questions are used to understand family behaviors and confirm or discard hypotheses made (Wright & Leahey, 2013). Circularity focuses on the interactions within the individual-nurse-family relationship and observations about family member interactions. It is useful to note how thoughts, feelings, and actions affect and influence member interactions. Circular communication shifts the focus so that clearer understandings about what is experienced in a particular situation are expressed in ways that others hear firsthand. Sharing effects of personal thoughts, feelings, and actions on others allows others to hear and sense agreement or disagreement, emotional pain, or uncertainty. The nurse listens carefully to what is said and how it is said to see if actions or behaviors are congruent. It is sometimes helpful to review a member's interactional patterns with other members and ask the individual to clarify more about his or her communication. The purpose of circular communication is to learn more about what the family is thinking and feeling during clinical and familial interactions. The reciprocal nature of communication becomes important and useful in planning intervention questions, as will be discussed later.

Circular communication goes two ways (Fig. 8.3). The nurse listens and reflects in a clear, open, and neutral way about what was heard. Then in a caring manner, the nurse assists the family members to respond to what has been said. For example, a mother and an older daughter are talking with the nurse about the ways their father/grandfather is reacting to his growing memory loss. The mother says, "I just cannot bear that he is so confused all the time. He repeats things over and over and seems to remember less every day." The nurse replies with a reflective statement, "He remembers less every day." "Yes," the mother continues, "he cannot remember if he has eaten his meals and is continually asking to eat. This is so distressing to me and it causes the children to get frustrated and sometimes be mean to him." The nurse turns to the daughter and facilitates circular communication: "Your mother is saying that you and your siblings get frustrated with your grandfather's forgetfulness and repetition." The nurse looks at the daughter and silently waits for her response. The daughter answers, "It upsets me to hear him say the same things over and over. He used to play games and sing with us when we were younger. He is not like the grandfather I used to know." The nurse goes on and clarifies meanings: "You are worried about your grandfather forgetting?" The conversation continues as they all express feelings, concerns, thoughts, and begin to understand each other's actions. The focus is on "I feel" and not accusatory. At conversation's end, the nurse has gained great insights into what is happening with this family. This information provides accurate information about members' responses to the person and the disease. Facilitating circular communication helps families. What is learned can be a foundation for goal setting, coping in new ways, and steps family members can take.

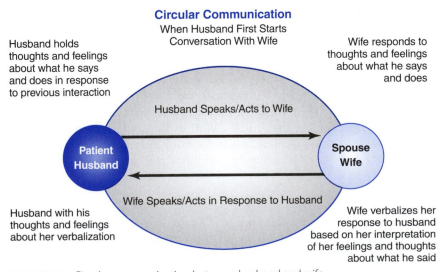

FIGURE 8-3 Circular communication between husband and wife.

Interventive Questions

A family-focused response that builds upon circular communication is a behavioral observation interventive question (Loos & Bell, 1990). For example, "What is it like for each of you when your father/grandfather is confused?" The mother and daughter look at each other. The mother answers, "It is difficult for me; I just want him to be happy and at peace, but my daughter and other children seem angry with him all the time." The daughter replies, "Mother, we want him to be happy, too; we are afraid when he gets angry and acts out. We do not know what to say to him. We are afraid of what he might do." With interventive questions, the nurse further facilitates communication between the daughter and the mother. This interaction suggests specific ways the nurse can follow up to provide needed education about the disease, safety concerns, respite care, and family stress management. Through communication, nurses can identify strengths to be commended and use these strengths to facilitate problem solving.

Family Nursing Practice and Assessment Processes

When conducting a comprehensive assessment, explore all relevant areas linked with the medical condition and family dynamics. Nurses often focus on physiological needs, but persons cannot be reduced to parts and individuals cannot be isolated from families. Therefore, the psychological, emotional, spiritual, and social aspects are also pertinent to medical care needs. Of course, as nurses we are always concerned about safety at home and in acute care settings.

Individuals have real lives outside health care settings; they are children, parents, spouses, partners, grandparents, cousins, aunts, and uncles. They are friends, neighbors, students, workers, housewives, and retirees. In their communities they are volunteers, civic leaders, coaches, local officials, and community leaders. They are people who others care about and they care about others. People have intimate and valued relationships that are part of their history and personal life stories. Health care settings are intrusions or interruptions in real life. Health and illness are often taken for granted until they become personal events. When health concerns arise, we often meet changes and transitions that last forever. Illness is often a threat, the possibility of a fear-filled future. The following sections describe ways to focus on care linked with the family unit.

Therapeutic Questioning

Nurses have long asked questions of individuals and families in their clinical practice. Starting in the 1950s, Hildegard Peplau (1952, 1997) suggested that focused attention be given through therapeutic relationships. Her perspective suggests that nurses take a reflective stance in nursing practice. An analysis approach to therapeutic questioning in interviewing, assessment, and interventions has now been developed (Wright & Leahey, 2013) based on the work of Tomm (1987, 1988). In their work Wright and Leahey articulated ways to skillfully formulate and use questions:

- Engage all family members and focus the meeting with the family.
- Assess the impact of the problem or illness on the family.
- Elicit family problem-solving skills, coping strategies, and strengths.
- Use "interventive" questioning to invite change.
- Request feedback about the meeting with the family.

Don't underestimate the power of using questions. Sincere questions curiously asked provide information, encourage reflection about experiences, and move people toward healing processes (Wright & Leahey, 2013). Well-thought-out intentional questions can successfully guide family discussion and imply directions for changes. Interventive questions used during assessments or stand-alone questions in health or illness discussions can help in the search for directions of meaningful change.

Conducting Family Interviews

The "15-minute family interview" (Wright & Leahey, 2013) provides a guide for you to actively engage family members in dialogue focused on perceptions of the illness experience. It is used as an introduction to start a relationship with the family; it is not designed to substitute for a full family assessment, but it is a beginning. The 15-minute interview can be completed with a care recipient and at least one other family member. This allows a meaningful but nonthreatening way to begin to listen and interact with families. This interview method can guide novices to master new skills. Assessments should always start with the specific needs individuals present as we can never assess everything possible. However, keep in mind that these presenting needs always have family factors to consider in planning nursing actions.

The 15-Minute Interview

When first learning to use a 15-minute interview, students or nurses might want to choose the individual and family member to interview as new experiences cause apprehension. Some nurses have little conversation with a family beyond answering direct questions, telling them they will ask the doctor, interacting during the admission session, providing care directions, or delivering discharge instructions, so this can be a bit frightening. Even nurses in home care report that even though they have conversations with families all the time, they do not think about having therapeutic conversations (Anderson & Friedemann, 2010; Anderson & Valentine, 1998).

When preparing for the 15-minute interview, consider where this will occur. Ideally, you will conduct this in a place where you will not be interrupted. You want to make sure everyone is comfortable before you begin and start with introductions. In this interview, it is a good idea to write the questions to be asked on a piece of paper before the interview (Box 8.3). They will be used after the introductions are made. Have some paper available to make notes.

BOX 8-3

15-Minute Family Interview Questions: Making a Family Connection

These eight therapeutic questions should be included in the 15-minute interview:

1. How can we be most helpful to your family and friends during your hospitalization (or care episode at home)?
2. What has been most or least helpful in your past hospitalizations or clinic visits?
3. What has been the greatest challenge facing you or your family members during this hospitalization, clinic, or home care visit?
4. Which of your family members or friends would you like us to share information with?
5. What do you need to best prepare you and your family members for discharge?
6. Who do you believe is suffering the most in your family in this hospitalization, clinic, or home care visit?
7. What is the one question you would like answered now in our meeting?
8. How have I been most helpful in this family meeting? How could we improve?

Source: Wright, L., & Leahey, M. (2013). *Nurses and families: A guide to family assessment and intervention* (6th ed., pp. 271–272). Philadelphia: F. A. Davis.

Nurses sometimes worry the first time they do a family interview, mainly for the following reasons:

- I do not know how the family will respond. Will they answer the questions? Will they think I am invading their privacy? Will they ask me something I don't know?
- I really do not know how to talk with families. I have never done this before.
- I usually avoid deep conversations with families.

Being prepared ahead of time helps. Knowing exactly what you will do with your planned questions helps. All new nurses experience some anxiety as they learn new things, but remember that individuals and family members are usually pleased to have conversations with nurses who are interested in them.

As you begin family conversations, focus on listening and truly hearing what is said. This can be difficult when you are nervous. What is the story they want you to hear? How can you acknowledge that you hear what is said? In what ways can you affirm the family and the concerns they express? Of course, courtesy and politeness are important. Open and welcoming introductions set the stage for what follows. An open and caring milieu or atmosphere can be infectious. Keep in mind that sometimes we can ask questions that people do not want to answer. If they refuse to answer a question, just skip it and go on. If it is really important, you might want to return to it later after you sense you have gained their confidence or trust. An initial encounter done with an ill-mannered approach can be damaging. But a friendly, sincere, and engaging approach can lead to a valued relationship. Initial impressions count! Those made in the first minutes count and can be lasting (Wright & Leahey, 2013). As you listen, commend—highlight good things about the family. Note the strengths you observe or hear as you talk together.

Nurses are often amazed at how well a family interview goes. Most families are pleased when someone talks with them and are thankful for time to share concerns and needs. The 15-minute interview provides an initial communication experience and provides opportunities to gain new insights, and gaining self-confidence through a successful interview experience and is a major step in talking and working with families. The 15-minute interview structure of engaging families can provide a memorable experience that offers insight into the value of thinking family for you. One question, item 7 in Box 8.3, gives you a chance to learn what others view as a priority need. Often, at the end of the interview, family members might say that this is the first time anyone ever asked them about what is happening and listened to what they had to say. So interview skills are important and can lead to therapeutic conversations and valued relationships.

Follow-Up to the 15-Minute Interview

After the 15-minute family interview, review the clinical record and see if the information gained has previously been noted. Often, it isn't there. Although nurses traditionally gather some information about families during admission assessments, it's not always documented.

After you have completed the interview and documented important information, take some time to reflect. Evaluate yourself. What is your response to the interview? Is there anything that caused you to respond negatively or in an extremely positive manner? If so, what caused this response in you? Mature family nurses recognize that the thinking family aspect of practice must occur before, during, and after caring events. At the end of the interview, you can begin thinking out loud with the family or other members of an interprofessional team about follow-up steps. What nursing actions are aligned with the information just obtained? What hypothetical steps with the family validate what you have heard the family share. Reflective evaluation, critical thinking skills, and clinical judgments based on nursing knowledge serve as guides for the planning of nursing actions and care to be delivered.

Using Interventive Questioning in Family Nursing

As previously mentioned, therapeutic questions are open-ended and elicit information that goes beyond mere facts or details. It is a skill to know what types of questions to ask and when to ask them. Questions can obtain various forms of information to help:

- Get a straight answer
- Direct the response of the individual-family
- Facilitate family's reflection about their lives
- Explain beliefs and behaviors
- Encourage family members to consider alternative ways to view or solve a problem

Interventive questions help the nurse identify the family's cognitive and emotional experiences linked with health or illness. Interventive questions provide ways to view member differences and similarities. Here are some examples of interventive questions:

- How is this illness affecting your family?
- Tell me about the ways (name a person) is managing the extra caregiving tasks.
- What seems to be the most troubling thing for your family in managing this situation?
- How does this illness situation most interfere with family life?
- When Mom is doing caregiving tasks, what do you think she is thinking about?
- While your Dad is struggling to walk with the walker, what changes in the household are each of you thinking are needed for his safety?

Interventive questions engage cognitive and emotional processes and often are less physically focused, but the answers provide a wealth of information about the family's response to the health or illness issue. Responses elicited can help members think about an issue from a different view. These questions can be used while a genogram or ecomap is completed. As the family tells their stories, nurses make sure that things are heard correctly and interpreted accurately. It is good to ask questions that provide needed clarification and double check what has been said. Key concerns get validated. Critical thinking and expert nursing knowledge are included in the analysis of the situation as clinical judgment is used to weigh potential actions in asking further questions or facilitating family interactions and change. Wright and Leahey (2013) and Loos and Bell (1990) offer extensive lists of differing types of interventive questions for your review.

Using Genograms in Family Nursing Practice

Genograms and ecomaps, tools discussed in earlier chapters, can be combined with your 15-minute interview and your formal family assessment. The genogram uses a family tree structure to document member relationships and other family information. Family members often get engaged as they provide family information and jointly share the record of family life patterns of three generations. Completing this tool gives the nurse and family time to share understandings of the family structure, relationships, critical family events, and health histories. The nurse can guide the genogram interview and information gathering so that it supports individual's medical needs, but also highlights important family health information. The structural map of a family case genogram is shown Figure 8.4.

Using Ecomaps in Family Nursing Practice

The ecomap, discussed in Chapter 5, highlights the family's connection to its environment and identifies the strengths of the bonds among individuals, family members, community

Wilson Family Genogram

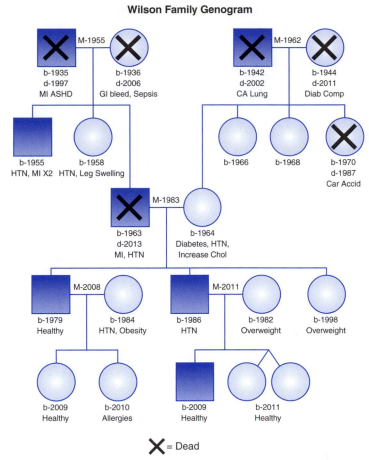

X = Dead

FIGURE 8-4 Wilson family genogram.

agencies, and other resources (Fig. 8.5). This tool provides information about ecological systems connected with the family microsystem (Denham, 2003). This visual representation shows family support networks, external stressors, and support agencies linked with the family unit. Information gained from an ecomap suggests the number, purposes, nature, and usefulness of member interactions with various community and social sectors. This ecological information can be used to evaluate the community resources needed for goal setting and planning nursing actions.

Additional Family Assessment Tools

Besides the tools and skills just described, three other commonly used family assessment tools may be used to guide a family assessment:

- Friedman's Family Assessment Model [Long Form] (1998)
- Hanson and Mischke's Family Systems Stressor-Strength Inventory [FS³I] (2001, cited in Hanson & Kaakinen, 2005)
- Friedemann's Assessment of Strategies in Families—Effectiveness [ASF-E] (1998)

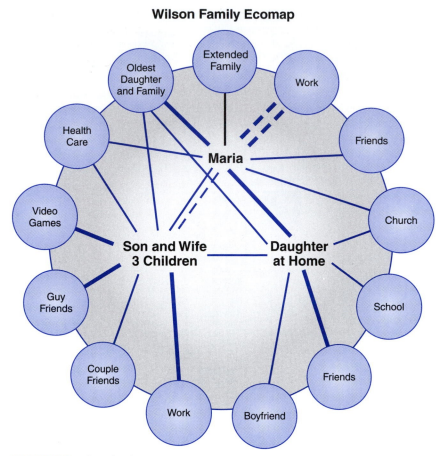

FIGURE 8-5 Wilson family ecomap.

Friedman's Family Assessment

Friedman's (1998) Family Assessment Model—Long Form (FAM) covers six broad categories: identification data, developmental stage and history, environmental data, family structure, family functions, and family stress and coping. Each category has several subcategories. Nurses assessing families decide which categories are most relevant as they tailor an assessment strategy. The topical areas can be a bit lengthy for a novice nurse and require the use of a written form for notes as the assessment is completed. Reviewing the full assessment form can provide some excellent ideas of family life for discussion. For example, if you are caring for a hospitalized person who will be available for several days, then you could select relevant topics and discuss different areas with care delivered on subsequent days. This allows discussion of many things, but avoids single long or drawn-out interviews. It can also be used successfully to engage different family members at various times. A cultural component is also included in this assessment.

Family Systems Stressor-Strength Inventory

The Family Systems Stressor-Strength Inventory (Hanson & Mischke, 2010) focuses on the stressful situations occurring in families and the strengths families use to maintain healthy family functioning. This assessment requires each person to complete an individual form before meeting the family nurse. Although some questions ask for facts, others ask members to describe things. The assessment is scored for each family member and the nurse notes if stressors require primary, secondary, or tertiary intervention. A primary care intervention might be suggesting birth control pills to a newly married couple who are both in school and do not feel ready for children at this time in their relationship. A secondary care intervention might engage a mother and her 15-year-old daughter with diabetes in a discussion about dietary and food selection to help avoid elevated glycemic readings. A tertiary care intervention could be a discussion about how family members will rotate caregiving shifts for their dying father. The written descriptions provide supplementary information that clarifies aspects of family life useful in developing a plan of care. This form of assessment could be useful in situations when working with family needs that extend over time.

ASF-E Assessment Inventory

Friedemann's ASF-E assessment inventory (1998) is based on a family nursing model called the Framework of Systemic Organization (1995). This model has a client-centered approach that focuses on strengths rather than problems. The assessment tool measures the family's basic organization and focuses on four targets or components of family life:

- Stability: how the family is organized and connections with each other
- Growth: the ways families adjust to change and unexpected happenings and individual family members development and growth
- Control: how the family adjusts to individual and family changes and considers family rules, roles, and ways of acting
- Spirituality: how the family keeps connected emotionally, ways different individuals seek meaning in life, and satisfaction with community activities and relationships

When the different family life target levels are calculated, the nurse and the family together determine areas in which the family wants to work. This includes setting goals and deciding on strategies aimed at what the family wants to happen. Scoring the ASF-E is a way to gain some understanding about the ways a particular family functions. Areas in which they might be stuck or not achieving health in the four target areas are identified and then the nurse assists the family to develop self-motivated change plans. Box 8.4 provides information about a family nurse leader in Switzerland and has developed many resources for teaching nursing students ways to work with families.

Other Family Tools

Family nurse researchers have developed instruments to assess various family concepts. Among these are family management style (Knafl & Deatrick, 2003), family coping (McCubbin et al., 1983), social capital in families (Looman, 2006), family functioning (Feetham & Humenick, 1982), family health promotion (Pender et al., 2010), and family health routines (Denham, 2003). Some of these ideas were introduced in Chapter 7, and more about their use is described later in this textbook.

Family Nursing Practice Models

Family nursing models are guides that emphasize family as the unit of care and consider ways individual members affect the health of the whole family and how families affect the individuals (Anderson, 2000; Wright & Leahey, 1984, 2013). Nurses who *think family*

BOX 8-4

Family Tree

Barbara Preusse-Bleuler, RN, MNS, (Switzerland)

Barbara Preusse-Bleuler, RN, MNS, is a lecturer and faculty member at the School of Health Professions, Institute of Nursing, Zurich University of Applied Sciences, Switzerland. Over the past 13 years, the university revolutionized nursing education to include bachelor's, master's, and doctoral programs. In 2000, Professor Preusse-Bleuler attended a program about Family Systems Nursing and the Calgary Family and Assessment Models taught by Dr. Kit Chesla at the Lindenhof Hospital and School in Berne. This experience profoundly influenced her and she developed a passion and vision for family nursing care. In the first Practice Development Project at the Lindenhof Hospital, guidelines and instruments were created to adapt the Calgary Models to Swiss nursing practices. Preusse-Bleuler discovered that the participatory approach of Action Learning and Action Research were effective tools for developing family nursing knowledge, attitudes, and skills with practicing nurses. This approach invited nurses to think systemically about families and illness and reflected a systemic way of working with nursing teams. From these experiences, Preusse-Bleuler wrote a handbook; developed instruments for effective skills training with self-learning; used peer-to-peer learning opportunities; designed education and training courses for beginning and advanced nurses; and developed sustainable implementation concepts for family nursing practice (all in the German language). In 2009, Preusse-Bleuler translated Wright and Leahey's *Nurses and Families: A Guide to Family Assessment and Intervention* into German with a second German edition in 2013. These products are being used to translate family nursing into various practice settings across several regions in Switzerland. Preusse-Bleuler's work has focused tirelessly on promoting family nursing in her teaching and supervision with the goal of ensuring that family nursing is an integral part of daily nursing practice in Switzerland.

---

intentionally include the family unit whether they are physically present or not. Become familiar with the various family theories and models and find one that best fits your personal beliefs. Experienced nurses often use more than a single theoretical perspective in their family work. As a novice family nurse, it is good to work from one theoretical approach. The model you select will serve as a guide for your family nursing practice

Family Health System Model

The Family Health System (FHS) model (Anderson, 2000; Anderson & Friedemann, 2010) gives some ideas about ways theory guides family nursing practice. This model builds on the work of other theories including Family Systems Theory (von Bertalanffy, 1968), the Illness Beliefs Model (Wright & Bell, 2009; Wright, Watson, & Bell, 1996), the Family Stress Theory (Anderson, 1994; Hill, 1958), and Change Theory (Watzlawick, Weakland, & Fisch, 1974). The FHS model (Anderson, 2000; Anderson & Friedemann, 2010; Anderson & Tomlinson, 1992) identifies family nursing care processes and shows not only how to *think family*, but also what to do when working with families across the continuum of care.

The FHS model (Fig. 8.6) provides an integrated approach to examine family health by considering the dynamics of families in five realms of family life: interactional, developmental, coping, integrity, and health realms (Anderson, 2000; Anderson & Tomlinson, 1992). These realms can be used to examine family life dynamics, strengths, and concerns across the life span. The overall goal of the FHS approach is improved health and functioning for family units. It is expected that assessments will address both family and individual health and that nursing care will reflect the family system and individual interactions. This care approach has been the basis for advanced practice nurses (APNs) at the Family

Family Health System Model

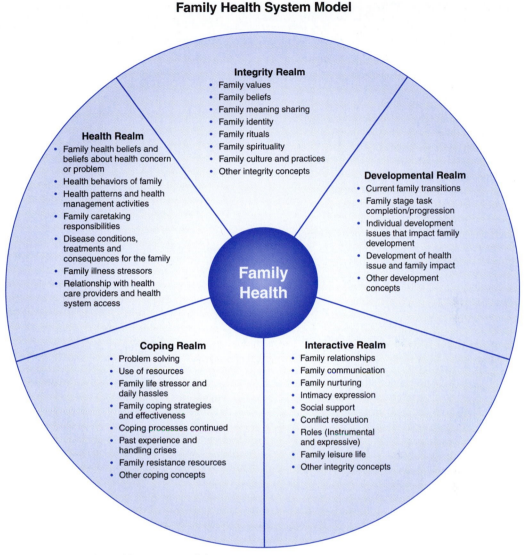

Integrity Realm
- Family values
- Family beliefs
- Family meaning sharing
- Family identity
- Family rituals
- Family spirituality
- Family culture and practices
- Other integrity concepts

Health Realm
- Family health beliefs and beliefs about health concern or problem
- Health behaviors of family
- Health patterns and health management activities
- Family caretaking responsibilities
- Disease conditions, treatments and consequences for the family
- Family illness stressors
- Relationship with health care providers and health system access

Developmental Realm
- Current family transitions
- Family stage task completion/progression
- Individual development issues that impact family development
- Development of health issue and family impact
- Other development concepts

Family Health

Coping Realm
- Problem solving
- Use of resources
- Family life stressor and daily hassles
- Family coping strategies and effectiveness
- Coping processes continued
- Past experience and handling crises
- Family resistance resources
- Other coping concepts

Interactive Realm
- Family relationships
- Family communication
- Family nurturing
- Intimacy expression
- Social support
- Conflict resolution
- Roles (Instrumental and expressive)
- Family leisure life
- Other integrity concepts

FIGURE 8-6 Family Health System model.

Nursing Center (Anderson & Valentine, 1998). The theoretical focus has been used in undergraduate and graduate family nursing programs, a framework in dissertation research (Byrd & Garwick, 2006), in community health agencies, and as a theoretical heuristic model for family nursing practice (Bomar, 2004).

The FHS model proposes that the five realms of family life are foundational to approaching the nursing care of families. Box 8.5 shows the family concepts that are included in each realm; other conceptual ideas may be added as nurses see fit. While considering the five realms, note the family strengths and areas of concern in each realm.

Box 8.6 provides a list of the assumptions underlying the FHS model (Anderson, 2000; Anderson & Tomlinson, 1992). This model encourages nurses to do three things:

1. View family as the expert on its life.
2. Engage the family system interaction with an attitude of respect for the family.
3. Believe that the family is giving their best effort to their family life.

BOX 8-5

Family Concepts of Five Realms of Family Life: Family Health System Model

1. Interactive processes
   - Family relationships
   - Family communication
   - Family nurturing
   - Intimacy expression
   - Social support
   - Conflict resolution
   - Roles (instrumental and expressive)
   - Family leisure life
   - Other interactive concepts
2. Developmental processes
   - Current family transitions
   - Family stage task completion/progression
   - Individual development issues that affect family development
   - Development of health issue and family impact
   - Other developmental concepts
3. Coping processes
   - Problem solving
   - Use of resources
   - Family life stressors and daily hassles
   - Family coping strategies and effectiveness
   - Coping processes utilized
   - Past experience with handling crises
   - Family resistance resources
   - Other coping concepts
4. Integrity processes
   - Family values
   - Family beliefs
   - Family meaning sharing
   - Family identity
   - Family rituals
   - Family spirituality
   - Family culture and practices
   - Other integrity concepts
5. Health processes
   - Family health beliefs and beliefs about health concern or problem
   - Health-promoting behaviors of family
   - Health patterns/practices and health management activities
   - Family caretaking responsibilities and impact
   - Disease conditions, treatments, and consequences for the family
   - Family illness stressors
   - Relationship with health care providers and health system access

---

In family-focused nursing, the individual-nurse-family partnership is used to promote family health through caring interactions that utilize family strengths to address health concerns. In the FHS model, the individual-nurse-family work values the family beliefs about the illness, and acknowledges the amount of family stress created by the health or illness situation and needs for providing care. It considers the ways family members interact with each other around family health issues and identifies the environmental

---

BOX 8-6

Assumptions of the Family Health System Model

1. Family health is systemic and process oriented.
2. Family health includes an interaction of biopsychosocial and contextual phenomena.
3. Family health incorporates the health of the collective and the interaction of the health of the individual with the collective.
4. The goal for intervention in family health includes an optimal response in each of these five realms of family experience.
5. All families have the capacity for transforming their quality of life and family health.
6. The interaction of the caring and informed family nurse and the family working together will facilitate movement toward family health.

---

influences and the resources available to the family. Individuals and families often need assistance as they manage the changes and transitions associated with health and illness.

The FHS model encourages family nurses to consider ways family interactions and beliefs influence integrity, coping, and development as they relate with each other, work together or function (e.g., decision making, problem solving), create meanings, resolve conflicts, manage stress, and improve health (e.g., family caregiving, family health promotion). Families use roles to achieve family tasks. Also, families have shared beliefs, rituals, and routines relevant to health and illness. The family health realms can be used to address all forms of care needs. By using family strengths, family nurses focus on things to address, change, or accomplish related to the family's health goals. With each individual situation, attention is given to examining family concerns and strengths in each of the FHS realms to achieve a family's desired outcomes and change. This model can prompt nurses to consider coordinated care across settings and include the family household, and not merely focus on the acute care setting.

Hospital to Home: Clinical Example Using the FHS in Family Care

Consider the goal of strengthening a family's ability to manage a health-related situation. A couple is taking their first child home from the hospital. The family nurse who worked with them during labor and delivery is planning two home visits the first week after discharge as the family requested. The nurse schedules the visit to ensure that both parents will be home. An earlier assessment indicated the couple has a strong caring relationship. The father wants to be involved in every step of his new son's care and his wife is breastfeeding. When the nurse visits the family home, assessment of the baby and mother are completed. However, the nurse also discusses concerns previously voiced by the couple during the hospitalization:

- Adjustment to life at home with the baby (developmental realm)
- Ways the baby is included in their lives and particular stressors (coping realm)
- Family rituals that are valued to be included in family life (integrity realm)
- Interactions with each other and extended family (interactive realm)
- Concerns linked with health promotion and health intervention (e.g., immunizations, healing after birth, pumping for extra milk, health questions) (health realm)
- Time for the couple relationship (interactive realm).

In assisting the family to organize their resources to deal with family issues from each realm, the nurse uses the FHS model to work with them in ways to address specific concerns and work toward achieving goals. The couple had addressed the first five areas previously mentioned, but they had not discussed the last concern. The nurse spoke with the couple about ways to keep their relationship strong. For example, they might arrange help to care for the baby so they could continue to have some time together. Research shows that couples who take regular date time weekly of at least 2 hours have more successful marriages (Gottman & Silver, 1999; Gottman & Silver, 2013). Working with families encourages nurses to provide holistic care.

Family Assessment Using the FHS Model

In the FHS approach, the individual-nurse-family partnership is used to identify the family's main concerns. The nurse starts with "thinking family" and uses interviewing, caring, and perceptive skills to establish a connection with family members. He realizes that the family members are the expert on their life and believes they try their best to manage health and illness. While listening during the initial contact, the nurse makes observations about member interactions. A 15-minute interview could be used. The genogram (see Fig. 8.4) and the ecomap (see Fig. 8.5) can be used to gather other family information. As the family story is told, identify strengths that permeate their lives. Write them down for later use and share when appropriate. For example, if the primary concern is stress with an illness (coping realm) or arrangement of care for an elderly member to stay at home (health realm), then these points are the focus of the care interventions. The FHS model can address many family life areas and care is always based upon family priorities using family strengths.

Family Health Interventions

The individual-nurse-family partnership is used to develop strategies aimed at goals. Family dialogue can help the nurse learn beliefs about things that will or will not work, what they are able and willing to do, and what is needed. As families talk, they often identify potential solutions without the nurse's guidance. During the family interaction, ensure neutrality, hypothetical thinking, and circularity. Check to see if there are care aspects that need to be coordinated. Using combined suggestions from the family and the nurse's expertise, set goals and make decisions about concrete intervention strategies that family members value.

Plans for family interventions are results of collaborative partnerships. Review findings from research literature to identify what evidence exists that supports family interventions (Melnyk & Fineout-Overholt, 2010). The number of intervention studies and evidence for family nursing continue to grow. For example, a demonstration project at a large medical center in Wisconsin studied 50 families managing different chronic illnesses (Anderson & Valentine, 1998, 2000). The results indicated that many families dealing with chronic illnesses discussed a need for a variety of interventions. Table 8.1 gives examples of these implemented family interventions. In this project, families were given a copy of the plan as a reminder of options they had developed (Anderson & Valentine, 1998). The family nurse verified and validated with the family their working care plans. Documentation of the plan in the patient/family record provided a record for the family nurse and others. Written comprehensive family assessment summaries may also be completed for report purposes.

Ongoing evaluation of progress toward achieving family goals or outcomes is essential. Were the goals met? If not met, why not? How effective was the family intervention? What did or did not work? What kinds of follow-up are needed (e.g., education, coaching, demonstrations)? It is important to check with the family at subsequent meetings or interactions about their progress toward the goals. Commend them for successes; encouraging and empowering support family unit efforts. Evaluation and continued planning are essential parts of continuing care. Consider family feedback, revision of care outcomes, or other

TABLE 8-1	*Family Interventions in Select Chronic Illnesses (Anderson & Valentine, 2000)*
Cancer	• Managing care demands and coverage, dying, fears, and loss • Unresolved family issues and plans after death • Sibling and health care professional (HCP) conflict • Equitable caregiving • Decrease strain on children's families • Home health nurse referral
Cardiac conditions	• Family difficulty, fears, stress, and anxiety impact on family life • Impending death and restructuring of life focus on quality • Health condition and focus on patient affecting marital quality • Broadening of social support • Fear of pain and depression • Grief and impact on family • Clarify and problem-solve family-HCP conflicts

Chronic pain	• Provide information about falls, illness, and medications
	• Promote clear understanding of disease process
	• Facilitate open communication in family
	• Problem-solve to coordinate care between home, acute care, and outpatient or physician care
	• Referral for home environment evaluation
	• Referral for home health nurse
	• Discuss with family:
	  • Nature of conflicts, sense of burden, and issues to problem-solve
	  • Independence maintenance

Dementia	• Explore division of labor by family members
	• Community support planning
	• Discuss with family:
	  • Disease process
	  • Develop communication tracking system,
	  • Address family stress concerns and future
	  • Wishes for death experience with family
	  • Advanced directives and quality of life (QOL)

Diabetes	• Develop plan to maintain caregiver health
	• Referrals, financial concerns, and home health nurse
	• Discuss with family:
	  • Family-HCP conflicts and problem-solve solutions
	  • Future trajectory of illness and meanings for illness
	  • Issues related to family communication

Continued

TABLE 8-1	*Family Interventions in Select Chronic Illnesses (Anderson & Valentine, 2000)—cont'd*
Primary family interventions— common to all chronic conditions	• Interventive questioning
	• Work out equitable distribution of care and caregiving plan
	• Depression evaluation
	• Strategies for social and community support
	• Referrals to HHN, financial concerns, respite, home environmental evaluation
	• Develop safety plan
	• Concrete family interventions
	• Managing care demands
	• Arrange care coverage
	• Unresolved family issues
	• Sibling and HCP conflict
	• Grief, fears, anxieties
	• Illness trajectory and resultant planning
	• Facilitate open communications
	• Role changes; family stress
	• Relationship quality changes and desires
Stroke	• Reframe personal attacks and soften with illness in mind
	• Increase social activities
	• Organize caregiving
	• Referral for depression evaluation
	• Discuss difficulties, roles changes, household functioning

nursing actions to incorporate over time. Evaluation enables systematic and timely analysis of progress toward meeting goals. Most families work hard to improve their family life and make needed adaptations to the health and illness situations and they are the experts at determining what worked and what did not. Through respectful listening, determine the best ways to help the family improve their life, alleviate suffering and emotional pain, promote health, and keep the family safe.

Terminating Relationships

Nurses do not always think about how they will end a relationship. In today's busy health care settings, persons are usually in and out of acute care settings quickly and it might not seem necessary to consider the relationship's end. However, even briefly formed ties need and deserve an appropriate ending. Once a bond has been formed, a need to acknowledge the separation that is to come exists. For example, if it is an inpatient setting in the United States, the discharge might be from hospital to home with follow-up care with a primary or specialty care practice. If more intensive care is required, the termination might result in a transfer to a step-down care setting, assisted living, nursing home, or home care agency. It is always important to acknowledge the individual and family members and assist them as they transition to the next stage of their care or health journey.

It is important to begin thinking of ways to build a culture of health in our nation (Lavizzo-Mourey, 2014). This implies taking a bigger picture of what defines health in our nation. The Robert Wood Johnson Foundation and others are encouraging us to consider ways costs, benefits, and effectiveness of treatment and prevention provide highly valued care. A culture of health could mean many things, but it begins in family households and communities. It involves living in ways that allow us to be and stay healthy. This involves caring in ways that not only address acute care needs, but see each care contact as a way to empower the family and motivate individuals. According to Hibbard, Stiockard, Mahoney, and Tusler (2004), achieving quality health outcomes must enlist activated persons who possess the following qualities:

- Believe personal roles are important.
- Have the needed confidence and knowledge to take action.
- Actually take action to maintain and improve health.
- Maintain actions to achieve outcomes even under stress.

A culture of health could include safe homes, violence prevention, proper use of medications, healthy weights, and physically active lives. Finding ways to increase personal activation has great potential for improving health outcomes (Greene & Hibbard, 2011); testing of family inclusion seems a logical nursing intervention.

Discussing things that might occur with the transfer, discharge, or departure provides a chance to ask additional questions and express concerns. Depending upon the depth of the relationship, a smooth termination with the family can include things such as brief letters to the family, commendations on strengths observed, compliments about progress made, wishes for sustained progress, and hope for the future (Wright & Leahey, 2013). If ongoing care is necessary, provide a review of the plan of care that needs further attention. Also furnish written and oral instructions, but ensure that they are created based on literacy, culture, and language needs, considering the resources that families have at home to be able to carry out the family interventions. A final conversation might include things like having them tell you about the most helpful thing in your work together or what they wished had been different. Responses can be insightful and help the nurse truly gain

---

BOX 8-7

Family Circle

A family is having trouble with their middle-school-aged son after being given family rules about coming home on time and completing family chore tasks. The parents are afraid that their son has befriended a group of older teens who are known to use drugs and alcohol. The parents think their family life is out of control and are not happy when their son disappears and does not contact them for a whole weekend. They are especially concerned because he has long had a history of attention deficit-hyperactivity disorder (ADHD) and has been in trouble in school. In addition, their family history indicates that alcoholism and addiction have been problems for many ancestors. When his mother takes him for his clinic visit, she says: "Our son is completely out of control and so is our family because of him." The family nurse wants to complete a family assessment during the visit.

1. Think about this family and identify areas you want to assess.
2. How can you use the 15-minute interview with this family?
3. List three interventive questions you might use.
4. What aspects of each family realm need addressing?
5. How will you go about discussing a plan to change the "sense of no control" this family is experiencing?

empathy for their challenges. The termination process involves some reflection by the nurse about what has been learned from this family interaction. Families have lessons to teach nurses. Thank the family and share what you have learned from them, and tell them what you will carry with you in your practice with other families, including differences learned from culturally diverse families. Evaluate yourself. What went well? What do you wish you might have done differently? Family nurses with years of practice can often recount lessons learned and wisdom they were taught by those receiving care. Take some time to work with others in your class to review the case study in Box 8.7. Talk together to decide the best ways to answer each of the questions.

Chapter Summary

Nurses often focus on the immediate needs of those in their care. Pressing demands that appear to require urgent attention are often given the priority. Holistic family care involves a larger perspective, one that includes the family unit, family relationships, and support systems. Nurses usually focus on the individual, but this does not regularly include an integrated individual-nurse-family approach. Sometimes nurses want to interact with families but they are uncertain where to begin or what to do. Thus, care often responds to expediency, immediacy, critical incidents, or unplanned interruptions. This chapter described many nursing skills and actions useful in establishing relationships and providing care with families. This chapter describes the importance of the individual-nurse-family relationship as an intentional relationship at the core of family nursing practice. A number of approaches, skills, and tools that family nurses can use in practice are described. The Family Health System model (Anderson, 2000; Anderson & Tomlinson, 1992) is used as an exemplar model to demonstrate one approach to family nursing. Thinking family employs a mind-set that facilitates nursing family care that integrates background knowledge about families, health and illness, caring, and the nursing process with family nursing assessment and intervention skills, evidence-based practice knowledge, and communication skills that promote family health.

REFERENCES

Anderson, K. H. (1997). Family Health System: Assessment and Intervention Guide. Unpublished tool. Eau Claire, WI: University of Wisconsin–Eau Claire.

Anderson, K. H. (2000). Family Health System approach to family systems nursing. *Journal of Family Nursing, 6*(2), 103–119. doi: 10.1177/107484070000600202

Anderson, K. H. (1998). The relationship between family sense of coherence and family quality of life after illness diagnosis: Collective and consensus views. In H. I. McCubbin, E. A. Thompson, A. I. Thompson, & J. E. Fromer (Eds.), *Stress, coping and health in families: Sense of coherence and resiliency* (pp. 169–187). Thousand Oaks, CA: Sage.

Anderson, K. H., & Friedemann, M. L. (2010). Strategies to teach family assessment and intervention through an online international curriculum. *Journal of Family Nursing, 16*(2), 213–233. doi: 10.1177/1074840710367639

Anderson, K. H., Nagy, S., Friedemann, M. L., & Buescher, A. (2011, June). *Nine categories of family interventions in chronic illness from family-focused studies.* Paper presented at the 10th International Family Nursing Association Conference, Kyoto, Japan.

Anderson, K. H., & Tomlinson, P. S. (1992). The Family Health System as an emerging paradigmatic view for nursing. *Image: Journal of Nursing Scholarship, 24*(1), 57–63.

Anderson, K. H., & Valentine, K. L. (1998). Establishing and sustaining a Family Nursing Center for families with chronic illness: The Wisconsin experience. *Journal of Family Nursing, 4*(2), 127–141.

Anderson, K. H., & Valentine, K. L. (2000, May). *Family health interventions: Helping middle-aged/older families with difficulty coping with chronic illness.* Paper presented at the 5th International Family Nursing Conference, Chicago, IL.

Antonovsky, A. (1994). The sense of coherence: An historical and future perspective. In H. I. McCubbin, E. A. Thompson, A. I. Thompson, & J. E. Fromer (Eds.), *Sense of coherence and resiliency: Stress, coping and health* (pp. 3–20). Madison: University of Wisconsin System.

Berkey, K. M., & Hanson, S. M. (1991). *Pocket guide to family assessment and intervention.* St. Louis: Mosby.

Bomar, P. (2004). *Promoting health in families: Applying family research and theory to nursing practice* (3rd ed.). Philadelphia: Saunders/Elsevier.

Byrd, M. M., & Garwick, A. W. (2006). Family identity: Black-white interracial family health experience. *Journal of Family Nursing, 12*(1), 22–37.

Cecchin, G. (1987). Hypothesizing, circularity, and neutrality revisited: An invitation to curiosity. *Family Process, 26,* 405–413. doi:10.1111/j.1545 -5300.1987.00405.xI

Clements, I. W., & Roberts, F. B. (1983). *Family health: A theoretical approach to family nursing care.* New York: John Wiley.

Denham, S. A. (2003). *Family health: A framework for nursing.* Philadelphia: F. A. Davis.

Doane, G. H., & Varcoe, C. (2005). *Family nursing as relational inquiry: Developing health-promoting practice.* Philadelphia: Lippincott Williams & Wilkins.

Feetham, S. L., & Humenick, S. S. (1982). The Feetham family functioning survey. In S. S. Humenick (Ed.), *Analysis of current assessment strategies in the health care of young children and child-bearing families* (pp. 249–268). Norwalk, CT: Appleton-Century-Crofts.

Friedemann, M. L. (1995). *The framework of systemic organization: A conceptual approach for nursing and families.* Thousand Oaks, CA: Sage.

Friedemann, M. L. (1998). Assessment of strategies in families—Effectiveness [ASF-E]. Retrieved from http://www2.fiu.edu/~friedemm/

Friedemann, M. L., Pagan-Coss, H., & Mayorga, C. (2008). The workings of a multicultural research team. *Journal of Transcultural Nursing, 19,* 266–273. doi:10.1177/1043659608317094

Friedman, M. M. (1998). *Family nursing: Research, theory, & practice* (4th ed.). Stamford, CT: Appleton & Lange.

Gottman, J. M., & Silver, N. (1999). *The seven principles for making marriage work.* New York: Three Rivers Press.

Gottman, J. M., & Silver, N. (2013). *What makes love last? How to build trust and avoid betrayal.* New York: Simon & Schuster.

Greene, J., & Hibbard, J. H. (2011). Why does patient activation matter? An examination of the relationship between patient activation and health-related outcomes. *Journal of General Internal Medicine, 27*(5), 520–526. doi: 10.1007/s11606-011-1931-2. Retrieved September 15, 2014 from http://link.springer.com/article/10.1007/s11606-011-1931-2#page-2

Hanson, S. M. H., & Kaakinen, J. R. (2005). Theoretical foundations for nursing of families. In S. M. H. Hanson, V. Gedaly-Duff, & J. R. Kaakinen (Eds.), *Family health care nursing: Theory, practice and research* (3rd ed., pp. 69–96). Philadelphia: F. A. Davis.

Hanson, S. M. H., & Mischke, K. B. (2010). Family systems stressor-strength inventory (FS^{3}I). In J. R. Kaakinen, V. Gedaly-Duff, D. P. Coehlo, & S. M. H. Hanson (Eds.), *Family health care nursing: Theory, practice and research* (4th ed.). Philadelphia: F. A. Davis.

Hartrick, G. A. (1997). A critical pedagogy of family nursing. *Journal of Nursing Education, 37*(2), 80–84.

Hibbard, J. H., Stiockard, J., Mahoney, E. R., & Tusler, M. (2004). Development of the Patient Activation Measure (PAM): Conceptualizing and measuring activation in patients and consumers. *Health Services Research, 39*(4), 1005–1026.

Hill, R. (1958). Social stresses on the family: Genesis features of stress. *Social Casework, 39,* 139–158.

Kaakinen, J. R., Gedaly-Duff, V., Coelho, D. P., & Hanson, S. M. H. (Eds.) (2014). *Family health care nursing: Theory, practice and research* (5th ed.). Philadelphia: F. A. Davis.

Kendall, J., & Tabacco, A. (2011). Parents and children together: In-home intervention for families with children with attention-deficit/hyperactivity disorder. In E. K. Svarsdottir and H. Jonsdottir (Eds.), *Family nursing in action* (pp. 185–216). Reykjavik: University of Iceland Press.

Knafl, K., & Deatrick, J. (2003). Further refinement of the Family Management Style Framework. *Journal of Family Nursing, 9*(3), 232–256.

Lavizzo-Mourey, R. (2014). Building a culture of health. Robert Wood Johnson. Retrieved September 15, 2014 from http://www.rwjf.org/en/about-rwjf/annual-reports/presidents-message-2014.html

Looman, W. S. (2006). Development and testing of the Social Capital Scale for families of children with special health care needs. *Research in Nursing & Health, 29*(4), 325–336.

Loos, F., & Bell, J. M. (1990). Circular questions: A family interviewing strategy. *Dimensions in Critical Care Nursing, 9*(1), 46–53.

McCubbin, H. I., McCubbin, M. A., Patterson, J. M., Cauble, A. E., Wilson, L. R., & Warwick, W. (1983). CHIP—Coping Health Inventory for Parents: An assessment of parental coping patterns in the care of the chronically ill child. *Journal of Marriage and the Family, 45,* 359–370.

McCubbin, M. A., & McCubbin, H. I. (1996). Resiliency in families: A conceptual model of family adjustment and adaptation in response to stress and crisis. In H. I. McCubbin, A. I. Thompson, & M. A. McCubbin (Eds.), *Family assessment: Resiliency, coping, and adaptation—Inventories for research and practice* (pp. 1–64). Madison: University of Wisconsin.

Melnyk, B., & Fineout-Overholt, E. (2010). Evidence-based practice in nursing & healthcare: A guide to best practice. Philadelphia: Lippincott Williams & Wilkins.

Miller, J. R., & Janosik, E. H. (1980). *Family-focused care.* New York: McGraw-Hill.

Nelms, T., & Eggenberger, S. K. (2010). The essence of the family critical illness experience nurse-family meetings. *Journal of Family Nursing, 16*(4), 462–486. doi:10.1177/1074840710386608

Pender, N. J., Murdaugh, C. L., & Parsons, M. A. (2010). *Health promotion in nursing practice.* New York: Prentice Hall.

Peplau, H. (1952). *Interpersonal relations in nursing.* New York: Putnam.

Peplau, H. (1997). Peplau's theory of interpersonal relations. *Nursing Science Quarterly, 10*(4), 162

Satir, V. (1967). *Conjoint family therapy.* Palo Alto, CA: Science and Behavior Books.

The White House. (2010). A more secure future: What the new health care law means for you and your family. Retrieved from http://www.whitehouse.gov/healthreform/healthcare-overview

Tomm, K. (1987). Interventive interviewing: Part II. Reflexive questioning as a means to self-healing. *Family Process, 26*(6), 167–183.

Tomm, K. (1988). Interventive interviewing: Part III. Intending to ask lineal, circular, strategic, or reflexive questions? *Family Process, 27*(1), 1–15.

von Bertalanffy, L. W. (1968). *General systems theory: Foundations, development, and applications.* New York: George Braziller.

Watzlawick, P., Weakland, J., & Fisch, R. (1974). *Changes: Principles of problem formulation and problem resolution.* New York: Norton.

World Health Organization, Regional Office for Europe. (2000). *The family health nurse: Context, conceptual framework and curriculum* (EUR/00/5019309/13). Copenhagen, Denmark: Author.

Wright, L., & Bell, J. (2009). *Beliefs and illness: A model for healing.* Calgary, Alberta, Canada: 4th Floor Press.

Wright, L. M., & Leahey, M. (1984). *Nurses and families: A guide to family assessment and intervention.* Philadelphia: F. A. Davis.

Wright, L. M., & Leahey, M. (1994). *Nurses and families: A guide to family assessment and intervention* (2nd ed.). Philadelphia: F. A. Davis.

Wright, L., & Leahey, M. (2013). *Nurses and families: A guide to family assessment and intervention* (6th ed.). Philadelphia: F. A. Davis.

Wright, L. M., Watson, W. L., & Bell, J. M. (1996). *Beliefs: The heart of healing in families and illness.* New York: Basic Books.

CHAPTER 9

Family and Nurse Presence in Family-Focused Care

Mary Bliesmer • Pat Earle • Sandra K. Eggenberger
• Norma Krumwiede • Sonja J. Meiers

"Nursing engages in a life-death journey, participates in birthing-living-playing-loving-dying as the very fabric of human existence. The moral and visionary compass for my journey comes not from the head but from the heart." Jean Watson (2007, p. 173)

CHAPTER OBJECTIVES

1. Differentiate between the ideas of nurse presence and family presence.
2. Describe the influence of nurse and family presence in various health and illness experiences.
3. Describe nursing actions that support family caring strategies and family presence.
4. Explain implications of being present with individuals, family members, and supportive others during nursing care encounters.

CHAPTER CONCEPTS

- Adaptation
- Family advocates
- Family balancing
- Family connecting
- Family emotions
- Family inquiry
- Family integrity
- Family presence
- Family vigilance
- Hope
- Nurse presence
- Satisfaction
- Vulnerability

Introduction

Presence can be viewed as "the difference that nursing makes" in promoting the health of individuals and families (Newman, 2008, p. 21). Presence refers to a commitment to another, full engagement or openness, interconnectedness, valuing another's dignity, and recognizing what is important to another (Melnechenko, 2003; Parse, 1998). Human presence can lessen the suffering and distress of another human through relationships and connections (Eggenberger & Nelms, 2007). Presence can also be considered from the perspective of being a family member who is connected to others in the family unit. Individual and family bonds must be respected by nurses who acknowledge the value and potential of connectedness and its powerful influence on health and illness. During times of illness, crisis, and uncertainty, family connections are intensified. Nurses who *think family* realize that members often want to be together at poignant points in life. The presence of a supportive family member can minimize the distress of an illness situation and maximize the health and healing potential of nursing care.

In 1995, a Family Nursing Research Team (FNRT) was formed at the School of Nursing at Minnesota State University, Mankato, to investigate how family nursing care links with family health and illness experiences (Fig. 9.1). The team aimed to develop practice knowledge that would assist nurses in supporting and caring for families. Family investigations explored health and illness experiences. The team also collaborated in teaching nursing students about the importance of nurse presence in health or illness care and partnered with other faculty colleagues in academic and practice settings. This chapter shares findings from this team's focused research program. Ways nurses can incorporate presence as they *think family* and provide family-focused nursing actions are described. The chapter includes an evolving case study that addresses the effects of a family tragedy. Examples of interpersonal relationships, availability, sensitivity, holism, intimacy, vulnerability, and adaptation are included. The case study highlights family presence and nurse presence as the family transitions through various health care settings. The ebb and flow of family strengths and the effects of nursing presence upon these transitions are described in the case study as Meloni's mother tells her story.

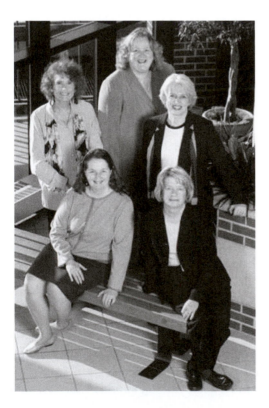

FIGURE 9-1 Family Nursing Research Team, Minnesota State University, Mankato.

The Concept of Presence

An early reference to presence defined this concept as "a mode of being fully available with a 'gift of the self'" (Paterson & Zderad, 1976, p. 132). Presence involves an interpersonal process that embodies sensitivity and availability (Finfgeld-Connett, 2006) and contributes to deep and valued relationships (Chinn & Kramer, 2008; Melnechenko, 2003). Being present is a way of being with another person in a manner that recognizes that person's values, meanings, and needs; it is an invitation to explore issues, concerns, and events as individuals choose (Parse, 1998). The power of presence becomes evident as one reflects on the importance of family presence in health and illness situations (Box 9.1).

Nurse Presence

The presence of a nurse is recognized as a nursing intervention or action, a relational skill of being with another, both physically and psychologically, during times of need (Dochterman & Bulechek, 2004; McMahon & Christopher, 2011). Nurse presence has been described as a key that opens the door to a relationship (Gardner, 1992), the essence of nursing (Koerner, 2007; Newman, 2008), and a way to embody caring during an illness experience (Finfgeld-Connett, 2008; Gardner, 1992; Snyder, Brandt, & Tseng, 2000). Nurse presence is a sincere human connection and a reciprocal exchange between nurses and persons (Hessel, 2009). During this interaction active listening, empathy, caring and compassion, attentiveness, intimacy, therapeutic touch, spiritual exploration, and recognition take place (Hessel, 2009). The presence of a nurse provides a space for relationship building. A nurse's accessibility may bring calm or peaceful feelings and even enable a spiritual or existential connection (Pavlish & Ceronsky, 2009).

Nurse presence is more than just treating physical needs; it means sharing the whole of human experience that can help others find meaning in their illness experience (Krumwiede et al., 2004; Meiers & Tomlinson, 2003; Nelms & Eggenberger, 2010). Research suggests that a nurse's presence and relationship can help families endure the illness experience (Iseminger, Levitt, & Kirk, 2009; Snyder et al., 2000), ease their suffering (Wright & Bell, 2009; Wright & Leahey, 2013), and create a healing environment (Wright & Bell, 2009). Nurse presence is facilitated through multiple interactions, clinical expertise, and availability in a health event or situation (Godkin, 2001). Nurse support occurs during a meaningful and healing relationship that affirms persons and their family members (DeLashmutt & Rankin, 2006). Presence allows nurses to go where people are in their experience, to learn

---

BOX 9-1

Describing the Concept of Presence

The term *presence* has been described in a number of ways and all of them can pertain to powerful ideas about nursing practice:

- Presence is an interpersonal process characterized by sensitivity, holism, intimacy, vulnerability, and adaptation to unique circumstances (Finfgeld-Connett, 2008).
- The consequences of presence influence its enactment in the future (Finfgeld-Connett, 2008).
- Presence has potential to enhance well-being for nurses and for individuals it can improve emotional and physical well-being (Finfgeld-Connett, 2008).
- Presence is a way of being with or being there for people as they describe experiences and meanings in the context of their lives (Gardner, 1985; Hessel, 2009).

about their experience as they define and live it, and to work with persons as they choose the meaning of the situation (Melnechenko, 2003). Nurse presence is described as a call to share and hear another's vulnerability and suffering (Miller & Douglas, 1998).

Case Study—Part 1: Family Life Before the Tragedy

Our family, as told from a mother's perspective, is a typical middle class family: neither rich nor poor. We raised our children in rural Minnesota, where I and three of the five children still live. We are a diverse family with varying personalities, interests, passions, likes and dislikes, values, professional interests, and love . . . most of the time, that is. While living the typical life, interesting things have happened along the way—big and small—and one tragic and totally shocking event occurred. Our family and the small community where we live were affected.

This story is about my daughter Meloni, the fourth of my five children. She is quiet, soft spoken, and very funny. She is a good mother, the kind all of us wish we could be, the type of mother who knows innately that children are more important than chores and more valuable than money. She spent many hours with her two sons, helping with their homework, building an igloo and then crawling in there with them, reading, snowmobiling, attending school activities, and volunteering in their classrooms while working full time. Meloni and her husband Stephen had the kind of marriage that many of us wish for our daughters and sons. Stephen was handsome, hardworking, a standout husband and father. He cared for his family with love and respect. He came from a close family with two girls and four boys. The family was well known and respected in their community.

Case Study—Part 2: Tragedy and the Engagement of Nurses

On a winter Friday evening, Stephen and his 11-year-old son Brad were attending the high school hockey game. Stephen headed home after taking Brad to a friend's house to spend the night. Meanwhile, Meloni and David, 13 years old, went to a local eatery for dinner. Meloni enjoyed her time with David . . . some kind of wonderful when a 13-year-old boy wants to go out with his mother! After watching the news, everyone went to bed not realizing their lives were about to change drastically! Meloni would never see David or Stephen alive again and she would courageously fight for 9 months to return to a somewhat normal life.

Meloni's mother continues: The sheriff came to my door earlier, but when no one answered, he left a message to call the sheriff in the town where my daughter and her family lived. The sheriff finally got in touch with my husband and told him the awful news. An intruder had broken into my daughter's home and shot and killed her husband. When she thought the intruder had left, she called softly across the hall to where her 13-year-old son was sleeping to bring a phone as she had been shot and critically wounded. David got on the phone and called 911, he barely got the words out about what happened when the intruder returned and shot and killed him. Meloni watched her firstborn bleed to death on the floor beside her. What followed was nothing short of miraculous. Meloni who had never been a rebel or fighter hung on, in part I'm sure, because her surviving son really needed her.

It was well below zero, a storm was coming. The roads were inaccessible due to the number of rescue vehicles blocking the way. An emergency helicopter was sent, but had to land at the local airport to which the ambulance took Meloni. She was transported to a trauma center 90 miles away where experienced experts were available.

The wonderful team of doctors, nurses, physical therapists, families and friends played important roles. I must accentuate the role that nurses played in caring for my daughter and our family. Although this was a busy unit, the nurses never appeared rushed. They acted as though Meloni was the most important person in the unit. They were attentive and explained everything. Staff members seemed always available. Communication was essential. A message board I used reassured me that nurses knew the location of a family member at all times. It is hard to put into words the security the nurses conveyed to the family as well as Meloni. Even when the nurses were not physically there, the family could feel their presence as family members remained at the hospital night and day.

Family Presence

During family life, members must face the inevitable times of illness, death, and painful life transitions. The presence of family members can be crucial to the wholeness of an individual. Knowing that a family member is available or nearby during times of trouble is often important to the individual managing an illness (Meleis, 2010). This comforts the individual in crisis as well as the family members who are distressed. A family's experience during illness can be filled with fear, anxiety, stress, and change. Families often feel helplessness, anger, sadness, and conflict as a family member navigates an illness experience (Alvarez & Kirby, 2006; Hughes, Bryan, & Robbins, 2005; Jones et al., 2004). A family's connection to the ill person often causes them to want to be nearby during acute, chronic, or terminal illness (Eggenberger, Meiers, Krumwiede, Bliesmer, & Earle, 2011; Eggenberger & Nelms, 2007; Krumwiede et al., 2004; Meiers, Eggenberger, Krumwiede, Bliesmer, & Earle, 2009; Meiers & Tomlinson, 2003).

When faced with serious or unexpected medical events, crisis with unexpected outcomes, uncertainties linked with surgery, fear associated with birth and death, and other critical points in time, family members support one another. The presence of a family member not only provides comfort, but the family unit is often more peaceful when they can be nearby. Even if discord and conflict surface, the family still needs to be together during a stressful illness experience (Eggenberger & Nelms, 2007). Despite divergent beliefs and perceptions, the distress and demands of an illness can seem more manageable when family is near.

Nursing literature is filled with facts about the importance of family presence for a hospitalized patient when nurses and other health providers perform invasive procedures (Basol, Ohman, Simones, & Skillings, 2009; Emergency Nurses Association, 2009; McClement, Fallis, & Pereira, 2009). Evidence indicates that family presence is important during times of acute illness requiring lifesaving measures such as cardiopulmonary resuscitation (Hung & Pang, 2011). Family presence can also facilitate positive health outcomes during chronic illness and life transitions (Chesla, 2010). Box 9.2 highlights a leading nursing scholar who has examined families during illness and nursing interventions focused on families. Even health promotion is better if individuals can learn along with someone who cares. Family's emotional bonds are ties to loved ones that call for closeness during illness and distress. Ill persons want to know their family is available. The need for presence appears to be a foundational family need experienced as family members protect, guide, support, and comfort one another (Doolin, Quinn, Bryant, Lyons, & Kleinpell, 2011; Eggenberger & Nelms, 2007). Family presence is an invisible and abiding attachment. Nurses who *think family* know that presence quells suffering and distress, silences some anxieties, and comforts in unfamiliar places.

Case Study—Part 3: Family Presence During Loss and Illness

My oldest son Bruce and his wife Jodi had arrived from California for a family visit unrelated to the tragedy that was unfolding. I awoke eager to spend time with them and the rest of the family. As I reached the bottom of the stairs, my husband met me and said that

> **BOX 9-2**
>
> **Family Tree**
>
> **Catherine Chesla, DNSc, FAAN (United States)**
>
> Catherine (Kit) Chesla, RN, DNSc, FAAN, is Professor and Shobe Endowed Chair for Ethics and Spirituality in the Department of Family Health Care Nursing at the University of California, San Francisco. For over 20 years she has been a mentor in family nursing education teaching family theory, intervention, and research methods to doctoral and family nurse practitioner (FNP) students. Her program of research focuses on understanding and intervening with families in which an adult member has a chronic illness, which has made her a groundbreaker in family research. She has conducted multiple studies with families living with type 2 diabetes in African American, Chinese American, Latino, and white families. She is involved in a community-based participatory, NIH-funded community-based project in San Francisco's Chinatown testing a family-focused cognitive behavioral intervention to assist Chinese immigrants in the management of their diabetes. Her team adapted an intervention to be culturally appropriate and tested its efficacy in this population. Chesla primarily focuses on family processes in chronic illness and moves knowledge to intervention testing. She has studied families from diverse backgrounds including African American, Chinese American, European American, and Latino. Her use of interpretive phenomenology in investigating these issues and her work with a large interdisciplinary team of nurses, psychologists, physicians, and dietitians who use quantitative approaches in the study of families and chronic illness make her a trailblazer in family nursing research. She exemplifies attention to the importance of family presence in the management of chronic illess. Her work has been widely published and she is a leading scholar in family nursing. She is a founding member of the International Family Nursing Association (IFNA), has served as a member of the Board of Directors and the 2013 Conference Committee, and is IFNA's current president.

this would be the most devastating day of my life. He told me to come into the kitchen and sit down. Bruce and Jodi were there. They shared the news of my son-in-law's death and the death of my grandson David! We piled into a car together as a family and headed over treacherous roads in –10 °F temperatures on the 90-mile drive to the trauma center. When we arrived, other family members were already there, filling the waiting room. We were all in shock, one of the first steps of the loss process. Disbelief followed. What does a mother and a family do with the reality of a horrible and awful atrocity?

After a while, we were allowed to see Meloni. The shock was almost unbearable. My beautiful daughter was bright yellow. She had gone from her usual weight of about 120 pounds to 180 pounds! I knew that this was a fluid accumulation, but my heart just wept. The anger that followed was palpable. Family members exhibited emotions differently. One was isolated. Another used chemicals. One argued loudly, the usual way of coping when things are out of control. One usually talkative member sat in total silence. Another spoke in measured responses, different from a typical critical approach. Tears. I, the "glass half full" type, was lulled into a sense that everyone was pulling together and putting petty differences aside. We were together—available. But, still, we were suffering and struggling as individuals and as a family.

Family Processes and Presence

Family presence throughout an evolving illness and tragedy is a process that can support family health. Family processes are a central element of the Family Health Model (FHM), and these interactions address ways family members work together (Denham, 2003). The FHM includes seven core family processes: communication, caregiving, cathexis, celebration, change, connectedness, and coordination, which are described further in Chapter 14. Over time, families develop individual and joint behaviors and actions. These behaviors serve as ways to organize daily life, health routines, and the many ways of being a family. Processes are central facets of family life and have potential to influence individual and family health and illness outcomes (Kaakinen, Hanson, & Denham, 2010; Weihs, Fisher, & Baird, 2002).

Family members available for each other during distress and suffering contribute valued meaning to relationships as they connect, give care, communicate about illness management, and coordinate needed actions (Denham & Looman, 2010; Weihs et al., 2002). Meaning is constructed through family relationships and their attachments (Frankl, 1992). Fidelity, devotion, faithfulness, loyalty, and regard are just some of the values aroused in family members by the presence of others (Kaakinen et al., 2010). These values, when nurtured, can bring a sense of care, peace, wholeness, and fulfillment. These values are supportive, act as deterrents to fears, help to overcome hopelessness, and promote a sense of well-being.

Nursing actions that support a family's processes have potential to improve health outcomes for individual members and the family as a whole (Chesla, 2010; Denham, 2003; Weihs et al., 2002). Nurses can encourage family beliefs that support healthy management of a chronic illness (Wright & Bell, 2009) and help family members cope (Knafl, Deatrick, & Havill, 2012; Knafl & Gillis, 2002). Nurses can facilitate communication and help resolve decisions and negotiations during difficult illness situations (Bakitas, Kryworuchko, Matlock, & Volandes, 2011; Wiegand, 2008). Also, presence and family involvement during an acute illness or end of life can decrease suffering and anxiety (Tschann, Kaufman, & Micco, 2003; Vandall-Walker & Clark, 2011).

Case Study—Part 4: Family Presence in Acute Care

Day by day, Meloni fought the pain of a torn liver, cardiac tamponade, a wound in the ileum requiring an ileostomy, a chest wound that dissected her breast, and an elbow so badly shattered that her left arm had to be amputated. She had more than 19 blood transfusions. Physical trauma was accompanied by deep emotional pain as she recalled her husband and son's brutal murders.

As the weeks and months passed, one daughter, one granddaughter, and I stayed close by Meloni. We needed to be together to support her and each other. We lived nearby, and we were at the hospital every day. We missed the day of Stephen and David's funeral. Family members from out of town left. I stayed at the hospital, sleeping in the waiting room most nights. It seemed that when I was unavailable something would go wrong. Of course, I really knew that it had nothing to do with whether I was there or not, but it felt strange and wrong to leave. Unbelievably, only once did I think that she would not make it through the night. As I sat by her bed, a student nurse told me it was "God's plan" that this had all happened. I told him there was no way I could believe in a loving God who would do this. Meloni made it through the night, but she remained in serious condition. I stayed at the bedside.

Family-Focused Care

Family-focused care invites the nurse into a pivotal place where nursing presence can be used to help families endure illness, face tragedy, and support health. Nurse presence has a relational nature that extends the reach from individuals seeking care to including relationships with family members. Nurses who *think family* recognize family is the recipient of their presence. They see this presence as an instrument for caring. Being present requires more than listening; it is a way of being that values the dignity and worth of others and shares deep connectedness (Hessel, 2009). Nurse presence can help unite family members and facilitate positive exchanges about beliefs as members support each other (Eggenberger et al., 2011; Krumwiede et al., 2004; Meiers et al., 2009; Wright & Leahey, 2013).

If nurses don't *think family* or use family-focused care approaches, then conversations with family groups and the presence of multiple family members can be viewed as burdensome. Yet, when nurses manage complex situations, they must address concerns of the family network. As nurses introduce themselves to an individual and family members, a relationship that can lead to therapeutic conversations begins (Wright & Leahey, 2013; Svavarsdottir, Tryggvadottir & Sigurdardottir, 2012). Therapeutic conversations acknowledge the experience from a variety of perspectives. Nurses who *think family* include family members in the care, address priorities, and use supportive communication (Hardin, 2012; Nelms & Eggenberger, 2010; Wright & Leahey, 2013). Family-focused care values members' needs for presence and encourages them to become partners in caring situations.

Nurses who *think family* view the family members as the care unit and include them in care delivery. For example, a Doctor of Nursing Practice (DNP) student at Minnesota State University, Mankato, tested an intervention to encourage family involvement (Van Heukelom, Bell, Eggenberger, & Bell, 2010). A family nursing intervention with four components was tested by the staff on a hospital unit:

- Family members were given a welcome letter during their unit orientation that stated they were valued partners in the care of their family member.
- A pad of paper was placed at the bedside for families to record their questions.
- Consistent introductions of nursing staff were made to persons and families.
- The nurse sat at the bedside for at least 2 minutes of focused time with each hospitalized person and the family during the first 4 hours of the nursing shift to ask specifically what they wanted to accomplish during that nursing shift.

Satisfaction surveys demonstrated some significant improvements noted in the scores. The student collaborated with the hospital unit to develop family-focused care.

Case Study—Part 5: Family and Nursing Presence Across Care Settings

The first days in the ICU, not knowing from minute to minute whether Meloni would live or die. . . . One day, I just lost it and cried and cried! A nurse put her arm around me and said, "This must be very tough for you. . . ." I appreciated the nurse's attentiveness not only to my daughter, but to me as well. One night a nurse woke me in the lounge to tell me Meloni was going to surgery again. I appreciated her thinking of me because if I had gone to the room and not seen her I would have freaked out! Knowing the nursing staff was consistently present and working with my daughter and the expert attending physicians was comforting.

It was a shock when Meloni was transferred out of intensive care. The nurses outside intensive care were not as attentive to her needs, or to mine. Next, Meloni was transferred to a tertiary medical center for consultation related to her liver damage. The presence of nursing here was similar to that in the previous institution. I requested a care conference. A nurse advocated for me and was present at the conference. After I requested it, this nurse found Meloni a room more conducive for our family to visit. Following acute care, Meloni was transferred to an intensive rehabilitation center for ongoing therapy. They expected her to do things on her own that I don't think she had done before. However, she was learning how to adapt to her new life at home again. There seemed to be more technical staff than professional staff. Nursing presence decreased, and less attention was paid to Meloni and our family.

Case Study—Part 6: Adaptation to a New Family Life at Home

Eventually, Meloni went back home—where the tragedy had happened. This surprised many people, but she said, "I will not let him take that from me too." Such strength and resilience! Amazing! The support of her friends was remarkable. Her home was cleaned by a business that dealt with the aftermath of such tragedies. It was refurnished before she returned home. She talked her brother into letting her drive around her property and country road. Nothing was going to keep her from seeing her remaining son grow up. However, the battle continued. She went to the hospital to have her ileostomy reattached and went home and developed MRSA (methicillin-resistant *Staphylococcus aureus*) infection, which responded well to antibiotics. She eventually went back to work part time at her position as the office manager of a small local tax firm.

Several years have passed. They have not all been easy. At the trial of the murderer, Meloni, gave a very moving Victim Impact Statement. She told the perpetrator that although people commented on how well she was handling it all, they didn't realize she cried herself to sleep each night. The murderer received two life sentences plus 20 years in prison. Meloni's remarkable friends and family supported her throughout it all. Although Brad had to stay with friends or at his uncle's home through the nine months of Meloni's hospitalization, he is a fine young man, kind, and never in any trouble. Meloni now has a kind, caring man in her life, an old classmate. However, the pain will always be felt from the evil a person inflicted on an entire family and community. Yet, the presence of family and nurses during a tragic experience is treasured by our family.

Family Nursing Research Team: Family Transitions and Illness Experiences

The Family Nursing Research Team (FNRT) at Minnesota State University, Mankato, conducted a series of studies to investigate the meanings of family presence during illness and identify the effect of nurses' presence during health, illness, and transitions (Eggenberger et al., 2011; Krumwiede et al., 2004; Eggenberger, Krumwiede, Meiers, Bliesmer, & Earle, 2004). Studies found several processes that families used to manage experiences (Box 9.3). These study findings suggest that nurses have great potential to positively support individual and family health as members use caring strategies to manage illness experiences. To illustrate processes and caring strategies this chapter includes quotes from family members who participated in this team's studies.

An early study by the FNRT described the health experience of families in a rural setting in Midwestern United States (Meiers et al., 2009). This study explored the processes that families in a rural setting used to maintain and regain health. These rural families experienced health as an ongoing process. Balancing family life in response to the inevitable transitions and changes linked with illness was an unending process. Examples of balancing include the following:

- Partnering with others to share the family work in the rural setting
- Being present for each other and the family during times of illness
- Prioritizing work and family time
- Creating space for family members
- Managing family decisions
- Modifying family routines and rituals

During times of transition, families continually balanced work and family, multiple commitments, individual and family needs, and resources. Transitions included birth, marriage,

	BOX 9-3

Family Nursing Research Team Investigations

FOCUS OF STUDY	HEALTH EXPERIENCE	KEY FINDINGS TO GUIDE FAMILY NURSING ACTIONS
Healthy families in rural setting	Healthy family transitions	Balancing the work of family Promoting health of family
Families managing neutropenia with cancer	Family with an acutely ill family member	Turbulent waiting Symptom management
Families and chronic illness	Chronic illness experience	Enduring transitions of illness Developing caring strategies Reintegration of a family
Aesthetic representations of family health experiences	Interpretation of family research findings with illness	Visual interpretations evoke emotion for families and family-focused care

growing independence of adolescents, separation through death or divorce, and financial threats and strains (Meiers et al., 2009). Figure 9.2 depicts the balancing processes and negotiations necessary as families develop a capacity for caring and managing uncertainty during times of transition.

During transitions, families continually readjusted unit life within the context of their evolving world (Meiers et al., 2009). Family members continued their work of family caring. Negotiating family relationships, roles, communication, boundaries, and member growth and maintaining family bonds were central elements for maintaining health and identity in these rural families. Interactive processes in the presence of family members influenced members' health during daily life and transitional times. Maintaining family integrity during transitions required enduring energy to balance competing needs. Families often desired and needed nurses' support and presence during transitional times. Many findings from this study support ideas suggested by the Family Health Model (Denham, 2003).

Family Caring Strategies

A study focused on families' cancer experiences showed the meanings of their caring strategies to manage events and symptoms resulting from a member's chemotherapy treatments during recovery (Krumwiede et al., 2004). The cancer diagnosis and following

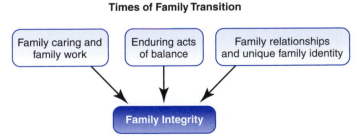

FIGURE 9-2 Times of transition and family presence.

cancer treatments caused families to develop new strategies as the ill family member was protected and integrity of the family unit supported. Families needed to gain a sense of power and control, understand perplexing situations, find answers to questions, and protect family members.

Family Uncertainty

Family uncertainty emerged as a significant concern for the family during the unsettling times with illness. Family caring strategies helped members search for the meanings in the illness events and find ways to support one another during periods of uncertainty. Seeking information was a consistent tactic. Family members responded to illness threats as they personally managed life demands. Families collectively monitored needs of ill members. Family strategies helped them access resources, manage demands, and advocate for their ill member. They sought information and guidance. They needed a sense of stability as they used coordinated efforts to guard and protect their families' integrity. Figure 9.3 depicts the caring strategies that helped families manage the anxiety when their ill member experienced neutropenia and chemotherapy was interrupted (Eggenberger et al., 2004). Nurses who *think family* can help expand caregiving capacities.

Family Inquiry

Family inquiry involves family efforts to gain information and knowledge to manage an illness (Eggenberger et al., 2004). It allows members to seek answers from multiple information sources and manage inconsistent or conflicting messages and get answers to questions. A nurse's presence may be needed to provide guidance for decision making and navigating an illness situation. A family managing a member's chemotherapy-induced neutropenia had frustrations and concerns about blood counts and conflicting information about neutropenia. A family member said: "It has been difficult to get answers. Our family has been confused at times. . . . we have not always even known what to ask. We do not know what to expect next."

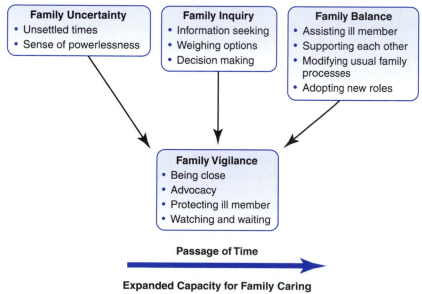

FIGURE 9-3 Managing family uncertainty.

As nurses help a family learn about an illness, manage symptoms, and make decisions, they support a protective family environment. Including family in education, coaching, communication, and decision making can help manage uncertainty (Chesla, 2010; McDaniel, Campbell, Hepworth, & Lorenz, 2005; Wright & Leahey, 2013). Intentionally including a family unit in discussions that focus on information, family beliefs, and family interpretation or meanings of events can support a family's caring strategies (Wright & Bell, 2009). Conversations with nurses, even brief interactions, support families during illness, increase satisfaction with care, and address concerns (Duhamel, Dupuis, & Wright, 2009; Svavarsdottir et al., 2012). Use of family meetings and conferences may help families to discuss the meanings of events and possible caring strategies (Griffin, 2010; Nelms & Eggenberger, 2010).

Family Balance

Balance addresses the ways family memebers simultaneously care for each other, the ill person, and their household needs. When illness occurs, family members cannot easily set aside usual demands. Symmetry of daily life is disrupted and conflicting demands may lead to imbalance. Nurses who *think family* help members coordinate caregiving roles as they aim for some normality and family integrity during troubled times.

Planning allows families to prepare for present and future needs (Kunerth, 2010). It is a proactive way to balance competing demands and manage obstacles. For instance, a family dealing with the chronic illness in a child with asthma had needs related to education, friends, leisure, and health care. One family member with a chronic illness stated, "I have a big calendar and on the big calendar go all kinds of things. We have a calendar for who is going where. We have a calendar on the fridge that everyone is supposed to put their stuff on. . . . We keep track of who needs a ride and when. I do the planning and organize for all the medical appointments and care."

Having preparatory tactics is a caring strategy that allows families to feel more confident when dealing with needs, transitions, and the complexity of care systems (Kautz & Van Horn, 2009). The use of intentional caring strategies helps the family manage the illness as well as individual and family lives.

Family Vigilance

With family vigilance, members create a healing and protecting environment for the member experiencing illness (Carr & Clarke, 1997; Dudley & Carr, 2004). Uncertainty from actual or potential threats can accentuate needs to stay close and connected. In Meloni's case, her mother said that she could not leave the hospital or her daughter's bedside. If a family member cannot be in close physical proximity, he may choose to stay connected through telephone, Skype, texting, e-mail, or other technology.

Family members have a strong need to be near a family member during an illness (Dudley & Carr, 2004). Families can protect their members, deal with hurtful comments, and prevent harmful actions by health professionals (Carr & Clark, 1997; Dewar, 2001; Kunerth, 2010). For example, the wife of a critically ill husband said, "I can't leave the room. I must be here in case anything happens. We [our family] all want to be here. It feels terrible when we leave. We want nurses to help us stay here" (Eggenberger & Nelms, 2007). The parents of a child hospitalized in a pediatric unit depended on the nurse's presence to support them: Just having someone to touch base with regularly, either by phone or in person at any time of the day to say, your baby's doing okay . . . to know when I leave at the end of the day and I'm not here I still feel like I have a connection to her. When you go, often you feel like you're abandoning them. . . . The nurse puts a bridge between home and hospital which is reassuring" (Meiers & Tomlinson, 2003).

The parents of an adult teenager with a chronic condition about to leave for college stated: "It is difficult to think that we may not be with him if he has a diabetic reaction or complication. We always watch his diet and symptoms closely, but now we are not sure what will happen when he is independent" (Eggenberger et al., 2011).

Nursing Actions to Support Family Presence Through Caring Strategies

A nurse who *thinks family* understands that family caring strategies support family vigilance and communicates ways families can connect during an illness experience. Nurses can support family vigilance by clearly communicating things the family can do to protect and be present. Family-focused nurses recognize that protection of a family member is a fundamental social process of family life (Boss, Doherty, LaRossa, Schumm, & Steinmetz, 1993). The family in an acute care setting is comforted when a nurse describes the following:

- When and how information about clinical status will be provided
- When to expect the nurse's return and how to find the nurse
- Ways they will be consistently updated with information
- When usual system routines occur and purposes of technological equipment
- Treatments and procedures in clear plain language
- Ways to participate in the care of their family member

Families recognize inclusion and value specific directions on ways to participate in the care of their ill member (Johnson et al., 2008). This information is especially important with a chronic condition, disability, or terminal illness. A nurse who is present supports family caring strategies by helping families to participate and explaining what to expect from health care professionals (Abraham & Moretz, 2012). In care situations, families need to know several things:

- When and who to call when questions arise or situations seem out of control
- Steps for follow-through and safety needs linked with medically prescribed treatments
- Ways family members can best be involved in care procedures
- Supportive actions that can empower the individual member and family
- Ways to locate necessary resources outside the household

Nurses who *think family* recognize that families balance multiple life aspects. These nurses initiate therapeutic conversations about the assistance and support needed by the ill person. Family members generally appreciate it when nurses anticipate their needs and provide useful information in clear and timely ways. Nurses who *think family* know that families living with a member who has a chronic condition face potential developmental changes as members age and conditions evolve. Family roles and illness demands change over time. Thus, nurses must assess, prepare, and plan for potential alterations in family processes.

As families wait, the nurse can give accurate timelines about when information will be available and updates on the status of treatments, tests, and surgery outcomes. On-going communication provides a protective environment. Nurse presence is comforting and gives a sense that care is continuous and coordinated. It says, you are not forgotten. You are important! A nurse who *thinks family* helps family members identify beliefs and communicate their values. These nurses know members are unique and respect rights to differing attitudes. Nurses who *think family* are present. They guide, teach, coach, counsel, and advise about health and illness. Box 9.4 introduces nurses from Thailand who

BOX 9-4

Family Tree

Chintana Wacharasin (Thailand)

Wannee Deoisres (Thailand)

Chintana Wacharasin, RN, PhD, is an Associate Professor at the Faculty of Nursing, Burapha University, Thailand, where she teaches the advanced practice of Family Systems Nursing to graduate nursing students at the master's and doctoral levels. Her interest in family nursing first began in her graduate studies at the University of Washington, where she learned to apply family nursing models with actual families. She has helped move family nursing in Thailand forward through several initiatives. In 2002, she co-developed the first master's program in Burapha University in 1997. In 2002, co-developed the First Family Nursing Conference in Thailand. She collaborated with colleagues at Khon Khen University to establish the Thai Family Nursing Society in 2004. Her current research focuses on examining family nursing interventions with families experiencing HIV-AIDS and thalassemia. She also developed a family health promotion program for families at all developmental stages. Dr. Wacharasin is the author of a textbook about Family Systems Nursing, *Theoretical Foundation for Advanced Family Nursing* (2007). She is the co-editor of the book *Family Nursing: Academic Articles for Continuing Education in Nursing Science 4* (2012) written in the Thai language. Along with Dr. Wannee Deoisres, she served as one of the co-chairs of the successful Eighth International Family Nursing Conference held in Bangkok in 2007. In 2005, she was honored with an Innovative Contribution to Family Nursing Award by the *Journal of Family Nursing*.

remain committed to nursing research and education that emphasizes the significance of nurses to families.

Family Connecting, Relating, Pondering, and Struggling

Families have other strategies for care and support of their members during chronic illness; these were identified in a study about family processes (Eggenberger et al., 2011). Interviews were conducted with families experiencing HIV-AIDS, multiple sclerosis, type 1 diabetes mellitus, ankylosing spondylitis, lymphoma, chronic obstructive pulmonary disease, and congenital muscular dystrophy. Four specific themes linked with family presence—connecting, relating, pondering, and struggling—were found when a member had a chronic condition (Eggenberger et al., 2011).

Connecting

The idea of connecting takes varied forms when member illness is a concern. Connecting is a way of making memories, commemorating shared lives, celebrating, or paying tribute to family identity. Chronic illness often creates a need for members to lean upon one another, draw strength from each other, and provide supportive care. Family bonds are central elements of family life and these connections are at the core of family units (Boss et al., 1993; Denham, 2003). For example, a wife with young children described family activities that created memories as her husband's symptoms of multiple sclerosis progressed (Eggenberger et al., 2011). She said, "I mean if there should ever come a time, and hopefully not, when Jon has a hard time walking . . . all these vacation memories with their dad, when he is walking, I just think are important, really important. . . ." Another ill father who was living with a chronic neuro-muscular disease limiting his physical function stated, "I coached my son's soccer team and thought, I don't know if I can do it in the future, so I better do it now." Memories are made from family connections and may feature their affection and value for each other.

Relating

Relating refers to efforts to continue family unit relationships among members as they face a chronic illness (Bell, 2011; Bell & Bell, 2012; Tollefson, Usher, & Foster, 2011). A father managing chronic degenerative musculoskeletal disease said, "We try to spend as much time together as a family as we can. We have to just put the disease over there and I try to continue being a helpful spouse and parent." Families describe intensified member relationships during long periods of waiting during cancer treatments (Eggenberger et al., 2011). Family members often use extreme efforts to maintain and build relationships when experiencing uncertainty, unknowns, and demands.

Families interact and relate with members, extended family, and their social networks while they manage chronic conditions. Members offer different perceptions, coping strategies, and understandings about what is occurring. They often interact in new ways as they maintain satisfying relationships. It is stressful to live with an ill person besieged by the physical, psychological, and logistical demands of a condition (Weingarten, 2013). A married couple described tensions while living with multiple sclerosis, "He [husband] thinks I worry too much. At times I want to talk about it more than he does. But I know I have to wait until he is ready and then I can explain my concerns." In contrast, the husband stated, "I don't see any purpose in talking about what the multiple sclerosis might do to my body until it happens. Why worry about what may not happen" (Eggenberger et al., 2011).

Families strive to develop trusting relationships with their care providers. A family dealing with chronic obstructive pulmonary disease wanted a provider to listen to their concerns about ongoing dyspnea. They often felt their story and voice were minimized. "It has been work to find a competent practitioner who cares about listening to us." Families that established a trusting provider relationship had a sense of comfort in this partnership. A family with a child with congenital muscular dystrophy shared their trust in a provider who understood their concerns, "She [their nurse practitioner] is always ready to listen to our anxieties when he gets a lung infection or fears when he starts school or a new activity." Families with a positive individual-nurse-family relationship felt supported and better able to handle the unknowns of a chronic illness (Eggenberger et al., 2011). "Just knowing we can call her [nurse] for guidance is a huge benefit. I am not sure how we could survive this without her help. It feels like she is always there for us. She helps our family understand what is happening." Nurses who *think family* sense that a medical diagnosis implies a life change and know that families and members have unique ways of addressing related needs.

Pondering

Family pondering occurs as members attempt to construct meaning and purpose. Families question and interpret the meanings of the illness. They wonder what a condition means for their family unit and member lives. They need to know how to manage illness symptoms. Families wonder how they will make space for this unexpected and unwanted assault and they puzzle over ways to establish new roles and processes as symptoms emerge and conditions change. Family members reflect on their history and their future as they seek to be prepared for the condition (Noble & Jones, 2005). Social networks provide assistance, guidance, and resources to manage demands. A family living with ongoing exacerbations of a chronic condition said, "The church and neighbors have been right there with us from the beginning" (Eggenberger et al., 2011).

Struggling

Families use much energy as they struggle with achieving wellness or managing disease. Struggling occurs as families attempt to resolve concerns over resources, services, financial assistance, or even diagnosing the problem (Neufeld, Harrison, Stewart, & Hugest, 2008). Family members often negotiate for medical appointments, pathology tests, medical treatments, test results, prescriptions, and equipment (Tong, Lowe, Sainsbury, & Craig, 2008). Family members make statements such as "It is all so much work. Sometimes we have trouble getting the children to their activities when my husband is not doing well. Trying to juggle work and appointments by myself is really difficult." Some families also struggle with care systems or staff to obtain adequate comfort needs (Tong et al., 2008). For instance, the wife of a family member with cancer who experienced hospitalization for an acute situation said, "At times it feels like the nurse looks right past us. What about me? I am his wife. I don't know why I am always the one who has to initiate the conversation." Parents of a junior high adolescent with a chronic illness shared their constant efforts: "We are so tired. We just lay there at night and listen to his breathing. We feel so blessed that he lived, but we never realized how hard this was all going to be. We have a hard time thinking about anything else besides him . . . yet we have jobs."

Family members struggle as they manage the conflicts and tensions that surround illness. A family shared their concerns with the extended family: "Sometimes they [extended family] just don't understand. They don't want to talk about the illness and future, yet I think that would help all of us" (Eggenberger et al., 2011). Witnessing a loved one's chronic illness is a continuous struggle with loss and letting go and differences in moving toward acceptance, and yet, developing an approach of being alongside the family is a foundation for nursing practice (Weingarten, 2013).

Living Within the Context of Chronic Illness

As families live with chronic illness, they experience individual and family vulnerabilities (Fig. 9.4). Family members wrestle with multiple unknowns as they work to manage uncertainties, care needs, symptoms, and unpredictability of illnesses. Although situations vary among families, many experience highly emotional times that tax their emotional and physical strengths. This stress can disrupt even the most organized households and exhaust resources.

Living with an illness means ongoing management, unpredictable outcomes, and family stress that occasionally erupts into conflict. Uncertainty can create arguments, disagreements, and disruptions that magnify suffering. Even organized and caring families with great resilience can become overly burdened with the demands of an illness. Persons with a chronic illness may perceive the illness differently from the family. They may respond with silence or turmoil. They can have difficulty managing without the presence of their family and sometimes with their presence. Nurses can help families cope and manage uncertainties (Duggleby et al., 2010; Knafl et al., 2012). Nurses who *think family* consider ways a chronic illness influences different members and work to strengthen family unit capacities to address these influences.

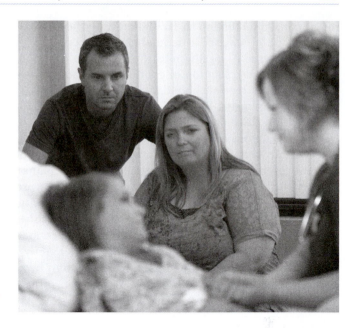

FIGURE 9-4 Family reintegration in chronic illness.

A nurse who *thinks family* is intentionally present and assists in the development of caring strategies. Families may find chronic illness leads to abiding family distress, suffering, conflict, and turmoil (Eggenberger et al., 2011). For example, Victor received a phone call from his physician: "The biopsy shows the tumor is malignant. You will need to come in next week to discuss the various treatment options. I will transfer you to my nurse and she will assist you." Victor was unsure whether malignant meant cancer or not. When the nurse answered the line, she said, "I need to arrange your appointment, but before we do that I am wondering if you have any questions about what the doctor just told you?" The nurse was able to translate the physician's message into clear language for Victor and help him understand that he did have cancer so that he could make sense of the diagnosis. When the nurse was sure Victor understood, her attention turned to his family and she asked if he needed her to talk with another family member.

Nurses who *think family* support their needs from the time of diagnosis through an ongoing process of family reintegration. The process of reintegration in chronic illness involves the family's capacity to function as follows:

- Adapt to reality and develop caring strategies to strengthen the family.
- Satisfy individual family member and family unit needs.
- Assist the family member with the chronic illness to manage the illness and related symptoms or complications.
- Manage the demands that the chronic illness places on everyday family life.

Reintegration begins with recognition of vulnerability and the realities aligned with a particular condition. Families need to be prepared for condition changes, challenges of illness management, and risks in living with change and uncertainty.

Family Integrity

Maintaining family integrity during times of illness is a goal for nursing because the family is the central social unit that manages the health and illness of its members (Litman, 1974). Family integrity is identified in the Nursing Intervention Classification system as an area for nursing intervention to facilitate family health (Bulechek, Butcher, & Dochterman, 2008). Family integrity is defined as family cohesion and unity (Bulechek et al., 2008, p. 345). A sense of togetherness through open communication and a tone of acceptance, forgiveness, and resolution of conflict demonstrate family integrity (Kautz & Van Horn, 2009). Families regulate boundaries and use values and meanings to support and maintain integrity (Tomlinson, Peden-McAlpine, & Sherman, 2012). Maintaining family integrity offers a supportive presence to members.

Nursing actions can assist a family in developing, maintaining, and regaining integrity. A nurse can help a family attain balance, vigilance, and inquiry to maintain integrity (Eggenberger et al., 2004). Assisting a family in planning, monitoring, communicating, and protecting their family member supports family processes (Eggenberger et al., 2011; Weingarten, 2013). A trusting individual-nurse-family relationship can support family integrity and aid in developing partnerships (Eggenberger & Nelms, 2007; Tomlinson et al., 2012). Nursing actions that address the connecting, pondering, struggling, and relating aspects of family support integrity. Family nurses can help create optimal health outcomes for the individual and family unit by maximizing their caring capacities (Weingarten, 2013).

Families as Advocates for Members with an Illness

The word *advocate* is derived from the Latin word *advocatus*, meaning to plead another's cause (Abate, 2002). Family members serve as advocates for members who can't speak for themselves, as may occur during times of acute illness (Krumwiede et al., 2004; Meiers & Tomlinson, 2003; Nelms & Eggenberger, 2010; Wiegand, 2008). A sudden hospitalization with a life-threatening illness can alter decision-making abilities. A person with a recent severe physical disability from an accident might need adjustments for living arrangements. Advocates who speak for them can help. Advocacy can be a proactive family response as they are vigilant in being protective and supporting the ill member (Dudley & Carr, 2004). During critical illness, families often speak with professional care providers on behalf of ill members. Family nurses help families make decisions, clarify treatments, and set future care directions (Meiers & Brauer, 2008).

Positive benefits can emerge in care situations when family is involved and advocates for its member (Kunerth, 2010). Offering support to families in negotiating the complexities of an illness or health care system can increase satisfaction and sense of personal power (Kautz & Van Horn, 2009; Neufeld et al., 2008). However, the need to continually advocate for the ill person can become a major source of stress for the family unit (Clabots, 2012). Families can become fatigued attempting to meet unending demands for advocacy and become overwhelmed when stress is continuous. Advocacy is integral to nursing practice, and thoughtful use of advocacy is an essential aspect of family-focused practice (Vaartio, Leino-Kilpi, Salantera, & Suominen, 2006). Nurses can help families communicate and coordinate as they negotiate health care systems.

Visual Interpretations Evoke Family Emotions

The emotional experience of a family living with an ill family member or enduring a tragic family event is powerful and often filled with suffering, conflicts, and despair (Wright & Bell, 2009). Illness experiences can deeply divide families, but they can also bring them together (Eggenberger & Nelms, 2007). Critical illnesses can be painful and threatening, but families can find ways to endure hardships and work together as a family (Eggenberger & Nelms,

2007; Krumwiede et al., 2004; Meiers & Tomlinson, 2003). Sometimes it is difficult to find words to fully describe emotions, responses, and reactions when undergoing great stresses. This was true for the Family Nursing Research Team (FNRT) at Mankato, Minnesota, and the team searched for new ways to communicate the power of a family's presence.

Art has been described as a path of inquiry and a way to generate understandings of human experience (Baumann, 1999; Munhall, 1994). Visual images give voice to data and may convey deeper meanings than the language of words (Richardson, 2000). Considering these assumptions, the FNRT commissioned two creative aesthetic expressions to convey the findings from grounded theory studies of families living with cancer (Krumwiede et al., 2004) and chronic illness (Eggenberger et al., 2011). The intent was to evoke viewer empathy about family presence during a member's illness. Nurses who *think family* during caring roles empathize as they share family emotions associated with illness, disease, and other tragic times.

Understanding the Family Experience of Neutropenia: Hope

A painting was created from the study about families managing chemotherapy-induced neutropenia (Eggenberger spacey et al., 2004). Families had responded to the cessation of chemotherapy because of decreased white blood cell count in their family member by taking precautions to prevent infection. Study families were vulnerable as they faced visible reminders of their member's mortality. The experience caused intensified connections with each other. Family members reported coming together, but also having a sense of aloneness with their thoughts and fears as they tried to protect their ill member.

Essie Mostaghimi, a professional artist, was commissioned by the nurse researchers to create a visual interpretation from the research findings (Fig. 9.5). This artist, with over 20 years' experience, described himself as an impressionist. Creation of an aesthetic expression of nursing research findings is an uncommon method for nurses, so the plan began with an open-ended dialogue between the researchers and the artist. This dialogue was an exchange of ideas about the emerging data themes, and some exemplary meaningful statements from the family interviews were discussed. At the end of the dialogue, both researchers and the artist attained a synergistic understanding of the significant themes. The artist was

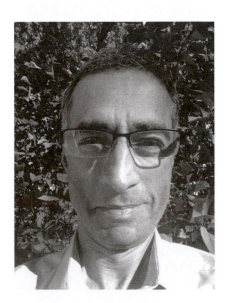

FIGURE 9-5 Artist Essie Mostaghimi.

prepared to move forward and create the visual work, an acrylic painting depicting his interpretation of the family data (Fig. 9.6). The visual artwork, titled *Understanding the Family Experience of Neutropenia: Hope,* was unveiled and a textual interpretation of the aesthetic expression created to blend the narrative text with the painting (Box 9.5).

Sculpture: The Other Side

The researchers then commissioned another artist, Jonathan Kamrath, whose disciplinary focus is mixed method sculpture (Fig. 9.7). Again, the researchers shared with the artist the major empirical findings and some narrative exemplars of the processes in the reintegration of families linked with chronic illness (Eggenberger et al., 2011). The artist used an interpretation process that resulted in a three-dimensional constructed door sculpture entitled *The Other Side,* depicting the family's life and goals, *The Dream,* before the diagnosis of the chronic illness, and *Life With Chronic Illness* portraying demands and concerns of the family as they experienced the chronic illness (Fig. 9.8). Textual description was composed by the artist to verbally interpret the work (Box 9.6).

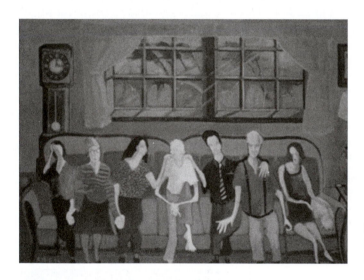

FIGURE 9-6 *Understanding the Family Experience of Neutropenia: Hope.*

BOX 9-5

Painting: Linking Art and Text

Understanding the Experience of Neutropenia: Hope

Essie Mostaghimi and the Family Nursing Research Team

A family is together on one long couch. The storm outside represents the turbulent times surrounding the cancer and neutropenia. However, the slivers of light continue to stream in and the storm does not destroy the family's hope. The shattered glass in the window represents disruption and the grandfather clock depicts time standing still while waiting for neutropenia to resolve. In the center of the painting, the family member with cancer is confined to a separate square on the couch and is dressed in white symbolizing innocence and neediness. Nonspecific faces represent differing family experiences, diverse family types, and changing family roles and relationships. Various out-of-perspective depictions, such as the twisted legs and thin elongated arms, represent pain and yearning throughout the cancer experience.

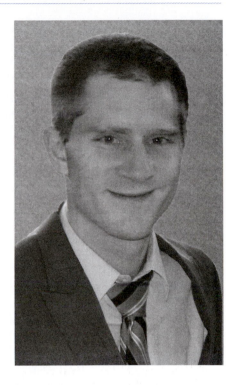

FIGURE 9-7 Artist Jonathan Kamrath.

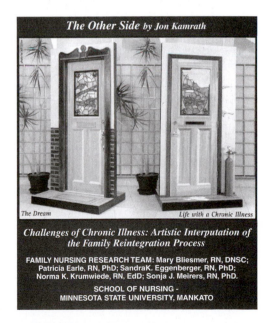

FIGURE 9-8 Challenges of chronic illness.

The aesthetic interpretation of research findings highlights the centrality of the family presence in the member's illness experiences. Throughout the trajectory of a chronic illness, the family experience is filled with uncertainty, distress, and suffering. Families want to care for their loved one, but they need knowledge, guidance, and coaching to maintain their relationships, caring strategies, and family health. The study findings suggest that nurse presence can ease some distress because it underpins and encourages the family in ways that support their ill member and each other.

> **BOX 9-6**
>
> **Sculpture: Linking Art and Text**
>
> **The Other Side by Jonathan Kamrath (2005)**
>
> *The Other Side* is a series of two individual, sequentially related pieces (*The Dream* and *Life With Chronic Illness*). Because these two separate pieces are physically joined, an interesting relationship of contrast is established between them. Although each piece needs to be interpreted within its relationship to the other, it is important to observe each as its own independent identity. One needs to first take in *The Dream*, noting its key features, then move to *Life with a Chronic Illness*. After observing each as its own complete unit, one can then appreciate the two together as a whole, taking note of the differences between the two (Meiers, Krumwiede, Eggenberger, Bliesmer, & Earle, 2007).

Transforming Health Care Systems to Embrace Family and Nurse Presence

Family care must be a target for quality improvement in health care systems (Abraham & Moretz, 2012; Black, Boore, & Parahoo, 2011; Institute for Patient-and Family-Centered Care, 2013). Real change in health care delivery encompasses more than technology and costs; it pertains to hearing the voiced needs of those receiving care, continuing care over time, and equipping families to manage health and illness. Health and illness largely occur when families are not in the presence of health professionals. How do we coordinate care so that it addresses needs in these long spaces between medical settings and the household production of health? What would change in health care if family were the focus?

Nurse leaders must guide from the front. Innovation is not just added technologies or aesthetics, but a focus on human relationships and optimal use of nursing skills and time. Family-focused nursing care involves actions that anticipate individual and family care needs beyond the doors of health care systems, agencies, and institutions. Family presence and nurse presence influences health outcomes and satisfaction with health care systems and nursing care (Abraham & Moretz, 2012; Duke & Scal, 2011; Moretz & Abraham, 2012). More attention to the development of human relational and communication skills is needed. Nurses who *think family* use the tool of nurse presence to intentionally focus on family and value it in all forms of care delivery.

The availability of community and societal support during health and illness experiences is critical to quality care. Excellent care delivery to fully satisfy needs must include the family unit as an intentional collaborative partner in care. Nurses who *think family* realize that families have active and primary roles in health and illness. Families need nurses who know how to be present and support the well-being and health of families so they can fulfill individual, familial, and societal roles and responsibilities in the best ways possible.

Individual and Family Satisfaction

Individuals and families do not always know what to ask for, but they know good care when they receive it. Satisfaction with care is a critical factor being measured in current health care arenas and nurse attention to families can make a difference in their satisfaction.

Current research suggests that nurses who are fully present for families and those who value the presence of a family positively influence satisfaction (Osborn et al., 2012). Including families, supporting family decision making, and allowing families control over care are factors that influence satisfaction (Osborn et al., 2012). As family influence in health care experiences and outcomes becomes more evident, family care is quickly becoming a target for satisfaction and quality improvement in health care systems (Osborn et al., 2012). Box 9.7 describes a team of researchers who strive to influence best practices by studying family nursing intervention for family caregivers. Initiatives to incorporate patients and family as partners in care align with the Institute of Medicine's pivotal report, *Crossing the Quality Chasm* (Institute of Medicine, 2001). Whether the concern is wellness, acute and chronic illness, end-of-life transitions, or other needs, nurse presence appears at the core of quality care, health outcomes, and satisfaction.

Measuring Satisfaction

The processes of eliminating barriers and building a family-focused institution for care delivery are wrought with challenges around ways to establish a culture focused on family and nurse presence (Abraham & Moretz, 2012). Satisfaction is not merely about measurement, but about relationships. It is not just about giving care, but about giving valued care. It is not only about outcomes, but also about perceived benefits.

Educational and practice perspectives are needed to develop visionary statements, strategic plans, and outcome measures that support individual-nurse-family partnerships. Policy changes, philosophies, missions, resource allocation, and practice expectations to embrace the significance of family and nurse presence are needed. Exemplars or role models,

---

BOX 9-7

Evidence-Based Family Nursing

Family Nursing Interventions: Family Caregivers of Seniors

In Canada, similar to the United States, an aging population is placing greater demands on family caregivers. The majority of caregiving comes from family members, and the burden of sickness and the time needed for caregiving place caregivers at risk for lessened quality of life and personal health problems. The Desjardins Research Chair in Nursing Care for Seniors and Their Families has conducted research for more than a decade on innovative nursing interventions for family caregivers. A stress management intervention is composed of five in-home visits and a follow-up visit a month later with specific objectives and activities for each meeting. Another intervention called "Taking Care of Myself" consists of ten 90-minute weekly sessions for six to eight caregivers. This family research team used theoretical frameworks to develop a four-step process for developing and testing their interventions. They involved caregivers in their processes and tailored interventions to satisfy needs of families. Many of the recommendations that came from this program of research were adopted as policy in 2009 after the Ministry of Health and Social Services and Ministry for the Family and Seniors invited the research team's opinions on best practices for families. The researchers note that families' complex interactions and needs, as well as those of individual members, need to be taken into account with any intervention.

Source: Ducharme, F. (2011). A research program on nursing interventions for family caregivers of seniors: Development and evaluation of psycho-educational interventions. In E. K. Svavarsdottir & H. Jonsdottir (Eds.), *Family nursing in action* (pp. 217–250). Reykjavik, Iceland: University of Iceland Press.

coaches, mentors, and educators who can demonstrate nursing presence are necessary. Students need opportunities to practice ways an individual-nurse-family partnership works as they strive to enhance presence. Leaders to guide others in the acquisition and use of techniques that enable families to practice wellness, care for ill members, and optimize the health of households are needed (Denham, 2003).

Creating Environments to Support Family Presence

Transforming health care organizational environments to support the presence of families is being recognized as a mechanism that supports quality improvement (Henriksen, Isaacson, Sadler, & Zimring, 2007; Karlsson, Tisell, Engström, & Andershed, 2011; Milford, Zapalo, & Davis, 2008). Unlike traditional health care environments, grounds and rooms are being remodeled and designed to be noninstitutional, aesthetically soothing spaces aimed at reducing anxiety and maximizing comfort (Evans & Thomas, 2011). Health care systems can focus on built environments that encourage family interactions, recognize family's protectiveness, and accommodate family's needs. Larger rooms that allow members to be close and private spaces that allow privacy can support family needs. A space for family meetings and decision making can support family presence. Room design and comfort measures (e.g., space, color, seating arrangements, refreshments, and artful distractions) influence comfort in the environment. Pleasant environments are restful during critical inpatient stays. For example, Figure 9.9 shows a large sofa and chair where family members can gather. The sofa converts to a sleeping area for the night. Keep in mind the rows of patients lying next to one another on the floor during the Crimean War long ago. The person who made the truly important difference at that time was the nurse with the light, Florence Nightingale. Although aesthetics can be comforting to the family, it is the nurse presence that makes difficult situations endurable, inconceivable tragedies bearable, and solace attainable.

Chapter Summary

This chapter explored nurse and family presence and the value of being with or being there for individuals and their family members over time and across care systems. It described the ways family presence is important to individual members at times of illness. Family

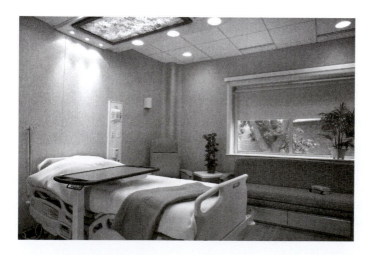

FIGURE 9-9 Hospital wellness room, Madelia, Minnesota.

presence implies a the need to consider not only the physically present family members, but also family bonds and connections during illness experiences. Nurse presence can open the door to genuine caring relationships with the family unit. Nurses who value presence recognize the need to acknowledge the unique nature of each situation. A nurse who is present can help families find meaning in illness experiences, identify strategies to support family capacity to care for members, and navigate the health and illness experiences. Nurses who *think family* use presence to assist individuals and family members to manage the stress, vulnerability, and uncertainty linked to illness. Presence is central to family–focused nursing practice and healing environments and may be a means to improve satisfaction with care.

REFERENCES

Abate, F. R. (Ed.). (2002). *Oxford American dictionary of current English*. New York: Oxford University Press.

Abraham, M., & Moretz, J. G. (2012). Implementing patient- and family-centered care: Understanding the challenges. *Pediatric Nursing, 38*(1), 44–47.

Alvarez, G. F., & Kirby, A. S. (2006). The perspective of families of the critically ill patient: Their needs. *Current Opinion in Critical Care, 12*, 614–618.

Bakitas, M., Kryworuchko, J., Matlock, D., & Volandes, A. E. (2011). Palliative medicine and decision science: The critical need for shared agenda to foster informed patient choice in serious illness. *Journal of Palliative Medicine, 14*(10), 1110–1116.

Basol, R., Ohman, K., Simones, J., & Skillings, K. (2009). Using research to determine support for a policy on family presence during resuscitation. *Dimensions in Critical Care Nursing, 28*(5), 237–247.

Baumann, S. L. (1999). Art as a path of inquiry. *Nursing Science Quarterly, 12*(2), 106–110.

Bell, J. M. (2011). Relationships: The heart of the matter in family nursing. *Journal of Family Nursing, 17*(3), 3–10.

Bell, L., & Bell, D. (2012). Positive relationships that support elder health and well-being are grounded in midlife/adolescent family. *Family & Community Health, 35*(4), 276–286.

Black, P., Boore, J. R. P., & Parahoo, K. (2011). The effect of nurse-facilitated family participation in the psychological care of the critically ill patient. *Journal of Advanced Nursing, 67*(5), 1091–1101. doi:10.1111/j.1365-2648.2010.05558.x

Boss, P. G., Doherty, W. J., LaRossa, W. R., Schumm, W. R., & Steinmetz, S. K. (Eds.). (1993). *Sourcebook of family theories and methods: A contextual approach*. New York: Plenum.

Bulechek, G. M., Butcher, H. K., & Dochterman, J. M. (2008). *Nursing interventions classification (NIC)*. St. Louis: Mosby.

Carr, J. M., & Clarke, P. (1997). Development of the concept of family vigilance. *Western Journal of Nursing Research, 19*(6), 726–739.

Chesla, C. A. (2010). Do family interventions improve health? *Journal of Family Nursing, 16*(4), 355–377. doi:10.1177/1074840710383145

Chinn, P., & Kramer, M. (2008). *Integrated theory and knowledge development in nursing* (7th ed.). St. Louis: Mosby.

Clabots, S., (2012). Strategies to help initiate and maintain the end-of-life discussion with patients and family members. *MedSurg Nursing, 21*(4), 197–203.

DeLashmutt, M., & Rankin, E. (2006). Finding spirituality and nursing presence: The student's challenge. *Journal of Holistic Nursing, 24*, 282–288.

Denham, S. A. (2003). *Family health: A framework for nursing*. Philadelphia: F. A. Davis.

Denham, S. A., & Looman, W. S. (2010). Families with chronic illness. In J. R. Kaakinen, V. Gedaly-Duff, D. P. Coehlo, & S. M. H. Hanson (Eds.), *Family health care nursing: Theory, practice and research* (4th ed., pp. 235–272). Philadelphia: F. A. Davis.

Dewar, A. (2001). Protecting strategies used by sufferers of catastrophic illnesses and injuries. *Journal of Clinical Nursing, 10*, 600–608.

Dochterman, J. M., & Bulechek, G. M. (Eds.). (2004). *Nursing interventions classification (NIC)* (4th ed.). St. Louis: Mosby.

Doolin, C., Quinn, L. D., Bryant, L. G., Lyons, A. A., & Kleinpell, R. M. (2011). Family presence during cardiopulmonary resuscitation: Using evidence-based knowledge to guide the advanced practice nurse in developing formal policy and practice guidelines. *Journal of the American Academy of Advanced Nurse Practitioners, 23*, 8–14. doi:10.1111/j.1745-7599.2010.00569.x

Dudley, S. K., & Carr, J. M. (2004). Vigilance: The experience of parents staying at the bedside of hospitalized children. *Journal of Pediatric Nursing, 19*(4), 267–275.

Duggleby, W., Holtslander, L., Kylman, J., Duncan, V., Hammond, C., & Williams, A. (2010). Meta-synthesis of the hope experience of family caregivers of persons with chronic illness. *Qualitative Health Research, 20*(2), 148–158.

Duhamel, F., Dupuis, F., & Wright, L. (2009). Families' and nurses' responses to the "one question questions": Reflections for clinical practice, education and research in family nursing. *Journal of Family Nursing, 15*(4), 461–485.

Duke, N., & Scal, P. (2011). Adult care transitioning for adolescents with special health care needs: A pivotal role for family centered care. *Maternal & Child Health Journal, 15*(1), 98–105. doi:10.1007/s10995-009-0547-1

Eggenberger, S. K., Krumwiede, N., Meiers, S., Bliesmer, M., & Earle, P. (2004). Family caring strategies in neutropenia. *Clinical Journal of Oncology Nursing, 8*(6), 617–621.

Eggenberger, S. K., Krumwiede, N., Meiers, S., Bliesmer, M., Earle, P., & Murray, S. (2004). Giving voice to family caring in cancer: Integrating visual art and research findings. *International Journal for Human Caring, 8*(3), 59–65.

Eggenberger, S. K., Meiers, S. J., Krumwiede, N. K., Bliesmer, M., & Earle, P. (2011). Family reintegration: A family health promoting process in chronic illness. *Journal of Nursing and Health Care of Chronic Illness, 3*, 283–292.

Eggenberger, S. K., & Nelms, T. P. (2007). Being family: The family experience when an adult member is hospitalized with a critical illness. *Journal of Clinical Nursing, 16*(9), 1618–1628.

Emergency Nursing Resources Development Committee (ENA). (2009). Emergency nursing resource: Family presence during invasive procedures and resuscitation in the emergency department. Retrieved from http://www.ena.org/IENR/ENR/Documents/FamilyPresenceENR.pdf

Evans, J., & Thomas, J. (2011). Understanding family requirements in the intensive care room. *Critical Care Nursing Quarterly, 34*(4), 290–296.

Finfgeld-Connett, D. (2006). Meta-synthesis of presence in nursing. *Journal of Advanced Nursing, 55*, 708–714.

Finfgeld-Connett, D. (2008). Qualitative convergence of three nursing concepts: Art of nursing, presence and caring. *Journal of Advanced Nursing, 63*(5), 527–534.

Frankl V. (1992) *Man's search for meaning: An introduction to logotherapy* (Lasch I, Trans. 4th ed.). Boston: Beacon.

Gardner, D. L. (1992). Presence. In G. M. Bulechek & J. C. McCloskey (Eds.). *Nursing interventions: Essential nursing treatments* (2nd ed., pp. 191–200). Philadelphia: W. B. Saunders.

Godkin, J. (2001). Healing presence. *Journal of Holistic Nursing, 19*, 5–21.

Griffin, T. (2010). Bringing change-of-shift report to the bedside: A patient- and family-centered approach. *Journal of Perinatal and Neonatal Nursing, 24*(4), 348–353.

Hardin, S. R. (2012). Engaging families to participate in care of older adult critical care patients. *Critical Care Nurse, 32*(3), 35–40. doi:http://dx.doi.org/10.4037/ccn2012407

Henneman, E. A., & Cardin, S. (2002). Family-centered critical care: A practical approach to making it happen. *Critical Care Nurse, 22*(6), 12–19.

Henriksen, K., Isaacson, S., Sadler, B., & Zimring, C. (2007). The role of the physical environment in crossing the quality chasm. *Joint Commission Journal on Quality & Patient Safety, 33*(11), 68–80.

Hessel, J. A. (2009). Presence in nursing practice: A concept analysis. *Holistic Nursing Practice, 23*(5), 276–281. doi:10.1097/HNP.0b013e3181b66cb5

Hughes, F., Bryan, K., & Robbins, I. (2005). Relatives' experiences of critical care. *Nursing in Critical Care, 10*(1), 23–30.

Hung, S. Y., & Pang, S. M. C. (2011). Family presence preference when patients are receiving resuscitation in an accident and emergency department. *Journal of Advanced Nursing, 67*(1), 56–67. doi:10.1111/j.1365-2648.2010.05441.x

Institute for Patient- and Family-Centered Care. (2013). Bibliographies/supporting evidence. Retrieved from http://www.ipfcc.org/advance/supporting.html

Institute of Medicine (2001). Committee on Quality of Health Care in America. *Crossing the quality chasm: A new health system for the 21st century.* Washington, DC: National Academies Press.

Iseminger, K., Levitt, F., & Kirk, L. (2009). Healing during existential moments: The "art" of nursing presence. *Nursing Clinics of North America, 44*(4), 447–459.

Johnson, B., Abraham, M., Conway, J., Simmons, L., Edgman-Levitan, S., Sodomka, P., Ford, D. (2008). *Partnering with patients and families to design a patient-and-family-centered health care system: Recommendations and promising practices.* Bethesda, MD: Institute for Patient- and Family-Centered Care.

Jones, C., Skirrow, P., Griffiths, R., Humphris, G., Ingleby, S., Eddleston, J., Gager, M. (2004). Posttraumatic stress disorder-related symptoms in relatives of patients following intensive care. *Intensive Care Medicine, 30*(3), 456–460. doi:10.1007/s00134-003-2149-5

Kaakinen, J. R., Gedaly-Duff, V., Coehlo, E. P., & Hanson, S. M. (2010). *Family health care nursing* (4th ed.). Philadelphia: F. A. Davis.

Kaakinen, J. R., Hanson, S. M. H., & Denham, S. A. (2010). Family health nursing: An introduction. In J. R. Kaakinen, V. Gedaly-Duff, D. P. Coehlo, & S. M. H. Hanson (Eds.), *Family health care nursing: Theory, practice and research* (4th ed., pp. 3–33). Philadelphia: F. A. Davis.

Karlsson, C., Tisell, A., Engström, A., & Andershed, B. (2011). Family members' satisfaction with critical care: A pilot study. *Nursing in Critical Care, 16*(1), 11–18. doi:10.1111/j.1478-5153.2010.00388.x

Kautz, D., & Van Horn, E. R. (2009). Promoting family integrity to inspire hope in rehabilitation patients: Strategies to provide evidence-based care. *Rehabilitation Nursing, 34*(4), 168–173.

Knafl, K., Deatrick, J. A., & Havill, N. L. (2012). Continued development of the family management style framework. *Journal of Family Nursing, 18*(1), 11–34.

Knafl, K., & Gilliss, C. L. (2002). Families and chronic illness: A synthesis of current research. *Journal of Family Nursing, 8*, 178–198.

Koerner, J. G. (2007). *Healing presence: The essence of nursing.* New York: Springer.

Krumwiede, N. K., Meiers, S. J., Bliesmer, M., Eggenberger, S. K., Earle, P., Murray, S., Rydholm, K. (2004). Turbulent waiting with intensified connections: The family experience of neutropenia. *Oncology Nursing Forum, 31*(6), 1145–1152.

Kunerth, L. (2010). *Caring processes that support families experiencing a chronic illness.* Unpublished master's thesis. Mankato, MN: Minnesota State University.

Litman, T. J. (1974). The family as a basic unit in health and medical care: A social-behavioral overview. *Social Science & Medicine, 8*(9–10), 495–519. doi:10.1016/0037-7856(74)90072-9

McClement, S. E., Fallis, W. M., & Pereira, A. (2009). Family presence during resuscitation: Canadian critical care nurses' perspectives. *Journal of Nursing Scholarship, 41*(3), 233–240. doi:10.1111/j.1547-5069.2009.01288.x

McDaniel, S. H., Campbell, T. L., Hepworth, J., & Lorenz, A. (2005). *Family-oriented primary care* (2nd ed.). New York: Springer.

McMahon, M. A., & Christopher, K. A. (2011). Toward a mid-range theory of nursing presence. *Nursing Forum, 46*(2), 71–82. doi:10.1111/j.1744-6198.2011.00215.x

Meiers, S. J., & Brauer, D. J. (2008). Existential caring in the family health experience: A proposed conceptualization. *Scandinavian Journal of Caring Science, 22*, 110–117.

Meiers, S., Eggenberger, S., Krumwiede, N., Bliesmer, M., & Earle, P. (2009). Enduring acts of balancing: Rural families creating health. In H. Lee (Ed.), *Conceptual basis for rural nursing* (3rd ed., pp. 110–125). New York: Springer.

Meiers, S. J., Krumwiede, N., Eggenberger, S. K., Bliesmer, M., & Earle, P. (2007). *The other side: Creation of a sculptural painting from a qualitative family study of chronic illness.* The Eighth International Interdisciplinary Conference: Advances in Qualitative Methods, September 21–24, Banff, Alberta, Canada.

Meiers, S. J., & Tomlinson, P. S. (2003). Family-nurse co-construction of meaning: A central phenomenon in family caring. *Scandinavian Journal of Caring Sciences, 17*, 193–201.

Meleis, A. I. (Ed.). (2010). Transitions theory: Middle range and situation—specific theories in nursing research and practice. New York: Springer.

Melnechenko, K. L. (2003). To make a difference: Nursing presence. *Nursing Forum, 38*(2), 18–24. doi:10.1111/j.1744-6198.2003.tb01207

Milford, C., Zapalo, B., & Davis, G. (2008). Transition to an individual-room NICU design: Process and outcome measures. *Neonatal Network, 27*(5), 299–305.

Miller, M. A., & Douglas, M. R. (1998). Presencing: Nurses commitment to caring for dying persons. *International Journal of Human Caring, 2*(3), 24–31.

Moretz, J., & Abraham, M. (2012). Implementing patient- and family-centered care: Part II—Strategies and resources for success. *Pediatric Nursing, 38*(2), 106–171.

Munhall, P. L. (1994). *Revisioning phenomenology: Nursing and health science research*. New York: National League for Nursing Press.

Nelms, T. P., & Eggenberger, S. K. (2010). Essence of the family critical illness experience and family meetings. *Journal of Family Nursing, 16*(4), 462–486.

Neufeld, A., Harrison, M. J., Stewart, M., & Hugest, K. (2008). Advocacy of women family caregivers: Response to nonsupportive interactions with professionals. *Qualitative Health Research, 3*, 301–310.

Newman, M. A. (2008). *Transforming presence: The difference that nursing makes*. Philadelphia: F. A. Davis.

Noble, A., & Jones, C. (2005). Benefits of narrative therapy: Holistic interventions at the end of life. *British Journal of Nursing, 14*(6), 330–333.

Osborn, T., Curtis, J., Nielsen, E., Back, A., Shannon, S., & Engelberg, R. (2012). Identifying elements of ICU care that families report as important but unsatisfactory: Decision-making, control, and ICU atmosphere. *Chest, 142*(5), 1185–1192.

Parse, R. R. (1998). *The human becoming school of thought*. Thousand Oaks, CA: Sage.

Paterson, J., & Zderad, L. (1976). *Humanistic nursing*. New York: John Wiley.

Pavlish, C., & Ceronsky, L. (2009). Oncology nurses' perceptions of nursing roles and professional attributes in palliative care. *Clinical Journal of Oncology Nursing, 13*(4), 404–412.

Richardson, L. (2000). Writing: A method of inquiry. In N. K. Denzin, & Y. S. Lincoln (Eds.), *Handbook of qualitative research* (2nd ed., pp. 923–948). Thousand Oaks, CA: Sage.

Snyder, M., Brandt, C., & Tseng, Y. (2000). Use of presence in the critical care unit. *AACN Clinical Issues, 11*(1), 27–33.

Svavarsdottir, E. K., Tryggvadottir, G. B., & Sigurdardottir, A. O. (2012). Knowledge translation in family nursing: Does a short-term therapeutic conversation intervention benefit families of children and adolescents in a hospital setting? Findings from the Landspitali University Hospital Family Nursing Implementation Project. *Journal of Family Nursing, 18*(3), 303–327.

Tollefson, J., Usher, K., & Foster, K. (2011). Relationships in pain: The experience of relationships to people living with chronic pain in rural areas. *International Journal of Nursing Practice, 17*, 478–485.

Tomlinson, P. S., Peden-McAlpine, C., & Sherman, S. (2012). A family systems nursing intervention model for a paediatric health crisis. *Journal of Advanced Nursing, 68*(3), 705–714.

Tong, A., Lowe, A. L., Sainsbury, P., & Craig, J. C. (2008). Experience of parents who have children with chronic kidney disease: A systematic review of qualitative studies. *Pediatrics, 121*, 349. doi:10.1542/peds.2006-3470

Tschann, J. M., Kaufman, S. R., & Micco, G. P. (2003). Family involvement in end-of-life hospital care. *American Geriatrics Society, 51*(6), 835–840.

Vaartio, H., Leino-Kilpi, H., Salantera, S., & Suominen, T. (2006). Nursing advocacy: How is it defined by patients and nurses, what does it involve and how is it experienced? *Scandinavian Journal of Caring Science. 20*(3), 282–292.

Vandall-Walker, V., & Clark, A. M. (2011). It starts with access! A grounded theory of family members working to get through critical illness. *Journal of Family Nursing, 17*(2), 148–181.

Van Heukelom, R., Bell, J., Eggenberger, S. K., & Bell, S. E. (2010, November). *Advancing family nursing practice: The Glen Taylor Nursing Institute for Family and Society.* Paper presentation at National Council for Family Relations at National Conference, Minneapolis, MN.

Watson, J. (2007). Conversations and reflections on my journey into the heart of nursing: Human caring-healing. In T. Hansen-Turton, S. Sherman, & V. Ferguson (Eds.). *Conversations with leaders: Frank talk from nurses (and others) on the front lines of leadership.* Indianapolis, IN: Sigma Theta Tau.

Weihs, K. L., Fisher, L., & Baird, M. (2002). Families, health and behavior. A section of the Commissioned Report by the Committee on Health and Behavior: Research, Practice, and Policy, Division of Neuroscience and Behavioral Health and Division of Health Promotion and Disease Prevention, Institute of Medicine, National Academy of Sciences. *Families, Systems & Health, 20*(1), 7–46.

Weingarten, K. (2013). The "Cruel radiance of what is": Helping couples live with chronic illness. *Family Process, 52*(1), 83–101. doi:10.1111/famp.12017

Wiegand, D. (2008). In their own time: The family experience during the process of withdrawal of life-sustaining therapy. *Journal of Palliative Medicine, 11*(8), 1115–1121.

Wiegand, D. L. M. (2006). Withdrawal of life-sustaining therapy after sudden, unexpected life-threatening illness or injury: Interactions between patients' families, health care providers, and the healthcare system. *American Journal of Critical Care, 15*(2), 178–187.

Wright, L. M., & Bell, J. M. (2009). *Beliefs: The heart of healing in families and illness.* New York: Basic Books.

Wright, L., & Leahey, M. (2013). *Nurses and families: A guide to family assessment and intervention* (6th ed.). Philadelphia: F. A. Davis.

CHAPTER 10

Family-Focused Care in Acute Illness

Sandra K. Eggenberger • Marcia Stevens

CHAPTER OBJECTIVES

1. Explore the family experience during acute illness.
2. Examine stress, uncertainty, and suffering that may occur in a family during an acute illness experience.
3. Review evidence that supports the presence of a family and family health during acute illness.
4. Describe nursing actions that support families during transitions in acute care illness.
5. Analyze environmental factors that support and challenge family-focused nursing practice in acute care settings.

CHAPTER CONCEPTS

- Acute care
- Acute care environments
- Bedside rounding
- Discharge
- Empowerment
- Family advisory council
- Family communication
- Family decision making
- Family interactions

- Family meetings
- Family processes
- Policies and visitation
- Satisfaction
- Stress
- Suffering
- Support
- Uncertainty

Introduction

Caring for patients in an acute care setting is the type of challenging practice that many nurses think about when envisioning their career. Nursing practice in this setting is often focused on meeting acute care needs of individuals, and is less centered on family needs. Yet, caring family members often accompany individuals in acute care settings and frequently they are distressed as they experience the illness and complex care provided to their loved ones. These family members need nurses who understand their experience and will develop a partnership that comforts them during this stressful time and prepares them for the future. This chapter describes the family experience during an acute care illness and the nursing actions needed to support families during illness trajectories. Barriers to family-focused nursing care in the acute care setting and ways to overcome them are addressed. Without nursing practice focused on the family, the individual with an illness could face readmissions, poor outcomes, and dissatisfaction (Bauer, Fitzgerald, Haesler, & Manfrin, 2009) and the family faces added stress and challenges (King et al., 2013). An exemplar case study of a family in which a family member experiences an acute illness is threaded throughout the chapter to illustrate ways family-focused nursing care can be provided.

Acute Care Settings

Acute care is needed for severe illness, traumatic injuries, disabilities, surgery, and complications of chronic conditions. Management of these situations may require admission to a medical unit, transfer to an intensive care unit (ICU), surgical intervention, or treatment in the emergency department. Persons admitted for acute care, along with family members, are anxious about their diagnosis, treatment, and outcomes. Even when procedures are elective, the experience can be stressful. The goal is to resolve the illness, injury, or other catastrophic dilemma as quickly and effectively as possible. Acute care stays are often brief but intense experiences. The equipment, treatments, interventions, numerous care providers, complex language used by care providers, and overall acute care culture are all unfamiliar to the patient and family.

The acute setting also poses unique challenges for the nurse. One must balance the acute care demands of the individual while partnering and communicating with the family throughout transitions that occur during an acute care stay (King et al., 2013; Strang, Henoch, Danielson, Browall, & Melin-Johansson, 2014). A nurse's focus on the complex care of the family member with the condition is a priority for both the patient and the family. Nurses' beliefs about the role of family members in acute care settings may be contrary to what the family expects, as the family attempts to fulfill roles as protector for their family member (Carr, 2014; Eggenberger & Nelms, 2007; Vandall-Walker & Clark, 2011; Wright & Bell, 2009). These beliefs may interfere with nurses' ideas about their capacity to provide family-focused care in acute care settings. Nurses focus on family often as background; families are often excluded, and may be viewed as a barrier to care delivery (Davidson, 2009; Davidson, Jones, & Bienvenu, 2012; Santiago, Lazar, Depeng, & Burns, 2014; Verhaeghe, Defloor, Van Zuuren, Duijnstee, & Grypdonick, 2005). Yet, nurses who *think family* understand that a nurse has profound power and influence over the tone and outcome of the experience for families and includes families as partners, develops relationships with family members, and addresses family concerns during the experience of an acute illness to improve care (Bell, 2011; Nelms & Eggenberger, 2010; Wright & Leahey, 2013).

Family Illness Experience During a Family Member's Acute Illness

Family-focused nursing care is important because illness is a shared family experience that can be overwhelming and threaten family health and the family's ability to support the member of the family with an acute illness (Azoulay et al., 2003; Davidson, Jones, & Bienvenu, 2012; Marshall, Bell, & Moules, 2010; McAdam, Dracup, White, Fontaine, & Puntillo, 2010; Williams, 2005). Hospitalization with an acute illness is stressful and brings worries, decision making, and changes in family processes such as family communication, bonds, and coordination. Family members of an acutely ill person experience multiple threats from the diagnosis of an illness, admission to an acute care setting, the environment, transitions, and complex hospital treatments. Concerns such as stress, uncertainty, and suffering often emerge during a family's experience with an acute illness (Davidson, Jones, & Bienvenu, 2012; Nelms & Eggenberger, 2010; Tong & Kaakinen, 2015).

Family Stress

Family stress can be described as the "pressure or tension in the family system—a disturbance in the steady state of the family" (Boss, 2002, p. 16). When faced with an acute illness, families are stressed because of changes in family life, threats to the individual and family, lives that are on hold, lack of information and communication, and waiting for answers (Davidson et al., 2007; Vandall-Walker & Clark, 2011). Diagnosis of an illness or admission to an acute care setting, a transfer, and discharge can increase stress as a family adjusts to the unknowns and changes (King et al., 2013; Stacy, 2012). Nurses who *think family* anticipate these times of family stress and offer support, explanations, and information.

The meanings of events and perceptions during an acute illness affect the degree of stress experienced (Boss, 2002; Davidson, 2010). Families try to gain some control in new situations by using behaviors they believe will fulfill their needs (Hardin, 2012). For example, a family questions nurses about care and treatments to better understand. Some family members might be hesitant to ask questions; others are abrupt, annoyed, and agitated. Nurses who are family focused initiate relationships and conversation with a family to understand their experience and perceptions (Bell, 2011; Hallsdottir & Svavarsdottir, 2012; Svavarsdottir, Tryggvadottir, & Sigurdardottir, 2012).

Individuals in a family unit may have views that differ from one another and cause conflict and overwhelm family members (Appleyard et al., 2000; Boss, 2002; Fontana, 2006). Some family members are angry, others are silent, some are conflictual, and still others work together (Warnock, Tod, Foster, & Soreny, 2010). Family members may argue with one another about who is helping more, who should make decisions, or who will be the leader of the family in supporting the family member with acute illness. Although an illness can bring a family closer together, it can also cause conflicts and disrupt a family and the usual functions, roles, and tasks (Cannon, 2011; Eggenberger & Nelms, 2010; Wiegand, 2008; Wiegand, Deatrick, & Knafl, 2008). Nurses who *think family* address the conflicts and recognize a family faces actual and perceived threats (Hardin, 2012). Actions by nurses must help families to communicate, resolve conflict, and reach consensus (Pastor-Montero et al., 2012). Nurses may not be able to solve all issues, but they can maximize care outcomes by providing clear and consistent explanations to a family, advocating for a family or individual family member while communicating and helping family members to interact and share their thinking (Fumagalli et al., 2006; Hardin, 2012; Khalaila, 2013). Table 10.1 identifies a few examples of research studies that explore stress during an acute illness and provide direction for family care.

Family Uncertainty

Distress of uncertainty is a central theme of the illness experience in acute care settings as family members withstand the unknowns of the health care environment, question illness outcomes, and struggle to make decisions and alter their family routines (Dupuis, Duhamel, & Gendron, 2011; Fontana, 2006; Trimm & Sanford, 2010; Vandall-Walker & Clark, 2011; Wiegand, 2008). Uncertainty has been defined as the inability to identify meanings of an illness event that influences abilities to manage situations

TABLE 10-1	*Literature Related to Family Stress With Acute and Critical Illness*

RESEARCH	FAMILIES STUDIED	FINDINGS	IMPLICATIONS: FAMILY-FOCUSED NURSING ACTIONS
Radfar, Ahmadi, & Fallahi Khoshknab (2013)	Family members of patients suffering from depression	Families work to tolerate a great amount of stress with depression. Psychological, physical, and financial factors impose turbulent life on families.	Reduce burden of family by providing knowledge about how to communicate with their family member. Offer emotional support resources to patients and families.
Davidson, Jones, & Bienvenu (2012)	Families who experienced critical illness	Family responses to critical illness include development of adverse, acute stress disorder and post-traumatic stress.	Optimal communication and inclusion in care can reduce family complications of stress. Refer families to support groups and follow-up care after critical illness experience.
Jones, Backman, & Griffiths (2012)	Families experiencing a critical illness	Post-traumatic stress occurs in relatives of critically ill individuals. An intervention of diaries may alleviate post-traumatic stress.	Provide patients and families with diaries during a critical illness.
Black, Boore, & Parahoo (2011)	Patients and families hospitalized with critical illness	Nurse-led facilitation designed to support family comfort and access to patient positively influenced patient psychological recovery from ICU.	Guide a family member in communicating with a critically ill patient.
Nelms & Eggenberger (2010)	Families experiencing a critical illness	Stress of critical illness is increased when communication is not therapeutic and maintained or exchange of information is inconsistent.	Nurse-family meetings can minimize the stress and distress of critical illness.
Davidson (2009)	Families experiencing a critical illness	Families experience stress and anxiety.	Family-centered care helps to meet the needs of families.

(Mishel & Clayton, 2008). Over the past decade, uncertainty has been described as a major and pervasive component of the illness experience that affects clinical outcomes (Hansen et al., 2012).

The uncertainty in illness theory proposes that uncertainty emerges in illness conditions when there is a lack of information, complexity, unpredictability, and ambiguity (Mishel, 1997; Mishel & Clayton, 2008). These issues certainly exist in the acute care setting. Acute illness causes family difficulties as they try to interpret information and deal with the unpredictability of outcomes (Mishel & Clayton, 2008). Nurses who *think family* prepare families for events that signal changes in treatment or condition and explain what matters to the patient and family in ways the family can understand (Hansen et al., 2012). Explaining symptoms and the possible effects of treatments must occur repeatedly with multiple family members who have various understandings at different times (Hansen et al., 2012). The complex system of care and multiple environmental transitions are challenging to the family. Various individuals in the system may use different words or interpret situations in their own way which may leave a family confused and mistrustful (Eggenberger & Nelms, 2007). Nurses who *think family* continually strive to clarify messages, treat concerns respectfully, and assist families in managing the unknowns and preparing for the future (Hardin, 2012; Stayt, 2009; Tapp, 2001; Van Horn & Kautz, 2007). Table 10.2 identifies a few examples of early and current research that explore uncertainty and provide direction for family care. Nurses who consistently exchange information with families, prepare them for upcoming events, and offer clarity can help families manage uncertainty during acute illness.

TABLE 10-2	*Research Related to Family Uncertainty During an Illness Experience*		
RESEARCH	**GROUPS STUDIED**	**OVERALL FINDINGS**	**IMPLICATIONS: FAMILY-FOCUSED NURSING ACTIONS**
Hansen et al (2012)	A synthesis of 15 qualitative studies exploring patient experiences with uncertainty during illness	Implications for nursing practice are evident in qualitative study findings.	Organize the trajectory of an illness through the health care system. Support patients through relationships. Provide knowledge through clear and accurate communication.
Eggenberger, Meiers, Krumwiede, Bliesmer, & Earle (2011)	Families with a family member living with various chronic illnesses	A process of family reintegration occurs within a context of uncertainty.	Include the family to reduce uncertainty. Assist family to manage the unknowns, plan for the future, and protect their ill family member. Acknowledge the struggle to adjust and manage trajectories.
Sammarco & Konecny (2010)	Latina breast cancer survivors	Latina population reported higher level of uncertainty when compared to Caucasian.	Address cultural differences in managing uncertainty. Anticipate unique needs based on culture.

Continued

TABLE 10-2	*Research Related to Family Uncertainty During an Illness Experience—cont'd*		
RESEARCH	**GROUPS STUDIED**	**OVERALL FINDINGS**	**IMPLICATIONS: FAMILY-FOCUSED NURSING ACTIONS**
Stone & Jones (2009)	Adult children of parents diagnosed with Alzheimer's disease	Sources of uncertainty include unpredictability of social relationships and potential family conflict.	Nurses need to assist family members to manage conflicts and their relationships.
Eggenberger & Nelms (2007)	Families experiencing critical illness	Uncertainty is a concern for family due to foreign environment, lack of understanding of treatment, and limited consistent information exchange. Increased uncertainty when family not included in the care of member or lacked connection with the nurse.	Explanations repeatedly to family members increase understandings. Clarify interpretations of other health care provides. Develop trusting relationship with family to minimize uncertainty. Engage in therapeutic conversations throughout illness. Prepare family for changes in environment, illness, or management.
Brashers (2003)	Individuals with HIV illness	Unpredictable interpersonal reactions contribute to uncertainty.	Address family perceptions and reactions to events of the HIV illness.
Northouse et al (2002)	Women with recurrent breast cancer and their family members	Family satisfaction with a family program that focused on giving information and uncertainty management techniques built on family strengths.	Identify and build on family strengths. Provide consistent exchange of information.
Sammarco (2001)	Younger breast cancer survivors below age 50	Negative correlation between perceived social support and uncertainty. Negative correlation between social network size and uncertainty. Negative correlation between uncertainty and quality of life.	Explore available social supports and access to social network. Consider patient and family's beliefs.

TABLE 10-2	Research Related to Family Uncertainty During an Illness Experience—cont'd		
RESEARCH	**GROUPS STUDIED**	**OVERALL FINDINGS**	**IMPLICATIONS: FAMILY-FOCUSED NURSING ACTIONS**
Mast (1998)	Breast cancer survivors	Uncertainty is stressful and pervasive. Uncertainty is a response to fear of recurrence, long-term treatment side effects.	Explore fears and discuss outcomes of treatment. Address perceived and actual threats.
Mishel (1997)	Individuals and family members living with acute and chronic illness	Social support decreases uncertainty. Uncertainty develops in acute and chronic illness. Reducing uncertainty in family members increases capacity to support ill member and decreases family's emotional distress.	Acknowledge uncertainty. Identify support in systems. Assist family members to maintain supportive network.

Family Suffering

Suffering in the acute care setting is most often attributed to the ill person; however, family members often hurt, worry, and feel the pain alongside their family member (Weingarten, 2012). Cassell defined "the state of severe distress associated with events that threaten the intactness of the person" (Cassell, 1991, p. 33). An individual with respiratory failure may be suffering with respiratory distress, but the family may also experience distress as they attempt to protect their loved one and despair as they observe the dyspnea. Suffering has been described as "physical, emotional, or spiritual anguish, pain or distress" (Wright, 2005, p. 3) that most certainly can occur in a family. Yet, family suffering may be overlooked when a priority is the family member with an acute illness. Family members have concerns about care outcomes, treatment decisions, and the changes that influence family life or threaten the family unit (Wright, 2005). Conflicts and tension often arise among members who hold different beliefs; nurses who fail to include or guide the family can actually magnify the suffering experience during acute care (Eggenberger & Nelms, 2007; Vandall-Walker & Clark, 2011). Suffering with a family member during an acute illness may not be eliminated, but it can be acknowledged and addressed, which makes a difference to the family (Martinez, D'Artois, & Rennick, 2007; Wright, 2005; Wright & Bell, 2009). See Table 10.3 for additional literature about suffering.

TABLE 10-3	*Literature Related to Family Suffering During an Illness Experience*	

AUTHORS	PREMISE AND FINDINGS	IMPLICATIONS: FAMILY-FOCUSED NURSING ACTIONS
Marshall, Bell, & Moules (2010)	Illness is viewed within family relationships. Relational suffering is a complex human experience that is a threat to wholeness and related to relationships with others (Marshall, 2007). Exploration of relational suffering in families with a family member experiencing mental illness.	A Family Systems Nursing Framework informed by the Illness Beliefs Model can examine beliefs to minimize suffering. Nurses who use therapeutic conversation to explore illness narratives and suffering experiences can soften relational suffering.
Verhaeghe, van Zuuren, Grypdonck, Duijnstee, & Defloor (2010)	Families focus efforts on making suffering bearable following a traumatic coma. Families attempt to protect entire family and loved ones from unnecessary suffering.	Supporting family members in their efforts to protect their loved ones should be encouraged. Encourage open and flexible visiting hours to allow families to protect.
Chintana (2010)	Family suffering with persons living with HIV infection and AIDS. Practice that fails to recognize the family as the unit of care invites unnecessary suffering. Developed and implemented a nursing intervention with the family.	Nursing interventions focused on developing nurse-family trusting relationships, exploring illness beliefs, promoting facilitating beliefs and challenging constraining beliefs, and affirming family strengths soften family suffering.
Eggenberger & Nelms (2007)	Families suffer as they face life-threatening illness of a family member. Nurses can magnify family suffering if they exclude and fail to connect with families.	Nurses who develop connecting relationships with families help families endure the suffering.
Isovaara, Arman, & Rehnsfeldt (2006)	Review explores family suffering related to war experiences. Families suffer from the physical and psychosocial disorders of veterans. Families function from a place of compassion.	Family must be viewed as a unique part of this experience.
Tapp (2001)	Families suffer as they manage their own distress and face life-threatening illness of a family member Emphasis on the relational elements of suffering is important to nursing pratice.	Nurse-family conversations created new understandings among family members that were helpful to the relationships, addressed concerns that contributed to suffering, and explored uncertainties with illness. Illness conversations with nurses can alleviate family suffering. Therapeutic conversations promote family healing.

Ecological Perspective of the Family Acute Illness Experience

An ecological perspective using the Family Health Model points out threats to family health in context of an acute illness (Denham, 2003). The daily routines of the family's members change to manage demands of the acutely ill member and that person's usual roles (Denham, 2003; Sacco, Stapleton, & Ingersoll, 2009). During the acute care event health routines of family members change as they attend to the ill member's personal needs. When a family waits for information, they sit long periods in waiting rooms and fail to attend to personal needs (Trochelman, Albert, Spence, Murray, & Slifcak, 2012). They lack sleep, may resort to eating meals from snack machines, forget their medications, and possibly postpone their regular medical treatments. During acute care, some usual family work continues, but advocacy for the ill member requires attention. Families try to balance usual life demands while satisfying ill member needs, offering protection and comfort, and managing personal concerns (Van Horn & Tesh, 2000). Families need a nurse's support while managing these demands.

Once the acute episode resolves, families often serve as caregivers when the individual returns home. Frequently the ill family member still requires care and family members need to be fully prepared to provide the necessary support (Popejoy, 2011). Preparing for discharge from the acute care setting often includes teaching that focuses on activity restrictions, diet, medications, and follow-up appointments. These details are important, but they may not be the family's most pressing needs (Popejoy, 2011). Yet, families may be reluctant to discuss concerns such as adequacy of health insurance and financial debt. How will they manage travel to follow-up medical visits or address the physical and emotional demands of care? Families need a system perspective of care, rather than an elemental patient-focused view (Hardin, 2012). Intentional planning for a coordinated acute care discharge is required to avoid possible readmissions and emergency care.

A nurse who is family focused also considers the context of the family home, even while the individual with an illness is hospitalized. Ill individuals may return to households where prior family routines are now barriers to health and deterrents to healing. For example, an individual with a recent cardiovascular event may require extensive changes in the family diet. With the illness event, the family must acquire new knowledge and skills (Bjornsdottir, 2002; Paterson, Kieloch, & Gmiterek, 2001; Popejoy, 2011). Families need support, education, and skills for home care that is often complex (Popejoy, 2011). Treatments often need to continue when an individual returns home and families need to know ways to support their family member. Family nurses can help members access clear information in timely ways, plan for realities, and guide problem solving for the acute stay and discharge home (Hansen et al., 2012; Popejoy, 2011; Weiss et al., 2007).

A family's home and household are rooted in a complex interdependent neighborhood of community and larger society systems. Families and their interdependent environments can provide resources for acutely ill persons, but resources across families are not all equal. A nurse who *thinks family* considers the unique environment and functions of each family member and plans. A family-focused nurse works with the family to seek resources and manage the challenges of a household environment during a family member's acute illness. An ecological perspective of the individual with an acute condition and the family's environment has potential to improve care, access to resources, and adjustment to transitions (Denham, 2003). Nurses continue to offer support and guidance as the family adjusts their environment and routines. Nurses worldwide are working to improve the health of families. Box 10.1 describes Dr. Chieko Sugishita, a leader in Japan who dedicated her career to transforming the care of families through research, education, and practice.

> **BOX 10-1**
>
> **Family Tree**
>
> **Chieko Sugishita, RN, PhD (Japan)**
>
> Chieko Sugishita, RN, PhD, provided bold leadership and tireless dedication to the early development of family nursing in Japan. Her efforts to build the science of family nursing began in 1971 as a research assistant at the University of Tokyo. For many years, she taught family health care as a lecturer, and in 1992, she was promoted to full professor and invited to lead the Department of Family Nursing at the University of Tokyo. In her leadership role at one of Japan's most prestigious universities, Dr. Sugishita carefully developed her strategic vision for advancing family nursing. She established it as an academic discipline, recruiting well-known researchers, aligning with strong political supporters, and developing graduate level education in family nursing. In 1994, she launched the *Japanese Journal of Research in Family Nursing* (JJRFN), which provided a forum for scholarly exchange. She was a leader in forming the first national family nursing organization of its kind in the world. On October 1, 1994 she organized and chaired the first national meeting of the Japanese Association for Research in Family Nursing (JARFN, <http://square.umin.ac.jp/jarfn/jarfn/index.html>) and served as its first president. JARFN currently has over 1,500 members and hosted the Tenth International Family Nursing Conference in Kyoto, Japan, in 2011. JARFN was one of the earliest nursing associations to be officially enrolled in the Japanese Scientific Academy. Dr. Sugishita nurtured a large community of family nursing researchers, educators, and practitioners and encouraged cross-fertilization of ideas by inviting family nursing colleagues from around the world to offer ideas in workshops and conferences. She encouraged small learning groups of Japanese nurses to travel abroad to visit programs of excellence in family nursing. In 2002 she translated the book *Beliefs: The Heart of Healing in Families and Illness* (Wright, Watson, & Bell, 1996) into Japanese language. She also published a Japanese undergraduate family nursing textbook. In 2005, at the Seventh International Family Nursing Conference in Canada, she was recognized for her significant pioneering contributions to family nursing. Dr. Chieko Sugishita died in 2007, but her influence continues to live on through her former students and colleagues who are current leaders.

Nursing Practice in Acute Care Settings

Evidence suggests nurses play pivotal roles in comforting the family, advocating for families, guiding families, and developing a connecting partnership with families during an acute illness experience (Bell, 2011; Butler, Copnell, & Willetts, 2014; Chesla & Stannard, 1997; Cypress, 2011; Eggenberger & Nelms, 2007; Meiers & Brauer, 2008; Meiers & Tomlinson, 2003; Soderstrom, Benzein, & Saveman, 2003; Svavarsdottir et al., 2012; Tomlinson, Peden-McAlpine, & Sherman, 2012; Wiegand, 2008). Nursing practice influences illness outcomes and prepares families for their support role (Chesla, 2010). Nurses guide a family to cope with the challenges of an illness and strive to meet the needs of the family.

The acute care experience has been studied for years and findings have identified that families need information, closeness, assurance, support, and comfort (Coulter, 1989; Leske, 1991; Molter, 1979). Families need nurses to provide a consistent exchange of information and guidance (Hardin, 2012; Nelms & Eggenberger, 2010). Families want to be near, watch over, and advocate for their ill member (Dudley & Carr, 2004; Eggenberger, Krumwiede, Meiers, Bliesmer, & Earle, 2004; Hardin, 2012; Khalaila, 2013). Families do not want to be left out; they want to be included in the care (Khalaila, 2013; Sacco et al., 2009). During acute situations, families are often faced with puzzling rituals, rules, technology, and strangers in an unfamiliar environment that is confusing and intensifies distress (Hupcey, 1998; Nelms & Eggenberger, 2010). This distress can be exacerbated when nurses view family as outsiders and allow them limited involvement and marginal control in decisions about what is happening (Vandall-Walker & Clark, 2011). Families want reassurance their family member is receiving optimal care.

Families need nurses who can provide quality care for their family member, but who are also able to develop relationships with the family unit. Yet, evidence suggests nurses might see needs for family involvement, but often feel ill prepared to develop caring relationships with them (Stayt, 2009). With multiple families' multiple needs, nurses may not be able to address every family concern, but a nurse can offer frequent honest information, support, and guidance with sensitivity in ways that meet the needs of families (Khalaila, 2013).

The nurse in the acute care setting faces several challenges to family-focused care. Technological advances, numerous care providers, and complex delegated medical tasks in this setting require nursing practice to integrate complex technical and relational skills to care for the physical needs of the ill individual and the emotional needs of the entire family (Eggenberger & Regan, 2010). A nurse collaborates within an interdisciplinary team whose members all strive to communicate with the families. A nurse in this setting must prioritize the care for an individual with an acute illness and the family who wants to know their family member is cared for with competence and compassion (Kaakinen, Coehlo, Steele, Tabacco, & Hanson, 2015). Family nurses encourage active roles by family members throughout the acute care stay and help them prepare for transitions. Nurses who are focused on the family invite them to participate: "Would you like to be involved in caring for your husband?" Knowledge and skills to assume caregiving roles are needed and family nurses assist them in making needed transitions. "Your husband will go home with this dressing, would you like to come closer and watch?" Nurses must assume that most families have questions, but they don't always know what or who to ask or are afraid to ask. A nurse acknowledges this difficulty, "At times it is difficult for a family to know what questions to ask, what is your most pressing concern right now?"

Families want and need nurses to initiate relationships with them (Bell, 2011). Nurses who are sensitive to family needs are trusted because they provide therapeutic interactions and initiate therapeutic conversations (Box 10.2) (Wright & Leahey, 2013). Nurses who *think family* focus on the patient and family experiences, rather than the patient alone. They are prepared for the distress that might result in the event of a life-changing acute illness. Nursing actions focused on the family in the acute care setting strive to promote health and well-being of the family unit. Patient-centered models and family-focused care have unique foci, approaches, beliefs, and practices for the nurse (Table 10.4). Box 10.3 describes a program of research in New Zealand that addresses family-focused care tied to community care and promotes a model of care focused on family health. Box 10.4 introduces Dr. Michiko Moriyama who has demonstrated outstanding global leadership in family nursing.

BOX 10-2

Questions to Begin a Therapeutic Conversation

Initiating conversations can be a challenge for nursing students and novice nurses. Asking open-ended questions is a good way to obtain information and share information with individuals and family members. Here are some examples of questions to ask:

- What kinds of questions do you have about the care that your family member will receive while you are here?
- Is this your first stay in this care center? If so I would like to tell you some things that will be useful.
- The words nurses and other health professionals use can be confusing; have you heard some terms that you would like to have better explained?
- What can I help you with the most right now?
- I understand this is a difficult time for you and your family. What is your main concern right now?

TABLE 10-4	Nursing Practice Comparison Between Patient-Centered Models and Family-Focused Care	
ELEMENTS OF NURSING PRACTICE	**PATIENT-CENTERED MODEL**	**FAMILY-FOCUSED CARE**
Focus of nursing practice	Outcomes for illness and injury focused on the individual as care recipient	Outcomes for individual and family unit focused on continuous coordinated care supporting health of individual and family.
Relational stance of the nurse	Relationship primarily directed toward ill person	Relationship directed toward individual with an illness and family unit.
Aims of nursing care actions	Therapeutic actions focus on the individual's acute needs with consideration of family involvement as background focus	Therapeutic actions aimed at individual's acute needs with intentional consideration of building a therapeutic individual-nurse-family partnership, including the family, and caring for the family.
Nurses' attitude	Emphasis on delegated tasks and independent nursing actions with ill person	Emphasis on delegated tasks and collaborative nursing actions with ill person and family unit.
	Focus of nursing care is problems linked with ill person	Focus of nursing care is health of ill person and family unit.
	Nurse directs care of ill hospitalized individual	Nurse shares responsibility for care of ill person with family unit and they collaborate in care of ill person and family unit.
	Nurses are expert decision makers who communicate with the family	Nurse involves ill person and family unit in decision making and communication while recognizing expertise of the family.
	Nurse prepares ill person for discharge with limited attention to family support or unique family needs	Nurse prepares ill person and family unit for discharge and considers concerns of both patient and family continuity of care and family health.
Nursing actions	Nurse cares for ill individual with a focus on disease or illness	Nurse cares for ill persons and family unit with a holistic focus on wellness, complication prevention, and self-management.
Significance of family involvement in care	Family viewed as background to the illness recovery	Family central to the care of the ill person and family health.
	Family included at times while focus is on the care of ill person	Family included with mutual goals on healing and wellness.
Acute care setting environment	Medical and health care providers are primary provider of direction for ill person's care	Families, nurse, and others care for the ill person and family unit and provide direction for care.

BOX 10-3
Evidence-Based Practice

Innovation in health care delivery is a national and global concern that needs to respond effectively and efficiently in ways that are not cost prohibitive. In the United Kingdom, they speak of "putting people first," in the United States there is conversation about "patient-centered medical homes," and in New Zealand the slogan is "better, sooner, more convenient." How can nurses be part of a changing workforce and contribute to innovative system reform? Needs for population health care suggest that it might be time to move away from primary, secondary, and tertiary thinking or care that primarily focuses on individuals. Dr. Merian Litchfield has long been interested in the predicament of young families living in complex health circumstances. Her initial studies allowed for home visits with naturally flowing conversations that created formats for future visits. Through these actions, she saw families transformed as they gained abilities to be proactive in their daily lives. She began to understand that family health was a process with partnerships, health factors, dialogue, and meanings.

The next phase of this research used case management. Specialty and family nurses formed a case team. They used caring relationships and fiscal responsibility in mentoring families with complex problems. Using a cooperative approach, the nursing teams used group meetings to discuss families' significant problems. They were addressed through what was called a "healthcare package," or HP. The teams gained an academic understanding about the ways family nursing practice improved health outcomes, increased satisfaction, addressed self-management concerns, and provided more integrated and effective care. In this care form, family nurses were leaders.

A third aspect of this program of research was to identify ways the family nurse role could make sense to various stakeholders including those in health care and community settings. A 3-year project with a rural deprived population used a participatory paradigm or partnership. Family health was viewed as neither fixed nor generalized. Nurses moved to become recognized parts of the community and visited with families whenever their health complexity became an issue. The family HP represented a collaborative interdisciplinary effort orchestrated by the family nurses and tailored to family needs. The essential aspects of this model are that it was people centered, integrated service design and delivery, was cost effective, offered a coherent skill mix and competencies, and encouraged professional nurse development. This care model used family nursing as the key factor in health care design. Family nursing honored the "humanness of the health circumstances" through this model, which was tested in New Zealand.

Source: Litchfield, M. C. (2011). Family nursing: A systematic approach to innovative health care delivery. In E. K. Svaversdottir & H. Jonsdottir (Eds.), *Family nursing in action* (pp. 285–307). Reykjavik, Iceland: University of Iceland Press.

Case Study Phase I: Introduction

To better understand the influence of nursing actions and family responses during an acute illness, an evolving case scenario of the May family will unfold throughout the chapter. The May family case study serves as an example of common situations experienced during an acute illness episode. Aspects of the case are described in each phase and then followed with discussion points that describe family experiences and particular family-focused nursing actions.

John May is 38 years old and is married to Sarah, who is 40 years old. They live in a suburban community of about 50,000 people. John is the chief executive of a large corporation and Sarah is a high school teacher. They have two children, 16-year-old son, Adam,

---

BOX 10-4

Family Tree

Michiko Moriyama, RN, PhD (Japan)

Michiko Moriyama, RN, PhD, is a professor of clinical nursing, at the Institute of Biomedical and Health Science, Division of Nursing Science, at Hiroshima University in Japan. She started the first Family Nursing Study Group at Yamaguchi Prefectural Hospital in Japan, where she developed and refined an innovative model for teaching practicing nurses the skills of family nursing through live demonstration, supervision, case consultation, and mentoring. She published books about the application of the Calgary Family Assessment and Intervention Models, produced five educational videotapes, and published articles in academic journals. Her current research focuses on caring for families with chronic illness and examining health care delivery systems. Dr. Moriyama has been a board member of the Japanese Society of Health Support Science, the Disease Management Association of Japan, Japan Society of Health Care Administration, and the Japanese Association for Research in Family Nursing (JARFN). She chaired the Tenth International Family Nursing Conference, June 24–27, 2011, hosted by JARFN in Kyoto, Japan (<http://www.ifnc2011.org/>). Three months before the conference was scheduled, Japan experienced a devastating earthquake and Dr. Moriyama provided competent, stabilizing leadership to ensure that the international meeting was a successful and well-organized event. The conference theme was "Making Family Visible: From Knowledge Building to Knowledge Translation." In 2005, Dr. Moriyama was awarded an Innovative Contribution to Family Nursing Award by the *Journal of Family Nursing* for her outstanding entrepreneurial and energetic leadership of family nursing in Japan.

---

and 14-year-old daughter Amanda. The family is close knit and spends much time together. Parents attend their children's sports activities and assist them with homework. They have lived in their home for a long while and have neighborhood friends who are like family. Members of the May family regularly see their physician, but no one has ever been hospitalized. Adam was hurt playing basketball a few months back and had stitches in the emergency room. Adam has asthma, which is well controlled with medication and preventive behaviors, and regularly sees his family physician.

John has a history of severe asthma and chronic hypertension; both conditions have been controlled for many years with several medications. John weighs 250 pounds, a large amount for his 5'10" height. He has been trying to lose weight and eat healthier. He smokes when under stress, but is trying to quit. Neither Sarah nor Amanda has health concerns. Their extended family lives in different states and is only seen on holidays or vacations. Joe May, John's father, died at a young age from a severe asthma attack. He was hospitalized with several episodes of respiratory problems before his death. Recently, John has been dealing with an ongoing respiratory problem and was treated with antibiotics by his family physician.

Case Application: Ecological Perspectives

The context of acute illness for the May family has many factors to consider. This family has lived in the same home and community for many years with few health problems. The family functions or interacts in ways members value. They have some health challenges but try to take precautions. John felt great loss when his father died and worries about what his family would do without him. The May parents work, but John's job provides most of the finances for their present lifestyle. His family encourages him to lose weight, quit smoking, and be more active.

Sarah worries about John's asthma and is fearful about his respiratory problems. She knows he takes his medicine and wants him to quit smoking. She worries what life would be like without him. She is nurturing and protective. Adam and Amanda see their father as the family protector. This family has health routines around self-care, safety, family care, mental health behaviors, family member caregiving, and illness care (Denham, 2003).

When nurses *think family*, they get to know families as unique social groups. They identify ways members care for one another. Once we learn about the May family it is important to understand the family unit and individuals. If you were assigned to their care, how might you consider the entire family unit's health? What strengths do you see? Are there areas of concern? What would a family-focused nurse notice and address?

Ideas of race, ethnicity, religion, culture, and education are not discussed in this case, but they might need attention in acute care. An interpreter may be needed if another language were spoken or a person were deaf. If a religion required special dietary practices, the nurse needs to know. Education level may require adjustments in communication, printed and verbal. Questions about work, school, community support, and resources might be appropriate. Learning about the family provides the nurse with a wealth of information to guide nursing actions.

Case Study Phase II: Acute Illness Requires Hospitalization

Sarah leaves for work before John and takes their children to school. Sarah receives a call from her husband, "I think you should come home. I stayed home from work today because I was feeling worse. I am feeling like I can't catch my breath." John is recalling his father's death and is frightened, but does not tell her. Sarah says she will be there soon. She arranges to leave her class with a substitute teacher and rushes home. John has been taking antibiotics for the last 5 days. His temperature is rising and he is having an increased shortness of breath. Sarah phones the physician when she arrives home and describes his condition. Sarah is advised to take him to the emergency department. John says, "Don't worry I will be okay," but he is anxious.

As they drive to the hospital little is said. John is having difficulty breathing and seems restless. When they arrive, Sarah is told to sit in the waiting room while he gets settled and the admission is completed. John is frightened, but says nothing. He waits in the examination area alone and wonders: What is wrong with me? What will happen? Why can't Sarah stay with me? What happened at the business meeting this morning? What will my children do if something happens?

Sarah sits in the waiting area. She thinks: I have information they need about John's medication, his history of hypertension, and his family history of asthma. What is happening? I am afraid. I need to arrange for Adam and Amanda to get to their sporting events this evening. I hope my students are okay with the substitute teacher. Why is no one telling me what is going on? I should be in there with John—why won't they let me?

Sarah feels very anxious. She is thinking about John's father, Joe, and his death at a young age. She questions: How would I manage without John? Should I call Adam and Amanda and tell them what is happening? What will I tell them? Yet, she sits silent as she waits to be invited into the room. After what seems like forever, Sarah asks the receptionist when she can see her husband. Finally, she is ushered to the room. Sarah looks at John with fear, but remains silent. Sarah asks the nurse, "What is wrong with my husband? Do I need to call my children?"

As the nurse leaves the room, she states, "The doctor will be here shortly to speak with you." John says he feels worse. Sarah says little because his shortness of breath seems worse. Sarah waits, holds his hand, and thinks about his condition last week. She wonders if she should have done something. Should she have acted sooner? She thinks about her son's and daughter's hockey games tonight. John said he had an important meeting at work. Why did he not get better with the antibiotics? Why is he so short of breath? Endless questions, fear, and anxiety overcome Sarah and John.

The physician finally arrives. John has been there a long time. Some tests are done and he is admitted to a medical-surgical floor. Sarah is grateful that the nurse asks her to stay in the room as he is settled. The nurse introduces herself, explains the plans of care for the diagnosis of pneumonia, and collects contact information from Sarah.

Case Application: Stress, Uncertainty, and Suffering With Acute Illness Hospitalization

The hospital environment and the hospitalization of a family member bring fear of the unknown, the stress of interrupted family activities, and an uncertain future that create emotional tensions for family members. Families often experience a sense of helplessness during acute care for a member and thoughts of losing the individual make them feel vulnerable. When families understand events they are reassured and less anxious. Nurses who *think family* explain purposes of equipment and treatments and answer questions. The nurse's deliberate actions to answer questions increase the family member's sense of control and gave her a sense of empowerment, the process of developing competence and a capacity to solve problems (Persily & Hildebrandt, 2008). Nurses in acute care settings know some usual treatments for particular diagnoses and anticipate predictable family questions. These nurses describe what will or might happen so that families are prepared and can act proactively.

Providing families with information, familiarizing them with environments, answering questions, and explaining roles and plans create trust and help build relationships (Svavarsdottir et al., 2012; Wright & Leahey, 2013). For instance, it helps to explain that the beeping of the intravenous equipment does not have the same meaning as the oximetry alarm. This helps family members understand that nurses respond to alarms with different levels of urgency. If a procedure is taking longer than expected, the family needs explanations so they don't think a complication has developed. For instance, including Sarah in the care helps establish a trusting therapeutic relationship and allows opportunities for Sarah to share important information she may have that is relevant to John's care. Nurses anticipate a family's concern and work to allay some of the usual family experiences with a hospitalization.

Family and persons with acute needs experience stress, uncertainty, and suffering during hospitalization (Van Horn & Kautz, 2007) and family members are often excluded from the care, creating additional distress (Hardin, 2012; Vandall-Walker & Clark, 2011). Reflect on this case from Sarah's point of view. Sarah had information that could be useful to the health care team. The separation during the admission caused some additional distress. Sarah was excluded. She might think the nurse uncaring and this decreases trust. The nurse missed an opportunity to develop a connecting relationship with this family by not providing introductions. The emergency department nurse failed to acknowledge Sarah's anxiety about John's condition. The unfamiliar setting and uncertainty about what was happening left many unanswered questions. This nurse could provide support by explaining what would happen and orienting them to the environment. Waiting for information with no updates increased Sarah's stress and limited her ability to make plans for her children's needs.

The nurse in the medical-surgical unit appears sensitive to family needs possibly because she is familiar with the evidence that suggests nurses can support families, assist them with stress, reduce uncertainty, and soften suffering experiences (Chesla, 2010; Davidson,

2009; Davidson et al., 2012; Eggenberger & Nelms, 2007; Hardin, 2012; Leahey & Svavarsdottir, 2009; Mitchell, Cahboyer, Burmeister, & Foster, 2009; Svavarsdottir et al., 2012; Wright, 2008). Individual-nurse-family interactions during acute care build connecting relationships and provide critical interventions that influence individual health and family unit (Bell, 2011; Svavarsdottir et al., 2012). Figure 10.1 depicts relationships among family needs, nursing actions, and care outcomes.

Case Study Phase III: Family Assessment and Communication

The nurse on the medical-surgical unit asks if Sarah and John would assist her in collecting information about the family. The nurse gathers the family together to collect family assessment data. The nurse generates a genogram, ecomap, attachment diagram, and circular communication pattern diagram to collect family assessment data about family illnesses, member relationships, and family communication patterns (Wright & Leahey, 2013). The nurse then moves to therapeutic questioning about primary concerns at this time. The nurse uses questions to collect family information: Tell me about the most difficult aspect of this illness for your family? What would be the most useful information for your family at this time? Tell me about concerns for your family? (Wright & Leahey, 2013). After the meeting, the nurse documents key information that is accessible to those caring for John and Sarah. In the acute care setting the nurse may use a brief assessment to document essential data of family structure and interactions and then further assess over time. (Université de Montreal, 2000).

Case Application: Family Assessment, Communication, and Documentation

Sarah is relieved that all contact and pertinent information is available to the health care team. Some units in the acute care setting may document family information on white boards, charts, or the electronic health record so that it is available for other health care providers. With multiple care providers and potential transfer to different care units, it is imperative for nurses not only to conduct family assessments early during admission, but also to document changes that occur. Assessment is an initial step to gain insight about unique family needs. As time goes by, note any other important information about family life, needs, and roles. Information documented about family care decisions is important and can promote coordinated care. Sharing information among the variety of caregivers over a 24-hour period or with the new staff when transfers to different units occur helps family members manage the stress of a transfer.

In the acute care setting family assessment that begins with a family meeting may provide the nurses with the opportunity to develop nurse-family relationships and gather necessary information to provide quality family-focused care. When family meetings are conducted on a consistent basis, the information obtained during the family meeting may provide the nurse and other health care providers with data to understand the family experience, support family coping, and guide family decision making through various acute care transitions (Khalaila, 2014; Nelms & Eggenberger, 2010). Family assessment was previously addressed in Chapter 5 of this textbook and family meetings to facilitate family assessment are explored further in Chapter 14.

Family-focused care can occur in short time periods; even brief moments can offer valued communication (Martinez et al., 2007). *Thinking family* means introducing yourself as new persons arrive in a room. Examples could include: "Hello. My name is Julie Jones and I am caring for John today. Would you share your name and relationship to John? I will check his blood pressure, then we can talk about what is going on." Recognize and commend the family for positive actions. An approach could be "You are doing a good job being here for your husband during this time." Praise can help family endure some strains and reinforces positive actions. Family members need to be encouraged. The 15-minute family interview (Wright & Leahey, 2009) and brief therapeutic conversations have been implemented in a variety of hospital units with positive outcomes (Benzein & Saveman, 2008; Martinez et al., 2007; Svavarsdottir & Jonsdottir, 2011; Svavarsdottir et al., 2012).

Open-ended questions facilitate explanations, facts, thoughts, and emotions. The Calgary Family Intervention Model describes linear intervention questions that inform a nurse about what members perceive as needs (Wright & Leahey, 2013). This model also includes circular questions in which a cycle of dialogue is used to facilitate change. These questions can focus on relationships and beliefs or uncover explanations. A circular question could be aimed at explanation, such as, "What has happened to your family since this illness?" Questions often focus on beliefs about the acute illness such as prognosis and treatment plans, spirituality, control, and family member roles (Wright & Bell, 2009). Nurses can ask: "Who in your family is most affected by this illness? How is this hospitalization affecting your family?"

An individual-nurse-family dialogue is purposeful and directs attention to concerns with the intent of alleviating suffering (Tapp, 2001). Many will readily share their story if given the chance. Saying "Tell me your biggest concern since you have been here" will help a nurse address the family's distress. When families believe they are heard, they will likely see the nurse as genuinely concerned. Every family interaction is an opportunity for the nurse to learn and address unique needs. Box 10.5 describes a practice situation where a nurse addresses the concerns of the individual with the illness and the family member. Use the questions to reflect on nurse-family-individual communication that is needed to ease distress.

Case Study Phase IV: Stress, Uncertainty, and Suffering in Deteriorating Condition

The next morning after Mr. May's admission, the nurse completes the initial assessment and greets John. The nurse observes John is dyspneic, has a heart rate of 120 beats per minute,

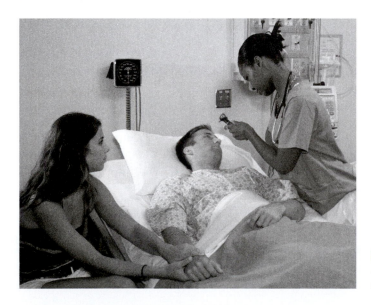

FIGURE 10-1 Relationships among family needs, nursing actions, and care outcomes.

BOX 10-5

Family Circle

Maria Sanchez is a 78-year-old Hispanic woman hospitalized for hematuria of unknown origin. A diagnostic work-up is being completed. This is the first time Maria has been hospitalized, and her adult daughter has been at her bedside since she was admitted. For the last 24 hours Maria has become increasingly withdrawn and has been lying curled up in bed. Tom, Maria's nurse, is thinking that she may be withdrawn because her arthritis is worse as she has not been taking her home remedy medications. Tom has been a nurse for more than 10 years and is viewed as competent by others. Tom notices that Maria has not changed position all morning and her lunch tray has not been touched. Tom figures that Maria is not able to fully comprehend the pain scale, because whenever he has asked her, she has consistently rated her pain at a 2 on the 0-to-10 scale. Maria has orders for ibuprofen and morphine when needed. Tom decides that he should give Maria the morphine to help get the pain under control so she can get up and moving. Maria's daughter, Josephine, insists that her mother not take the morphine. Tom is thinking the daughter will eventually see the benefits of the morphine when her mother is feeling better and able to move around. He wants to give Maria the medicine.

Practice Questions:

- What should Tom do in this situation?
- If the Maria only reports a 2 on the pain scale, should Tom assume that something else is going on?
- Should Tom give the ibuprofen first?
- Is it possible that Maria does not really understand the question or what is meant by a pain scale?

Family-Focused Practice Questions:

- Josephine, does your mother speak and understand English?
- Maria, would it be okay if I had one of our staff interpreters help me better understand what is happening with your pain?
- Maria and Josephine, I would like to get to know you better. Can you tell me more about what happened at home before you came to the hospital?
- Maria and Josephine, I am wondering what questions you would like me to answer.

and a temperature of 102.6°F. Bilateral adventitious sounds in the lungs are heard. The physician is notified and orders received. An electrocardiogram shows ventricular tachycardia. Blood gases are drawn. Results indicate hypoxia, hypercarbia, and acidosis. John's symptoms show increasing respiratory failure. The physician orders John's immediate transfer to the intensive care unit (ICU).

John's nurse contacts Sarah to tell of John's transfer and describes the reasons. Sarah had gone home late last night to be with her children. She had arranged to take the next few days off from work and made transportation arrangements for the children. She had explained to them what was happening and tried to answer questions. They are frightened and wanted to stay home from school and go to the hospital with her. She insisted that they needed to keep up with their classes. Adam and Amanda think they should be at the hospital, but respect their mother's request. Sarah called John's family last night and told them he was hospitalized.

After the phone call from the hospital staff, Sarah immediately left home. She arrives at the ICU as the nurses are completing John's transfer assessment. A nurse asks her to sit in the waiting room until they are finished. Sarah's fear escalates. She thinks: *What are they doing? Why has he been transferred to the ICU? This must mean his condition is really bad. Why didn't that nurse tell me anything?* Sarah lets herself think the painful thought, *does this mean he could die? Maybe I should have let Adam and Amanda stay home today.*

She thinks, *I need to call John's mother. I promised to let her know if things changed.* Sarah had told John's older brother and younger sister about the hospitalization. She called her family as well. She had reassured everyone that things were under control and that they need not come because they live far away and have complicated lives. Now she worries that she did the wrong thing. Sarah did not want to upset them, but what if something is terribly wrong?

Although it seemed like hours, only 10 minutes passed before a nurse greeted Sarah: "My name is Julie. I am the registered nurse caring for your husband today. I will be with you and him. I want to explain what is happening and answer questions. This must be difficult for you." The nurse asks Sarah to come with her to John's room. She explains the equipment being used to monitor John. She points to a chair where Sarah can sit near her husband. The nurse explains that the doctor will be in later this morning and that a specialist has also been called to consult.

The nurse begins to develop a relationship with Sarah. She acknowledges the stress linked with this experience. The nurse explains that the ICU staff is here to provide the care needed. Sarah shares concerns about their children, "What shall I tell our children? Maybe I should notify John's mother and his family." Sarah wonders who else she needs to call. The nurse says, "This must be frightening." The nurse asks other questions about her family and children, inquires about her work, and asks if she has other questions. Together they develop a plan related to communicating with the children and family members. The nurse tells Sarah to ask questions when things are unclear.

Case Application: Stress, Uncertainty, and Suffering With Deteriorating Condition

A change in the condition of an ill family member can magnify the distress and suffering of the family as they face daunting threats of an illness and environment with the unknowns and uncertainty of future outcomes. Nurses who reach out, include, welcome, comfort, and advocate are supportive, but those who fail to acknowledge, exclude, and limit their interactions add to family distress (Nelms & Eggenberger, 2010; Vandall-Walker & Clark, 2011). Family stress and uncertainty can be diminished through early and ongoing communication, supportive interactions, and collaborative partnerships (McMillan & Small, 2007). Nurses play crucial roles in helping a family endure difficult acute experiences and maintain a healthy family (Appleyard et al. 2000; Van Horn & Kautz, 2007).

Case Study Phase V: Family Presence During a Serious Illness

In the next 36 hours, John's condition continues to deteriorate. Sarah has notified their extended family and suggested that they should come. Sarah's mother has arrived and is staying at their home to help care for the children. John's older brother is bringing his mother and they will arrive soon. John's younger sister, a single parent, has decided she cannot leave her young children or job. This sister likes to be in charge and control things. She calls the ICU desk often to check on John's condition and gets angry when they refuse to give information. She texts Sarah continually and wants to know what is happening. Sarah is guarded, watchful, and trying to protect John. Sarah's suffering is evident to the ICU nursing staff. Sarah calls her mother to ask if she would take the car, pick up Adam and Amanda from school, and drive them to the hospital.

Adam and Amanda were scared when their grandmother arrived at school. Adam asked many questions on the ride to the hospital. Amanda sat silently and looked out the window. The silence was heavy. When they arrive, John's nurse takes a few minutes to speak with them before they go to his room. They barely hear what she says because of their anxiety. Finally, the children are allowed to see their father, but he barely acknowledges their presence. Adam and Amanda spend about 5 minutes in the ICU room with their father and mother. The nurse explains some things about what is happening. Tears are streaming down Sarah's cheeks. Adam is brave and asks, "Will my father be okay?' The nurse responds, "We are doing everything we can to help him. He needs to rest and give things time to work." The nurse asks them if they have questions and tries to answer simply. She explains equipment to the children and helps them speak with their father. They return to the waiting area to sit with their grandmother and wait.

Sarah says, "I need to stay strong for them. They need me." Sarah says to the nurses, "He seems to be getting worse, no matter what you do. I don't know how much more we can take. I am not sure what to say when the children ask me if he will die." John's nurse realizes that Sarah is struggling with fears and asking difficult questions without answers. The nurse listens intently and tries to answer questions truthfully. The nurse uses caring and clinical judgments to communicate with Sarah.

John's family and Sarah's siblings arrive at the hospital and gather in the waiting room. Different family members are at John's bedside around the clock. John's brother is troubled by his sister as she is texting him with questions. John's mother is overheard saying, "We need to transfer him to a different hospital because they are not doing enough here." John's older brother states, "John would not want all of these machines." The extended family is large and takes up much of the space in the waiting area. Tensions are rising and some members seem at odds with others. More than 24 hours pass.

Some nurses welcome the family's vigilance but others are troubled by their presence. Nurses' statements include, "John's family is always here. I wonder how we can offer more support. I am going to ask them to join me for a family conference to discuss what is happening." One nurse says, "John's family just needs to go home and let us take care of him. They always want to be in the room when we have things to do. Go home, get some rest, and leave the caregiving to us." Nurses who are not family focused often perceive the family as a barrier to care, rather than the partner.

John's condition deteriorates to respiratory failure; the rapid response team is called, and eventually an intubation is required. One nurse tries to move Sarah and one of her siblings out of the ICU and into the waiting room despite their protests. Sarah states, "We must be here! We want John to know we are here!" A nurse responsible for the family during the procedure says, "I understand. You should be here if you think that is important." She shows them a place to stand near the bedside and explains what is occurring as cardiopulmonary resuscitation begins.

John's children have been talking with their grandmother in the waiting room. They make their way back into the ICU while the response team is in action. Amanda begins to cry and Adam stands at the doorway silently. One nurse asks the children to leave. Another nurse, the one that had spoken with them earlier, puts her arm around Amanda and talks to them. She explains what is happening. This nurse helps Sarah comfort her children and make a decision about their presence and observation of what is happening.

Case Application: Family Presence During Invasive Procedures

Families want to be vigilant and support their ill member, especially in the acute care setting (Dudley & Carr, 2004; Vandall-Walker & Clark, 2011). Being together as a family often decreases distress of the family and supports the ill member of the family. Nurses who *think family* support the family's presence during invasive intubation procedure and explain what they observe. A family-focused care setting has policies to support family presence that are beneficial to families (Abraham & Moretz, 2012; Doolin, Quinn, Bryant, Lyons, & Kleinpell, 2011). Current research indicates that most families want to be present during treatments, invasive procedures, and cardiopulmonary resuscitation (CPR) (Davidson et al., 2007). Box 10.6 provides selected evidence related to family presence. Additional information about the importance of family presence is provided in Chapter 9.

Many family members want the option to stay with their member during resuscitation efforts, and current practice has turned to family inclusion (American Association of Critical Care Nurses, 2010; Emergency Nurses Association, 2009, 2010). Family members present during cardiopulmonary resuscitation report that they would do so again because it helps remove doubts and eases distress (American Association of Critical Care Nurses,

---

BOX 10-6

Perceived Benefits and Barriers of Family Presence

Perceived Benefits of Family Presence From the Family Perspective

- Reduces fear and anxiety among family members.
- Dispels dread of the unknown and guilt with not being present at the bedside.
- Enhances feelings of usefulness (e.g., providing information to health care team, offering support and comfort to patient).
- Supports the family feelings of needing to protect and being connected to their family member.
- Fosters the appreciation for the efforts of the health care team to ensure "everything possible" is being done and allays some doubts.
- Allows opportunity to speak with patient and possibly say thoughts and good-byes.

Perceived Barriers to Family Presence From Health Care Providers' Perspective

- Fears that distraught family members may distract the staff from providing care needed by the ill patient.
- Concerns that family members' distress would hamper their performance and increase own emotional response.
- Increased risk of litigation by family members.
- Lack of space in the room and lack of staff to provide support for family members.
- Rights of confidentiality and privacy of patient violated.
- Experience may be too traumatic for family and have lasting ill effects.

Perceived Benefits of Family Presence From Health Care Providers' Perspective

- Reminds staff to care for a patient with privacy, dignity, and respect.
- Prompts staff to recall the patient is a person who is a member of a family.
- Encourages professional behavior and holistic care to a patient during a crisis situation.
- Allows a family member to recognize staff's efforts to care for the patient and advocate for the patient.
- Offers the nurse an opportunity to educate the family, support the family, and reaffirm the role of the family as a support network.

Source: Adapted from American Association of Critical Care Nurses (2010). AACN Practice Alert: Family presence during resuscitation and invasive procedures. Retrieved May 17, 2012 from http://www.aacn.org/WD/Practice/Docs/PracticeAlerts/Family%20Presence%2004-2010%20final.pdf; Duran, C. R., Oman, K. S., Abel, J. J., Koziel, V. M., & Szymanski, D. (2007). Attitudes toward and beliefs about family presence: A survey of healthcare providers, patients' families, and patients. *American Journal of Critical Care, 16*(3), 270–282; Halm, M. (2005). Family presence during resuscitation: A critical review of the literature. *American Journal of Critical Care, 14*(6), 494–512.

2010; Duran, Oman, Jordan, Koziel, & Szymanski, 2007; Meyers, Eichhorn, Guzzetta, Clark, & Taliaferro, 2000). Encouraging family presence can increase family satisfaction with the health care system with this practice (American Association of Critical Care Nurses, 2011; Davidson et al., 2007; Roberti & Fitzpatrick, 2010). Families and health professionals report the benefit of family presence. Yet some professionals continue to be concerned that family presence is too anxiety-provoking for families; research has not supported these perceptions (Duran et al., 2007; Emergency Nurses Association, 2010; Halm, 2005). Research suggests that acute care policies often do not support the evidence (American Association of Critical Care Nurses, 2011; Emergency Nurses Association, 2009). A nurse who *thinks family* understands practice guidelines related to family member presence and supports family visitation and presence and works to develop policies that advocate for families (American Association of Critical Care Nurses, 2011; Davidson et al., 2007; Emergency Nurses Association, 2009).

Research findings suggest children and families need to be together during stress and crises, and recommendations suggest that nurses should include them in acute care of adults (Clarke & Harrison, 2001; Kean, 2010). Helping parents decide what information to share and including them during acute care is important (Kean, 2010; Knutsson, Samuelsson, Hellstrom, & Berghbom, 2008). Yet, resources for children visiting adults during acute care and critical illness are limited. Nurses who *think family* advocate for children and discuss the best ways to include them in care. A family nurse prepares a child for the acute setting, communicates in a developmentally appropriate way, and provides a child-friendly environment.

Case Study Phase VI: Information Exchange and Family Conflicts

John's condition remains unstable. The family has difficulties communicating about future plans. Tension builds as members share their beliefs. Sarah thinks she understands her husband's wishes about quality of life and use of extraordinary measures. She has spoken with the physician and has a grasp of the current state of John's condition and the potential outcomes. John's brother says, "He said he never wanted to live on machines." With further discussion the conflict increases and soon the family sits in separate parts of the waiting room in silence. Sarah comments to the nurse, "We have always been a strong family that could talk about everything. I just don't understand what has happened to us. We seem to be in such different places."

The nurse decides to work toward arranging a family meeting in which the family can explore their thinking and move toward decisions. She wants to encourage understanding, identify strengths to commend, and find ways to build consensus. The nurse says to Sarah, "A family meeting can help share thinking and beliefs. It is a way to provide additional information to the whole family and offer support to move forward. I would be there to help your family. Would this be useful for you and your family at this time?"

Case Application: Family Decision Making

Numerous decisions need to be made during an illness and many require family involvement. Decision making may focus on issues related to treatment choices; deciding what, where, and when to obtain health services; and decisions about withdrawal of life support and organ donation (Jacobowski, Girard, Mulder, & Wesley, 2010). Even when individuals discuss preferences or provide written documentation about their choices, they often need support and guidance to navigate the distresses associated with the decision (Luce & White, 2007;

Wiegand, 2008). Nurses assist by providing complex information in simple terms, using drawings to explain and clarifying goals. Decision points occur throughout an illness with many opportunities for nurses to guide and partner with family members (Bakitas, Kryworuchko, Matlock, & Volandes, 2011; McBride Robichaux & Clark, 2006) (Box 10.7).

Nurses who *think family* can assist at various decision points by providing information and clarifying possible outcomes of a selected path, or they can discuss what could occur if no treatment is obtained. Yet, beliefs of family members related to decisions and how to care for their ill family member may differ. Usual communication processes may be disrupted and open expression of emotions in caring ways may be challenging for some family members. Nurses are often present during these difficult times and family-focused nurses remain with the family to help communication continue and be sure all voices are heard (Warnock et al., 2010). Best practice models include informed choices, shared decision making, support for decisions, and dialogue (Bakitas et al., 2011).

Yet, in the acute care setting some myths and misunderstandings about the Health Insurance Portability and Accountability Act (HIPAA) exist and hamper nurse-family communication. In 1996, HIPAA regulations were implemented to protect personal health information, ensure that individuals had access to health insurance, and streamline some administration processes. HIPAA was never intended to dictate policies that hamper family assessment, prevent family inclusion, or withhold necessary information from family members. Individuals can give permission for information sharing. If the patient is incapacitated, a health care provider may share information with family, friends, or others as long as professional judgment is used to determine what is in the best interest of the person (Office of Civil Rights, Department of Health and Human Services, 2012).

Case Study Phase VII: Transfers in Acute Care Settings and Discharge to Home

After several days in the ICU, John is finally able to breathe on this own. The weaning process is frightening, but the nurse provides continuous information, shares specific plans,

---

BOX 10-7

Families' Needs Related to Decision Making in Acute Care

Decision making can be a challenging task during an inpatient admission for an acute care concern. Here are some features of nursing care that family members would likely find helpful when a member has an acute condition needing attention.

- Families need a nurse who develops trusted relationships with them so they can partner in decision making.
- Families want a nurse who guides them in supporting the family member with an illness and helping them make decisions about their role.
- Families value a nurse advocating for them throughout hospitalization.
- Families need a nurse to provide information that is easy to understand on a consistent basis.
- Families want a nurse who helps them balance the needs of multiple family members.
- Families need health care providers to give them time to make decisions.
- Families appreciate guidance at various decision points.
- Families need a nurse who helps them plan for transitions.
- Families value guidance in creating the opportunities for shared decision making.

and interprets information. The nurse tells Sarah and John, "Our plans are to adjust the settings on the machine and watch how the changes are tolerated. I will stay close to watch the machinery and John. Let me know if you question anything you see or hear." The nurse continually reassures them that John is improving. She gives specific information and explains steps in the progression of care. The nurse supports Sarah's decision to remain vigilant and stay near her husband. Each time John is assessed, the nurse shares the meaning of what is found with Sarah. When Amanda and Adam visit again with Sarah's mother, the nurse speaks to them, answers questions, and explains in words they understand.

With time, John is transferred back to the medical floor. He expresses his sense of relief with improvement, "I am so glad to be better, maybe I can get some sleep." Sarah is anxious about the transfer. She thinks, Will these nurses watch John closely? I trusted those nurses in the ICU; they were so helpful. Now I have to get acquainted with these new nurses. They do not seem as visible as those in ICU. No one has spoken to me yet and the transfer happened an hour ago.

The nurses on the medical floor are prepared for Sarah's anxiety with the transfer. In a short time, the nurse introduces herself and explains plans. She says, "I am the nurse caring for John. Sometimes family members worry what will happen when their loved one moves out of the ICU into a unit like this. What questions do you have that I can answer right now?" The nurse reassures Sarah, "I plan to keep my eyes on John, check his progress often, and keep you informed. Let me be certain we have your family contact information. If it is okay, I would like to briefly review the genogram we have in John's records to be sure that I have a good understanding of your family."

As days go by, John's condition continues to improve and he is soon ready for discharge. Before that time, nurses have spent time with John and Sarah reviewing purposes of medications and side effects. They have explained about asthma risks and spoken about prevention. They spoke about home environments and irritants that trigger asthma. Tobacco cessation was explained and information about local resources provided. Also, the importance of balancing work, family roles, and health was discussed. The concerns of the children have been explored.

Sarah says, "We are happy to go home. Nurses have been so good about teaching us, answering questions, and taking care of our needs." John's home plan calls for several days of rest and then work from home for 2 weeks before returning to his office. Sarah says, "I am glad we have clear instructions written so we understand. We know what to do at home." The nurse talks with Sarah about balancing personal care needs with those of the family. Sarah replies, "We will be so glad to have John home. We know what to watch for and how to create some new routines for healthier lives."

Case Application: Preparing for Transfers Within and Discharge From Acute Care Setting

Transfer and discharge planning occur throughout an acute care stay. As transfers between units occur, the family nurse addresses the stress that can occur with transfers and need for coordinated care. Communication with health care providers about family needs and past experiences is important. In the May family, nurses collaborated with others to ensure that discussions and issues were not overlooked. As the discharge was planned, needs of the entire family were considered. As Sarah drove John home, they and the children discussed their experience and their feelings of relief that John was returning to health as well as some of their fears and concerns. The nurse had prepared them for stress and uncertainty of returning to roles and responsibilities. The May family also discussed the ways they had been treated during their acute care experiences.

Delivery of Family-Focused Care: Environmental Factors in Acute Care Setting

Economic and social policies influence ways nursing care is delivered. The public is more selective about where to receive care, but health insurance plans, preferred providers, and cost of co-payments drive some decisions. People expect high-quality nursing care (Box 10.8). Health care consumers make decisions based on published outcomes, satisfaction scores, and provider rankings. The Hospital Consumer Assessment of Healthcare Providers and Systems (HCAHPS) Survey is one such publication. This survey is mandated by the Centers for Medicare and Medicaid Services (CMS) and hospital reimbursement is linked to the HCAHPS scores (CMS.gov). Publicly reported data guides individuals concerning where to seek care.

Quality measures are important ways to evaluate nursing actions. The quality of nurse-patient communication and satisfaction with health care experiences are areas measured by acute care institutions. The acute care environment is a complex system in which family care can thrive or barriers can prevent care delivery (Table 10.5). Take time to consider environmental factors that can be viewed as supportive and barriers to individuals with an acute illness and their families.

Moving Family-Focused Care in Acute Care Settings Forward

Individual-nurse-family collaborations are used to manage the barriers and obstacles that prevent safe quality care. Collaborations are grounded in trusting relationships that acknowledge, affirm, and support family units during acute care. Nurses who *think family* work with supervisors and administrators to identify best ways to satisfy family needs, lead family meetings, and conduct bedside reports, family rounding, and family interventions. Several current initiatives in nursing practice aim to move family care forward.

BOX 10-8

Elements of a Hospitalization That Improve Family Care

The Institute for Healthcare Improvement (2011) recently published a White Paper compiling evidence to advance recommendations that are most apt to improve family experiences during hospitalization and increase patient response scores to the Hospital Consumer Assessment of Healthcare Providers and Systems (HCAHPS) survey question related to willingness to recommend the hospital to others. These recommendations are identified here:

- Leadership with a focus on the family
- Engagement of staff and providers in the values of family-focused care
- Respectful partnerships with patients and family members
- Access to care without long and unreasonable delay
- Coordinated evidence-based care shared by all team members including patient and family

Source: Adapted from Balik, B., Conway, J., Zipperer, L., & Watson, J. (2011). *Achieving an exceptional patient and family experience of inpatient hospital care.* IHI Innovation Series White Paper. Cambridge, MA: Institute for Healthcare Improvement. Retrieved from www.IHI.org

TABLE 10-5	*Supportive Environmental Factors and Barriers to Family-Focused Care*

ENVIRONMENTAL FACTORS TO SUPPORT FAMILY-FOCUSED CARE	ENVIRONMENTAL BARRIERS TO FAMILY-FOCUSED CARE
Leadership, organization, and culture are focused on family care that is publicly verifiable and rewarded. Family is included in measurement, learning, and improvement in practice with family feedback as a routine practice.	Nurses with heavy workloads and high stress levels may convey their stress and create inabilities to partner with families (Åstedt-Kurki, Paavilainen, Tammentie, & Paunonen-Ilmonen, 2001). Families are often largely unheard and unrecognized.
Family members are treated as partners in care and the information they offer is perceived as useful and important for planning safe and quality care.	Family members are viewed as visitors.
Staff is committed to the shared values of family-focused care. Staff experiences in working with families increase their personal satisfaction levels.	Staff is not educated or prepared to provide or value family-focused care. Staff members lack work satisfaction with families.
Teamwork is essential with staff being recruited for the values they display regarding the mission of family-focused care.	Cooperation and equality among team members are inconsistent related to family care.
All care situations are anchored in respectful partnerships with family members. Care is based on a customized and interdisciplinary care plan with family members consistently educated.	Limited appreciation or understanding of family experience with a hospitalization. Limited documentation of family involvement in the electronic health record or other clinical documentation systems used.
Physical environment promotes healing (9 p.m. lights are dimmed, door to patient room is closed, phones and pagers are on vibrate, use of ear plugs, portable white noise machines for room, face masks, blinds block out light). Manage noise in environment as much as possible. However, family's presence is supported. Physical environment meets the nutritional, sleep, exercise, and routine needs of family members.	The architectural hospital design is not conducive to family participation in care; stress of the noise or lighting (i.e., window blinds not closed, overhead lights on, monitoring equipment screens face patient, door remains open to hallway).
Policies support engagement by family members (i.e., family visiting policies enable family to spend the night in comfort and include children as visitors).	Visiting policies are strictly adhered to and family members experience discomfort when they are "outside the policy" (e.g., staying after hours).
Continual information exchange with the family that is understandable and targeted toward educational level of family members. Honest and open approach to providing information that is truthful. Ongoing and consistent family meetings to dialogue, explore, and address concerns.	Information is not tailored to the health literacy needs of family members and is inconsistently provided by clinicians. Limited information exchanges and family meetings only during times of crisis.
Family members are able to retain family relationships and remain close to family members by participating in care routines comfortable for them and the hospitalized individual.	Staff members fail to identify what parts of patient care family members feel comfortable providing, or wish to provide, and what parts they prefer the staff to complete.

Continued

TABLE 10-5	*Supportive Environmental Factors and Barriers to Family-Focused Care—cont'd*

ENVIRONMENTAL FACTORS TO SUPPORT FAMILY-FOCUSED CARE	ENVIRONMENTAL BARRIERS TO FAMILY-FOCUSED CARE
Family members share their priorities and usual routines to assist the health care team in focusing on the family's perceptions of priorities of care rather than only those of the health care team.	Nurses disregard family routines, such as when someone likes to take a shower or if a family member always cares for someone at home.
Family members need to be comfortable in the hospital environment to reduce distress and suffering (e.g., massage, music, aromatherapy, art therapy, pet therapy, gardens and soothing sound of water, nutritional support).	Hospital policy does not allow for complementary therapy services nor does it foster innovative and cost-effective approaches to supporting family comfort and usual household routines while in the hospital.
Questions by family members are encouraged and answered regularly with information given in clear language or with use of drawing pictures to illustrate.	Family questions go unanswered unless family clearly seeks information.
Family decisions are honored and families participate in decision making to the level they feel comfortable.	Reluctance of health care providers to engage families in decision making.
Family members feel cared for, respected, welcome, and know that help will be given when it is needed.	Family members feel anxious because they feel largely ignored.
Family advisory councils actively participate with hospital administrators and nursing staff to improve family care experiences.	Hospital staff and nurses make decisions without consideration of the family experience during hospitalization in the acute care settings.
Innovative programs are used to educate staff about how to deliver family-focused care.	Programs assume that nurses already know about family care and fail to offer continuing education in these areas.
Peer recognition programs that honor providers who embrace the values of family-focused care (selected by peers and by family members in follow-up surveys).	No recognition is given to those who address family care needs.
The nursing team uses hourly rounding to ensure that needs for each patient and family are met.	Hourly rounding is conducted by staff without training about ways to interact with family members.
Family care rounding is regularly conducted by physicians/interdisciplinary team and nurses at prescheduled times so family members can be included in decision making about care management.	Family care or rounding policies are not in place and family members are not included in care management or decision-making activities.
Communication mnemonics used for all staff to deliver consistent messages and be proactive in communication approaches (e.g., AIDET: acknowledge, introduce, duration, explain, and thank).	Communication format not formalized within the setting, leaving opportunity for inadequate and inconsistent messages.
Regular and consistent family meetings bring family members together with nursing staff to discuss experiences.	Family information needs are not clearly met through structured communication programs and family needs are inconsistently addressed during hospitalization.

Family Policies and Visitation

Policies about family visitation in acute care settings have been changing in recent years. Some hospitals are viewing families as a respected part of the health care team, rather than merely seeing them as visitors (Leape et al., 2009). This changed perspective is based on research findings that indicate that when families' partnership in care management of acute illness is improved, continuity of care is enhanced, and hospital readmissions are reduced (Bauer et al., 2009). These mutually important outcomes resulted in improved satisfaction and reduced medical errors (Wiggins, 2008). Unrestricted family visitation increases patient comfort and satisfaction for the hospitalized person, and family members report increased satisfaction, decreased anxiety and uncertainty, improved communication, and better patient/family teaching (American Association of Critical Care Nurses, 2011; Vandall-Walker & Clark, 2011).

The Institute for Patient- and Family-Centered Care has formulated a set of guidelines to change hospital visiting policies and practices. The core concepts of these guidelines are respect and dignity, information sharing, participation, and collaboration (Johnson et al., 2008). However, nurses continue to report inconsistent visitation policies, and hospital units continue to restrict the patient's access to designated support persons during acute care experiences, especially serious ones (American Association of Critical Care Nurses, 2010; Davidson et al., 2007; Vandall-Walker & Clark, 2011). Research evidence supports the idea that family and other care partners should be allowed to visit 24 hours a day, even during serious illness.

Family Presence During Invasive Procedures and Cardiopulmonary Resuscitation

Nurses identify needs for policies, procedures, and educational programs that support family-focused care during crisis events such as cardiopulmonary resuscitation and invasive procedures (Halm, 2005). Although many nursing organizations have taken bold moves to support family presence, more actions are still needed to be sure practice is based on evidence. In 1993, the Emergency Nurses Association (ENA) adopted a resolution to support family presence during invasive procedures and resuscitation. In 1994, their first position statement was completed and a resource was developed to address family presence (ENA, 2009, 2010). Ideas about family presence have also been included in the American Heart Association (2005) guidelines for cardiopulmonary resuscitation. In 2010, the American Association of Critical Care Nurses (2010, 2011) published a practice alert that identifies the increasing evidence for the practice of family presence during resuscitation and invasive procedures. The vision of the National Hospice and Palliative Care Organization (2008) clearly focuses on including families and a position statement on palliative care is also directed toward standards of practice that meet individual and family needs.

Family Participation in Rounds and Change of Shift

Family participation in interdisciplinary rounds and bedside change-of-shift reports has gained momentum in recent years. Communication with families during pediatric and end-of-life care is a common nursing practice (Committee on Hospital Care, 2003). However, the routine incorporation of families into regular rounds and change-of-shift reports on all hospital units is only beginning. Nurses need education and practice sessions to make family participation in rounds and shift reports effective and feasible (Anderson & Mangino, 2006; Santiago, Lazar, Depeng, & Burns, 2014). When rounds with families are available, it is useful to inform families about them in verbal and written formats. Some early findings suggest bedside rounds increase satisfaction with communication (Anderson & Mangino, 2006; Rappaport, Ketterer, Nilforoshan, & Sharif, 2012). Family participation offers times for bidirectional communication and clarification of information (Davidson et al., 2007; Rappaport et al., 2012). More research is needed to fully understand the benefits of family participation in rounds in different areas of acute care (Jacobowski et al., 2010) and the most meaningful ways to include family in rounds. Family rounds can be implemented through various processes such as those suggested in Box 10.9.

Family Support Groups

In 2001, the Committee on Early Childhood, Adoption, and Dependent Care of the American Academy of Pediatrics clearly highlighted the need for family support programs. Recommendations included needs to consider family significance, recognize the family as part of the community, and enhance their strengths. Family support sessions in adult acute care settings have now expanded to areas such as palliative care (Henriksson, Benzein, Ternestedt, & Andershed, 2011), family caregivers in mental health (Chien, Chan, Morrissey, & Thompson, 2005), and chronic illness (Munn-Giddings & McVicar, 2006) where research has provided positive results. Support groups can improve dissemination of clear information, offer support, reduce burdens, and increase abilities to manage stress and have the potential to increase communication between health care providers and family members, reduce uncertainty and family concerns, and help family

---

BOX 10-9

Processes to Include in Family Rounds

The following items are ideas to consider when planning to include family rounds in daily nursing practice:

- Staff members are provided with written handouts and educational practice sessions prior to implementation of family rounds.
- Family rounds structure includes interdisciplinary team at the bedside with a number of family members.
- Family rounds occur daily.
- Nurse explains the family rounds to the family in verbal and written formats.
- Nurse helps to bring the family to the bedside.
- Interpreters are available when needed.
- Core physicians and providers provide a summary of the family member's care needs for the family using understandable language.
- Nurse provides pertinent information to the family and health care team.
- Family has the opportunity to ask questions.
- Follow-up family meetings are offered to provide additional support, answer additional questions, and encourage communication among family members.

_____

Source: Adapted from Anderson, C. D., & Mangino, R. R. (2006). Nurse shift report: Who says you can't talk in front of the patient? *Nursing Administration Quarterly, 30*(2), 112–122; Jacobowski, N. L., Girard, T. D., Mulder, J. A., & Wesley, E. (2010). Communication in critical care: Family rounds in the intensive care unit. *American Journal of Critical Care, 19*(5), 421–430; Rappaport, D. I., Ketterer, T. A., Nilforoshan, V., & Sharif, I. (2012). Family-centered rounds: Views of families, nurses, trainees, and attending physicians. *Clinical Pediatrics, 51*(3), 260–266.

members know that health professionals understand (Sabo et al., 1989; Sacco et al., 2009). Technology can also facilitate online education and support systems for families (Xu et al., 2014). Family satisfaction may increase with regular involvement in support groups during and following an acute care experience. Nurses who *think family* can participate with their employing agencies to determine what support groups are most useful.

Family Advisory Councils

Family advisory councils being implemented in a variety of organizations to strengthen family care may help solidify family-focused care in the acute care setting (Halm, Sabo, & Rudiger, 2006). These councils engage acute care staff in family partnerships and provide a mechanism to improve care processes that help nurses better understand family needs. Inviting families to be family faculty is another useful tactic. Family members have developed presentations for acute care staff on such topics as improving communication, healing partnerships, and family experiences. Family narratives have been shown to influence care (Children's Hospital of Philadelphia, 2013).

Family-Nurse Meetings

Bringing families together as a group to talk about their experiences, beliefs, and thinking has been a successful strategy that provides insight and comfort (Cypress, 2011; Robinson & Wright, 1995). Family meetings have potential to decrease uncertainty and suffering (Nelms & Eggenberger, 2010), increase satisfaction (Alvarez & Kirby, 2006), and facilitate decision making (Wingate & Wiegand, 2008). Families report that these meetings help them better understand the struggles of other family members and establish trusting relationships critical to quality care (Appleyard et al., 2000; Lynn-McHale & Deatrick, 2000; Nelms & Eggenberger, 2010). Inviting conversation during family meetings acknowledges families' needs and offers intentional therapeutic conversation (Wright & Leahey, 2013). Family meetings can help identify specific concerns, manage stress, and gain understandings. Conducting family meetings at regularly scheduled times, rather than only during crisis decision points, has potential to offer an intervention that families and providers value (Hannon, O'Reilly, Bennett, Breen, & Lawlor, 2012).

Family Documentation with Electronic Records

Implementation of the electronic health record (EHR) has provided the opportunity for point-of-care information and the ability to access information promptly. Inclusion of family information is often an "add-on" to the patient record and it is only included if the nurse providing care views it as important. When assessment of family is not addressed in the standardized flow sheet generated by the EHR, it is unlikely that the nurse will document the family as part of the patient's care system, rendering the family invisible. The EHR has had great benefit for health care institutions' need to collect data and record outcomes. On the other side, its implementation has been shown to have limited usefulness in improving acute care nurses' clinical judgment or improving team communication (Kelley, Brandon, & Docherty, 2011).

The EHR is a tool that will remain, so it is essential that nurses incorporate family information in the chart. Investigators suggest that the EHR does not make the individual-family-nurse relationship visible or promote provider communication about those issues that matter the most to families, such as their involvement in care (de Ruiter, 2007, 2011).

Regardless, if the standardized forms do not address the family, nurses can still describe family-related care in narrative notes or documentation. When documentation includes family assessment data and aspects of the family and illness experience, then it is most likely that the concerns of a family will be addressed.

Strategies to ensure that care remains family focused include the use of family stories, short narratives in which family experience is shared. For example, a family may provide daily updates, concerns, or questions. A social narrative to share their story with care providers could be useful. This intervention could capture family preferences, experiences, and needs. Family information that is part of a record could be viewed by those providing care and used to facilitate decision making and planning care strategies.

A Family-Focused Environment

The design and aesthetics of acute care hospitals in the United States include innovative colors, attractive lighting, prerecorded music, waterfalls, and healing gardens for viewing or walking. Such features have been demonstrated to positively affect patient outcomes (Center for Health Design, 2012; Ulrich et al., 2008). Innovative nurse-designed hospital work environments that improve efficiency and safety and add features that mitigate stress for patients and families are becoming more commonplace (Kreitzer & Zborowsky, 2009). Often these settings include private, single-bed hospital rooms with space for family members. Private rooms are more conducive to family involvement in patient care. Education centers, chapels, meditation areas, spaces for family members to meet and remain overnight, laundry areas, small kitchenettes, and in-room dining could be considerations. Furniture arrangements in waiting areas can facilitate privacy and socializing for family groups. Efforts to address hospital designs should consider needs of families because health care structures and environments can affect quality of care, satisfaction, and efficacy (Center for Health Design, 2012; Trochelman et al., 2012).

Chapter Summary

Whether it is a hospitalized child, adult, or older adult, each family presents with needs, strengths, and challenges that require attention and care during a distressing experience that affects the entire family. The stress and uncertainty of illness influence the entire family. Communication, roles, and the disruption of usual routines add to the distress of acute illness. Even if a family is not physically present, family members are important to the individual's health care outcomes. Nurses have pivotal roles in communicating with and comforting family, advocating for decision-making processes, and reducing family suffering in acute illness. Despite the complex and hurried demands of acute care settings, family nurses connect with, advocate for, and respect all; they individualize care and partner with the family so they can cope with demands and support their ill family member. Nurses who *think family* intentionally practice with a focus on the individual with the illness and their family.

REFERENCES

Abate, F. R. (Ed.) (2002). *Oxford American dictionary of current English*. New York: Oxford University Press.

Abraham, M., & Moretz, J. G. (2012). Implementing patient- and family-centered care: Part 2— Understanding the challenges. *Pediatric Nursing, 38*(1), 44–47.

Alvarez, G. F., & Kirby, A. S. (2006). The perspective of families of the critically ill patient: Their needs. Current Opinion in Critical Care, 12, 614–618.

American Academy of Pediatrics, Committee on Hospital Care. (2003). Family-centered care and the pediatrician's role. Pediatrics, 112(3), 691–696.

American Association of Critical Care Nurses. (2010). AACN Practice Alert: Family presence during resuscitation and invasive procedures. Retrieved May 17, 2012 from http://www.aacn.org/WD/Practice/Docs/PracticeAlerts/Family%20Presence%2004-2010%20final.pdf

American Association of Critical Care Nurses. (2011). AACN Practice Alert: Family visitation in the adult ICU. Retrieved May 16, 2012 from http://www.aacn.org/WD/practice/docs/practicealerts/family-visitation-adult-icu-practicealert.pdf

American Heart Association. (2005). 2005 American Heart Association Guidelines for Cardiopulmonary Resuscitation and Emergency Cardiovascular Care. Circulation, 112, IV1–203.

Anderson, C. D., & Mangino, R. R. (2006). Nurse shift report: Who says you can't talk in front of the patient? Nursing Administration Quarterly, 30(2), 112–122.

Appleyard, M. E., Gavaghan, S. R., Gonzalez, C., Ananian, L., Tyrell, R., & Carroll, D. L. (2000). Nurse-coached intervention for the families of patients in critical care unit. Critical Care Nurse, 20(3), 40–48.

Åstedt-Kurki, P., Paavilainen, E., Tammentie, T., & Paunonen-Ilmonen, M. (2001). Interaction between adult patients' family members and nursing staff on a hospital ward. Scandinavian Journal of Caring Science, 15(2), 142–150.

Azoulay, E., Pochard, F., Chevret, S., Arich, C., Brivet, F., Brun, F. , . . . French Famirea Group. (2003). Family participation on care to the critically ill: Opinions of families and staff. Intensive Care Medicine, 29(9), 1498–1504.

Bacon, F. (1996). In B. Vickers (Ed.), Francis Bacon: The major works. Oxford, England: Oxford University Press.

Bakitas, M., Kryworuchko, J., Matlock, D., & Volandes, A. E. (2011). Palliative medicine and decision science: The critical need for shared agenda to foster informed patient choice in serious illnesss. Journal of Palliative Medicine, 14(10), 1110–1116.

Balik, B., Conway, J., Zipperer, L., & Watson, J. (2011). Achieving an exceptional patient and family experience of inpatient hospital care. IHI innovation series white paper. Cambridge, MA: Institute for Healthcare Improvement. Retrieved from www.IHI.org

Bauer, M., Fitzgerald, L, Haesler, E., & Manfrin, M. (2009). Hospital discharge planning for frail older people and their family. Are we delivering best practice? A review of the evidence. Journal of Clinical Nursing, 18, 2539–2546.

Bell, J. (2011). Relationships: The heart of the matter in family nursing. Journal of Family Nursing, 17(1), 3–10.

Benzein, E. G., & Saveman, B. I. (2008). Health-promoting conversations about hope and suffering with couples in palliative care. International Journal of Palliative Nursing, 14, 439–445.

Bjornsdottir, K. (2002). From the state to the family: Reconfiguring the responsibility for long-term nursing care at home. Nursing Inquiry, 9(1), 3–11.

Black, P., Boore, J. P., & Parahoo, K. (2011). The effect of nurse-facilitated family participation in the psychological care of the critically ill patient. Journal of Advanced Nursing, 67(5), 1091–1101. doi:10.1111/j.1365-2648.2010.05558.x

Boss, P. (2002). Family stress management: A contextual approach (2nd ed.). Thousand Oaks, CA: Sage.

Butler, A., Copnell, B., & Willetts, G. (2014). Family-centred care in the paediatric intensive care unit: an integrative review of the literature. Journal of Clinical Nursing, 23(15/16), 2086–2100. doi:10.1111/jocn.12498

Cannon, S. (2011). Family-centered care in the critical care setting: is it best practice? Dimensions of Critical Care Nursing, 30(5), 241–245. doi:10.1097/DCC.0b013e3182276f9a

Carr, J. M., & Clarke, P. (1997). Development of the concept of family vigilance. Western Journal of Nursing Research, 19(6), 726–739.

Carr, J. M. (2014). A middle range theory of family vigilance. MEDSURG Nursing, 23(4), 251–255.

Cassell, E. J. (1991). The nature of suffering the goals of medicine. Oxford: Oxford University Press.

Center for Health Design. (2012). The Center for Health Design Pebble Project overview. Retrieved from the Center for Health Design Web site at http://www.healthdesign.org/sites /default/files/Pebble Project Brochure.pdf

Chesla, C. (2010). Do family interventions improve health? *Journal of Family Nursing, 16*, 355–377. doi:10.1177/1074840710383145

Chesla, C. A., & Stannard, D. (1997). Breakdown in the nursing care of families in the ICU. *American Journal of Critical Care, 6*(1), 64–71.

Chien, W. T., Chan, S., Morrissey, J., & Thompson, D. (2005). Effectiveness of a mutual support group for families of patients with schizophrenia. *Journal of Advanced Nursing, 51*(6), 595–608.

Children's Hospital of Philadelphia. (2013). Family-centered care at the Children's Hospital of Philadelphia. Retrieved February 26, 2013 from http://www.chop.edu/service/family-centered-care/family-centered-care1.html

Chintana, W. (2010). Families suffering with HIV/AIDS: What family nursing interventions are useful to promote healing? *Journal of Family Nursing, 16*(3), 302–321. doi:10.1177/1074840710376774

Clarke, C., & Harrison, D. (2001). The needs of children visiting on adult intensive care units: A review of the literature and recommendations for practice. *Journal of Advanced Nursing, 34*(1), 61–68.

Coulter, M. (1989). The needs of family members of patients in critical care units. *Critical Care Nursing, 5*, 4–10.

Curtis, J. R., Engelberg, R. A., Wenrich, M. D., Shannon, S. E., Treece, P. D., & Rubenfeld, G. D. (2005). Missed opportunities during family conferences about end-of-life care in the intensive care unit. *American Journal of Respiratory Critical Care Medicine, 171*(8), 844–849.

Cypress, B. S. (2011). Family conference in the intensive care unit: A systematic review. *Dimensions of Critical Care Nursing, 30*(5), 246–255. doi:10.1097?DCCob013e318227701

Davidson, J. E. (2009). Family-centered care: Meeting the needs of patients' families and helping families adapt to critical illness. *Critical Care Nurse, 29*(3), 28–34.

Davidson, J. E. (2010). Facilitated sensemaking a strategy and new middle-range theory to support families of intensive care unit patients. *Critical Care Nurse, 30*(6), 28–39. doi:10.4037/ccn2010410

Davidson, J., Jones, C., & Bienvenu, O. (2012). Family response to critical illness: Postintensive care syndrome-family. *Critical Care Medicine, 40*(2), 618–624.

Davidson, J. E., Powers, K., Hedayat, K. M., Tieszen, M., Kon, A. A., Shepard, E., & Armstrong, D. (2007). Clinical practice guidelines for support of the family in the patient-centered intensive care unit: American College of Critical Care Medicine task force 2004–2005. *Critical Care Medicine, 35*(2), 605–622.

Denham, S. A. (2003). *Family health: A framework for nursing.* Philadelphia: F.A. Davis.

Department of Health and Human Services (DHHS). (2011). National Strategy for Quality Improvement in Health Care. Retrieved on May 28, 2012 from http://www.healthcare.gov/law/resources/reports/quality03212011a.html#na

de Ruiter, H. P. (2007). Quantifying nursing: Caring or catastrophe? *Creative Nursing, 13*(2), 10.

de Ruiter, H. P. (2011). The invisibility of family in the electronic patient record. Paper presented at the International Family Nursing Conference, June 25, 2011.

Doolin, C., Quinn, L. D., Bryant, L. G., Lyons, A. A., & Kleinpell, R. M. (2011). Family presence during cardiopulmonary resuscitation: Using evidence-based knowledge to guide the advanced practice nurse in developing formal policy and practice guidelines. *Journal of the American Academy of Advanced of Nurse Practitioners, 23*, 8–14. doi:10.1111/j.1745-7599.2010.00569.x

Dossey, B. M., & Keegan, L. (2013). *Holistic nursing* (6th ed.). Burlington, MA: Jones & Bartlett.

Dudley, S. K., & Carr, J. M. (2004). Vigilance: the experience of parents staying at the bedside of hospitalized children. *Journal of Pediatric Nursing, 19*(4), 267–275.

Duhamel, F., Dupuis, F., & Wright, L. (2009). Families' and nurses' responses to the "one question questions": Reflections for clinical practice, education and research in family nursing. *Journal of Family Nursing, 15*(4), 461–485.

Dupuis, F., Duhamel, F., Gendron, S. (2011). Transitioning care of an adolescent with cystic fibrosis: Development of systemic hypothesis between parents, adolescents, and health care professionals. *Journal of Family Nursing, 17*(3), 291–311.

Duran, C. R., Oman, K. S., Abel, J. J., Koziel, V. M., & Szymanski, D. (2007). Attitudes toward and beliefs about family presence: A survey of healthcare providers, patients' families, and patients. *American Journal of Critical Care, 16*(3), 270–282.

Eggenberger, S. K., Krumwiede, N., Meiers, S., Bliesmer, M., & Earle, P. (2004). Family caring strategies in neutropenia. *Clinical Journal of Oncology Nursing, 8*(6), 617–621.

Eggenberger, S. K., Meiers, S. J., Krumwiede, N. K., Bliesmer, M., & Earle, P. (2011). Family reintegration: A family health promoting process in chronic illness. *Journal of Nursing and Health Care of Chronic Illness, 3*, 283–292.

Eggenberger, S., & Nelms, T. (2007). Being family: The family experience when an adult member is hospitalized with a critical illness. *Journal of Clinical Nursing, 16*, 1618–1628.

Eggenberger, S. K. , & Regan, M. (2010). Expanding simulation to teach family nursing. *Journal of Nursing Education, 49*(10), 550–558. doi:http://dx.doi.org/10.3928/01484834-20100630-01

Emergency Nurses Association. (2009). Emergency nursing resource: Family presence during invasive procedures and resuscitation in the emergency department. Des Plaines, IL: Author. Retrieved from http://www.ena.org/Research/ENR/Documents/FamilyPresence.pdf

Emergency Nurses Association. (2010). Position statement: Family presence during invasive procedures and resuscitation in the emergency department. Des Plaines, IL: Author. Retrieved from http://www.ena.org/SiteCollectionDocuments/Position%20Statements/FamilyPresence.pdf

Fontana, J. S. (2006). A sudden, life-threatening medical crisis: The family's perspective. *Advances in Nursing Science, 29*(3), 222–231.

Fumagalli, S., Boncinelli, L., Lo Nostro, A., Valoti, P., Baldereshi, G., Di Bari, M., . . . Marchionne, M. (2006). Reduced cardiocirculatory complications with unrestrictive visiting policy in an intensive care unit: Results from a pilot, randomized trial. *Circulation, 113*, 946–952.

Gardner, G., Woollett, K., Daly, N., & Richardson, B. (2009). Measuring the effect of patient comfort rounds on practice environment and patient satisfaction: A pilot study. *International Journal of Nursing Practice, 15*(4), 287–293.

Halm, M. (2005). Family presence during resuscitation: A critical review of the literature. *American Journal of Critical Care, 14*(6), 494–512.

Halm, M. A., Sabo, J., & Rudiger, M. (2006). The patient-family advisory council keeping a pulse on our customers. *Critical Care Nurses, 26*(5), 58–67.

Hannon, B., O'Reilly, V., Bennett, K., Breen, K., & Lawlor, P. G. (2012). Meeting the family: measuring effectiveness of family meetings in a specialist inpatient palliative care unit. *Palliative & Supportive Care, 10*(1), 43–49.

Hansen, B. S., Rørtveit, K., Leiknes, I., Morken, I., Testad, I., Joa, I., & Severinsson, E. (2012). Patient experiences of uncertainty—A synthesis to guide nursing practice and research. *Journal of Nursing Management, 20*(2), 266–277. doi:10.1111/j.1365-2834.2011.01369.x

Hardin, S. R. (2012). Engaging families to participate in care of older adult critical care patients. *Critical Care Nurse, 32*(3), 35–40. doi: http://dx.doi.org/10.4037/ccn2012407

Henriksson, A., Benzein, E., Ternestedt, B., & Andershed, B. (2011). Meeting needs of family members with life-threatening illness: A support group program during ongoing palliative care. *Palliative and Supportive Care, 9*, 263–271.

Heyland, D., Rocker, G., Dodek, P., Kurtogiannis, D., Konopad, E., Cook, D., . . . Callaghan, C. (2002). Family satisfaction with care in the intensive care unit: Results of a multiple center study. *Critical Care Medicine, 30*, 1413–1418.

Hinkle, J. L., & Fitzpatrick, E. (2011). Needs of American relatives of intensive care patients: Perceptions of relatives, physicians and nurses. *Intensive & Critical Care Nursing, 27*(4), 218–225. doi:10.1016/j.iccn.2011.04.003

Hirsch, A. M., Hoeksel, R., Dupler, A. E., & Kaakinen, J. R. (2010). Nurses and families in adult medical-surgical settings. In Kaakinen, J. R., Gedaly-Duff, V., Coehlo, E. P., & Harmon Hanson, S. M. (Eds.), *Family health care nursing: Theory, practice, and research* (4th ed.). Philadelphia: F. A. Davis.

Horner, S. (1997). Uncertainty in mothers' care for their ill children. *Journal of Advanced Nursing, 26*, 658–663.

Hughes, F., Bryan, K., & Robbins, I. (2005). Relatives' experiences of critical care. *Nursing in Critical Care, 10*(1), 23–30.

Hupcey, J. E. (1998). Establishing the nurse-family relationship in the intensive care unit. *Western Journal of Nursing Research, 20*(2), 180–194.

Institute of Medicine. (2001). Crossing the quality chasm: A new health system for the 21st century. Retrieved December 21, 2012 from http://www.iom.edu/Reports/2001/Crossing-the-Quality-Chasm-A-New-Health-System-for-the-21st-Century.aspx

Isovaara, S., Arman, M., & Rehnsfeldt, A. (2006). Family suffering related to war experiences: An interpretative synopsis review of the literature from a caring science perspective. *Scandinavian Journal of Caring Sciences, 20*(3), 241–250.

Jacobowski, N. L., Girard, T. D., Mulder, J. A., & Wesley, E. (2010). Communication in critical care: Family rounds in the intensive care unit. *American Journal of Critical Care, 19*(5), 421–430.

Johnson, B., Abraham, M., Conway, J., Simmons, L., Edgman-Levitan, S., Sodomka, P., . . . Ford, D. (2008). Partnering with patients and families to design a patient- and family-centered health care system: Recommendations and promising practices. Bethesda, MD: Institute for Patient- and Family-Centered Health Care.

Jones, C., Backman, C., & Griffiths, R. (2012). Intensive care diaries and relatives' symptoms of posttraumatic stress disorder after critical illness: A pilot study. *American Journal of Critical Care, 21*(3), 172–176. doi:10.4037/ajcc2012569

Kaakinen, J. R., Gedaly-Duff, V., Coehlo, E. P., & Harmon Hanson, S. M. (2010). *Family health care nursing* (4th ed.). Philadelphia: F. A. Davis.

Kaakinen, J. R., Coehlo, D. P., Steele, R., Tabacco, A. & Hanson, S. H. (2015). *Family health care nursing: Theory, practice, and research.* Philadelphia: F. A. Davis.

Kean, S. (2010). Children and young people visiting an adult intensive care unit. *Journal of* Advanced Nursing, 66(4), 868–877.

Kelley, T. F., Brandon, D. H., & Docherty, S. L. (2011). Electronic nursing documentation as a strategy to improve quality of patient care. *Journal of Nursing Scholarship, 43*(2), 154–162.

King, B., Gilmore-Bykovskyi, A., Roiland, R., Polnaszek, B., Bowers, B., & Kind, A. (2013). The consequences of poor communication during transitions from hospital to skilled nursing facility: A qualitative study. *Journal of the American Geriatrics Society, 61*(7), 1095–1102.

Knafl, K. A., Deatrick, J. A., Knafl, G. J., Gallo, A. M., Grey, M., & Dixon, J. (2013). Patterns of family management of childhood chronic conditions and their relationship to child and family functioning. *Journal of Pediatric Nursing, 28*(6), 523–535. doi:10.1016/j.pedn.2013.03.006

Knutsson, S., Samuelsson, I. P., Hellstrom, A. L., & Berghbom, J. (2008). Children's experiences of visiting a seriously ill/injured relative on an adult intensive care unit. *Journal of Advanced Nursing* 61(2), 154–162. doi:10.1111/j.1365-2648.2007.04472.x

Kreitzer, M. J., & Zborowsky, T. (2009). Creating optimal healing environments. In M. Snyder & R. Lindquist (Eds.), *Complementary and alternative therapies in nursing.* New York: Springer.

Leahey, M., & Svavarsdottir, E. K. (2009). Implementing family nursing: How do we translate knowledge into clinical practice? *Journal of Family Nursing, 15*(4), 445–460. doi:10.1177/1074840709349070

Leape, L., Berwick, D., Clancy, C., Conway, J., Gluck, P., Guest, J., . . . Isaac, T. (2009). Transforming healthcare: A safety imperative. *Quality and Safety in Health Care, 18,* 424–428.

Leske, J. S. (1991). Overview of family needs after critical illness: From assessment to intervention. *AACN Clinical Issues, 2*(2), 220–228.

Li, H., Melnyk, B. M., & McCann, R. (2004). Review of intervention studies of families with hospitalized elderly relatives. *Journal of Nursing Scholarship, 36*(1), 54–59.

Litchfield, M. C. (2011). Family nursing: A systematic approach to innovative health care delivery. In E. K. Svaversdottir & H. Jonsdottir (Eds.), *Family nursing in action* (pp. 285–307). Reykjavik, Iceland: University of Iceland Press.

Luce, J. M., & White, D. B. (2007). The pressure to withhold or withdraw life-sustaining therapy from critically ill patients in the United States. *American Journal of Respiratory and Critical Care Medicine, 175,* 1104–1108.

Lynn-McHale, D. J., & Deatrick, J. A. (2000). Trust between family and health care provider. *Journal of Family Nursing, 6,* 210–230.

MacLean, S., Guzzetta, C. E., White, C., Fontaine, D., Eichhorn, E., Meyers, T. A., & Desy, P. (2003). Family presence during cardiopulmonary resuscitation and invasive procedures: Practices of critical care and emergency nurses. *American Journal of Critical Care, 12*(3), 246–257.

Marek, K. D., Adams, S. J., Stetzer, F., Popejoy, L., & Rantz, M. (2010). The relationship of community-based nurse care coordination to costs in the Medicare and Medicaid programs. *Research in Nursing and Health, 33,* 235–242.

Marshall, A., Bell, J., & Moules, N. (2010). Beliefs, suffering, and healing: A clinical practice model for families experiencing mental illness. *Perspectives in Psychiatric Care, 46*(3), 197–208. doi:10.1111/j.1744-6163.2010.00259.x

Martinez, A. M., D'Artois, D., & Rennick, J. (2007). Does "the 15-minute (or less) family interview" influence nursing practice? *Journal of Family Nursing, 13,* 157–178.

Mast, M. (1998). Survivors of breast cancer: Illness uncertainty, positive reappraisal, and emotional distress. *Oncology Nursing Forum, 25*(3), 555–562.

McAdam, J. L., Dracup, K. A., White, D. B., Fontaine, D. K., & Puntillo, K. A. (2010). Symptom experiences of family members of intensive care unit patients at high risk for dying. *Critical Care Medicine, 38*(4), 1078-1085. doi:http://dx.doi.org/10.1097/CCM.0b013e3181cf6d94

McBride Robichaux, C., & Clark, A. P. (2006). Practice of expert critical care nurses in situations of prognostic conflict at the end of life. *American Journal of Critical Care, 5,* 480–491.

McCabe, C. (2003). Nurse-patient communication: An exploration of patients' experiences. *Journal of Clinical Nursing, 13*(1), 41–49.

McMillan, S. C., & Small, B. J. (2007). Using the COPE intervention for family caregivers to improve symptoms of hospice homecare patients: A clinical trial. *Oncology Nursing Forum, 34*(2), 313–321.

Meiers, S. J. (2003). Family-nurse co-construction of meaning: A central phenomenon of family caring. *Scandinavian Journal of Caring Science, 17,* 193–201.

Meiers, S. J., & Brauer, D. J. (2008). Existential caring in the family health experience: A proposed conceptualization. *Scandinavian Journal of Caring Science, 22,* 110–117.

Meterko, M., Mohr, D. C., & Young, G. J. (2004). Teamwork culture and patient satisfaction in hospitals. *Medical Care, 42*(5), 492–498.

Meyers, T. A., Eichhorn, D. J., Guzzetta, C. E., Clark, A. P., & Taliaferro, E. (2000). Family presence during invasive procedures and resuscitation: The experience of family members, nurses, and physicians. *American Journal of Nursing, 100*(2), 32–42.

Mishel, M. H. (1997). Uncertainty in acute illness. *Annual Review of Nursing Research, 15,* 57–80.

Mishel, M. H., & Clayton, M. (2008). Theories of uncertainty in illness. In J. M. Smith & P. R. Liehr (Eds.), *Middle range theory for nursing* (2nd ed.). New York: Springer.

Mitchell, M., Chaboyer, W., Burmeister, E., & Foster, M. (2009). Positive effects of a nursing intervention on family-centered care in adult critical care. *American Journal of Critical Care, 18*(6), 543–553.

Molter, N. C. (1979). The needs of relatives of critically ill patients: A descriptive study. *Heart and Lung, 8,* 332–339.

Munn-Giddings, C., & McVicar, A. (2006). Self-help groups as mutual support: What do carers value? *Health and Social Care in the Community, 15*(1), 26–34.

National Hospice and Palliative Care Organization. (2008). Position statement on access to palliative care in critical care settings: A call to action. Alexandria, VA: Author. Retrieved from http://www.nhpco.org/files/public/NHPCO_PC-in-ICU_statement_Sept08.pdf

Nelms, T. P., & Eggenberger, S. K. (2010). Essence of the family critical illness experience and family meetings. *Journal of Family Nursing, 16*(4), 462–486.

Northouse, L. L, Walker, J., Schafenacker, A., Mood, D., Mellon, S., Galvin, E., . . . Fretman-Gibb, L. (2002). A family-based program of care for women with recurrent breast cancer and their family members. *Oncology Nursing Forum, 29*(10), 1411–1419. doi:10.1188/02.ONF.1411-1419

Office of Civil Rights: Health and Human Services Department. (2012). A health care provider's guide to the HIPAA privacy role: Communicating with a patient's family, friends or others involved in the patient's care. Retrieved on May 22, 2012 from http://www.hhs.gov/ocr/privacy/hipaa/understanding/coveredentities/provider_ffg.pdf

Pastor-Montero, S. M., Romero-Sanchez, J. M., Paramio-Castro, O., Lilo-Crespo, M., Castro-Yuste, C., Toledano-Losa, A. C., . . . Frandsen, A. J. (2012). Tackling parental loss, a participatory action research approach: Research protocol. *Journal of Advanced Nursing, 61*(11), 2578–2585.

Paterson, B., Kieloch, B., & Gmiterek, J. (2001). They never told us anything: Postdischarge instruction for families of persons with brain injuries. *Rehabilitation Nursing, 26*(20), 48–53.

Persily, C. A., & Hildebrandt, E. (2008). Theory of community empowerment. In M. J. Smith & P. R. Liehr (Eds.), *Middle range theory of nursing* (2nd ed., pp. 131–144). New York: Springer.

Picker Institute. (2012). Improving healthcare through the patient's eyes. Retrieved May 28, 2012 from http://pickerinstitute.org/

Planetree. (2012). The Planetree Model. Retrieved May 28, 2012 from http://planetree.org/

Popejoy, L. L. (2011). Complexity of family caregiving and discharge planning. *Journal of Family Nursing, 17*(1):61–81. doi:10.1177/1074840710394855

Rappaport, D. I., Ketterer, T. A., Nilforoshan, V., & Sharif, I. (2012). Family-centered rounds: Views of families, nurses, trainees, and attending physicians. *Clinical Pediatrics, 51*(3), 260–266.

Roberti, S. M., & Fitzpatrick, J. J. (2010). Assessing family satisfaction with care of critically ill patients: A pilot study. *Critical Care Nurse, 30*(6), 18–26. doi:10.4037/ccn/2010448

Robichaux, C. M., & Clark, A. P. (2006). Practice of expert critical care nurses in situations of prognostic conflict at the end of life. *American Journal of Critical Care, 15*(5), 480–491.

Robinson, C. A., & Wright, L. M. (1995). Family nursing interventions: What families say makes a difference. *Journal of Family Nursing, 1*, 327–345.

Sabo, K. A., Kraay, C., Rudy, E., Abraham, T., Bender, M., Lewandowski, W., & Dawson, D. (1989). ICU family support group sessions: Family members' perceived benefits. *Applied Nursing Research, 2*(2), 82–89.

Sacco, T. L., Stapleton, M. F., & Ingersoll, G. L. (2009). Support groups facilitated by families of former patients: Creating family inclusive critical care units. *Critical Care Nurse, 29*(3), 36–45.

Sammarco, A. (2001). Perceived social support, uncertainty, and quality of life of younger breast cancer survivors. *Cancer Nursing, 24*(3), 212–219.

Sammarco, A., & Konecny, L. M. (2010). Quality of life, social support, and uncertainty among Latina and Caucasian breast cancer survivors: A comparative study. *Oncology Nursing Forum, 37*(1), 93–99.

Santiago, C., Lazar, L., Depeng, J., & Burns, K. A. (2014). A survey of the attitudes and perceptions of multidisciplinary team members towards family presence at bedside rounds in the intensive care unit. *Intensive and Critical Care Nursing, 30*(1), 13–21. doi:10.1016/j.iccn.2013.06.003

Sharkey, T. (1995). The effects of uncertainty in families with children who are chronically ill. *Home Healthcare Nurse, 13*(4), 37–42.

Soderstrom, I., Benzein, E., & Saveman, B. (2003). Nurses' experiences of interactions with family members in the intensive care unit. *Scandinavian Journal of Caring Sciences, 17*, 185–192.

Stacy, K. M. (2012). Withdrawal of life-sustaining treatment: A case study. *Critical Care Nurse, 32*(3), 14–24. doi:http://dx.doi.org/10.4037/ccn2012152

Stayt, L. C. (2009). Death, empathy and self-preservation: The emotional labour of caring for families of the critically in adult intensive care. *Journal of Clinical Nursing, 18*, 1267–1275.

Stone, A. M., & Jones, C. L. (2009). Sources of uncertainty: Experiences of Alzheimer's disease. *Issues in Mental Health Nursing, 30*, 677–686.

Strang, S., Henoch, I., Danielson, E., Browall, M., & Melin-Johansson, C. (2014). Communication about existential issues with patients close to death-nurses' reflections on content, process and meaning. *Psycho-Oncology, 23*(5), 562–568. doi:10.1002/pon.3456

Svavarsdottir, E. K., & Jonsdottir, H. (2011). *Family nursing in action.* Reykjavik, Iceland: University of Iceland Press.

Svavarsdottir, E. K., Tryggvadottir, G. B., & Sigurdardottir, A. O. (2012). Knowledge translation in family nursing: Does a short-term therapeutic conversation intervention benefit families of children and adolescents in a hospital setting? Findings from the Landspitali University Hospital Family Nursing Implementation Project. *Journal of Family Nursing, 18*(3), 303–327.

Tapp, D. M. (2001). Conserving the vitality of suffering: Addressing family constraints to illness conversations. *Nursing Inquiry, 8*(4), 254–263.

Tinsley, C. J., Hill, B., Shah, J., Zimmerman, G., Wilson, M., Freier, F., & Abd-Allah, S. (2008). Intensive care unit experience of families during cardiopulmonary resuscitation in pediatrics. *Pediatrics, 122*, 799. doi: 10.1542/peds.2007-3650

Tomlinson, P. S., Peden-McAlpine, C., & Sherman, S. (2012). A family systems nursing intervention model for paediatric health crisis. *Journal of Advanced Nursing, 68*(3), 705–714.

Tong, V., & Kaakinen, J. R. (2015). Family nursing in acute care adult settings. In J. R. Kaakinen, D. P. Coehlo, R. Steele, A. Tabacco, & S. M. Harmon Hanson (Eds.), *Family health care nursing: Theory, practice, and research* (5th ed.). Philadelphia: F. A. Davis.

Trimm, D. R., & Sanford, J. T. (2010). The process of family waiting during surgery. *Journal of Family Nursing, 16* (4), 435–461. doi:10.1177/1074840710385691

Trochelman, K., Albert, N., Spence, J., Murray, T., & Slifcak, E. (2012). Patients and their families weigh in on evidence-based hospital design. *Critical Care Nurse, 32*(1), 1–11. doi:10.4037/ccn2012785

Ulrich, R. S., Zimring, C., Zhu, X., DuBose, J., Seo, H. B., Choi, Y. S., . . . Joseph, A. (2008). A review of the research literature on evidence-based healthcare design. *Health Environments Research & Design Journal, 1*(3), 61–125.

Université de Montreal (2000). *Family genograph*. Montreal, Quebec, Canada.

Vandall-Walker, V., & Clark, A. (2011). It starts with access! A grounded theory of family members working to get through critical illness. *Journal of Family Nursing, 17*(2), 148–181. doi:10.1177/1074840711406728

Van Horn, E. R., & Kautz, D. (2007). Promotion of family integrity in the acute care setting: A review of the literature. *Dimensions of Critical Care Nurse, 26*(3), 101–107.

Van Horn, E., & Tesh, A. (2000). The effect of critical care hospitalization on family members: stress and responses. *Dimensions of Critical Care Nursing, 19*(4), 40–49.

Verhaeghe, S., Defloor, T., Van Zuuren, F., Duijnstee, M., & Grypdonick, M. (2005). The needs and experiences of family members of adult patients in an intensive care unit: A review of the literature. *Journal of Clinical Nursing, 14*(4), 501–509.

Verhaeghe, S., van Zuuren, F., Grypdonck, M., Duijnstee, M., & Defloor, T. (2010). The focus of family members' functioning in the acute phase of traumatic coma. Part Two: protecting from suffering and protecting what remains to rebuild life. *Journal of Clinical Nursing, 19*(3–4), 583–589. doi:10.1111/j.1365-2702.2009.02964.

Warnock, C., Tod, A., Foster, J., & Soreny, C. (2010). Breaking bad news in inpatient clinical settings: Role of the nurse. *Journal of Advanced Nursing, 66*(7), 1543–1555. doi:10.111/j.1365-2648.2010.05325.x

Warren, N. (2012). Involving patient and family advisors in the patient and family-centered care model. *MEDSURG Nursing, 21*(4), 233–239.

Weihs, K. L., Fisher, L., & Baird, M. (2002). Families, health and behavior. A section of the Commissioned Report by the Committee on Health and Behavior: Research, Practice, and Policy, Division of Neuroscience and Behavioral Health and Division of Health Promotion and Disease Prevention, Institute of Medicine, National Academy of Sciences. *Families, Systems and Health, 20*(1), 7–46.

Weingarten, K. (2012). Sorrow: A therapist's reflection on the inevitable and the unknowable. *Family Process, 51*(4), 440–455.

Weiss, M. E., Piacentine, L. B., Ancona, J., Gresser, S., Toman, S., & Vega-Stromberg, T. (2007). Perceived readiness for hospital discharge in adult medical-surgical patients. *Clinical Nurse Specialist, 21*, 31–42.

Wiegand, D. (2008). In their own time: the family experience during the process of withdrawal of life-sustaining therapy. *Journal of Palliative Medicine, 11*(8), 1115–1121.

Wiegand, D. L. (2006). Withdrawal of life-sustaining therapy after sudden, unexpected life-threatening illness or injury: Interactions between patients' families, healthcare providers, and the health care system. *American Journal of Critical Care, 15*(2), 178–187.

Wiegand D. L., Deatrick J. A., & Knafl K. A. (2008). Family management styles related to withdrawal of life-sustaining therapy from adults who are acutely ill or injured. *Journal of Family Nursing, 14*(1), 16–32. doi:10.1177/1074840707313338.10.1177/1074840707313338

Wiggins, M. S. (2008). The partnership care delivery model: An examination of the core concept and the need for a new model of care. *Journal of Nursing Management, 16*, 629–638.

Williams, C. (2005). The identification of family members' contribution to patients' care in the intensive care unit: A naturalistic inquiry. *Nursing in Critical Care, 10*(1), 6–14.

Wineman, N. M., O'Brien, R. A., Nealon, N. R., & Kaskel, B. (1993). Congruence in uncertainty between individuals with multiple sclerosis and their spouses. *Journal of Neuroscience Nursing, 25,* 356–361.

Wingate, S., & Wiegand, D. L. (2008). End-of-life care in the critical care unit for patients with heart failure. *Critical Care Nurse, 28*(2), 84–94.

Wolf, Z. R., Miller, P. A., & Devine, M. (2003). Relationship between nurse caring and patient satisfaction in patients undergoing invasive cardiac procedures. *MEDSURG Nursing, 12*(6), 391–396. Retrieved May 12, 2012 from http://findarticles.com/p/articles/mi_m0FSS/is_6_12/ai_n18616793/?tag=content;col1

Wright, L. M. (2005). *Spirituality, suffering, and illness: Ideas for healing.* Philadelphia: F. A. Davis.

Wright, L. (2008). Softening suffering through spiritual care practices: One possibility for healing families. *Journal of Family Nursing, 14*(4), 394–411.

Wright, L. M., & Bell, J. M. (2009). *Beliefs and illness: A model of healing.* Calgary, Alberta, Canada: 4th Floor Press.

Wright, L. M., & Leahey, M. (2009). *Nurses and families: A guide to family assessment and intervention* (4th ed.). Philadelphia: F. A. Davis.

Wright, L., & Leahey, M. (2013). *Nurses and families: A guide to family assessment and intervention* (6th ed.). Philadelphia: F. A. Davis.

Wright, L. M., Watson, W. L., & Bell, J. M. (1996). *Beliefs: the heart of healing in families and illness.* New York; Basic Books.

Xu, Y., Testerman, L., Owen, J., Bantum, E., Thornton, A., & Stanton, A. (2014). Modeling intention to participate in face-to-face and online lung cancer support groups. *Psycho-Oncology, 23*(5), 555–561. doi:10.1002/pon.3449

CHAPTER 11

Family-Focused Care and Chronic Illness

Sharon A. Denham

Sharon A. Denham

CHAPTER OBJECTIVES

1. Explain chronic illness experiences from individual and family perspectives.
2. Examine special family concerns associated with chronic disease management.
3. Describe ways nurses prepare families to satisfy various member needs associated with chronic illness.
4. Discuss management of family stressors associated with living with uncertainty.
5. Use family-focused care to support and overcome barriers when child and adult members have a chronic illness.

CHAPTER CONCEPTS

- Care coordination
- Chronic illness
- Collaboration
- Family health routines
- In-time
- Non-normative
- Normative
- Off-time

Introduction

This chapter considers the complex care needs linked with chronic illness and families' diverse experiences in living with chronic illness over time. Chronic conditions are not static; they often change. A major goal is self-management so that complications are delayed or prevented. Although nurses are often well prepared to address the acute conditions, many are less familiar with long-term needs related to chronic conditions. Acute illnesses usually have rapid onset and symptoms are often short-lived. Those suffering with an acute illness may heal and resume prior activities, suffer from disabilities or limitations, or die. Acute conditions disrupt life, can be traumatic, and put stress on family members, but situations are usually temporary and more quickly resolved.

On the other hand, chronic health conditions typically last more than a year and have no cure. The World Health Organization (2002) defines chronic disease as health problems that require ongoing management over a period of years or decades. Common chronic conditions are asthma, diabetes, cerebral palsy, multiple sclerosis, and cancer. Chronic conditions often require unusual attention and intrude into all aspects of family life. Many can be self-managed with medications and lifestyle changes. Persons with chronic conditions often live active healthy lives for many years. Persons living with conditions, such as asthma or diabetes can mostly live healthy lives when diseases and risk factors are managed. However, some chronic conditions such as multiple sclerosis, amyotrophic lateral sclerosis, and lupus can progressively worsen over time. Persons with disabilities can be severely challenged to accomplish some daily tasks and some require a continuous caregiver. Many veterans of the Vietnam, Afghanistan, or Iraqi wars experienced severe injuries and live with significant physiological limitations often accompanied by post-traumatic stress syndrome. Veterans may live decades with needs that tax a family's abilities and resources.

Although nurses often agree that family is important in chronic care management, their formal education does not always prepare them to see needs of family units. Caregiver support is often discussed for parental care of dependent children or dying persons, but less attention is given to the chronic care needs of adults. Nurses often *think family* with the elderly population or conditions such as Alzheimer's disease. Less attention is given to chronic conditions such as Down syndrome where persons can live into their 50s and outlive aged parents. Family needs of decades or a lifetime with a chronic condition are rarely considered. Changes with developmental stages and adaptations over time are needed. Maintaining high-quality family household life can deplete resources with some types of chronic illness.

Nursing concerns and system matters potentially linked with chronic care needs are addressed using the Family Health Model (Denham, 2003). A case study of the Zimanske family, a family living with a rare genetic condition, is threaded throughout this chapter. Their story provides ways to view multiple concerns associated with chronic disorders. Their experience begins at their son's birth and continues through diagnosis, disease progression, and after his death. Their story demonstrates how diagnosis of a chronic condition saturated their family life. Chronic conditions change, require different forms of attention, and can create hardships. This chapter describes ways family unit problems can be paired with member's chronic conditions.

Defining Chronic Illness and the Associated Needs

Care of chronic illness is part of daily life for many families across the nation and throughout the world. Getting older makes the odds of having two or more conditions greater. In 2005, chronic disease was the cause of 70% of Americans' deaths and accounted for more than 50% of all deaths (Kung, Hoyart, Xu, & Murphy, 2008). When many individuals live with multiple chronic conditions, the overall health of the nation's people is worsened (Institute of Medicine, 2012). Threats can be enormous when multiple members from a single household have several chronic conditions.

In the United States, health is generally viewed using a deficit perspective. Morbidity and mortality rates are key indicators of a nation's health. Health is a construct that includes physical, mental, spiritual, and social dimensions. With family and population health we look beyond merely saving lives and consider the quality of those lives. Many factors influence chronic conditions such as disease stage at diagnosis, age of affected person, competing family needs, access to care, and availability or lack of needed resources. Nurses who *think family* know chronic conditions permeate lives, far beyond biological and pathophysiological disease traits. Nursing is often defined as attending to an individual's experience and response to health and illness (American Nurses Association, 2010). Thus, family-focused nursing care with chronic illness is attending to the family's experience and members' responses to chronic illness.

Chronic illnesses sometimes lead to earlier deaths and severely impacts the individual and family's quality of life, altering their ability to perform usual activities of daily living, interrupting education, and limiting the ability to work and engage in neighborhood and community activities. Socioeconomic conditions, the place where one lives, and the ways persons interact, perform activities of daily living, solve problems, and deal with disruptions are often additional factors linked with chronic illness and its management.

Nurses who *think family* consider familie's capacities to care for members with chronic conditions, regardless of whether the diagnosed person is young or old. When infants, children, or teens have a chronic disease diagnosis, the condition and medical treatments usually change over time. For example, a person diagnosed with type 1 diabetes has a vastly different medical treatment when age 35 than when first diagnosed at 11 years old. Keeping pace with changes in best medical practices is something those living with chronic conditions and their family unit's might need to support their changing care needs.

Family nurses realize that whenever they meet persons with chronic conditions in a clinical situation, it is a chance to assess the condition, answer questions, give updated information, and address family quality-of-life concerns. Visits are times to update treatments, ascertain needed resources, and assess thinking that might differ from best care management. For example, before the late 1970s, good diabetes management occurred with what was at times impure insulin that varied with batches. Insulin needles were boiled and reused. Dietary exchange food lists were used. Urine was regularly checked by individuals for glycosuria. Today's treatment of diabetes involves regular blood glucose monitoring, hemoglobin A_{1C}, disposable fine-gauge needles, and lifestyle management. Counting carbohydrates, choosing low-calorie high-nutrient foods, managing portion size, and balancing dietary intake and physical activity are stressed today. Although family health routines are important to diabetes management, family is not always present or intentionally included in the education (Denham, 2003).

Chronic Conditions in Adults

Persons diagnosed with a chronic illness as children will still have the condition as they get older. Thus, when children with type 1 diabetes become adults they are likely to experience two or more complications as they age. In adulthood, the most common chronic conditions are cardiovascular disease, risks related to hypertension and obesity, and arthritis (Chen, Baumgardner, & Rice, 2011; Halfon & Newacheck, 2010). Chronic conditions can be accompanied by long-standing pain, severe disabilities, impaired senses, and depression or other mental health conditions. When individuals have more than one chronic condition the term multimorbidity is applied. Chronic conditions can greatly compromise life and make disease management extremely challenging. The lived experience of chronic illness affects person and family unit, extended kin, and friends. *Thinking family* linked with chronic care requires nurses to focus on disease management from a household perspective.

Conditions once only seen in pediatrics, such as congenital heart defects and cystic fibrosis (CF), are now adult diseases as these persons live longer (Halfon & Newacheck, 2010). The Adult Congenital Heart Association estimates there are 750,000 adults with the diagnosis. The Cystic Fibrosis Foundation (2010) reported that in the 1950s children rarely lived to attend grade school. Now the median predicted age of survival is 38 years. Although the exact conditions and age of onset vary, many share common clinical experiences throughout the disease trajectory and various demands are made on family members.

Chronic Conditions in Children

In general, children are likely to have chronic conditions that are genetic or environmental in nature. Childhood diseases mostly result from congenital abnormalities, neonatal exposures, or impairments due to unintentional injuries, whereas adults have chronic conditions from cumulative effects of lifestyle risks, environmental exposures, and degenerative conditions (Halfon & Newacheck, 2010). Major advances in health care services, technologies, and medicines have occurred. Management of chronic conditions that were once life limiting has changed; as people with chronic illness live longer disease prevalence has grown (Cohen et al., 2011; Tennant, Pearce, Bythell, & Rankin, 2010). For example, children who, in the past, might have died in infancy now survive once-fatal conditions such as extreme premature birth, congenital heart disease, cystic fibrosis, and infectious diseases. Chronic childhood conditions lead to developmental vulnerability and dependence on adults for caregiving, and are manifested as different types, prevalence, and patterns of chronic disease (Halfon & Newacheck, 2010). Other common childhood conditions are obesity, allergies, asthma, learning disorders, and emotional problems (Bethell et al., 2011). Children with severe chronic conditions have complex care needs with great family demands (Capen & Dedlow, 1998). Some problems that result include the following:

- Lack of availability of qualified caregivers
- Lack of privacy with care providers in the home
- Focus on equipment rather than the child
- Needs for emergency backup
- Lack of respite care
- Complications when the child gets intercurrent illnesses
- The need for special educational services
- The absence of health coverage for expensive regimes

Compelling demands and enduring stressors place great burdens on family units. Increasingly, chronic conditions once considered adult diseases (e.g., hypertension, type 2 diabetes) now occur in children as a result of lifestyle factors.

Management of Chronic Conditions

A wide range of chronic conditions exist with varying levels of severity and health impacts. Individuals with chronic conditions are daughters and sons, sisters and brothers, parents, grandparents, and members of nuclear, blended, cohabiting, single-sex, or other nontraditional families.

Care Coordination

Care coordination is of utmost importance in chronic disease management. Families find that many necessary activities become extraordinary tasks that they are unprepared to handle. Nurses working with families when a member has a chronic condition need to assist them to learn ways to share in care management. Ill persons and family members need knowledge and support about the disease and skills to manage care. Families need to know how to care for their member, but also how to care for themselves. The vigilance needed to respond to care needs can be exhausting. Conditions change over time and so teaching and counseling must be attuned to current science and best practices.

Family Involvement in Care

Nurses often speak about patient education, and when the condition is chronic then family education is needed as well. Chronic conditions are family matters! Problems confronted affect the multimember household. Family and individual needs vary even when the diagnosis is the same. Nurses who *think family* are not just sensitive to the individual's pathophysiological changes, but also to socioemotional changes in the family unit. Altered treatment plans, variations in medical management, and caregiver fatigue are problems to be faced. Families need attention, too (Box 11.1).

Research evidence is available to guide individual's medical treatment from disease-focused perspectives. Growing amounts of evidence related to the benefits of technology and medical treatments in the care and management of chronic conditions are available (Clifford & Clifton, 2012; Smith, Soubhi, Fortin, & O'Dowd, 2012; Venter, Burns, Heffors, & Ehrenberg, 2012). For example, we know much about the pathophysiology of diabetes and best practices for management with diet and medication. However, we have long known that situational factors of eating and inappropriate food offers from others challenge one's abilities to adhere to prescribed diets (Ary, Toobert, Wilson, & Glasgow, 1986). Newer findings suggest that adherence to prescribed medicine regimens is poor (Cramer, 2004).

The importance of a whole person approach to medical care is in its infancy (Hayes, Naylor, & Egger, 2012). Managing chronic illness touches every part of daily lives and affects household members differently. Therefore, *thinking family* means giving attention to the following:

- The family responses to chronic illness (Knafl, Deatrick, & Havill, 2012)
- The importance of care coordination (Maeng, Martsolf, Scanlon, & Christianson, 2012)
- The relevance of time in chronic care management (Barclay-Goddard, King, Dubouloz, & Schwartz, 2012)

Individuals and families need help that fosters resilience and maintains as much normality as possible.

Financial Costs

Annual costs of medical care of chronic illness represents 75% of U.S. total annual health care spending, or approximately $1.5 trillion (Institute of Medicine, 2012). Evidence-based interventions are needed to attend to preventable conditions using lifestyle changes, such as eating nutritious foods, increasing physical activity, and stopping tobacco use. Public health practices and policies that support promising societal approaches for change are needed. Roles of families in prevention of some chronic conditions cannot be ignored. Nurses who *think family* are eager to teach family units about preventable risks, wellness, and lifestyle actions that promote individual and family health. When evidence to support

---

BOX 11-1

Family Challenges With Chronic Conditions

For a single diagnosis such as asthma or diabetes, the family must navigate many challenges over many years:

- Multiple doctors' visits
- Medical directions of multiple specialists
- Costs of medications, treatments, and travel to receive care
- Potential hospitalization
- Separation from peers, school or work absences
- Physical and emotional challenges of the disease

current practices is lacking, then we need innovation and new conceptual models to guide care. When it comes to chronic illness, we need to be creative and rethink care delivery so information sharing, skill acquisition, and medical services are delivered in the ways needed by family units. Long-held medical model thinking and traditional patterns of care delivery have focused on episodic care, mending acute care problems, and attending to single person needs. These attitudes are not always useful approaches for meeting chronic care needs. Chronic care management needs highly coordinated, evidence-based, family-focused care that prevents complications, reduces exacerbations, and addresses family households and family unit needs.

Chronic Conditions and Family Nursing Care

The Zimanske family serves as an exemplar case for this chapter to help readers better understand the many needs of a family living with chronic illness. This chapter explains differences in family care needs when illness is chronic rather than acute. Nurses who *think family* provide care to those with evolving chronic conditions. This Zimanske case study provides insights into how a childhood chronic condition affects members of the family unit differently over time.

Case Study: Family Perspective of Chronic Illness

For the Zimanske family, life changed with the diagnosis of a chronic condition for its youngest member, Michael (Box 11.2). Theresa, Michael's mother, explains, "We were married, had a suburban home, two kids, a camper in the driveway. . . . Then, one day, everything changed for us." Michael's diagnosis of Schimke immune-osseous dysplasia (SIOD) came after months of health challenges and tests (Box 11.3). Life for this family was referred to as life before the diagnosis and life after the diagnosis. Life before the diagnosis included plans for Michael and his older sister to grow up, experience youthful life activities, graduate from high school, begin families of their own, and grow old with their parents. According to Theresa, life after the diagnosis meant:

- Understanding the condition
- Managing disease effects on his and our physical, emotional, and social well-being
- Coming to terms with the possibility that he would not live the life we had imagined
- Living with dramatic changes in the experience of family life

Theresa explained that the family manages the illness but also contends with the logistics attached to the illness: "Michael's total health care picture was intricately connected to the well-being of our whole family, both physically, emotionally, and socially."

Stress and Coping

Ideas of stress and coping have been studied since the 1930s as researchers were interested in ways that families contended with the loss of income and stress of unemployment during the Depression Era (Angell, 1936; Cavan & Ranck, 1938). Research identified that well-organized and cohesive families before the depression were the most capable of dealing with the stress of economic losses and family struggles. Early work on family stress factors was done by Rueben Hill (1949). Hill's early work (refer to Chapter 7) was about the ways

BOX 11-2

Family Circle

Michael, son of Theresa and Don Zimanske, brother of Jessica Zimanske, was diagnosed in 1999 with SIOD at the age of 7 following a 2-year diagnostic process, which began at his kindergarten physical examination. At the age of 5, Michael was the fastest runner on his T-ball team. By age 9, he was physically confined to a wheelchair, but his resilient spirit was not. Michael traveled a medical path that constantly changed due to the progressive symptoms caused by SIOD with a life-limiting prognosis that did not define him or his family. Seeking treatment he challenged medical providers to see beyond his diagnosis and see him as a boy with family and friends in a life outside of medical trauma and disease. In 2005, after suffering severe complication due to SIOD, Michael went to his heavenly home. He left a legacy of hope, which resulted in the Be the Change campaign, completely inspired by the life of a change-maker, Michael Zimanske.

After reading this chapter, answer these three questions:

1. Identify three ways using family-focused care when caring for persons with chronic illness differs from care guided solely by the medical model perspective.
2. Describe three areas of resilience you have identified in the Zimanske family.
3. Give an example of how nurses who use family-focused care can attend to the individual with a chronic illness in a way that positively promotes coordinated care.

Identify two similarities and two differences between Michael's family's needs and another family where an adult has a chronic illness.

BOX 11-3

Schimke Immune-osseous Dysplasia (SIOD)

According to Genetics Home Reference (ghr.nlm.nih.gov, GeneReviews), Schimke immune-osseous dysplasia (SIOD) is a rare, autosomal recessive condition characterized by short stature, kidney disease, and weakened immune system. This rare inherited condition, 1 in 3 million births, causes multiple hyperpigmented macules, characteristic facial features, progressive renal failure, decreased white blood cell count, recurrent infections, atherosclerosis, and reduced blood flow to the brain leading to cerebral ischemia (Boerkoel et al., 2001; Lucke et al., 2006; NIH, 2014). Those with the disease have normal intellectual and neurological development for a time. Kidney disease often leads to renal failure and end-stage renal disease. A shortage of T cells that help the body fight infection causes a person to be more susceptible to illness. Individuals with SIOD may develop atherosclerosis, cerebral ischemia and strokes, hypothyroidism, and hypoplastic pelvis. Abnormalities of hip bone development may lead to limitations in mobility and require hip replacements. Kidney transplantation may be required as a result of renal disease, and bone marrow transplantation may be indicated. SIOD is progressive, incurable, and often fatal. Few individuals with this condition survive beyond 20 years with some dying in early childhood and those with milder late-onset forms of SIOD surviving into adulthood with treatment of renal disease.

families coped with separation and reunion during wartime. His ideas have remained virtually unchallenged over time (Box 11.4).

Stress can lead to a family crisis when usual coping mechanisms are not effective in resolving problems. Stress is linked with events that upset usual family life patterns and affect members' roles, behaviors, and emotional strengths. Crises shake the family foundation and often create great levels of disorganization. When chronic disease management occurs, it calls into action abilities to organize and manage effectively. If members view the stress

---

BOX 11-4

Assumptions Linked With Stress

Reuben Hill's (1949) original stress model made several assumptions:

- Unplanned and unexpected events can be more stressful than those anticipated.
- Stressors focused on one family member versus the whole family have different forms of related stress.
- Severity of stress makes a difference.
- Stressors that occur within the family (e.g., serious illness) are more stressful than events that occur outside the family (e.g., war, economic recession).
- Perceptions of stress are increased when no prior experience in handling a situation exists and reduced if the family believes they can handle the situation.
- Stressors that are ambiguous are more challenging than ones that are more predictable or less ambiguous.

---

of situations in controllable parts, they seem more successful in managing. Families that receive a diagnosis of a chronic illness in a member may experience various types of stress and may need help in coping.

Meanings of Events

Stress and coping often focus on ways people process meanings of events and readjust to changing situations. A number of highly valued conceptual care models can help nurses describe, explain, and predict individual and family's response to chronic illness (Antonovsky, 1979; Lazarus, 1993; Selye, 1976). The ways situations are perceived and unique responses can influence whether an illness is viewed as stressful or a crisis. When families are overwhelmed or exhaust their resources, they are in a crisis state (Boss, 1988). Loss often occurs with chronic conditions. One form of loss, called ambiguous loss, occurs when there is no closure and people get stuck or are unable to move on with their lives (Boss, 2000). For example, how does one deal with the uncertainty of a soldier missing in action? Or not knowing whether your loved one died in the tragedy of the Twin Towers on September 11, 2001? How does an adult child cope with a parent with cognitive loss or a parent cope with an adult child with schizophrenia? Sadness, emotional suffering, ambivalence, and misgivings are often experienced. Doubts, fears, and heartaches get resolved differently. Family nurses are attuned to life transitions caused by chronic illnesses. Nurses who *think family* target family strengths and areas of resilience.

Family Resilience

The ability to withstand and rebound from adversity is called resilience; it is a positive way to manage stress. Family resilience focuses on the ability to "rally in times of crisis, to buffer stress, reduce the risk of dysfunction, and support optimal adaptation" (Walsh, 2012, p. 175). Resilience views families not as dysfunctional or damaged but as capable and able to skillfully survive stressors. Resilience and family strengths are important to individuals, family units, and the communities where they live (Box 11.5).

When nurses take a resilience perspective, they focus on family members as part of a resourceful whole. This is particularly important for families with chronic conditions. It helps when nurses recognize the family as capable of thriving despite the challenges, while still acknowledging the difficulties faced on a day-to-day basis. Resilience enables families to respond favorably even in the most troubling or difficult situations and suggests areas for

> ### BOX 11-5
> #### Traits of Resilient Families
>
> - Ability to adapt to stressful situations
> - Actions that demonstrate care for one another
> - Capacity to communicate openly and honestly with one another and manage conflicts
> - Flexibility in assuming needed roles and responsibilities
> - Connections to larger social and community groups that are enriching

assessment and nursing actions (Simon, Murphy, & Smith, 2005). Resilience is not static—it is a dynamic quality sensitive to the changes across time at the individual and family level (McCubbin & McCubbin, 1989). As families face long periods of stress, strain, or transition, a pileup effect can cause difficulty in adapting. Families can use strengths, hardiness, and abilities to adapt but they need adequate resources and supports. Nurses can assist the family to resolve problems, make wise decisions, and manage crisis situations.

Focus on Strengths

The traditional deficit or problem-focused care models rely on symptom management and attempts to fix what is wrong. Stress assessment must include the individual and family members, and identify specific factors that are troubling or are strengths to build upon. Resilience suggests that focus on family strengths provides a useful way to direct nursing actions. Multiple factors influence responses to individual needs and family members can pool their strengths to them. Some families might need referrals for additional support. As nurses *think family* they help them identify problems and gain skills to cope effectively. If pain is a problem, nurses can help family units identify ways, besides medications, to manage symptoms. A critical appraisal of the use of family resilience in chronic pain management found that focusing on strengths offers helpful strategies (West, Usher, & Foster, 2011). The individual-nurse-family partnership can be used to identify needs, set goals, plan care, and evaluate outcomes.

Family Models

Many theories and conceptual models help nurses understand chronic conditions and functional needs. Several relevant care models have been introduced (Chapters 7 and 8). The Family Management Style Framework (FMSF) (Knafl & Deatrick, 2003; Knafl et al., 2012) is especially useful for thinking about care management of a child with a chronic condition. This model has been applied to family management of lethal congenital childhood conditions (Rempel, Blythe, Rogers, & Ravindran, 2012), families caring for older adults with dementia (Beeber & Zimmerman, 2012), and sudden death of a family member (Wiegand, 2012). Family management style is the way family members define the situation, manage conditions, and view consequences (Knafl & Deatrick, 2003). Definition of the situation includes beliefs about cause, seriousness, and predictability of the illness. Views of the ease or difficulty in managing a condition and normality are considered. Management behaviors include values and priorities related to illness management and the extent a family has developed routines and strategies to manage. Perceived consequences are views about the balance between illness management, other life aspects, and future implications (Knafl et al., 2012). Nurses can use the FMSF to realistically identify strengths and needs in chronic disease management.

The Family Health Model (FHM) discussed in earlier chapters uses an ecological view to identify interdependent factors linked with chronic illness. The model's three domains, contextual, functional, and structural, can be used to assess, plan coordinated care with multiple family members, identify appropriate nursing actions, and evaluate individual and family outcomes in different realms of family life (Denham, 2003). As you read about the Zimanskes' experience, consider ways the FHM can guide family thinking. For example, the family context enables the nurse to learn about the family household, financial concerns, needed member resources, transportation to medical visits, and community resources. Assessment of the functional domain helps the nurse learn about member roles, communication styles, family strengths, and ways the chronic condition influences member interactions. The structural aspect can help the nurse identify which usual family routines might be disrupted and plan new ones for managing the chronic illness. The FHM can guide nurses as they assist families in managing stress, developing resilience factors, and optimizing their family management style (Box 11.6). Nurses can use the FHM to collaborate with family units to manage care needs.

Diagnosis

For the Zimanske family, the diagnosis of SIOD affected every aspect of family life. Michael was small at birth, born 6 weeks prematurely, but otherwise considered healthy and normal. His size, sensitivity to light, and poor feeding were initially viewed as factors linked with early birth. His parents, Theresa and Don, and sister Jessica welcomed him with hope for a "normal" family experience in Minnesota's suburbs.

Michael was a healthy toddler, visited his primary care provider regularly for well-child checks, and had few minor illnesses. At his kindergarten checkup, the pediatrician noticed Michael had not grown since the last visit and ordered bone radiographs. Later that week, Michael visited his dentist and had x-ray films of his teeth, part of a normal dental evaluation. Noting abnormal development of Michael's teeth and jawbones, the dentist referred the family

---

BOX 11-6

Evidence-Based Practice and Chronic Conditions

Family-focused nurses realize that ideas about chronic care are based upon evidence. Consider these two examples:

1. What are the relationships between having a child with a chronic condition and family functioning?
   Based on a secondary data analysis from six independent studies, families of children with and without chronic conditions do not differ significantly from one another in the usual ways families manage daily activities. However, risk factors identified that seem to result in greater family difficulties when coping with chronic illness include older child age at diagnosis, fewer children in the home, and lower household income (Herzer et al., 2010).
2. Does family-centered care improve outcomes for children with chronic conditions and families?
   A systematic review of evidence related to families of children with chronic conditions found positive associations between family care and improved efficiency in service use, health status, satisfaction, access to care, communication, systems of care, ways families function, and family outcomes (Kuhlthau et al., 2011).

to the University of Minnesota Medical Center for further evaluation. A genetics consult led to additional tests and the discovery of proteinuria, suggesting abnormal kidney function. The geneticist found Michael's abnormal findings in several body systems that seemed unrelated. Standard genetic testing failed to identify any genetic conditions. The geneticist found Michael's abnormal findings in several body systems that seemed unrelated (Fig. 11.1).

THERESA: "From the age of 5 to 7, we were chasing separate issues that were like pieces of a puzzle that didn't fit. There were so many specialists, so many issues, and no one could figure out how they were connected. The challenge for us as a family was that each specialist was only seeing part of the picture. The nephrologist told us that Michael's kidney function was declining and he would probably eventually need a kidney transplant. The orthopedist focused on Michael's worsening hip pain and sent us all over the cities to see different bone specialists. Michael's geneticist said there must be some reason that all of this was happening to Michael and she was determined to find an answer."

As the geneticist traveled around the country to professional conferences, she made a point to ask physicians if they had seen a case like Michael's. Finally, at a conference in Texas, she met a research team who knew of a child with similar issues in Canada. This patient had been diagnosed with SIOD. After additional testing, Michael was finally diagnosed with SIOD at 7 years. Imagine the stress this family faced in 2 years of searching for a diagnosis. The diagnosis explained the medical issues, but the illness journey had just begun. Once Michael was diagnosed, his older sister and parents faced dramatic life changes (see Box 11.3).

Chronic Conditions and Ecological Perspectives

The Family Health Model (FHM) can help the nurse understand multiple interactive factors relevant to the Zimanske family's health concerns (Denham, 2003). This ecological perspective reminds us that family members have relationships within and outside the household and these interactions influence family health over time (Bronfenbrenner, 2005). This perspective allows nurses to identify interdependent family health factors linked with

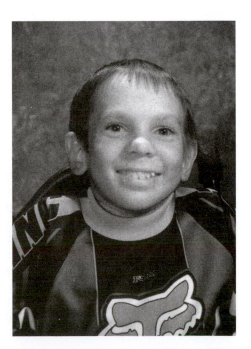

FIGURE 11-1 Michael: A child and family live with a chronic condition.

chronic conditions (Denham, 2003). The Zimanske family faced many frustrations in deal-ing with unconnected health care providers who never spoke to each other as they sought a diagnosis. Each was capable in their area of expertise, but they didn't connect the various symptoms. Family frustration and anxiety were high as they dealt with uncertainties from a growing pile of questions.

Other Factors Affecting Families With Chronically Ill Members

Most care for individuals with chronic conditions occurs in the home and community. When a medical model of care is used, illness care management focuses on prescribed med-ical regimens and adherence. From an ecological perspective, care management refers to daily life experiences. Family-focused care requires the nurse to consider ways care man-agement fits or does not fit into the family life and what negotiations are necessary (Baile, Tacchi, & Aaron, 2012; Sperry, 2011). Although families spend time with health profes-sionals, more time is spent in their household interacting with social networks within their community. Problems and decisions are often handled alone. Family nurses consider ways time is regularly organized and how activities, resources, responsibilities, and roles are used to manage the disease. Family members have many conflicting responsibilities and may lack needed resources or supports. Some families can experience a pileup of troubling fac-tors over time. For example, diabetes management requires altered meal schedules, food choices, physical activities, and medical care, and affects social aspects. If family members don't understand or refuse to support the member with a chronic disease, then this person may have more difficulty making the needed lifestyle changes.

Sociopolitical Factors

Social and political factors have influenced the ways families manage chronic conditions. Several poignant examples of issues that affect families raising children with chronic health conditions are available (Ray, 2003). For example, resources for management of certain conditions are often allocated based on eligibility criteria. Treatment for a mental health concern may require the family to paint an extremely dire picture that exaggerates, em-phasizes, or embellishes facts about behaviors. Often individuals cannot receive emergency mental health care unless the person is suicidal or threatening others.

Federal or state policies that budget for community-based services may affect care access for some persons with chronic conditions. Choices far removed from families' lives can sig-nificantly influence the availability of supports. Availability of health insurance or cash or access to health care professionals or specialists affects the care individuals receive. Often seemingly unrelated systems and processes affect families' abilities to care for their members.

Societal norms that recognize maternal caregivers may overlook roles of fathers or other caregivers of children with chronic conditions; they may be less visible and receive less sup-port (Ray, 2003). In the United States, although the Family and Medical Leave Act (FMLA) of 1993 requires large employers to provide employees job protection and unpaid leave for medical reasons, this is unevenly applied by states' parental leave policies. Employer's discretion could mean ineligibility for medical leave without losing your job. Laws have been unevenly applied for GLBT (gay, lesbian, bisexual, transsexual) persons, civil partners, foster or adoptive parents, and grandparents who provide care for those that are ill. Social and political contexts—from an ecological perspective—can influence ways families provide chronic care in different ways.

School attendance takes up a large part of children's days, a time when they are sepa-rated from the family household and subject to potentially different societal, physiological, and psychological pressures. School attendance can be affected in direct proportion to the severity and visibility of a chronic condition. The following are some of the factors influencing school experiences:

- Openness of teachers to learn about a child's needs
- Comfort of the school system to manage the child's condition
- Intensity of medication or treatment needs during the school day
- Child's abilities to participate with others
- Child's self-care needs (e.g., hygiene, meals, mobility, disruptive behaviors)
- Perceptions and tolerance for differences by teachers, school administration, and classmates
- Availability of health care assistance

Adults might experience similar concerns as they try to remain employed. Children and adults with medically complex conditions often require frequent medical visits to multiple providers. Absenteeism can mean falling behind in learning for children and job loss for an adult. This expensive care can be a financial burden to families. Care needs can hinder school attendance or cost lost work time.

Importance of School for Children With Chronic Conditions

Michael's ability to attend school and be with friends was important to his quality of life. Staying in school, as his condition progressed, was a growing challenge. As more severe neurological problems developed, he became less able-bodied. SIOD affects the vascular system and persons with this condition often develop arteriosclerosis and cerebral ischemia due to decreased blood flow to the brain. For Michael, this meant transient ischemic attacks (TIAs).

THERESA: "One day the school nurse called and told us that when Michael was writing, the pencil kept dropping out of his hand, and he was slurring his speech. We took him to the emergency department and found out he was having TIAs. This meant seeing a whole new set of specialists. He was put on new medication to prevent blood clots. The TIAs were minor and he quickly returned to normal after the attacks, but the TIAs were progressive. This is when everyone got scared to have him around. I thought, 'Should he be playing? Should he be going to school?' But we knew that for Michael's best quality of life, he needed to go to school and be with friends. I made a deal with the school. I quit my current job and found one closer to the school so I would never be more than 5 minutes away. If anything happened they could call me and I would be there. I was his transportation. He had to go to school."

Stigma Associated With Chronic Illnesses

Nurses who *think family* acknowledge the reality of social norms and stereotypes. Stigma is a predominant social attitude toward people who are different, including those with chronic conditions (Seligman & Darling, 2007). Some chronic conditions are more visible than others. For example, persons with mental illness experience stigma comparable to persons with AIDS or ex-convicts (Baldwin, Schultz, Rogers, & Rogers, 2011). Mental illness or cognitive disabilities make a person "stand out" due to unusual behaviors or speech. For example, persons with schizophrenia or psychosis may hear and respond to voices unseen by others. Those with cognitive disabilities may act younger than actual ages. Even some health professionals often hold more negative attitudes toward persons with disabilities (Seligman & Darling, 2007).

Stigma is a product of social norms and stereotypes. It affects families of individuals with chronic conditions by what has been described as "courtesy stigma" (Goffman, 1963).

BOX 11-7

Family Tree

Darunee Jongudomkarn, RN, PhD (Thailand)

Dr. Jongudomkarn is an Associate Professor in the Faculty of Nursing at Khon Kaen University in Thailand, and served as the director of the master's degree program in Family Nursing (2003–2010). In 2003, she led a study about the competency needs of family nursing and developed a curriculum to guide all master's level family nursing programs in Thailand. Her efforts successfully preserved the education and advanced practices of family nursing in Thailand. Her scholarly work with families focuses on pain management, quality of life, gender, and women's health. She has published an integrative review of family nursing interventions in Thailand as well as several other family nursing articles in the Thai language. She and her colleagues have developed the Khon Kaen University Pediatric Pain Assessment Tool, the Khon Kaen University Family Quality of Life Scale, and the Khon Kaen University Family Health Nursing Model. In 2003, Dr. Jongudomkarn established the Family Nursing Society of Thailand, one of only two national family nursing organizations in the world: http://www.thaifamilynurse .org/index.php/en/. This organization has over 300 members. In 2007, she was awarded an Innovative Contribution to Family Nursing Award from the *Journal of Family Nursing* at the Eighth International Family Nursing Conference to honor her foundational leadership in family nursing in Thailand.

This refers to avoidance, rejection, or ridicule that extends to others associated with a person who is viewed differently. Parents and siblings of children with disabilities may be viewed as troubled or burdened, or brave and courageous, by persons who have not met the family (Seligman & Darling, 2007). *Thinking family* implies being considerate of disparate appearances or actions and seeking understanding about the troubling aspects that encircle families when a member has chronic illness. It is important that nurses understand that families vary widely and things like cultural and the nation where one resides influences the ways nursing care is delivered (Box 11.7).

Facing Stigma in Daily Life

When he was in elementary school, Michael's skeletal issues with his hips became a focus around which he would plan his daily activities. THERESA: "Because of hip pain, he knew he could only walk a certain amount each day, so he would plan his day in the mornings before he got out of bed. He would slide around on the floor at home to save his ability to walk for school and other activities. Eventually he got a scooter. Then the Big Day came in fourth grade when he had to go to school in a wheelchair. He wanted his friends to treat him the same but it actually turned out to not be a big deal. One day I watched from a distance as Michael and his friends made their way down the school hallway. They were tripping all over him, laying on his chair and playing. I thought, 'I need to talk with the teachers and ask the kids to be careful around him.' One day I went to a playground and watched him. I could see his school friends saw Michael and not the wheelchair. This was a good thing. It was a learning process for all of us."

Family Functioning With a Chronically Ill Member

Using an ecological point of view helps us understand that when a member has a chronic condition family units must make adaptations to medical and lifestyle needs. Chronic conditions often alter relationships and roles. A mother with a chronic condition may not parent in ways others imagine. Family roles and responsibilities may be altered when a member has a chronic condition. Family nurses recognize that the person with chronic needs can influence family stress. Nurses who *think family* assess family processes, member interactions, and individual roles when planning nursing actions and working with individuals to set goals for care outcomes.

Theresa described a provider interaction: "As we were leaving the room, right after receiving the diagnosis, our doctor turned to us and said, 'I feel it's necessary to tell you that most marriages involved in chronic illness situations like this end in divorce.' I thought, what else? My husband and I didn't talk all the way home. We were overwhelmed with information." A misperception by some providers and families is that a member with a chronic condition is harmful to marriages and families (Eddy & Walker, 1999). In the 1980s, research about children with disabilities was guided by assumptions that a child with a chronic condition was tragic and detrimental to family health and marriage (Risdal & Singer, 2004). Some care providers still believe they assist families by preparing them for negative outcomes. However, current research underscores the idea that family responses to chronic conditions range widely with positive adaptations and strengthened families (Risdal & Singer, 2004). Nurses who focus on family strengths can be most helpful to families.

Providing Useful Nursing Actions

Stress can be associated with chronic conditions. Nurses who *think family* realize that the most effective way to support a family unit is by identifying strengths. These are used to identify strategies for adapting in the unique ways needed to manage chronic conditions. Theresa recommends using a positive approach to family members. For example, a nurse could say, "Through our discussions, I see you are a loving, supportive couple. I believe you will endure the challenges of this diagnosis." This recognizes the positive relationship strengths, commends the family, and lends hope for an uncertain future.

The family not only faces uncertainties with an initial chronic diagnosis, but must also deal with changes as the chronic condition shapes the developing person, family unit, and daily family life. Children with chronic conditions may not progress through typical stages and may fail to meet developmental milestones at the same pace as peers (Larkin, Jahoda, McMahon, & Pert, 2012). Chronic conditions can influence child development and physical or cognitive limitations (Friedman, Holmbeck, DeLucia, Jandasek, & Zebracki, 2009). Adults living with chronic conditions can experience similar concerns and need family supports. Future uncertainty can weigh heavily on a family's future. Healthy children aspire to leave the family home as they enter adulthood; children with chronic conditions may have different timelines. Leaving home and independence, particularly if the condition has cognitive or physical limitation issues, may be impossible for some children with chronic conditions and create great disabilities for older persons as well. The uncertainty of a chronic condition may interfere with things like activities of daily living, education and employment, caregiving tasks, and family vacations

Living With Optional Plans

THERESA: "With every planned event, we always had a plan B because of Michael's changing and progressive condition. His sister often took the brunt of this constantly altered activity. Our daughter grew accustomed to taking 'the back seat' in family decisions. Choosing where to sit at a Twins baseball game, we could not consider preferred seating because we had to sit in the wheelchair section. Family outings and vacation choices were made based on wheelchair accessibility. Even decisions about daily chores needed to be altered. Our daughter understood but at times she struggled with the fairness of the choices."

Life span developmental theory considers the timing of normal or usual developmental stages and identifies if the event occurrence is on-time or off-time (Mortimer, 2012). Transitions that do not occur at an expected time are considered off-time and might require special focus. Family development theory refers to transitions through normative events versus non-normative ones that might occur due to chronic conditions (Gavazzi, 2011). Chronic conditions can delay or alter family milestones. Launching is the time when families help young adults transition to independence; they marry, attend college, or acquire one's own apartment. If events can never occur or are off-time, they are viewed as non-normative. Family nurses can teach family members ways to plan for on-time and off-time transitions and milestones.

THERESA: "At age 5, Michael was the fastest runner on his T-ball team and by age 9 he was confined to a wheelchair. With chronic illness some things seem to stand still, frozen in time while other things are fast forwarded. The patient and family deal with both at the same time; wishing for what was and coping with what is. It was a delicate balance between allowing Michael to be age appropriate and attend events like school dances and a Friday night movie with friends, as we considered the "what-ifs" of his multilayered, life-limiting disease."

In families in which a child has a chronic condition, launching into adulthood can be delayed or complicated. In families in which an adult has a chronic condition, normative events such as retirement, grandparenting, or experiencing an "empty nest" might happen off-time or not at all. Daily life can be filled with unexpected things as activities are interrupted; frustration and conflict must be faced. Nurses who *think family* help them evaluate resource needs and support them through transitions, whether on-time or off-time.

Obstructed Routines of Families With Chronically Ill Members

An ecological perspective is useful in thinking about daily life in family households and ways systems can be supportive or threatening. The Family Health Model explains ways family health routines and rituals are important in daily life (Denham, 2003). A chronic condition often requires adaptation or modification of old routines and structuring of new ones. Some routines change dramatically and new ones must be created. Routines are habits or daily practices done regularly without conscious thought and it is hard to change things we do not think about. Routines are like our skin, we may not notice them until they are disrupted—they are part of usual life. They might be protective or give a sense of security or normality. Some chronic conditions call for radical changes that can seem as painful as removing skin. A family meal of fried chicken, mashed potatoes, gravy, and homemade biscuits for Sunday dinner may be the family tradition, a family health routine. This is more than a meal, it is part of family identity—what we do as a family. If dietary modifications are needed, then this routine and others might need to be altered. Routines can be underlying causes for chronic conditions, part of self-management, and very difficult to alter.

What family routine changes might be needed if an adult is diagnosed with type 2 diabetes? Is this different from a family with a child diagnosed with type 1 diabetes? What happens if a member must be fed through a gastrostomy tube or needs daily hemodialysis? What kinds of changes are called for in these families? Family-focused care uses intentional actions to assess, set goals, and plan daily routines. Routines have many threads, being woven from our culture, values, beliefs, attitudes, and motivation. Deconstruction of old routines and establishment of new ones must be planned in far greater detail than went into creating the original routine. Altering routines is a family matter that requires coordination and willingness to change. Family members usually want to help, but may not know the best things to do. In some families, members can be highly resistant, create temptations to ignore desired care needs, and even be subversive (Denham, Manoogian, & Schuster, 2007; Manoogian, Harter, & Denham, 2010). Some family members do not view the needed changes as their problem. Nurses who *think family* recognize these challenges and collaborate to identify the best ways to meet needs.

Reconstructing Family Health Routines

Nurses who *think family* focus on family health routines as they partner with families to set goals, plan actions, and reconstruct new life aspects to effectively address medical needs linked with chronic conditions. Individual-nurse-family collaboration can foster conversations around routines tied to dietary requirements or restrictions. Favoring a positive stance can help family units create action plans with measurable goals to achieve. For example, dietary changes are challenging and have deeply associated linkages with family lives. Food consumption revolves around beliefs and associated values and eating with others occurs regularly. It is a social activity and changes need to consider social aspects. Family meals are not easily altered. In order to make effective changes, families need information, skills, motivation, goals, and plans for action.

THERESA: "Social activities dramatically changed. Birthday party invites for Michael and sleepover events got complicated and eventually stopped. My friendships got limited because there wasn't free time. My husband worked overtime whenever possible to support us. This was especially important when I started working part-time to be home with Michael and took multiple leaves of absence without pay as his illness progressed. The disease meant Jessica had to handle things at home—phone calls, housekeeping chores, and others in my constant absence. Mother-daughter time with Jessica was altered because I was so often away with Michael. On Jessica's 16th birthday, I was at the hospital with Michael. My husband and I were consistently apart because of medical appointments. One year the flowers my husband bought for our wedding anniversary were delivered to the hospital because I was there with Michael.

The Zimanske family tried to maintain family routines that enabled them to manage Michael's condition and retain as much normality as possible. Michael played T-ball and golf with adaptations as his physical condition changed. He had to give up dreams to play football but learned to love wheelchair basketball. When he was in the hospital, Michael's sister attended social activities and church functions (Fig. 11.2). She had supportive relationships beyond the family." While adaptations were made, things were seldom easy.

Family Member Care for Self

THERESA: "Consistently I was told by medical providers that I needed to take care of myself. How could I do that? When Michael was in the hospital, most days the first opportunity for a meal was at night with only vending machines available. Often the only sleeping option was a plastic, not-so-easy-to-recline chair next to Michael's bed. My blanket was often a sheet from Michael's bed because I couldn't find anything else."

Nurses can anticipate some needs of the family, especially for those spending the night with a child, and help provide a healing environment each day. In the clinic, ask family members how many appointments they have that day. Be concerned about how much time they spend in the clinic. Stress affects family members' abilities to comprehend information and cope. Chronic fatigue can be masked but it adds barriers.

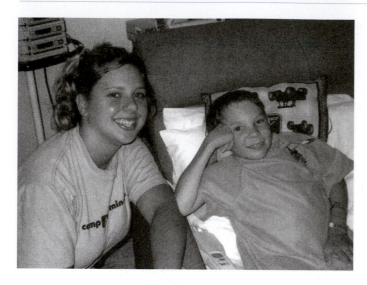

FIGURE 11-2 Michael and his sister Jessica.

The nurse who *thinks family* recognizes ways care environments limit family's abilities to continue family health routines. This requires more than passing suggestions; it requires intentional dialogue to ascertain needs. Caring for a chronically ill member puts others at risk for sleep deprivation, poor nutritional intake, fatigue, and general neglect of their physical, emotional, and social needs. Nurses who *think family* genuinely respect family's comfort needs and know some situations can be overwhelming. They know it is not always easy to ask for help. Care environments can look like well-oiled machines with clinicians continually attending to tasks. This might be mysterious and confusing as families seeking services erroneously interpret actions. Nurses can explain, show care and kindness, and communicate.

Family Stress and Uncertainty With Chronic Conditions

Family response to chronic conditions depends upon unique family unit factors (e.g., age of onset, course, outcome, degree of incapacitation, complications, supports). Chronic conditions can have acute onset, such as in congenital conditions or traumatic brain injury, or a gradual onset such as muscular dystrophy (Rolland & Walsh, 2006). The course of a chronic condition may be progressive, constant, continuous, relapsing, or episodic. Outcomes may result in comorbid conditions, a shortened life span, or death, or may not affect the life span at all. Disabilities can occur in cognition, movement, sensation, and social interactions. While many have few daily limitations from a chronic condition, others may have some form of stress and others have incapacitation of some degree. Coping and planning are affected by ambiguity about the future and the time that will elapse before things change (Rolland & Walsh, 2006). Family care addresses the diverse ways a specific condition manifests over time and the expressed needs of a particular family (Fig. 11.3). In the Zimanske family, Michael's illness had a gradual onset, and symptoms emerged over time as his condition worsened.

Living With a New Normal

THERESA: "Normal was like a roller-coaster during Michael's diagnostic process with many ups and downs. Normal abruptly stopped when the rare disease was named. There is nothing normal about a health care experience. Michael deserved and needed normal in

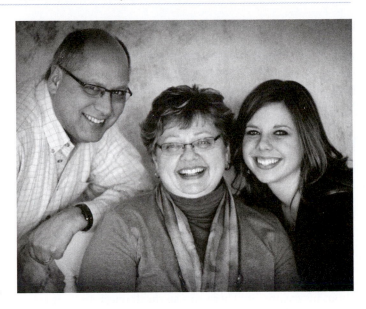

FIGURE 11-3 Michael's family.

the midst of abnormal. One of my roles was to provide him and my family with some normal. This meant medical providers had to help because we were most often in their environment and not ours. Patient-centered care coordination was vital to keeping some normality in our life. Sometimes medical providers pretended our life was normal and gave little thought about our needs. This often upset schedules. At times Michael was uncooperative because he felt unheard and not valued. Having blood draws three times a week isn't normal. Going to dialysis 4 days out of 7 is not normal. Michael needed medical providers to acknowledge and say to him, this is not normal. This is a big deal. I needed relationships I could trust and depend on to redefine normal."

Given the rare occurrence of Michael's condition, the family did not know what to expect. How long would he live? How would his changing conditions affect us? Michael's condition was progressively incapacitating and fatal. It was important for nurses to consider what uncertainty means to the family. Nurses who *think family* know they cannot always provide an answer or a solution, but honesty, trust, and availability to listen are important.

Living With a Fatal Diagnosis

THERESA: "Consider what the word fatal means to a family. Ask what questions we have. Uncertainty is lessened with honest conversation. Admitting uncertainties and limitations develops strong relationships between providers and family. Trust is needed. Sometimes medical providers made assumptions and judgments about us. We sometimes found out through frustrating conversations that some knew nothing about Michael's rare disease. Some admitted their limitations. For example, they might say, 'I never heard of this diagnosis' or 'I don't have any experience with this disease.' But if they made a promise to get educated, this suggested that they wanted to be our partner. Trusting your caregiver allows patients and families the freedom to admit their limitations and creates a relationship that contains no judgments or assumptions. It establishes an honest climate of 'I will give my best, but I'm not perfect' between persons in the health care relationship. Honesty becomes the one thing each can be certain of."

Nurses who *think family* avoid stereotypes and assumptions about family situations. These nurses are authentic, face situations, do not placate people with thoughtless actions, and welcome questions even when they lack answers. Nurses who *think family* reflect on what it must be like living in the other's shoes. They listen and help find needed information. Nurses who *think family* respect the experience of those receiving care and realize they have expert knowledge about the person receiving care. One's national origin has great influence on the ways family care is understood and important for nurses to recognize when caring for individuals that have immigrated from other places (Box 11.8).

Uncertainty

THERESA: "On Halloween, Michael developed an infection. We knew that if he had any fevers we had to catch it right away or the problem would become serious. That night we went to the emergency department, he was really sick. He had an infection and his kidneys were shutting down. He went to get an MRI (magnetic resonance imaging) scan and afterward he had a big stroke. He thought his name was Robert. They started talking about dialysis. They were trying to adjust his medications, but no one really knew what to do. SIOD is such a rare disease that there was no treatment guidance. It was a guessing game. They said they could 'try this' or 'try that,' but there were no guarantees. We were asked to make decisions about his treatment. There was so much uncertainty. It was horrible. That's when I learned I had to trust my gut. We were going on faith now and we had to trust in God."

"Michael's condition became increasingly unstable. He received dialysis and was in the hospital much of the time with unstable blood pressure, increasing numbers of strokes, and complications with fluid status. He attended school a few hours a day when he was not in the hospital. The school adjusted his individualized education plan (IEP) to lower expectations for his academic achievement. This is when things started to shift personally for us as a family. Now, the question was 'Will he survive?' We had to rethink how we were going to treat him medically, emotionally, and physically."

Although Michael's case is about a rare illness, similar things also happen with other more common chronic conditions. Uncertainty is characteristically a part of the experience. Letting families voice concerns, listening to what is said, and managing awkward silences are part of family care.

BOX 11-8
Family Tree

Margareth Angelo, RN, PhD (Brazil)

Dr. Margareth Angelo is a Professor and Director of the Department of Maternal-Child and Psychiatric Nursing at the University of São Paulo, Brazil. For over 20 years she has taught family nursing intervention and research methods to undergraduate and graduate students. She is the founder and coordinator of the Group of Studies on Family Nursing. This group brings together teaching, research, and clinical activities related to the family phenomena such as the health-illness situation, family nursing interventions, family nursing education, and qualitative research methods. Dr. Angelo has authored several book chapters and numerous articles published in national and international nursing journals. She has received awards and international recognition for her work in family nursing development in Brazil. Her academic work includes international exchange activities and research collaboration, developed as a visiting professor at universities in Latin America and Europe, and mentorship of graduate students from Portuguese- and Spanish-speaking countries. In 2010, she worked with others at the School of Nursing to host a First International Symposium on Family Nursing in São Paulo, Brazil. In 2012, she was elected to the Board of Directors for the International Family Nursing Association.

Hearing the Story

Families with members who have a chronic condition need nurses who understand the family's story. Families gain expertise over years of caring for members with chronic conditions. Some stories are not favorable. They tell of misunderstandings, confusion, lack of knowledge, failure, or other difficulties managing conditions. The best way to learn about living with a condition is to ask families to share their story. These actions are important and certainly aligned with providing competent nursing care, but they are not all that people seeking care expect. Hearing family stories provides a way to learn about an experience from the perspective of those who have lived with it. This point of view seeks to capture the larger perspective of many relevant things. Nurses who *think family* make time to hear the unique family experiences and are available to hear stories.

Forming Relationships

Nurses who *think family* ask questions: "What was it like for you when you learned about this diagnosis?" "How has your family managed to maintain normalcy?" Family nurses can listen to the telling of unique family stories that give clues about disease management and family needs. This takes time, but it helps build trust, encourages mutual understanding, and offers empathy. Building trust may not involve words. Consider Theresa's description:

THERESA: "What began as a watch-dog time period to ensure my son got a couple hours of uninterrupted sleep in the hospital turned into a life-altering situation. We were often in the hospital more than at home, and sleep became a treasured commodity. Michael's best sleep was from 5 a.m. to 7 a.m. However, he was often awakened for things that could easily be done later. So I started to place my chair outside the door of his hospital room during that time and monitored who and why they wanted to enter. I realized this was the only quiet time I got in a 24-hour period. So I used the time to read, pray, collect my thoughts, and prepare for the day ahead. Hospital nurses and staff would walk by; some said good morning and others just glanced at me. I'm sure many wondered what that woman in the hallway was doing. One morning a nurse who walked by me every morning brought her office chair and placed it next to mine in the hallway. She demonstrated that she saw me and my needs. She viewed a person, a woman burdened and in need of something more than the typical morning chit-chat. In the relationship we developed, she became a trusted friend and offered a few minutes of normal. Inside every disease are real people who need the medical community to assist them to remain in the world outside the hospital and clinic walls."

Asking the family to tell their story helps the nurse align care processes with family's perceived needs. Although nurses may define health as the absence of disease, a family of persons with chronic conditions may define health based on expectations. For example, Michael's confirmed diagnosis meant he would lose functions over time and a new family life trajectory needed to develop. Anticipatory guidance for a healthy 10-year-old includes increased independence over time. Anticipatory guidance for Michael's family likely varied from the norm as he grew older and experienced decreasing levels of independence.

THERESA: "Although we wanted to believe Michael's outcome would be different from the prognosis given, we had to quietly prepare for life without him. There is little way to prepare for such a tremendous loss. It means what some nurses would define as denial becomes a critical part of our coping. Some days we had to pretend our life was normal. Only in a relationship with us would you know we still talked with him about college, his hope to drive a big caterpillar on road construction, and his desire to marry. Our definition of Michael's health, physical and emotional, had a life-limiting scope, but we viewed each day through a lens of hope and possibility. Our realignment was painful, exhausting, and often confusing. It was important to discuss our spiritual beliefs with medical providers during ongoing and escalating needs."

Changing Perceptions

Time plays important roles in ways quality of life is understood. Research highlights the notion of response shift to chronic conditions as a reconceptualization in the meaning of an illness experience (Barclay-Goddard et al., 2012). This means that perception of well-being or life quality is different from others. For example, a man with a spinal cord injury may initially consider life quality low because he can't walk or function as he did before the injury. Over time, this situation may be reframed. A "good life" might be viewed as abilities to participate in family or social activities, times when one is pain free, or finding new life meanings through compassion and spirituality (Barclay-Goddard et al., 2012).

THERESA: "This disease abruptly invaded Michael's life. The rest of our life continued. The world events still continued around us. School activities continued. Our daughter's softball practices, her games—those continued. To me, his mother, it seemed as though one day I was buying him cleats for T-ball team and a few days later he was to be fitted for a wheelchair."

Being a healthy family before illness meant work, raising healthy children, and finding time for fun. After diagnosis, this family re-formed ideas of a healthy family to include Michael's changing condition. They learned to live with vulnerabilities and uncertainty in new ways. They found new meanings, celebrated successes, and rethought normal. Through many adaptations the family demonstrated they were a resilient family enduring the unmanageable and impossible.

Preparing For and Acknowledging Changes Over Time

Michael's renal status worsened and he needed a kidney transplant. Family members were evaluated as a suitable match for a kidney donor. Theresa was ruled out due to high blood pressure. His father discovered he had a mitral valve problem requiring heart surgery. His aunt was identified as a match and the planning for transplant began. Dates for the transplant were canceled due to Michael's medical status, infections, and cardiac instability.

THERESA: "Finally, a date was set for the transplant. It was a hopeful time. We battled to get to this point and it finally came. We walked in that day not knowing what would happen—it was stress times a million. My sister was in one operating room and my son in another. It was an amazing and fearful time. There is nothing to prepare a family for something like this. How do you thank someone for a gift like this? No Hallmark card that says 'Thanks for the kidney' exists. Michael and his aunt did well and were able to leave the hospital within a week."

If you were a nurse working with this family, what kinds of things would you say? Would you take time to listen as they shared fears and thankfulness? Family nurses learn to be with others during uncomfortable times. Being vulnerable is not easy but it can build trust and relationships.

Michael returned to school. However, the immunosuppressive medications required caused him to have frequent and more severe strokes. Nurses are often unaware of the severe side effects of antirejection drugs and the unique challenges faced by individuals and families after transplant and these drugs are taken. His immune system was suppressed or compromised, and he was no longer able to attend school.

THERESA: "This was a turning point for us. In my heart, I began to wonder, 'Is this the beginning of the end?' You get to a tipping point logically, where you know this little boy and his body can't sustain this. For the first time, I saw Michael giving up. He would say, 'I want to stay on the couch.' I would tell him how important it was to keep up his strength so that he could return to basketball. He said, 'I don't want to go back to basketball.' We were teetering between reality, hope, and possibility."

Michael's immune status worsened and he was not able to be in public without risking infection. The family was confined to minimize risk of infection exposure. Families go through difficult times filled with new risks, vagueness, and wariness.

THERESA: "We were grateful to be home as a family. Family and friends left food at the door but couldn't come inside. It was a sacred time for our family."

Nurses seldom hear the stories about what happens when families go home. Medical staff members seldom learn what occurs after discharge following successful organ transplant. Families are alone as they experience fears, diminished hopes, and frightening times.

Calling on Family Strengths

Resilience is positive functioning and maintenance of competence despite risk or adversity (Supkoff, Puig, & Sroufe, 2012). Identifying family strengths can help a family satisfy needs associated with chronic illness. For example, cancer is a disease of both young and old—yet, little is known how best to support extended families and grandparents as these emotional experiences are faced (Box 11.9). Family stories identify problem solving that has worked in the past. Rather than identify shortcomings, family nurses can identify positive observations and offer praise for successfully accomplishing tasks. Commendations involve the nurse "noticing, drawing forth, and highlighting previously unobserved, forgotten, or unspoken

---

BOX 11-9

Experiencing Cancer Within a Family

When a child experiences cancer, the family also experiences the illness. It is a family affair. Many children experience cancer and spend many days at inpatient settings. The many painful and invasive treatments are challenges. Family routines are disrupted, emotional distress occurs, member roles change, great uncertainty is faced, and financial hardship often happens. Families manage endless transitions as the child goes through various stages of treatment, illness trajectories, remissions, and relapse. Too often the effects of childhood cancer are not fully appreciative of the effects this illness also has on the family. A comprehensive program of family, psychological, and relational research was used in Alberta Children's Hospital in Calgary, Canada, to offer a collaborative intervention. The pediatric hematology/oncology/blood and marrow transplant program and the Faculty of Nursing at the University of Calgary formed a partnership that used research findings to influence the nursing curriculum. Relational implies that all human experience occurs within the context of relationships that are systemic and interactional. A large amount of literature about cancer exists; however, little has examined the experiences of grandparents of the diagnosed child. Grandparents have strong emotional experiences while they offer support but receive none themselves. Little was known about how care or practice could be effectively changed. This research is ongoing. Conflicting evidence has shown an equal number of studies find parents and family suffering as a result from the illness, while others do not find this true and find families are strengthened. Comprehensive study of relational factors is being undertaken to determine what causes results and what influences long-term care that families receive. This research and its findings are portals for changes in practice. Reducing the human suffering experienced from an illness condition such as childhood cancer should be part of the treatment plan. Finding better ways to make this happen is an important part of exceptional care guided by evidence-based practice.

family strengths, competencies, or resources" (Limacher & Wright, 2003, p. 132). Nurses who *think family* use commendations to encourage family, acknowledge strengths, and praise accomplishments.

Family nurses facilitate positive reframing of hurdles faced by families. They encourage family to talk about positive adaptations, meanings they are discovering in difficult situations, and ways hope is perceived. These are unique experiences. By asking open-ended questions, listening, and reflecting on what families say, nurses can gain new insights. What strengths are described? What kinds of nursing actions can be used to help families adapt? Nurses can acknowledge and help families celebrate thriving in difficult situations.

Overcoming Barriers During Chronic Illness

A common barrier with chronic illness is a tendency to focus on individual symptoms and problems. Individual- and problem-focused care often addresses things not at the top of the family's list of identified needs (Peyrot et al., 2005). A study of quality of life in children with quadriplegic cerebral palsy found that parents and providers had different views of what was most important to a child's quality of life (Morrow, Quine, Loughlin, & Craig, 2008). While professionals focused on weight gain, families focused on the child feeling loved. In the study, health professionals referred to burdens of the child's condition on parents, whereas parents viewed the child's condition as a part of life and a source of joy despite anxieties generated (Morrow et al., 2008). Ask questions about family priorities.

Empowerment

Over time, the amount of trust and decision making families and nurses share will change. Family empowerment is an interactive process that mobilizes resources to satisfy needs (Box 11.10). Empowerment involves nonjudgmental collaboration and willingness to shift responsibilities over time at the pace most appropriate from a family's perspective (Hulme, 1999). Families often have a high level of dependence on health professionals. The Zimanske family was unfamiliar with the condition and overwhelmed with the diagnosis. They left the hospital in a state of disbelief and emotional shock. They needed information in small doses and follow-up from the providers. Family needs time to think things over, react, and grieve. The pace of information delivery is often based on care providers' needs rather than family need. Unfortunately, busy medical practices and time-focused clinicians usually give all information at once. Little time is allotted for questions or responses. Families face critical news and are sent on their way still in shock. Care management changes, complications occur, and exacerbations bring new questions. Nurses often assume people know what to do. But many are poorly taught about conditions, and information is not parceled as needed, but given as a single giant dose.

The participatory phase of family empowerment is a challenging time as the balance of power is shifted to the family. The nurse questions the family about their needs as the condition progresses. Individuals with a chronic condition and their families become experts and know more about some things than clinicians. A successful shift in this balance of power requires nurses to listen, reflect, and collaborate.

In the collaboration phase, the family is encouraged to become assertive and less reliant on health professionals (Hulme, 1999). Family can independently negotiate roles and responsibilities in family life. The family begins to normalize the chronic condition and adapt. Families might move through empowerment steps in a nonlinear fashion. Nurses who *think*

BOX 11-10

Four Phases of Empowerment

Research with families dealing with chronic conditions suggests that many families progress through these four phases of empowerment:

- Professional dominated empowerment
- Participatory empowerment
- Challenging empowerment
- Collaborative empowerment

Source: Hulme, P. A. (1999). Family empowerment: A nursing intervention with suggested outcomes for families of children with a chronic health condition. *Journal of Family Nursing, 5*(1), 33–50.

---

family are tuned to family's actions, reactions, words, and requests as medical expertise and family expertise are combined.

Care Coordination

A challenging barrier to family-focused care and chronic illness management is the fragmentation of care delivery. Various care systems, numerous specialists, and little communication among providers cause care management to be puzzling and exhausting for families. Families need assistance with care coordination. It might help to schedule visits to multiple specialists in the same facility on the same day rather than scheduling multiple returns. Family case managers can help navigate systems and manage care needs such as acquisition and management of equipment, medication adherence, appointment coordination, and efficient use of resources. Families managing chronic conditions need empowering partnerships that put them at the helm of disease and life management.

Various definitions of care coordination make discussion of the topic a challenge (McDonald, Sundarum, Bravata, & Lewis, 2007). We discuss care coordination through a family nursing lens and use nursing processes. Thinking family reminds us that care coordination begins with assurance that family is an active participant. Coordinated care implies that roles pertinent to needs are effectively communicated and information about methods for performing self-care management tasks is provided. Nurses who *think family* develop family relationships that effectively coordinate care. Things like family identity, cultural preferences, self-care abilities, motivation, and personal beliefs affect care management. Collaboration is needed to ensure that gaps or care duplication is avoided. Competing plans increase the risks of treatment errors and poor outcomes.

Care coordination recognizes that meeting with clinicians is disruptive and plays havoc with daily lives. Although medical visits are essential, they are not easily handled. Information from practitioners often differs. Sometimes it seems that the left hand does not know what the right is doing. Optimal coordination involves synchronizing treatments, medical visits, and medications to meet individual and family needs.

THERESA: "Care coordination worked well with Michael's primary pediatric clinic. From the time of diagnosis they wanted to be the liaison between multispecialty care the syndrome demanded. We developed a specific protocol for appointments, which gave stability to weekly and sometimes daily laboratory draws and security in emergency scenarios. That gave us more family time at home, less time on the road, and more normal routines and schedules. Care coordination didn't go well between the specialty care departments and was a big challenge. Each specialty operated independent of the other and did not serve Michael as a patient or us as a family. It should flow as a team from one to another, each area of care taking responsibility and using their medical expertise and injecting that into the total collaborative process."

Family-focused care coordination should minimize visits or schedule them in ways that best fit the family schedule. This might mean negotiating appointments so a child can attend soccer practice or enable a father or grandparent to attend clinic appointments. Nurses who *think family* know communication about care needs must be family communication. Setting reasonable and manageable goals for families is more than doctor visits, treatment, and medicine.

Family Difficulties in Changing Routines

Individuals and families are concerned with symptom control, clinical progress, and usual routines. Life schedules need to accommodate prescribed treatments so they improve quality of life. Adults with heart disease may need to decrease work, assume a less stressful job, or exercise to improve cardiac health. Persons with diabetes may need their family to support them by altering family health routines, physical activity, and medical management. Not all family members may be supportive and not all families are well organized and positively functioning. Changes increase stress if they alter finances, reduce personal time, alter dietary choices, or limit social life. Families are not always willing to alter personal lifestyles, especially when they don't understand reasons. Lifetime changes can be viewed as burdens. The weight of caregiving can fall on single persons. Nurses can't solve family problems, but they can give appropriate help and useful support. *Thinking family* means helping with integration of new family health routines, accessing needed resources, and setting goals for the most effective care outcomes.

Caring for the Caregivers of Those With a Chronic Illness

THERESA: "I had a routine mammogram that indicated changes. I received a call one afternoon from the gynecologist. Michael came into the kitchen, where I was talking on the phone. He could tell by my face that something was wrong, and he thought it was bad news about him. I put the phone down and said, 'Michael, it's okay—it's not about you.' Then the news hit me: I had breast cancer. I thought, 'Now what am I going to do?' I hung up the phone and told Michael about it first. He said, 'Now I can take care of you, Mom.'"

Theresa had a double mastectomy and a series of surgeries to repair a skin flap. She was unable to physically care for Michael for several months because of the recovery process and pain from these surgeries.

THERESA: "It was a time that our family really needed a strong partnership with care providers. We lived in deep fear. It was especially hard for Jessica. She was 16 and dealing with her brother's progressive condition, her mother's breast cancer, and her father's heart condition. There was much emotion in our home—it became unrecognizable as our home because we are not like that as a family. I dug my heels in deeper. 'This will not be us!' As a family, we committed to getting through this. We needed a commitment from our care providers that they would be with us through the process."

Caregiver fatigue is a barrier to care with chronic illness. Caregivers experience caregiving difficulties and emotional pain. This has been called compassion fatigue in the literature and occurs when an empathic relationship results in a psychological response to progressive and deep-seated stress to prolonged care needs and exhaustion in the caregiver (Lynch & Lobo, 2012). Self-care is important for caregivers. Family nurses can help caregivers anticipate the long haul of chronic illness and help them prepare mentally and practically for future needs (Rolland & Walsh, 2006). Chronic illness is often in the foreground of family life.

THERESA: "In January 2005, Michael developed a fever. He knew when his temperature got to a certain point, we had to go to the hospital. He said, 'I'll do whatever it takes to stay home tonight.' I think he knew that this would be his last night at home—I saw a resolve in him, and there was no fear. I recall him sitting in front of the television watching cartoons with a cool towel on his head, eating popsicles to keep his temperature down until morning. We knew he would be admitted in the morning and it was serious. That night I went into his bedroom and sat on his bed. I had drain tubes in from my surgery. I just stared at him. He woke up and said, 'What are you doing?' 'Just checking,' I said. That was the last night he was home—he never came home again. He was admitted to the hospital for treatment of a severe infection."

Theresa stayed at his bedside. Don went to work. Jessica continued school. After a month passed, it was determined Michael needed a bone marrow transplant and chemotherapy. He went into the operating room for a procedure.

THERESA: "Don and I were in the waiting room when a nurse came out of the operating room to tell us that Michael had a massive heart attack on the table just as the procedure started. They had resuscitated him, but they feared that in the process he had a stroke and they were not sure he would survive. They told us to call anyone who wants to see him and tell them to be here within the hour. We called Jessica and other family members. My family took turns staying with us, holding vigil. Michael survived the day but never woke up. We ultimately decided to stop treatment and he was peaceful."

Michael died at the age of 13 years. Since his death, Theresa has spent time in a program she calls Be the Change. Through this program she shares her story with nurses, medical students, physicians, and anyone who will listen. She is a strong advocate for what families need when a member has a chronic illness. Learn more about her, Michael, and their family story at her Web site <http://bethechangemn.com/>.

Chapter Summary

Theresa notes, "I believe that when health care providers see and hear the real human beings that are involved in the medical story, a stronger connection is made." Family-focused care in chronic conditions requires nurses to see and hear the people experiencing the condition. The family is always intricately connected to chronic conditions that last for years. Nurses who *think family* understand the connected relationships between family units, their household, and communities as chronic conditions are managed. Family nurses give intentional attention to supporting the family to plan goals and develop strategies linked with conditions. Prior lifestyles are interrupted and new ways need to be structured to meet disease and family needs. Family nurses use coordinated care to meet needs linked with the changes over time as living with the condition evolves. Nurses listen to the family's story, respect their expertise, and form partnerships with them. Thinking family assists families household members to best manage long-standing situations over time.

Chapter Recognitions

Early work on Chapter 11 was initiated by Wendy Looman, PhD, RN, CNP, an Associate Professor at the School of Nursing at the University of Minnesota in Minneapolis. Dr. Looman has great expertise and extensive scholarship in areas of special health care needs of children. Mary Erickson, DNP, RN, CNP, a long-time employee at Children's Hospitals and Clinics of Minnesota, also made important contributions. A special expression of gratitude is owed to Theresa Zimanske for generously sharing her family story about Michael and allowing us to share how his chronic condition warranted family-focused care.

REFERENCES

American Nurses Association (2010). *Nursing's social policy statement: The essence of the profession.* Silver Spring, MD: Nursesbooks.org.

Angell, R. C. (1936). *The family encounters the depression.* New York: Charles Scribner.

Antonovsky, A. (1979). *Health, stress, and coping.* San Francisco: Jossey-Bass.

Ary, D. V., Toobert, D., Wilson, W., & Glasgow, R. E. (1986). Patient perspectives contributing to nonadherence to diabetes regimen. *Diabetes Care, 9*(2), 168–172.

Baile, W. F., Tacchi, P., & Aaron, J. (2012). What professionals in healthcare can do: Family caregivers as members of the treatment team. In R. C. Talley, R. McCorkle, & W. F. Baile (Eds.), *Cancer caregiving in the United States. Research, practice, policy* (Pt. 1, pp. 103–124). New York: Springer. doi 10.1007/978-1-4614-3154-1_6

Baldwin, M. L., Schultz, I. Z., Rogers, S., & Rogers, E. S. (2011). Stigma, discrimination, and employment outcomes among persons with mental health disabilities. doi:10.1007/978-1-4419-0428-7_3. Retrieved from http://www.springerlink.com/content/uj14117168838407/fulltext.pdf

Baradaran-Heravi, A., Morimoto, M., Lucke, T., & Boerkoel, C. F. (2011). Schimke immunoosseous dysplasia. *Gene Reviews.* Retrieved July 24, 2012 from http://www.ncbi.nlm.nih.gov/books/NBK1376/

Barclay-Goddard, R., King, J., Dubouloz, C., & Schwartz, C. E. (2012). Building on transformative learning and response shift theory to investigate health-related quality of life changes over time in individuals with chronic health conditions and disability. *Archives of Physical Medicine and Rehabilitation, 93*(2), 214–220. doi:10.1016/j.apmr. 2011.09.010

Beeber, A. S., & Zimmerman, S. (2012). Adapting the family management style framework for families caring for older adults with dementia. *Journal of Family Nursing, 18*(1), 123–145. doi: 10.1177/1074840711427144

Bethell, C., Kogan, M. D., Strickland, B. B., Schor, E. L., Robertson, J., Newacheck, P. W. (2011). A national and state profile of leading health problems and health care quality for US children: Key insurance disparities and across-state variations. *Academic Pediatrics, 11*, S22–S33.

Boerkoel, C. F., Takashima, H., Stankiewicz, P., Garcia, C. A., Leber, S. M., Rhee-Morris, L., & Lupski, J. R. (2001). Periaxin mutations cause recessive Dejerine-Sottas neuropathy. *American Journal of Human Genetics, 68*(2), 325–333.

Boss, P. (1988). *Family stress management.* Thousand Oaks, CA: Sage.

Boss, P. (2000). *Ambiguous loss: Learning to live with unresolved grief.* Cambridge, MA: Harvard University Press.

Bronfenbrenner, U. (2005). The bioecological theory of human development. In U. Bronfenbrenner (Ed.), *Making human beings human: Bioecological perspectives on human development* (pp. 3–15). Thousand Oaks: Sage.

Capen, C. L., & Dedlow, R. (1998) Discharging ventilator-dependent children: A continuing challenge. *Journal of Pediatric Nursing, 13*(3), 175–184.

Cavan, R. S., & Ranck, K. H. (1938). *The family and the Depression.* Chicago: University of Chicago Press.

Chen, H-Y., Baumgardner, D. J., & Rice, J. P. (2011). Health-related quality of life among adults with multiple chronic conditions in the United States, Behavioral Risk Factor Surveillance System. *Preventing Chronic Disease, 8*(1), A09. Retrieved from http://www.cdc.gov/pcd/issues/2011/jan/09_0234.htm

Child and Adolescent Health Measurement Initiative (2012). Exploring health conditions in the 2009/10 NS-CSHCN. Data Resource Center, supported by Cooperative Agreement

1_U59_MC06980_01 from the U.S. Department of Health and Human Services, Health Resources and Services Administration (HRSA), Maternal and Child Health Bureau (MCHB).

Clifford, G. D., & Clifton, D. (2012). Wireless technology in disease management and medicine. *Annual Review of Medicine, 63*, 479–492. doi:10.1146/annurev-med-051210-114650

Cohen, E., Kuo, D. Z., Agrawal, R., Berry, J. G., Bhagat, S. K., Simon, T. D., & Srivastava, R. (2011). Children with medical complexity: An emerging population for clinical and research initiatives. *Pediatrics, 127*(3), 529–538.

Cramer, J. A. (2004). A systematic review of adherence with medications for diabetes. *Diabetes Care, 27*(5), 1218–1224.

Cystic Fibrosis Foundation Patient Registry: Annual data report 2010. Retrieved on June 25, 2012 from http://www.cff.org/

Denham, S. A. (2003). *Family health: A framework for nursing.* Philadelphia: F. A. Davis.

Denham, S. A., Manoogian, M., & Schuster, L. (2007). Managing family support and dietary routines: Type 2 diabetes in rural Appalachian families. *Families, Systems, & Health, 25*(1), 36–52.

Eddy, L. L., & Walker, A. J. (1999). The impact of children with chronic health problems on marriage. *Journal of Family Nursing, 5*(1), 10–32.

Fogt, E. J., Dodd, L. M., Jenning, E. M., & Clemens, A. H. (1978). Development and evaluation of a glucose analyzer for a glucose-controlled insulin infusion system (Biostator). *Clinical Chemistry, 24*(8), 1366–1372.

Friedman, D., Holmbeck, G. N., DeLucia, C., Jandasek, B., & Zebracki, K. (2009). Trajectories of autonomy development across the adolescent transition in children with spina bifida. *Rehabilitation Psychology, 54*(1), 16–27.

Gavazzi, S. M. (2011). Family development theory. In S. M. Gavazzi (Ed.), *Families with adolescents.* New York: Springer. doi:10.1007/978-1-4419-8246-9_3

Goffman, E. (1963). *Stigma: Notes on the management of spoiled identity.* Englewood Cliffs, NJ: Prentice Hall.

Halfon, N., & Newacheck, P. W. (2010). Evolving notions of childhood chronic conditions. *Journal of the American Medical Association, 303*(7), 665–666. doi:10.1001/jama. 2010.130

Hayes, C., Naylor, R., & Egger, G. (2012). Understanding chronic pain in a lifestyle context: The emergence of a whole-person approach. *American Journal of Lifestyle Medicine, 6*(2), 421–428. doi:10.1177/1559827612439282

Herzer, M., Godiwala, N., Hommel, K. A., Driscoll, K., Mitchell, M., Crosby, L. E., . . . Modi, A. C. (2010). Family functioning in the context of pediatric chronic conditions. *Journal of Developmental and Behavioral Pediatrics, 31*(1), 26–34.

Hill, R. (1949). *Families under stress.* New York: Harper & Row.

Hulme, P. A. (1999). Family empowerment: A nursing intervention with suggested outcomes for families of children with a chronic health condition. *Journal of Family Nursing, 5*(1), 33–50.

Institute of Medicine. (2012). *Living well with chronic illness: A call for public health action.* Washington, DC: National Academy of Sciences.

Jardine, E. (1998). Core guidelines for the discharge of the child on long term assisted ventilation in the United Kingdom. *Thorax, 53*, 762–767.

Knafl, K. A., & Deatrick, J. A. (2003). Further refinement of the Family Management Style Framework. *Journal of Family Nursing, 9*(3), 232–256.

Knafl, K. A., Deatrick, J. A., & Havill, N. L. (2012). Continued development of the family management style framework. *Journal of Family Nursing, 18*(1), 11–34. doi:10.1177/1074840711427294

Kuhlthau, K. A., Bloom, S., Van Cleave, J., Knapp, A. A., Romm, D., Klata, K., . . . Perrin, J. M. (2011). Evidence for family-centered care for children with special health care needs: A systematic review. *Academic Pediatrics, 11*(2), 136–143.

Kung, H. C., Hoyart, D. L., Xu, J., & Murphy, S. L. (2008). Deaths: Final data for 2005. *National Vital Statistics Report, 56*(10). Retrieved July 23, 2012 from http://www.cdc.gov/nchs/data/nvsr/nvsr56/nvsr56_10.pdf

Larkin, P., Jahoda, A., McMahon, K., & Pert, C. (2012). Interpersonal sources of conflict in young people with mild to moderate intellectual disabilities at transition from adolescence to adulthood. *Journal of Applied Research in Intellectual Disabilities, 25*, 29–38.

Lazarus, R. S. (1993). Coping theory and research: Past, present, and future. *Psychosomatic Medicine, 55*, 234–247.

Limacher, L. H., & Wright, L. M. (2003). Commendations: Listening to the silent side of a family intervention. *Journal of Family Nursing, 9*, 130–150.

Lucke, T., Tsikas, D., Kanzelmeyer, N. K., Boerkoel, C. F., Clewing, J. M., Vaske, B., Ehrich, J.H., & Das, A. M. (2006). Vaso-occlusion in Schimke-immuno-osseous dysplasia: Is the NO pathway involved? *Hormone and Metabolic Research, 38*(10), 678–682.

Lynch, S. H., & Lobo, M. L. (2012). Compassion fatigue in family caregivers: A Wilsonian concept analysis. *Journal of Advanced Nursing, 68*(9), 2125–2134 (online issue). doi:10.1111/j.1365-2648.2012.05985.x

Manoogian, M. M., Harter, L. M., & Denham, S. A. (2010). The storied nature of health legacies in the familial experience of type 2 diabetes. *Journal of Family Communication, 10*, 1–17.

Maeng, D. D., Martsolf, G. R., Scanlon, D. P., & Christianson, J. B. (2012). Care coordination for the chronically ill: Understanding the patient's perspective. *Health Services Research, 47*(5), 1960–1979. doi:10.1111/j.1475-6773.2012.01405.x

Margolan, H., Fraser, J., & Lenton, S. (2004) parental experience of services when their child requires long-term ventilation: Implications for commissioning and providing services. *Child: Care, Health & Development, 30*(3), 257–264.

McCubbin, M. A., & McCubbin, H. I. (1989). Families coping with illness: The resiliency model of family stress, adjustment and adaptation. In C. B. Danielson, B. Hamel-Bissel, & P. Winstead-Fry (Eds.), *Families, health & illness: Perspectives on coping and intervention*. St. Louis: Mosby.

McDonald, K. M., Sundarum, V., Bravata, D. M., & Lewis, R. (2007). Closing the quality gap: A critical analysis of quality improvement strategies. *Care Coordination* (Vol 7). Report No. 04(07(0051-7). Rockville, MD: Agency for Healthcare Research and Quality

Morrow, A. M., Quine, S., Loughlin, E. V. O., & Craig, J. C. (2008). Different priorities: A comparison of parents' and health professionals' perceptions of quality of life in quadriplegic cerebral palsy. Archives of Diseases in Childhood, 93, 119–125. doi:10.1136/adc.2006.115055

Mortimer, J. T. (2012). The evolution, contributions, and prospects of the Youth Development Study: An investigation in life course social psychology. *Social Psychology Quarterly, 75*(1), 5–27.

Moules, N. J., Laing, C., Morck, A., & Toner, N. (2011). Stepping into the middle: Family research in pediatric oncology. In E. K. Svavarsdottir & H. Jonsdottir (Eds.), *Family nursing in action* (pp. 271–284). Reykjavik, Iceland: University of Iceland.

Noyes, J. (2007). Comparison of ventilator-dependent child reports of health-related quality of life with parent reports and normative populations. *Journal of Advanced Practice Nursing, 58*(1), 1–10.

National Institutes of Health. (2014). Schimke immune-osseous dysplasia. Retrieved September 4, 2014 from **ghr.nlm.nih.gov**/condition/**schimke-immuno-osseous-Dysplasia**

Patterson, J. (1988). Families experiencing stress: The family adjustment and adaptation response model. *Family Systems Medicine, 5*(2), 202–237.

Peyrot, M., Rubin, R. R., Lauritzen, T., Snoek, F. J., Matthews, D. R., & Skovlund, S. E. (2005). Psychosocial problems and barriers to improved diabetes management: Results of the crossnational Diabetes Attitudes, Wishes, and Needs (DAWN) Study. *Diabetic Medicine, 22*, 1379–1385.

Ray, L. D. (2003). The social and political conditions that shape special-needs parenting. *Journal of Family Nursing, 9*(3), 281–304.

Rempel, G. R., Blythe, C., Rogers, L. G., & Ravindran, V. (2012). The process of family management when a baby is diagnosed with a lethal congenital condition. *Journal of Family Nursing, 18*(1), 35–64. doi:10.1177/1074840711427143

Risdal, D., & Singer, G. H. (2004). Marital adjustment in parents of children with disabilities: A historical review and meta-analysis. *Research & Practice for Persons with Severe Disabilities, 29*(2), 95–103.

Rolland, J. S., & Walsh, F. (2006). Facilitating family resilience with childhood illness and disability. *Current Opinion in Pediatrics, 18*, 527–538.

Seligman, M., & Darling, R. B. (2007). Effects on the family. In M. Seligman & R. B. Darling (Eds.), *Ordinary families, special children* (3rd ed., pp. 181–217). New York: Guilford.

Selye, H. (1976). *The stress of life* (rev. ed.). New York: McGraw-Hill.

Simon, J. B., Murphy, J. J., & Smith, S. M. (2005). Understanding and fostering family resilience. *The Family Journal, 13*(4), 427–436. doi:10.1177/1066480705278724

Smith, S. M., Soubhi, H., Fortin, M., & O'Dowd, T. (2012). Interventions for improving outcomes in patients with multimorbidity in primary care and community settings (review). *Cochrane Database of Systematic Reviews, 4*, CD006560. doi:10.1002/14651858.CD006560.pub2

Sperry, L. (2011). Spiritually competent practice with individuals and families dealing with medical conditions. *The Family Journal, 19*(4), 412–416. doi:10.1177/1066480711417236

Supkoff, L. M., Puig, J., & Sroufe, L. A. (2012). Situating resilience in developmental context. In M. Ungar (Ed.), *The social ecology of resilience: A handbook of theory and practice* (pp. 127–142). New York: Springer. doi:10.1007/978-1-4614-0586-3_12

Tennant, P. W., Pearce, M. S., Bythell, M., & Rankin, J. (2010). 20-year survival of children born with congenital anomalies: A population-based study. *Lancet, 375*, 649–656. doi:10.1016/S0140-6736(09)61922-X

Venter, A., Burns, R., Hefford, M., & Ehrenberg, N. (2012). Results of a telehealth-enabled chronic care management service to support people with long-term conditions at home. *Journal of Telemedicine and Telecare, 18*, 172–175.

Walsh, F. (2012). Facilitating family resilience: Relational forces for positive youth development in conditions of adversity. *Social Ecology of Resilience, 4*, 173–185. doi:10.1007/978-1-4614-0586-3_15

West, C., Usher, K., & Foster, K. (2011). Family resilience: Towards a new model of chronic pain management. *Collegian, 18*(1), 3–10.

Wiegand, D. L. (2012). Family management after the sudden death of a family member. *Journal of Family Nursing, 18*(1), 146–163. doi:10.1177/1074840711428451

World Health Organization (2002). Innovative care for chronic conditions: Building blocks for action: Global report. Geneva: WHO.

CHAPTER 12

Family-Focused Care to Meet Population Needs

Sue Ellen Bell • Kelly Krumwiede

CHAPTER OBJECTIVES

1. Compare and contrast individual, family, and population-based health care.
2. Apply an ecological lens to identify multiple levels of health risks associated with human health.
3. Identify the relationships between population-based health and vulnerable populations, health disparities, and social determinants of health.
4. Explore societal health challenges from multiple perspectives.
5. Analyze the evidence that supports the need for population-based care.

CHAPTER CONCEPTS

- Department of Health and Human Services
- Distributive justice
- Environmental health
- Government regulations
- Health care costs
- Health disparities
- Health equity
- Health Resources and Services Association
- Healthy People Initiative
- Indian Health Service
- Medicaid
- Medicare
- Population health
- Prevention
- Social justice
- State Children's Health Insurance Program
- Surgeon General
- Vulnerability

Introduction

The culture in the United States is strongly influenced by individualism and competition, but it is also useful to understand the importance of population needs. Population needs pertain to those of the larger society. Families are made up of individuals who live in neighborhoods, communities, and larger societies. An ecological lens can help identify the many interactions and interdependent complexities of populations, society, and people. All are dynamic. They are affected by many environmental risks (e.g., natural hazards, disasters, legislative policies, politics). Distributive justice, government regulations, professional guidelines, standards of care, health promotion, prevention, and at-risk groups are all linked with population health. Social determinants of health, culture, vulnerable populations, and disparities also influence health and illness.

Individual care is tailored to meet the unique health needs of one person and generally aims at cure. Medical care addresses diagnosis, treatment, and rehabilitative options performed by physicians and health care practitioners and uses pharmaceuticals, treatments, radiation, and surgery to achieve results. Care evaluation generally involves measuring satisfaction levels and seeing if treatments improved health. Although these findings are useful for individuals, they do not solve population problems. Health care delivery tends to focus on provision of medical services and payments for individual disease treatment with little focus on the impact of the environment or society on families or their communities. This chapter explores ways the lives of individuals and families intersect with the larger society. Some relevant ideas introduced in Chapter 3 are built on in this chapter. Instead of thinking about health care as "fixing" problems, this chapter considers ways to prevent them.

A Brief History of Population Health in the United States

Since the late 1800s, medicine and medical education have been focused primarily on the internal environments of care. Diagnostic tools such as the stethoscope, radiograph, microscope, spirometer, electrocardiograph, and chemical or bacterial tests allowed body assessment (Starr, 1982). Treatments were a few effective medications, immunizations, and surgery. Little medical information was available to nonmedical persons. The American Medical Association asserted its influence and physician authority was the rule. Nurses' practice was directed by physician orders. Tasks (e.g., medication delivery, injections, intravenous fluids, vital signs, documentation) were their primary work. Independent nursing actions were few. Nurses attended to activities of daily living and provided physical or psychological comfort measures. Patients were dependent on the medical team for all cures.

In 1945, the Hill-Burton Act, a law signed by President Truman, appropriated funds for building hospitals across the nation. Long underserved people such as African Americans began to demand health care equity; it was 1963 before hospitals in the South were required to treat black persons. Nurses started to focus on cultural differences and varied responses among those getting care. After World War II and the Vietnam War, new immigrants came to the United States. These immigrants held health care beliefs at odds with the Western views of health and treatments for illness (Bell & Whiteford, 1987; Fadiman, 1997; Tripp-Reimer & Thieman, 1981). Since the 1990s, the push has been for equal health care outcomes, not just equal access (Shi & Stevens, 2010).

Transitions in Caring Practices

Nurses discovered that applying the same interventions to all individuals regardless of culture did not result in the same health outcomes. Nurses began to develop ethnonursing methods (Leininger, 1970, 1990; Tripp-Reimer, 1982), a way to see cultural influences and treat people differently. Cultural competence is now an essential skill for nurses and researchers have found various ways to measure it (Schim, Doorenbos, Miller, & Benkert, 2003). Cultural safety assures accessible and equitable health care for all, as power differences cause health beliefs and behaviors to affect care delivery (Papps & Ramsden, 1996; Polaschek, 1998; Richardson & Carryer, 2005). The social context of illness and health includes system level factors (e.g., politics, government, religion, economics) that cause disadvantages for some (Powers & Faden, 2006; Shi & Stevens, 2010). Politics and power influence health and illness, so blame shouldn't be placed entirely on the victim of ill health (Doutrich, Arcus, Dekker, Spuck, & Pollock-Robinson, 2012).

Medical Interventions

Rates of surgical and medical interventions have varied geographically; studies of this type are called area studies (Song et al., 2010). Medical care is often influenced by availability of hospital beds, numbers and types of practitioners, and access to imaging machines (Baker, Fisher, & Wennberg, 2008; Wennberg, Bronner, Skinner, Fisher, & Goodman, 2009). A study of physicians in Morrisville, Vermont, found that they performed tonsillectomies more often than others in the state. Tightened constraints on tonsillectomies significantly lowered the rate. Rates of carotid endarterectomies, cesarean sections, and hysterectomies also differed geographically. For example, coronary angiography was performed at a 53% higher rate in Florida than Colorado. Reviews found that the number of specialists in the region was an important factor in higher use (Hannan, Wu, & Chassin, 2006). We live in a global society and the needs of people vary from place to place and diverse community needs must be considered (Box 12.1).

Insurance and Policy

As a result of these area studies, insurers and others called for consistency in medical treatment across the country. Efforts to identify best practices were initiated. Insurers saw consistency as a way to control costs. Efforts were made to correct medical practice variations through use of medical practice guidelines (Schneider, 2014), which raised concerns that individuals needed to be empowered to work with medical care providers in deciding best treatment options.

BOX 12-1

Family Tree

Maria do Céu Barbieri Figueiredo (Portugal)

Maria do Céu Barbieri Figueiredo, RN, MSc, PhD, is a nursing professor at the University of Porto Nursing College in Portugal. Her interest in family nursing was first nurtured by Dr. Dorothy Whyte, supervisor of her master's degree at the University of Edinburgh, United Kingdom. In 2004, she was awarded a PhD in Nursing Science at the University of Porto, where she had examined the nursing care needs of families of children with heart defects using a systemic family approach, based on the Calgary Family Assessment and Intervention Models (Wright & Leahey, 2013). She has helped move family nursing in Portugal forward through several initiatives that include dissemination of the Family Health Nurse conceptual framework of the World Health Organization (2000) in collaboration with the Nursing National Association of Portugal (Ordem dos Enfermeiros). She organized the first family nursing postgraduate education program in Portugal and has supervised several dissertations and theses with a family nursing focus. She provided leadership for the First (2008), Second (2009), Third (2010), and Fourth (2012) International Symposium in Family Nursing in Porto, Portugal, and co-edited e-books with papers presented in these symposia. Dr. Maria do Céu Barbieri Figueiredo serves as a member of the Family Nursing Practice Committee of the International Family Nursing Association and is Portugal's representative to the Collaborative Family Health Nursing Project under way in Europe. Her research currently focuses on the family nursing approach in community care and cultural adaptation and validation of instruments for use in family nursing.

Infrastructure Elements and Environmental Health

Health policy has mostly focused on decreasing cost and improving access, insurance, and services. To date, nurses have had little influence in these areas. Health is mostly influenced by personal lifestyle choices, the environment, and living or working conditions. A 2008 series called "Unnatural Causes: Is Inequality Making Us Sick?" showed how people's homes and where they work are backdrops to illness and life expectancy (California Newsreel, 2008).

Starting in the 1970s, researchers identified many environmental influences (e.g., lead, smoke, asbestos, mercury, radon, DDT, polychlorinated biphenyls [PCBs], other persistent organic pollutants [POPs]) as risk factors that can lead to illness and disease (Schneider, 2014). In public health, talk about upstream and downstream risks and solutions for health problems is common. Upstream risks are the source of the problem and the complex social and economic concerns related to health and illness prevention. Downstream risks are closely related to the illness or medical event leading to medical intervention or hospitalization. Much of U.S. health care delivery, including nursing, is based on downstream thinking, but upstream thinking focuses on solutions (e.g., behavior, environment, policy, social factors). Upstream solutions have the potential to prevent poor health.

Various environmental areas are places where interventions can influence a more healthy population:

- The social environment
  - Culture—such as the influence of entertainers on lifestyle choices
  - Economy—lack of resources may limit healthy choices and treatment options
  - Religion—certain practices can increase health risks
  - Politics—beliefs in a certain set of principles and the push to ensure the large majority follows their beliefs
  - Policy—creation of laws and regulations that require the population to follow a specific set of behaviors
- The physical environment
  - Air—high clean air standards that ensure the population isn't at risk for health problems
  - Water—standards that prevent pollution and support sufficient access to the population
  - Land—laws and regulations that ensure that, while private property rights are maintained, property owners do not create hazards for others
  - Food—inspections to ensure that growers, processors, and importers do not put the population at risk
  - Homes—standards that ensure homes are constructed to withstand the weather and other hazards, such as earthquakes, and regulations to ensure that homes don't have internal pollution problems, such as mold and asbestos, that are health risks
  - Worksites—Occupational Safety and Health Administration (OSHA) regulations to ensure reduced risk of employee injury
  - Recreation—regulations and standards to ensure that recreational facilities do not put patrons at risk
- The global environment
  - Emergency response—state and federal agencies that respond to ensure population safety in a disaster
  - Travel—regulations that ensure communicable diseases do not cross national borders
  - Immigration—laws that restrict persons who may harm citizens from entering the country

Recent episodes of terrorism, increased violence in some large population centers, chronic diseases, and pathogens resistant to antibiotics are also risks. These threats call for shifts from individual to more family- and population-focused care. See Table 12.1 for a list of some current laws that regulate population health.

Population Health Perspectives

In the United States, medical care expenditures greatly supersede those for population or public health care. Rather than focus on health promotion and disease prevention, money is primarily spent for intensive and expensive individual care after being stricken by illness or disease (Robert Wood Johnson Foundation, 2011). Yet, many underlying causes of death are preventable. In 2010, the leading causes of death were mostly chronic diseases, unintentional injuries, Alzheimer's disease, renal disease, pneumonia/influenza, and suicide (Centers for Disease Control and Prevention, 2013). Risk factors for the 10 leading causes of death were tobacco use, diet, physical inactivity, and alcohol consumption. Upstream thinking would mean aiming to prevent the disease from occurring rather than treating the disease after diagnosis.

The health of populations is often measured by life expectancy, infant mortality rate, and other death rates. Of the world's nations, the United States has the 50th highest life expectancy but spends more on medical care than any other country (Robert Wood Johnson Foundation, 2009). High rates of violence, political instability, and AIDS are partially responsible for the low life expectancy in many nations at the bottom of the life expectancy ranking, but the United States does not have these problems. Some might say the United States spends more but has lower beneficial returns or that some people get too much care and others not enough. Nations that provide health care to all and focus on population health have the highest number of estimated life years. Life expectancy, distribution of care services, and long-term costs could change with a greater prevention focus.

TABLE 12-1	*Examples of U.S. Environmental Legislation to Improve Population Health*
LEGISLATIVE ACT	**AUTHORITY**
Clean Air Act (1970)	Regulated hazardous air pollution emissions
Occupational Safety and Health Act (1970)	Regulated safety and emissions standards within the workplace
Toxic Substances Control Act (1976)	Mandated testing of substances for human safety prior to marketing
Resource Conservation and Recovery Act (1976)	Outlawed open dumps
	Regulated hazardous waste from petroleum refining, pesticide manufacturing, and some pharmaceutical production from "cradle to grave"
Environmental Protection Agency (1992)	Ruled that environmental tobacco smoke was a carcinogen
Food Prevention Plan (2007)	Created an integrated FDA plan for prevention, intervention, and response to foodborne illnesses
The FDA Food Safety Modernization Act (FSMA) (2011)	Shifted the focus of U.S. regulators from reaction to prevention of foodborne illnesses

Primary, Secondary, and Tertiary Prevention

In population health, there are three levels of prevention:

- Primary prevention describes actions taken before the problem exists, such as immunizations, purification of water, sewage treatments.
- Secondary prevention aims for early detection and prompt intervention if a problem is found, such as through screening tests (e.g., mammography and colonoscopy).
- Tertiary prevention acts to minimize further complications once a problem is identified, such as diabetes education after diagnosis, medical management, and use of pharmaceuticals.

Traditional medical care mostly aims at tertiary prevention, which tends to be expensive. Secondary prevention can often involve expensive testing or screening. Primary or upstream prevention is the least expensive.

Access to Medical Care

Some medical treatments are very expensive and not always fully covered by health insurance. Wealth and health have been repeatedly linked through research (Anderson et al., 2008; Avendano, Glymour, Banks, & Mackenbach, 2009). Wealth means healthier living conditions, ability to buy more nutritious foods, lower stress, and access to better services (Baum, Garofalo, & Yali, 1999; Bird et al., 2010). Longer life is linked with higher socioeconomic status. These factors affect the vulnerability of individuals, families, and communities. Stage of life, culture, health literacy, and the abilities to speak, read, and write English also influence health risks and outcomes. Neighborhood affects access to clean water, social support, and safety. In 2011, Japan's families experienced a giant tsunami that killed nearly 16,000 people and destroyed homes and reordered lives of those living 6 to 7 miles away. Drs. Nojima and Hohashi are teaching nurses in this nation ways to give family-focused care (Box 12.2).

Fairness in the Distribution of Goods and Services

The burden of lower life expectancy and higher rates of infant mortality falls disproportionately on the poor. Health disparities exist when certain groups do not have the same health opportunities as others and often result from unequal distribution of social goods. For example, we do not choose the family we are born into and so we acquire by default the heritage of our families. Health equity means fairness in the distribution of services and resources so that all can achieve optimal health. Equity cannot be guaranteed because each patient situation is different, but fair apportionment of resources is the optimal goal. Nations address these needs differently.

Social Justice

A book about social justice noted needs to address the underlying social determinants vital to overall population health (Powers & Faden, 2006). Social justice implies that principles of fairness exist and people deserve equal chances. Some think social justice should be a fifth metaparadigm concept in nursing due to its importance in achieving population health (Schim, Benkert, Bell, Walker, & Danford, 2007). Social justice implies many ideas. For example, distributive justice refers to initiating and supporting action to meet public needs, especially of vulnerable populations (Grace, 2009). Formal systems and laws exist to help decide who gets goods (e.g., food, shelter, clean environment,

> **BOX 12-2**
>
> **Family Tree**
>
> **Sayumi Nojima, RN, PHN, DSN (Japan)**
>
> Sayumi Nojima, RN, PHN, DSN, is the vice president at Kochi Prefectural University. After receiving a doctoral degree of Science in Nursing from the University of California, San Francisco, she joined the Faculty of Nursing at Kochi Women's University and started a master's program that focused on advanced practice and the preparation of certified nurse specialists in family nursing. Dr. Nojima developed the Family Empowerment Nursing Model, which has been extensively used in nursing education and practice in Japan. She is the Chief Editor (with Hiroko Watanabe) of the *Japanese Journal of Family Nursing* (Kango Kyokai Publisher). Dr. Nojima has served for many years as a board member of the Japanese Association for Research in Family Nursing (JARFN) and was the vice president of JARFN (2004–2013). In 2011, Dr. Nojima was awarded an Innovative Contribution to Family Nursing Award from the *Journal of Family Nursing* at the Tenth International Family Nursing Conference in Kyoto, Japan.
>
> **Naohiro Hohashi, PhD, RN, PHN (Japan)**
>
> Naohiro Hohashi, PhD, RN, PHN, is a Professor of Health Care Nursing and Department Director, Kobe University Graduate School of Health Sciences. Dr. Hohashi has research and practice expertise with a wide range of subjects, from inpatient (at hospitals) to outpatient and at-home (community) and is guiding a program leading to certification in Family Health Nursing in Japan. He has conducted comparative research on how the family is affected by culture and values in Japan, Hong Kong, and North America. Dr. Hohashi has developed the Concentric Sphere Family Environment Model and the Family Environment assessment tool to measure family functioning. Dr. Hohashi currently serves on the Board of Directors of the Japanese Association for Research in Family Nursing (JARFN). In 2014, he was identified as Transcultural Nursing Scholar of the Transcultural Nursing Society. Dr. Hohashi has created multiple collegial relationships with members of the International Family Nursing Association.

health care) and services. Nurses who *think family* can advocate for fair distribution of available resources.

Governments and people disagree about what is fair; national consensus seems impossible. In the United States, self-reliance and individual freedom are valued. Distributive justice is usually viewed as equal access and equal shares but not necessarily equal outcomes. Public health advocates think fair distribution can occur only when all have an "even playing field." Agreement about inequalities must be addressed before resource distribution will change. Health care financing has implications for the health outcomes of the nation's families.

Lifestyle Behaviors

Major causes of illness and disease, in the United States and other developed nations, are mostly linked with behaviors or lifestyle choices. Lifestyle risk factors are attributed to tobacco use, high blood pressure, overweight, physical inactivity, alcohol abuse, and unhealthy dietary intake (Danaei et al., 2009). In 2010, heart disease and malignant neoplasms accounted for 47% of all deaths (Murphy, Xu, & Kochanek, 2012). Other contributors to disease are genetic composition (at least 20% of all infant deaths), microbial agents (6%), and toxic agents (4%) (Mokdad, Marks, Stroup, & Geberding, 2004). When large groups of people act in similar ways, these risks are viewed as social determinants of health. For example, the placement of sugary products near the checkout aisle becomes an environmental factor that influences buyers' choice. Even knowing that items are unhealthy, people may be highly motivated to choose impulsively the less healthy items.

Population Health Costs

Upstream interventions that occur before the disease or disability are the most effective means for extending life and influencing spiraling health care costs. In 2012, the Institute of Medicine called for doubling the spending on public health. Finances in medical care are focused on acute care and heroic cures for those already sick and fail to promote balanced treatment of personal or community-based prevention (Institute of Medicine, 2012). Current health care systems are inadequately prepared to address population health needs and this can have serious negative consequences for the nation's families.

Population-Based Health Actions

A population is a collection of individuals with shared personal or environmental characteristics (Minnesota Department of Health, 2001). They might share a common culture, ethnicity, language, values, norms, or risk factors. Individual care only improves care for a single person. A population approach considers broader factors that mold health and lead to illness or disease in the larger population.

Imagine you are a nurse in a critical care unit and for the past 6 months you have noticed more adults being admitted for myocardial infarction (MI). Downstream thinking means that lifesaving measures and medical management take place in an inpatient setting for the person with a MI. Upstream thinking asks: Why are MIs occurring at an increasing rate? Upstream thinking keeps records of those with an MI to see what similarities might explain the increase. Results can help answer the question and could lead to preventing the problem. For example, several years ago New York State implemented a comprehensive smoking ban that reduced the number of hospital admissions for MI (Juster et al., 2007). Nurses who *think family* understand the implications of public health measures and help enact policies to make important changes (Box 12.3).

An example of population-based care that demonstrates the interventions at each level of practice is The Heart of New Ulm project, started in 2008 (Hearts Beat Back, 2010). This project, led and financed by a hospital health care system in Minnesota, used many community partnerships. New Ulm, a small city south of Minneapolis, has many residents of German ancestry. Leaders recognized that beer, brats, and butter were often on the menu of the local families. The project aimed to reduce numbers of heart attacks over 10 years (Hearts Beat Back, 2010). Health-screening programs and a variety of community-based programs were available to assist residents to decrease their risks by improving their diets and physical activity, eliminating tobacco use, and addressing social behaviors. Community education programs (e.g., cooking classes, sharing recipes, grocery shopping tours, tobacco

---

BOX 12-3

Population-Based Health Practices

Population health considers three levels of practice to change risky behaviors, improve life expectancy, decrease infant mortality rate, and decrease death rates from preventable diseases and injuries:

- Individual-focused interventions (e.g., vaccinations, lifestyle behaviors)
- Community-focused interventions (e.g., safe air and water, housing, safe places to walk)
- System-focused interventions (e.g., homeland security, relief after disasters, prevention of type 2 diabetes and obesity and their complications)

cessation series, chronic disease management classes) were available. Community efforts promoted physical activity (e.g., walking/running events and clubs, dance classes, bike riding, aerobic exercise classes). Environmental changes such as constructing sidewalks to improve walking opportunities, creating parks, and initiating tobacco use restriction policies were instituted. Online resources, blogs, and phone applications were created to support local activities and share successes. They took the perspective that health is a shared community responsibility.

Social Determinants of Health

Population health addresses environmental and lifestyle factors of the community to increase survival and decrease morbidity. Social determinants, both economic and social conditions, influence a population's state of health (Box 12.4). Risk assessments are a first step toward change; then policies, programs, or projects are planned with strategies for implementation and evaluation (Centers for Disease Control and Prevention, 2011b). Coalitions and partnerships designed for programs that focus on prevention, health promotion efforts, and medical care interventions must be successful.

Health Care Services

In the United States, health care expenditures were about $2.6 trillion in 2010 compared to $256 billion spent in 1980, and only 3% of this money went for population health (Kaiser Health Foundation, 2012). The question of whether this health care system is actually a sick care system was discussed in a film called "Escape Fire: The Fight to Rescue American Healthcare." Stakeholders and businesses that benefit from the current system will vigorously work to oppose a transition to a prevention-based system; however, the market, being what it is in this country, will adjust once cost savings and opportunity for other types of service providers increase.

Plans to enact the Affordable Health Care Act (ACA) are under way. The ACA focuses on primary and secondary prevention and lifestyle factors and is designed to benefit all

---

BOX 12-4

Health Determinants for Individuals, Families, and Communities

The following factors influence health and illness of individuals, families, and population groups residing in various geographical regions:

- Biology (genetics, family history, physical and mental problems)
- Behaviors (alcohol abuse, tobacco use, lack of regular exercise, level of health literacy, stress management)
- Social environment (e.g., relationships with family, friends, neighbors, and others; faith communities; schools; government agencies; safety; availability of resources; culture; media; and public transportation)
- Physical environment (e.g., weather, climate change, buildings, recreational settings, neighborhoods, housing, pollutants, agriculture, toxic substances)
- Access to affordable and quality health care
- Policymaking (e.g., smoking bans, tax increases on tobacco sales, litter ordinances, seatbelt laws)

Source: Healthy People 2020. (2011). *About healthy people*. Retrieved from http://www.healthypeople.gov/2020/about/default.aspx

U.S. citizens with investments in wellness, disease prevention, and public health emergencies. The federal government aims to partner with states and communities to control such health problems as obesity, health disparities, tobacco use, vaccine-preventable illnesses, and HIV/AIDS. The goal is to increase the effectiveness of public health and improve access to behavioral health services. Family nurses could lead in the coordination of care across home, community, and institutional settings. Investment in prevention and community programs that increase physical activity, improve nutrition, and prevent tobacco use could mean $5.60 is saved for every dollar spent, a savings of $16 billion in 5 years (Levi, Segal, & Juliano, 2009). Problems of high blood pressure, overweight, and obesity are preventable. Obese persons are four times more likely to suffer from progressive knee osteoarthritis and other arthritis. Approximately 20% of all cancer cases can be attributed to obesity (Wolin, Carson, & Colditz, 2010). Currently, it is difficult to have programs or initiatives that focus on preventive care (Mayes & Oliver, 2012). Some raise concerns that you can't see benefits of preventive actions for years or decades.

The ACA is providing vulnerable or at-risk individuals and families access and payment for medical care (Box 12.5). Some health promotion and disease prevention activities targeted toward the family and community are included. Several primary and secondary prevention services for adults and children are also covered (Box 12.6). Persons covered by Medicare also have preventive services covered (Box 12.7). This is the first time medical coverage for prevention has been legislated.

Differences in Health Care Delivery

Nurses who work within the medical approach focus their care on treating disease and illness in acute care settings for individuals; nurses with a public health approach focus on population needs and societal deficits that may cause disease. Both medical and public health approaches are essential for family-focused care. Nurses need familiarity with medical approaches, but also need to recognize ways population care can be integrated. Those

---

BOX 12-5

Major Policy Changes in the Affordable Health Care Act (2010)

The Affordable Health Care Act:

- Prohibits health insurers from refusing coverage based on patients' medical histories and pre-existing conditions.
- Prohibits health insurers from charging different rates based on patients' medical histories or gender.
- Repeals insurance companies' exemption from antitrust laws.
- Establishes minimum standards for qualified health benefit plans.
- Covers adult children under parents' health insurance until the age of 26.
- Requires most employers to provide coverage for their workers or pay a surtax on the workers' wages up to 8%.
- Expands Medicaid to include more low-income Americans by increasing Medicaid eligibility limits to 133% of the federal poverty level and by covering adults without dependents as long as neither population segment falls under the narrow exceptions outlined by various clauses throughout the proposal.
- Provides a subsidy to low- and middle-income Americans to help buy insurance; this change will require most Americans to carry or obtain qualifying health insurance coverage or possibly face a surtax for noncompliance.

BOX 12-6

Preventive Services Under the Affordable Care Act

After September 23, 2010, the following preventive services are covered without having to pay a copayment, co-insurance, or meet a deductible when provided by an in-network provider:
Adults (16 preventive services):

- Abdominal aortic aneurysm (one time screening for men who have ever smoked)
- Alcohol misuse (screening and counseling)
- Aspirin (use for men and women of certain ages)
- Blood pressure screening (all adults)
- Cholesterol screening (adults of certain ages or high risk)
- Colorectal cancer screening (adults over 50)
- Depression (adults)
- Type 2 diabetes (screening for adults with high blood pressure)
- Diet counseling (adults at risk for chronic disease)
- HIV screening (adults at higher risk)
- Immunizations (doses, ages, populations vary)
- Obesity (screening and counseling for all adults)
- Sexually transmitted diseases prevention counseling (adults at high risk)
- Tobacco use (screening all adults and cessation interventions for tobacco users)
- Syphilis screening (adults at higher risk)

Women and pregnant women (private plans began covering August 1, 2012):

- Well-woman visits
- Gestational diabetes screening (for women 24 to 28 weeks pregnant and those at high risk)
- Human papillomavirus (HPV) DNA testing (women 30+ years testing every 3 years)
- Sexually transmitted infections (STI) counseling (sexually active women)
- HIV screening and counseling (sexually active women)
- Contraception and contraceptive counseling (FDA-approved methods, sterilization procedures, education, and counseling)
- Breastfeeding support, supplies, and counseling (pregnant and postpartum women)
- Interpersonal and domestic violence screening and counseling

Children (27 services):

- Alcohol and drug use (assessments for adolescents)
- Autism screening (18 and 24 months)
- Behavioral assessments (0 to 11 months, 1 to 4 years, 5 to 10 years, 11 to 14 years, 15 to 17 years)
- Blood pressure screening (0 to 11 months, 1 to 4 years, 5 to 10 years, 11 to 14 years, 15 to 17 years)
- Cervical dysplasia screening (for sexually active females)
- Congenital hypothyroidism screening (for newborns)
- Depression (screening for adolescents)
- Developmental screening (children under 3 years and surveillance throughout childhood)
- Dyslipidemia (higher risk for lipid disorders/0 to 11 months, 1 to 4 years, 5 to 10 years, 11 to 14 years, 15 to 17 years)
- Fluoride chemoprevention (supplements for children with no fluoride in water)
- Gonorrhea (preventive medication for the eyes of all newborns)
- Hearing screening (all newborns)
- Height, weight, and body mass index (0 to 11 months, 1 to 4 years, 5 to 10 years, 11 to 14 years, 15 to 17 years)
- Hematocrit or hemoglobin screening
- Hemoglobinopathies (sickle cell screening for newborns)
- HIV screening (adolescents at high risk)

Continued

BOX 12-6

Preventive Services Under the Affordable Care Act—cont'd

- Immunization vaccines birth to 18 years (doses, recommended ages, and populations vary)
- Iron supplements (children 6 to 12 months at risk for anemia)
- Lead screening (children at risk of exposure)
- Medical history for all children throughout development (0 to 11 months, 1 to 4 years, 5 to 10 years, 11 to 14 years, 15 to 17 years)
- Obesity screening and counseling
- Oral health risk assessment (0 to 11 months, 1 to 4 years, 5 to 10 years)
- Phenylketonuria (PKU) screening for genetic disorder in newborns
- Sexually transmitted infection (STI) prevention and counseling for adolescents
- Tuberculin testing (0 to 11 months, 1 to 4 years, 5 to 10 years, 11 to 14 years, 15 to 17 years)
- Vision screening for all children

BOX 12-7

Preventive Services Covered by Medicare

Several preventive services qualify for those insured through a Medicare plan:

- Tobacco cessation counseling
- Screenings (bone mass, cervical cancer, cholesterol, diabetes, HIV, breast cancer, prostate cancer, others)
- Influenza shots, pneumonia shots, and hepatitis B shots

Medical nutrition therapy to help people manage diabetes or kidney disease

---

getting medical care return to households and communities and are affected by social determinants of health.

Vulnerable Populations and Family Health

Focus on vulnerable populations is needed for global, social, political, economic, and ethical reasons (Shi & Stevens, 2010). These high-risk groups have great health needs due to poor physical and mental health (Shi & Stevens, 2010). As factors relevant to health disparities are considered, three populations are identified (Aday, 1993, 2001):

- Physically vulnerable—high-risk mothers and infants, chronically ill and disabled, persons with AIDS/HIV
- Psychologically vulnerable—mentally ill and disabled, alcohol or substance abusers, those at risk for suicide or homicide
- Socially vulnerable—abusing families, homeless, immigrants, refugees

Vulnerability can be linked with situations such as HIV status and teen pregnancy, experiences individuals might have prevented if risky sexual behaviors were avoided (Shi & Stevens, 2010). Moral judgments and political factors play roles in perpetuating some disparities. For instance, when condoms or birth control pills are available without shame, many will access them. Gaps in wealth and power can also create vulnerability. Vulnerability is created and resolved through social actions.

Vulnerability and Public Policy

Vulnerability is influenced by norms, attitudes, beliefs, and values of individuals and families living in communities and also by social and health policies. When broad social agreement occurs, points of view become laws at local, state, and national levels. In 2012, 20 grade school children and six staff members were fatally shot at Sandy Hook Elementary School in Newtown, Connecticut. National debates about laws to limit or prohibit gun ownership and screening followed. Although some support laws for background checks and limited magazine rounds of ammunition, many citizens and the National Rifle Association oppose any restrictions to the constitutional right of Americans to bear arms. Opponents of gun control measures cite statistics indicating increased gun violence in communities with the most restrictive gun laws. U.S. homicide rates from firearms is 3.3 deaths per 100,000 people yet other countries with restrictive gun laws have much lower rates (e.g., Canada with 0.5 death per 100,000; United Kingdom with 0.1 death per 100,000) (United Nations Office on Drugs and Crimes, 2012). Moral people often disagree about the ways violence should be addressed. Although one group believes reducing ownership of guns will reduce gun violence, an opposing group believes the cure lies in resolving the underlying community problems that encourage violence.

Some societal views about disease are prone to stigma and victim blaming (Mechanic & Tanner, 2007). Links between socioeconomic disparities, life expectancy, and health risks are often viewed as personal deficiencies or attributes (Shi & Stevens, 2010). Individuals are blamed for poor health choices. People begin life with diverse circumstances not always under their control. For example, when persons are discharged from an acute setting with a particular medical diagnosis, the same written and oral instructions are often given to college graduates and grade school dropouts. Reading, language, and innate intelligence influence understanding, ability to follow instructions, and care outcomes; instructions need to account for these factors.

Public and Family Health

Public health is defined as "the practice of preventing disease and promoting good health within groups of people, from small communities to entire countries" (American Public Health Association, 2011, para. 1). Public health nursing is defined as "the practice of promoting and protecting the health of populations using knowledge from nursing, social, and public health sciences" (American Public Health Association, 1996, para. 1). In public health, the population is the client, but work with individuals, families, and systems also occurs. Individual care is only a small portion of practice. Public health nurses usually work in a particular geographical region to improve individual and family health. Public health nurses aim to improve the quality of life for a particular population and the greater society. Equity in service delivery despite age, gender, race, and ethnicity is the goal.

Core Functions of Public Health

Three core functions—assessment, policy development, and assurance—guide public health practice that protects individuals and families in a societal context (Institute of Medicine, 1988). Assessment refers to data collection; monitoring population health status, needs, and problems; and dissemination of information. Assessment might identify trends for children with asthma in a particular community and find the reasons for risks. Policy development refers to leadership in developing national, regional, state, and local policies or statutes.

Nurses work toward policy development to eliminate environmental factors that make asthma worse. An upstream focus is to decrease air pollutants. Assurance refers to making sure that high-priority services are available. Nurses who *think family* measure the usefulness and effectiveness of intervention programs. Assurance makes sure public health workers and nurses provide competent care. Besides these core functions, 10 essential public health services also serve to guide practice (Box 12.8).

Social Determinants That Influence Family Health

Social determinants include socioeconomic factors such as social class, family income, levels of education, and employment. These factors influence the affordability and location of where families live. Where people live affects other life aspects, such as quality of schools, per-hour wages, safety, violence, and food access. Overcrowding and unsanitary conditions can increase exposure to diseases. Air pollution increases risks for asthma and lung disease.

Probably one of the best ways to influence good health is good nutrition. Several societal factors work against good nutrition and include lack of access to nutrient-dense foods, social relationships and marketing that influence poor food choices, use of processed and prepackaged foods, routine snacking, and busy lifestyles whereby families rarely eat meals together and are likely to eat meals outside the home. Families who share fewer than three mealtimes a week have poorer health outcomes (Neumark-Sztainer, Eisenberg, Fulkerson, Story, & Larson, 2008). Nurses who *think family* can help families improve nutrition by teaching the basics of good nutrition, label reading, meal planning, food shopping, budgeting, preparing fruits and vegetables, and home cooking. Surprisingly, in some households no one knows how to prepare meals without prepackaged, processed foods.

Widespread concerns about mental health exist. According to the National Institute of Mental Health (NIMH), some form of mental illness affects about 60 million Americans (1 in 4 adults; 1 in 10 children). Worldwide, 4 of the 10 leading causes of disability are linked with mental disorders. The World Health Organization (WHO) predicts that by 2020, major depressive illness, including depression, bipolar disorder, and borderline personality disorder, will be the leading cause of disability for the world's women and

---

BOX 12-8

Ten Essential Public Health Services

The strength of the public health service rests on its capacity to deliver effectively the following services:

- Monitor health status to identify community health problems.
- Diagnose and investigate health problems and hazards in the community.
- Inform, educate, and empower people about health issues.
- Mobilize community partnerships to identify and solve health problems.
- Develop policies and plans that support individual and community efforts.
- Enforce laws and regulations that protect health and ensure safety.
- Link people to needed personal health services and ensure the provision of health care when otherwise unavailable.
- Ensure a competent public health and personal health care workforce.
- Evaluate effectiveness, accessibility, and quality of personal and population-based health services.
- Research for new insights and innovative solutions to health problems.

children. Children and adolescents are often affected with autism, attention deficit disorder, anxiety disorders, eating disorders, and psychosis (National Institute of Mental Health, 2013). Without adequate treatment, the social consequences are overwhelming. Costs linked with untreated mental illness are shocking. Stigma and misunderstandings about mental disorders lead to delays in diagnosis and care, particularly for the uninsured, minority, low income, and elderly groups (National Institute of Mental Health, 2005). Families are generally ill equipped to manage severe conditions. Stigma often leads to resistance to treatment, resulting in poorly managed conditions and school failures, homelessness, physical or emotional abuse, alcohol and substance abuse, unstable employment, and crime (National Alliance of Mental Health, 2005). Nurses who *think family* consider social determinants when they give individual and family care.

Theoretical Frameworks for Family and Societal Health Care

Nurses can use theoretical models to address such qualities as resilience (Rew & Horner, 2003), health promotion (Pender, Murdaugh, & Parsons, 2011), and self-efficacy (Bandura, 1997). Other frameworks can address community and vulnerability (Fig. 12.1). For example, the Vulnerability Model (Flaskerud & Winslow, 1998) identifies resource availability, relative risks, and health status. Community unemployment, poverty, violence and crime, schools, community organizations, and availability of grocery stores and farmers' markets need to be examined. The Chronic Care Model (CCM) is a way to examine system interactions linked with disease management (Wagner, Austin, & Von Korff, 1996). Research using the CCM has demonstrated some improvement in care outcomes (Wallace, 2011).

Nurses who *think family* know household and social factors need to be assessed. When care is planned, wellness, health promotion, prevention, and care management issues can be considered based upon vulnerability. Students and nurses often recognize individual responsibility without considering social implications. Failure to include social determinants ignores circumstances and living environments and may prevent selection of the most effective interventions. Review the Family Circle case and talk with others in your class about the choices, priorities, and decisions that need to be made (Box 12.9).

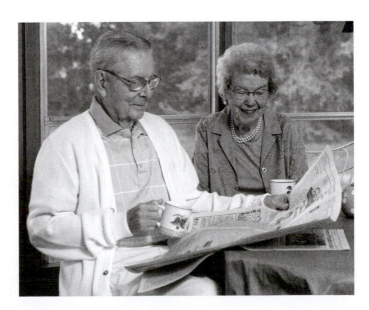

FIGURE 12-1 Family-focused care is necessary to meet the needs of vulnerable populations.

BOX 12-9

Family Circle

Last night you heard a national evening news report that caught your attention. This morning, the headline of your local newspaper contains the same statement in large letters. You read the headline: "For the first time, a generation of Americans is expected to live shorter lives than their parents."

1. What kinds of things do you think this article would disclose?
2. What do these headlines mean to you, your family, and Americans?
3. What upstream family and population efforts are needed to turn this tide?
4. What actions might a family or population-focused nurse take to prevent the potential downstream outcomes?

The Role of the Government in Population Health and Its Financing

The idea that government should share some responsibility for health care has a long history. It goes back at least to the Greek city-states, where citizens' taxes supported public physicians. The idea of compulsory participation in a health insurance system is old. In 1798, a Marine Hospital Service was created and owners of merchant ships contributed 20 cents a month into a sickness fund for each employed seaman (Starr, 1982). In the 19th century, labor unions required workers to join relief funds to cover disease and injury treatment. Some payers, policy makers, providers, and purchasers have vested interests in perpetuating the current medical delivery system that favors treatment over prevention. Leadership is needed to help citizens identify benefits of focusing on health promotion and disease prevention. Family nurses can do this with individuals as health counseling and education are tailored to household and community needs.

Department of Health and Human Services

In the United States, the Department of Health and Human Services (DHHS) is the main agency dealing with the issues of poverty, vulnerability, and health disparities. An Office of the Secretary and 11 operating divisions provide a wide range of health services (Box 12.10). These agencies perform many tasks and services such as research, food and drug safety testing, and grant issuing. About half of U.S. citizens receive some form of government-supported health care.

The Surgeon General

In the United States, the Surgeon General is appointed by the president and is the head of the Public Health Service Commission Corps. This is the most widely recognized and respected voice of public health issues. The Surgeon General sees that the public is provided with information about personal health and the nation's health, reports important medical findings, suggests steps that should be taken to increase health, and oversees the nation's 6,500 uniformed health officers who serve around the world.

Health Resources and Services Administration

Each state and most cities in the United States have their own Department of Health but the federal government takes the lead in defining health activities and goals to improve the nation's health. The Health Resources and Services Administration (HRSA) is made

---

BOX 12-10

Department of Health and Human Services Offices

Agencies of DHHS:
- Health Resources and Services Administration (HRSA)
- Food and Drug Administration (FDA)
- Administration on Aging (AoA)
- National Institutes of Health (NIH)
- Centers for Disease Control and Prevention (CDC)
- Substance Abuse and Mental Health Services Administration (SAMHSA)
- Indian Health Services (IHS)
- Office of the Inspector General (OIG)
- Agency for Healthcare Research and Quality (AHRQ)
- Administration for Children and Families (ACF)
- Agency for Toxic Substances and Disease Registry (ATSDR)
- Centers for Medicare and Medicaid Services (CMS)

---

up of six bureaus and 10 offices (Box 12.11). Several operating divisions of HRSA provide leadership and financial support (Table 12.2). HRSA grants assist uninsured, those with HIV/AIDS, pregnant women, mothers, and children. Financial supports to train health professionals and improve rural community care systems target four goals:

1. Improve access to quality care and services.
2. Strengthen the health workforce.
3. Build healthy communities.
4. Improve health equity.

BOX 12-11

Bureaus and Offices of the Health Resources and Services Administration

The Health Resources and Services Administration has six bureaus:
- Bureau of Clinician Recruitment and Service
- Bureau of Health Professionals
- Bureau of Primary Health Care
- Healthcare Systems Bureau
- HIV/AIDS Bureau
- Maternal and Child Health Bureau

The Health Resources and Services Administration has 10 offices:
- Office of Planning, Analysis, and Evaluation
- Office of Rural Health Policy
- Office of Regional Operations
- Office of Special Health Affairs
  - Office of Health Equity
  - Office of Global Health Affairs
  - Office of Strategic Priorities
  - Office of Health Information, Technology, and Quality
  - Office of Emergency Preparedness and Continuity of Operations
- Office of Women's Health

TABLE 12-2	Operating Divisions of the Department of Health and Human Services

DIVISION	PURPOSE
Administration for Children and Families (ACF)	Promotion of the economic and social well-being of families, children, individuals, and communities
Administration on Aging (AoA)	Development of a comprehensive, coordinated, and cost-effective system of home and community-based services that helps elderly individuals maintain their health and independence in their homes and communities
Agency for Healthcare Research and Quality (AHRQ)	Improvement of the quality, safety, efficiency, and effectiveness of health care for all Americans
Agency for Toxic Substances and Disease Registry (ATSDR)	Assessment of hazardous waste sites, health consultation concerning specific hazardous substances, response to releases of hazardous substances, and education and training concerning hazardous substances
Centers for Disease Control and Prevention (CDC)	Creation of the expertise, information, and tools that people and communities need to protect their health through health promotion; prevention of disease, injury, and disability; and preparedness for new health threats
Centers for Medicare and Medicaid Services (CMS)	Administration of Medicare, Medicaid, and the Children's Health Insurance Program
Food and Drug Administration (FDA)	Regulation of medical products, tobacco, food safety, global regulatory operations and policies
Health Resources and Services Administration (HRSA)	Improvement of access to quality health care services for people who are uninsured, isolated, or medically vulnerable through strengthening the health workforce, building healthy communities, and improving health equity
Indian Health Service (IHS)	Promotion of the physical, mental, social, and spiritual health of American Indians and Alaska Natives to the highest possible level
National Institutes of Health (NIH)	Discovery and dissemination of fundamental knowledge about the nature and behavior of living systems and the application of that knowledge to enhance health, lengthen life, and reduce the burdens of illness and disability
Office of the Inspector General (OIG)	Performance of audits, evaluations, investigations, and law enforcement efforts relating to HHS programs and operations
	Promotion of economy, efficiency, and effectiveness of HHS programs and prevention or identification of fraud, waste, and abuse
Substance Abuse and Mental Health Services Administration (SAMHSA)	Reduction of the impact of substance abuse and mental illness on America's communities

The government sponsors programs to ease the effects of race, class, educational status, and poverty on health outcomes. Examples include the Healthy People Initiative, Medicare and Medicaid programs, Head Start, and the Children's Health Insurance Program.

Healthy People 2020

The United States has goals and objectives that aim to decrease and eliminate illness and health care disparities. The Healthy People Initiative has produced four national reports on the health status of the nation and proposes health objectives for 10-year periods. Progress has been made in reducing coronary heart disease, cancer, incidence of AIDS, and syphilis. Healthy People 2020 (2011) includes four overarching goals aligned with public health, and none include direct medical care delivery (Box 12.12). Attainment of these goals would increase the overall health of the diverse U.S. citizens. Nurses who *think family* are aware of these objectives and include them in their practice. Family nurses know that their role includes using time with individuals as a way to target disparities and vulnerabilities linked with family units.

Medicare, Medicaid, and Other Benefits

Since the 1960s, laws have established several large health care programs. The programs provide health care access and payment for special groups who might otherwise forfeit medical care. In 1965, Medicare funding was signed into law to provide health care for citizens over age 65. Medicare Part A covers inpatient hospital care, hospice, home health care, and skilled nursing. Medicare Part B covers doctors, health provider services, home health, and durable medical equipment. Medicare Part C offers health care plans from private insurers. Medicare Part D helps cover the cost of prescription drugs. Many people do not pay for Medicare Part A, but most pay for Medicare Parts B, C, and D. The monthly Social Security income varies based on wages earned and age at the time of retirement. Intended only as a supplement to retirement income, it provides a meager living for those with no savings or pensions, and for those individuals health care coverage takes a large portion.

In 1965, Medicaid, another national health program for low-income persons, was created. State participation in Medicaid is voluntary; however, all states have participated since 1982. In some states, Medicaid is subcontracted to private companies, but others directly pay providers. States and counties vary in Medicaid provision but in most cases the benefit is closely regulated, time limited, and intended for the poor. Some families have difficulty finding medical providers or dentists who will accept Medicaid because reimbursement to providers in some areas does not cover the cost of providing the care. Sick individuals often use high-cost local emergency departments as a safety net. Pharmaceutical choices and payments are regulated by a state formulary that identifies what can or cannot be prescribed.

In 1930, the Veterans Health Administration was established and is the largest integrated health care system. The Veterans Health Administration is divided into regions with

---

BOX 12-12

Healthy People 2020 Goals

Healthy People 2020 tracks 1,200 objectives in 42 topic areas aimed at accomplishing four goals:

- Attain high-quality, longer lives free of preventable disease, disability, injury, and premature death
- Achieve health equity, eliminate disparities, and improve the health of all groups
- Create social and physical environments that promote good health for all
- Promote quality of life, healthy development, and healthy behaviors across all life stages

medical centers and community-based outpatient clinics. Most veterans receive services free or with modest copayments. In 1921, the Snyder Act provided health services to Native American tribes. Today, the Indian Health Service (IHS), a division of the DHHS, has an annual appropriation near $4 billion and provides care to nearly 2 million Native Americans (Shi & Stevens, 2010). The IHS provides care for well over 500 tribal groups. Native Americans also qualify for health care funding through Medicare and Medicaid.

State Children's Health Insurance Program

The state Children's Health Insurance Program (CHIP) was enacted as part of the Balanced Budget Act of 1997 (Centers for Medicare and Medicaid Services, 2012). CHIP provides health coverage for children whose families earned too much to qualify for Medicaid benefits but who were still uninsured because of limited income. Like Medicaid, the federal government matches state spending; however, these funds are capped nationwide and each state receives an allotment. Millions of children are enrolled in Medicaid, and CHIP extends coverage to millions more. Yet, many eligible children are still not covered. Family-focused care implies that the complex needs, abilities, and availability of resources will be considered (Box 12.13).

Health Policy Development and Nurses' Roles

Public policies aim to influence individual, family, population, and institutional behaviors. Health policy begins with agenda setting to guide disease prevention and health promotion initiatives at the local, state, and national levels (Milstead, 2013). Governments respond

---

BOX 12-13

Evidence-Based Family Nursing

Clear communication with persons who have low literacy or low health literacy is important. Although information abounds and is easily accessible on the Internet, it is important that those needing specific information can understand it. A project titled Get a Head Start on Asthma developed a family-centered Web-based asthma education program for an urban multisite Head Start program. This is a federally funded child development program for low-income culturally diverse families with preschool children. A partnership was formed with low-income English, Hmong, and Spanish-speaking parents of preschool children (ages 3–5 years). Four project phases were assessment, review of 300 existing Web sites, development of a CD-ROM, and Web site development. Four literacy areas were addressed: functional literacy (acceptable reading level), language literacy (translation), health literacy (simple terminology), and computer literacy (ease of use, access). The goal was to address literacy levels of different families. Many knowledge gaps about asthma were identified. Many families did not have access to computers or the Internet or have any experience using computers. Web site design considered graphic layouts, color, graphics, aesthetics, information density, ease of navigation, and abilities with computer technologies. Asthma education was developed for diverse cultural and linguistic backgrounds. Parents needed support to gain better computer literacy skills. Study findings indicated that Web-based interventions have potential for family nurses to assist families with children with asthma, but also to help families with other chronic conditions.

Source: Garwick, A., Seppelt, A., & Belew, J. L. (2011). Addressing family health literacy to create a family-centered culturally relevant web-based asthma education project. In E. K. Svavarsdottir & H. Jonsdottir (Eds.), *Family nursing in action* (pp. 251–266). Reykjavik, Iceland: University of Iceland Press.

to identified problems with legislation, regulation, and programs. Government officials have responsibility to safeguard public health, but local citizens can engage in advocacy that shapes health policy. Nurses can have strong voices and communicate needs to local representatives and elected officials.

The world of health care is a vineyard of intertwined systems that rarely, if ever, interact or communicate with one another. Policies are written by government agencies, independent provider groups, foundations, and advocacy groups. The policy process includes program implementation and involves such national agencies as the Centers for Medicare and Medicaid Services (CMS). Other state and local health departments, hospitals, and health care delivery systems are part of the process.

Changes in public attitudes and values are often the impetus for policy changes. The Centers for Disease Control and Prevention (2011a) reports that tobacco use is responsible for more deaths than HIV infection, illegal drug use, alcohol use, motor vehicle injuries, suicides, and murders combined. The CDC considers tobacco use to be the leading preventable cause of death in the United States. Although no federal bans have been issued on smoking or production of tobacco products, most states have established laws that ban tobacco use in workplaces, restaurants, businesses, and bars, and on college campuses. Some states have increased their tobacco taxes, making it more difficult to continue tobacco use or for teens to buy tobacco products (U. S. Department of Health and Human Services, 2012). Federal and state laws limit the sale of tobacco products to adults. Yet, the American people continue to use tobacco products, often starting use as early as adolescence.

Public health and other nurses can provide information pertinent to public policies at a variety of stages (Milstead, 2013). Nursing is viewed as one of the most trusted occupational groups. Legislators are willing to meet with and listen to nurses, especially through annual state and national Nursing Day on the Hill venues. Nurses who *think family* can be strong advocates for the nation's families. Legislators often have nurses on their staffs to help answer policy issues from their constituents. Registered nurses and student nurses can write their legislators about pending legislation affecting nurses and health care. Organizations such as the American Nurses Association, the National League for Nursing, the American Association of Colleges of Nursing, and the National Student Nurses Association often send newsletters and e-mails asking nurses to write to their senators and representatives about pending legislation. Nurses who *think family* can be advocates for family health and emphasize the links with individual and community needs.

Family nurses can learn about policy through formal coursework and education. It is useful to stay abreast of current issues affecting individual and family health. Policy internships in Washington, D.C., are available and one can become a member of an advocacy group. Some believe that population health should be a key concern linked to all national policies (Mayes & Oliver, 2012). This means that all policies would focus on the specific ways health needs should be included or addressed. Family nurses can be change agents and important advocates in bringing concerns to local government and regional representatives. Civic responsibility can entail knowledge of one's neighborhood and acting for positive health outcomes where you live.

Chapter Summary

This chapter discusses community and population perspectives. Ways in which individual, family, and societal health are linked are described. Nurses caring for individuals in acute and primary care settings can easily overlook the ecological factors and influences of larger environments. Thinking family implies awareness of how the ecological contexts of neighborhood, community, and society are integral parts of health and illness risks. As individuals and families live in their households, they meet the upstream opportunities to promote health and prevent disease. People are influenced by many factors outside their volition. Levels of motivation, locus of control, and other personal factors play health and illness roles, but environmental and social factors outside their control are also influential. Nurses who *think family* recognize that they can empower those they meet to consider the larger picture of what makes people healthy and ways they get sick. If the goal is family-focused care, then it is essential for nurses to see that families are equipped to think beyond "medicalized care" as their only resource. Family-focused nurses are adept at assisting individuals to access what they need in their community. Family nurses can teach families how to advocate for fair distribution of health services. Family nurses who are knowledgeable about the community and population health can be leaders in moving away from a sick care system.

REFERENCES

Aday, L. A. (1993). Equity, accessibility, and ethical issues—Is the U. S. health care reform debate asking the right questions? *American Behavioral Scientist, 36*(6), 724–740.

Aday, L. A. (2001). *At risk in America: The health and health care needs of vulnerable populations in the United States* (2nd ed.). San Francisco: Jossey-Bass.

American Nurses Association. (2007). *Public health nursing: Scope and standards of practice.* Silver Spring, MD: Author.

American Public Health Association. (1996). *Definition and role of public health nursing.* Washington, DC: Author.

American Public Health Association. (2011). *What is public health? Our commitment to safe, healthy communities.* Retrieved from http://www.apha.org/NR/rdonlyres/C57478B8-8682-4347-8DDF-A1E24E82B919/0/what_is_PH_May1_Final.pdf

Anderson, A. F., Carson, C., Watt, H. C., Lawlor, D. A., Avlund, K., & Ebrahim, S. (2008). Life-course socio-economic position, area deprivation and type 2 diabetes: Findings from the British women's heart and health study. *Diabetic Medicine, 25*(12), 1462–1468.

Avendano, M., Glymour, M. M., Banks, J., & Mackenbach, J. P. (2009). Health disadvantage in U.S. adults aged 50 to 74 years: A comparison of the health of rich and poor Americans with that of Europeans. *American Journal of Public Health, 99*(3), 540–548.

Baker, L. C., Fisher, E. S., & Wennberg, J. E. (2008). Variations in hospital resource use for Medicare and privately insured populations in California. *Health Affairs, 27*(2), 123–134. Epub 2008 Feb 12.

Bandura, A. (1997). *Self-efficacy: The exercise of control.* New York: W. H. Freeman.

Baum, A., Garofalo, J. P., & Yali, A. M. (1999). Socioeconomic status and chronic stress: Does stress account for SES effects on health? *Annals of New York Academy of Sciences, 896,* 131–144.

Bell, S. E., & Whiteford, M. B. (1987). Tai Dam health care practices: Asian refugee women in Iowa. *Social Science and Medicine, 24*(4), 317–325.

Bird, C. E., Seeman, T., Escarce, J. J., Basurto-Davila, R., Finch, B. K., Dubowitz, T., Heron, M., . . . Lurie, N. (2010). Neighborhood socioeconomic status and biological "wear & tear" in a nationally representative sample of U.S. adults. *Journal of Epidemiology and Community Health, 64*(10), 860–865.

California Newsreel. (2008). *Unnatural causes: Is inequality making us sick?* Retrieved from http://www.unnaturalcauses.org

Centers for Disease Control and Prevention. (2011a). *Smoking and tobacco use: Tobacco-related mortality.* Retrieved from http://www.cdc.gov/tobacco/data_statistics/fact_sheets/health_effects/tobacco_related_mortality

Centers for Disease Control and Prevention. (2011b). *Healthy places: Health impact assessments.* Retrieved on from http://www.cdc.gov/healthyplaces/hia.htm

Centers for Disease Control and Prevention. (2013). *Leading causes of death.* Retrieved from http://www.cdc.gov/nchs/fastats/leading-causes-of-death.htm

Centers for Medicare and Medicaid Services. (2012). *Financing and reimbursement*. Retrieved on from http://www.medicaid.gov/Medicaid-CHIP-Program-Information/By-Topics/Financing-and-Reimbursement/Financing-and-Reimbursement.html

Central Intelligence Agency. *Country comparison life expectancy at birth*. Retrieved from https://www.cia.gov/library/publications/the-world-factbook/rankorder/2102rank.html

Danaei, G., Ding, E. L., Mozaffarian, D., Taylor, B., Rehm, J., Murray, C. J. L., & Ezzati, M. (2009). The preventable causes of death in the United States: Comparative risk assessment of dietary, lifestyle, and metabolic risk factors. *PLOS Medicine 6*(4), e1000058. doi:10.1371/journal.pmed.100005

Doutrich, D., Arcus, K., Dekker, L., Spuck, J., & Pollock-Robinson, C. (2012). Cultural safety in New Zealand and the United States: Looking at a way forward together. *Journal of Transcultural Nursing, 23*(2), 143–150.

Fadiman, A. (1997). *The spirit catches you and you fall down*. New York: Farrar, Straus, & Giroux.

Flaskerud, J. H., & Winslow, B. W. (1998). Conceptualizing vulnerable populations health-related research. *Nursing Research, 47*(2), 69–78.

Garwick, A., Seppelt, A., & Belew, J. L. (2011). Addressing family health literacy to create a family-centered culturally relevant web-based asthma education project. In E. K. Svavarsdottir & H. Jonsdottir (Eds.), *Family nursing in action* (pp. 251–266). Reykjavik, Iceland: University of Iceland Press.

Grace, P. J. (2009). *Nursing ethics and professional responsibility*. Sudbury, MA: Jones & Bartlett.

Hannan, E. L., Wu, C., & Chassin, M. R. (2006). Differences in per capita rates of revascularization and in choice of revascularization procedure for eleven states. *BMS Health Services Research, 16*(6), 35. Published online March 16, 2006. doi:10.1186/1472-6963-6-35

Health Resources and Services Administration. (1995). *Medically underserved areas and populations (MUA/Ps): Guidelines for MUA and MUP designation*. Retrieved from http://bhpr.hrsa.gov/shortage/muaps/index.html

Healthy People 2020. (2011). *About healthy people*. Retrieved from http://www.healthypeople.gov/2020/about/default.aspx

Hearts Beat Back. (2010). *The heart of New Ulm*. Retrieved from http://www.heartsbeatback.org/project

Institute of Medicine. (1988). *The future of the public's health in the 21st century*. Washington, DC: The National Academies Press.

Institute of Medicine, Board on Population Health and Public Health Practice. (2012). *For the public's health: Investing in a healthier future*. Retrieved from http://iom.edu/Reports/2012/For-the-Publics-Health-Investing-in-a-Healthier-Future.aspx

Juster, H. R., Loomis, B. R., Hinman, T. M., Farrelly, M. C., Hyland, A., Bauer, U. E., & Birkhead, G. S. (2007). Declines in hospital admissions for acute myocardial infarction in New York state after implementation of a comprehensive smoking ban. *American Journal of Public Health, 97*, 2035–2039. doi:10.2105/AJPH.2006.099994

Kaiser Health Foundation. (2012). *National health expenditures, 2010*. Retrieved from http://www.kaiseredu.org/Issue-Modules/US-Health-Care-Costs/Background-Brief.aspx

Leininger, M. M. (1970). *Nursing and anthropology: Two worlds to blend*. New York: Wiley.

Leininger, M. M. (1990). Ethnomethods: The philosophic and epistemic bases to explicate transcultural nursing knowledge. *Journal of Transcultural Nursing, 1*(2), 40–51.

Levi, J., Segal, L. M., & Juliano, C. (2009). *Prevention for a healthier America: Investments in disease prevention yield significant savings, stronger communities*. Washington, DC: Trust for America's Health.

Mayes, R., & Oliver, T. R. (2012). Chronic disease and the shifting focus of public health: Is prevention still a political lightweight? *Journal of Health Politics, Policy, and Law, 37*(2), 181–200.

Mechanic, D., & Tanner, J. (2007). Vulnerable people, groups, and populations: Societal view. *Health Affairs, 26*(5), 1220–1230.

Milstead, J. A. (2013). *Health policy and politics: A nurse's guide* (4th ed.). Sudbury, MA: Jones & Bartlett.

Minnesota Department of Health. Division of Community Health. (2001). *Public health interventions: Applications for public health nursing practice*. St. Paul: Minnesota Department of Health.

Mokdad, A. H., Marks, J. S., Stroup, D. F., & Geberding, J. L. (2004). Actual causes of death in the United States, 2000. *Journal of the American Medical Association, 291*, 1238–1245.

Murphy, S. L., Xu, J., & Kochanek, K. D. (2012). Deaths: Preliminary data for 2010. *National Vital Statistics Reports, 60*(4), 1–69.

National Institute of Mental Health (NIMH). (2005). *Mental illness exacts heavy toll, beginning in youth.* Retrieved from http://www.nimh.nih.gov/science-news/2005/mental-illness-exacts-heavy-toll-beginning-in-youth.shtml

National Institute of Mental Health (NIMH). (2013). *Child and adolescent mental health: Statistics.* Retrieved from http://www.nimh.nih.gov/statistics/index.shtml

Neumark-Sztainer, D., Eisenberg, M. E., Fulkerson, J. A., Story, M., & Larson, N. I. (2008). Family meals and disordered eating in adolescents—Longitudinal findings from project EAT. *Archives of Pediatrics and Adolescent Medicine, 162*, 17–22.

Papps, E., & Ramsden, I. (1996). Cultural safety in nursing: The New Zealand experience. *International Journal of Qualitative Health Care, 8*(5), 491–497.

Pender, N., Murdaugh, C., & Parsons, M. (2011). *Health promotion in nursing practice* (6th ed.). Upper Saddle River, NJ: Pearson Prentice Hall.

Polaschek, N. R. (1998). Cultural safety: A new concept in nursing people of different ethnicities. *Journal of Advanced Nursing, 27*(3), 452–457.

Powers, M., & Faden, R. (2006). *Social justice: The moral foundations of public health and health policy.* New York: Oxford University Press.

Rew, L., & Horner, S. D. (2003). Youth resilience framework for reducing health-risk behaviors in adolescents. *Journal of Pediatric Nursing, 18*(6), 379–388.

Richardson, R., & Carryer, J. (2005). Teaching cultural safety in a New Zealand nursing education program. *Journal of Nursing Education, 44*(5), 201–208.

Robert Wood Johnson Foundation. (2009). *Paradox of plenty.* Retrieved from http://www.rwjf.org/pr/product.jsp?id=45108

Robert Wood Johnson Foundation. (2011). *How does an investment in prevention improve public health?* Retrieved from http://www.rwjf.org/healthpolicy/publichealth/product.jsp?id=73313

Schim, S. M., Benkert, R., Bell, S. E., Walker, D. S., & Danford, C. A. (2007). Social justice: Added metaparadigm concept for urban health nursing. *Public Health Nursing, 24*(1), 73–80.

Schim, S. M., Doorenbos, A. Z., Miller, J., & Benkert, R. (2003). Development of a cultural competence assessment instrument. *Journal of Nursing Measurement, 11*(1), 29–40.

Schneider, M. (2014). *Introduction to public health* (4th ed.). Sudbury, MA: Jones & Bartlett.

Shi, L., & Stevens, G. D. (2010). *Vulnerable populations in the United States* (2nd ed.). San Francisco, CA: Jossey-Bass.

Song, Y., Skinner, J., Bynum, J., Sutherland, J., Wennberg, J. E., & Fisher, E. S. (2010). Regional variations in diagnostic practices. *New England Journal of Medicine, 363*(1), 45–53. Epub 2010 May 12.

Starr, P. (1982). *The social transformation of American medicine.* New York: Basic Books.

Tripp-Reimer, T. (1982). Barriers to health care: Variations in interpretation of Appalachian client behavior by Appalachian and non-Appalachian health professionals. *Western Journal of Nursing Research, 4*(2), 179–191.

Tripp-Reimer, T., & Thieman, K. (1981). Traditional health beliefs/practices of Vietnamese refugees. *Journal of the Iowa Medical Society, 71*(12), 533–535.

United Nations Office on Drugs and Crimes (UNODC) (2012). *UNODC crime statistics.* Retrieved from *http://www.unodc.org/unodc/en/data-and-analysis/homicide.html*

United States Department of Health and Human Services. (2012). *Preventing tobacco use among youth and young adults: A report of the Surgeon General.* Retrieved from http://www.surgeon-general.gov/library/preventing-youth-tobacco-use/full-report.pdf

Wagner, E. H., Austin, B. T., & Von Korff, M. (1996). Organizing care for patients with chronic illness. *Milbank Quarterly, 74*(4), 551–544.

Wallace, P. (2011). Population health in action: Successful models. In D. B. Nash, J. Reifsnyder, R. J. Fabius, & V. P. Pracilio (Eds.), *Population health: Creating a culture of wellness* (pp. 241–256). Sudbury, MA: Jones & Bartlett.

Wennberg, J. E., Bronner, K., Skinner, J. S., Fisher, E. S., & Goodman, D. C. (2009). Inpatient care intensity and patients' ratings of their hospital experiences. *Health Affairs, 28*(1), 103–112.

Wolin, K. Y., Carson, K., & Colditz, G. A. (2010). Obesity and cancer. *Oncologist, 15*(6), 556–565. Published online May 27, 2010. doi:10.1634/theoncologist.2009-0285 PMCID: PMC3227989.

Wright, L., & Leahy, M. (2013). *Nurses and families: A guide to family assessment and intervention* (6th ed.). Philadelphia: F. A. Davis.

CHAPTER 13

"Doing For" and "Being With"

Patricia K. Young • Susan Lampe

CHAPTER OBJECTIVES

1. Differentiate between the constructs of "doing for" and "being with."
2. Explain nursing actions linked with "doing for" and "being with."
3. Explain the aspects of relationship-based family nursing practice.
4. Analyze perceived barriers to cultivating caring relationships.
5. Define the scope of caring in family nursing practice.
6. Examine personal strengths and limitations that enhance or threaten caring relationships.

CHAPTER CONCEPTS

- "Being with"
- Burnout
- Caring
- Caring barriers
- "Doing for"
- Intentional care
- Mindfulness
- Personal barriers
- Refection
- Self-care skills

Introduction

This chapter discusses a conflict often found in nursing that pertains to ideas about "doing for" and "being with" those receiving care in clinical care situations. Task-oriented nurses are busily doing nursing activities, trying to fulfill expected roles and meet employer's expectations. Most work favors the "doing for" task-oriented actions, but this aspect of care is different from "being with" a person. "Being with" is about sensitively providing care. Some nurses might say that "being with" not only uses nursing skills and competencies, but it helps them form individual-nurse-family relationships. Technology can help extend the scope of care, but it is not the same as the presence of a nurse. Those seeking care want someone who cares, listens, and is available.

Since the 1980s, much has been published about the importance of nurses' caring roles. Many have discussed values and meanings associated with giving nursing care. In a busy world, clinical practice is often reduced to tasks. Work is measured by outcomes, compliance with regulations, and meeting accreditation standards. Sometimes nurses are uncertain about the limits of professional boundaries. You might ask, "How can nurses give care without being too friendly or overly involved? What about invading a family's privacy?" At the end of a workday, nurses might be unsure about how they will find time to truly give care.

Many people become nurses because they want to help others. However, the demands of daily work leave little time to do extra things. Getting family members involved just seems like an additional burden. How do you fit family members into an already too busy day? Nurses are often asked to "do more with less." Complete more tasks. Prioritize care. Achieve the desired outcomes. Most activities seem to focus on "doing for." All of the tasks and activities distract nurses from "being with" those who need their care. Nurses who *think family* know the difference between "doing" and "being." They are adept at enacting both. Listening, thinking, and reflecting are tools for "being." This chapter identifies what nurses can do to strengthen the caring aspects of practice. Ideas about "being with" and the development of meaningful relationships are explained.

Understanding the Concepts

The ideas of "doing for" and "being with" seem to reflect different ways to provide care. In nursing practice, more attention seems to be given to "doing for." But "being with" is just as important. These two caring expressions are central to nursing values in providing family-focused care (Fig. 13.1).

"Doing For"

"Doing for" involves tasks and action. This work includes the person needing care and their family members. "Doing for" implies action, busyness. Some might say the opposite of "doing for" is doing nothing. That is not what is implied here.

"Doing For" the Person

Virginia Henderson (1991), a nursing theorist, focused many of her ideas on "doing for." She said nurses' roles were to assist the sick to accomplish tasks they are unable to do

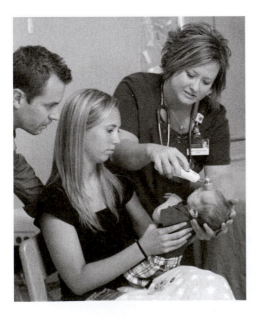

FIGURE 13-1 "Doing for" and "being with" are two important concepts in ways of providing care.

independently. This view is about performing activities for individuals and was often emphasized in the 1960s. "Doing for" describes the actions nurses take to provide care to a person to promote or maintain health, recover, manage an illness or disease, or even have a peaceful death. "Doing for" is done with psychomotor skills. These actions include taking vital signs, giving medications, helping with personal hygiene, monitoring intravenous fluids, and changing dressings. Consider the following examples:

- A nurse cares for the physical needs (e.g., bath, nutrition, elimination, vital signs) of an unconscious person. "Doing for" is direct care given when a physical limitation exists, such as wearing a cast or dealing with hemiparesis from a stroke.
- While changing a dressing the nurse is completing a procedure and teaching a family member how to do needed tasks. "Doing for" can benefit the person and the family.

"Doing For" the Person's Family

Think about a family that does not understand what is happening with a member. The nurse will "do for" the person and family by giving needed care. At the same time, the nurse evaluates what questions the family might have. Family nurses know that recognizing and acknowledging family has great potential for healing (Wright & Leahey, 1999). Family nurses know it is important that families be able to manage care at home. They want to be sure that family units have the knowledge and skills needed. In ambulatory care settings, "doing for" might be health teaching or giving counseling. Families need to know what to do when persons have complex or extensive care needs. They might even be concerned about things nurses think of as usual care (e.g., bathing, grooming, toileting, diet, activity, medications). "Doing for" is more than just taking care of the obvious care needs. Think about a family that has a child with a developmental disability. "Doing for" could mean the nurse acts as an advocate and speaks to a physician on their behalf. Nurses who *think family* notice unique family situations and anticipate future needs. These nurses provide needed information and help locate resources. "Doing for" can also imply the nurse reflects about family care needs and helps family members get information they need.

"Being With"

"Being with" can mean sitting quietly with individuals or families without visible actions—doing nothing. However, this is only partially true. "Being with" involves sharing an emotional presence. This includes listening, seeking to understand a point of view, and learning what matters most. "Being with" might mean assisting family members to understand an elder's point of view in an end-of-life decision.

Being Emotionally Present and Listening

"Being with" is somewhat like the idea of presence. To be present means that the nurse is available and willing to connect with another human being (Benner & Wrubel, 1989). It is a way of recognizing a shared humanity and is different from being aloof, when one is physically present but one's thoughts are elsewhere. Nurses can use eye contact, body language, and tone of voice to enhance a sense of presence or "being with." For example, a new mother may need emotional support and health teaching for breastfeeding. A spouse of an individual with newly diagnosed diabetes may need to learn to give insulin. "Being with" means the nurse listens to concerns. Questions are answered. Empathy is given. Nurses who *think family* know that coaching usually requires a caring presence.

"Being with" is not passive or a one-way activity. "Being with" is a skill that can be learned. Some nurses maintain that "being with" individuals or a family is the essential core of nursing practice (Hartrick Doane, 2002; Idczak, 2007). When nurses focus on "being with" they are in tune and alert for opportunities to notice and respond to individual and family cues. "Being with" implies an open mind and willingness to understanding other perspectives, providing a calm, reassuring presence during a crisis. This presence means listening to needs in a situation because needs for individuals and families differ. Dame Cicely Saunders, an English nurse, physician, medical social worker, and writer, is best known for her role in beginning the hospice movement. She taught that "being with" was a key element in the care of the dying. Presence is important for building trust through an individual-nurse-family relationship. Nurses learn how to treat pain, care for those who are dying, and empathize with those who are suffering by being present.

Understanding Others

Family members know how a member responds to pain. They can share information about what impedes treatment, care management, or rehabilitation; one another's food preferences and physical activity; each other's medical history; and how other members view illness experiences. Family members can discuss reasons why self-care practices are not being done. To "be with" a woman newly diagnosed with breast cancer, the nurse may ask her to share feelings about the diagnosis. As the nurse listens, she may describe her fears and concerns, providing an opportunity for the nurse to explain or answer troubling questions. The nurse might note some of her inner strengths and offer positive feedback. Dr. Erla Svavarsdottir has worked extensively at Landspitali University Hospital in Reykjavik, Iceland to involve families of those experiencing chronic conditions (Box 13.1).

Learning What Matters to the Person and the Family

Therapeutic relationships are built by "being with" individuals. Showing respect and building trust come through "being with" those needing care services. Learning "little things," like the preference for tea rather than coffee, can demonstrate care and empathy. Nursing presence implies care that can be experienced by others. A classic study about expertise in

---

BOX 13-1

Family Tree

Erla Svavarsdottir, PhD (Iceland)

Erla Kolbrun Svavarsdottir, PhD, RN, is a professor and academic chair of Family Nursing, Faculty of Nursing, School of Health Sciences, at the University of Iceland. She established the clinical specialization of Family Systems Nursing at the master's and doctoral levels. She also serves as the head of the Section of Research and Development in Family Nursing at Landspitali University Hospital in Reykjavik, Iceland. Dr. Svavarsdottir completed her doctoral program in 1997 at the University of Wisconsin–Madison under the supervision of Dr. Marilyn McCubbin. She has provided sustained leadership in cutting-edge knowledge translation efforts in family nursing as co-principal investigator of the Landspitali University Hospital Family Nursing Implementation Project (2007–2011). This landmark 4-year project implemented Family Systems Nursing on every unit of a large university hospital in Reykjavik. Dr. Svavarsdottir has worked extensively with Icelandic researchers on family intervention research projects with families of children and adolescents experiencing cancer, asthma, diabetes, anorexia, and bulimia. She received an Innovative Contribution to Family Nursing Award in 2005 from the *Journal of Family Nursing* for her outstanding leadership in family nursing in Iceland. In 2009 she chaired the Ninth International Family Nursing Conference held in Reykjavik, Iceland. She is co-editor of a family nursing textbook called *Family Nursing in Action* (2011) and co-authored a chapter in this book. Dr. Svavarsdottir has served on the Board of Directors for the International Family Nursing Association.

nursing practice said that families have vital secrets that are important for optimal individual care (Benner, Hooper-Kyriakidis, & Stannard, 1999). When student nurses established connections with children in their care, they were better prepared to connect with others in the future (Coetzee, 2004). Family nurses are likely to have similar experiences with adults. Opening oneself to human relationships is at the core of nursing practice (Hartrick Doane, 2002). Nurses who only concentrate on "doing for" can overlook the uniqueness of the individuals, families, and situations found through "being with" others.

The Practice of "Doing For" and "Being With"

Consider this excerpt from the novel *Cutting for Stone* (Verghese, 2009). A surgeon, Dr. Stone, is reading a letter he received from a patient's mother—a patient who had died recently in the emergency department. The mother wrote:

> *Dr. Stone—My son's terrible death is not something I will ever get over, but perhaps in time it will be less painful. But I cannot get over one image, a last image that could have been different. Before I was asked to leave the room in a very rough manner, I must tell you that I saw my son was terrified and there was no one who addressed his fear. The only person who tried was a nurse. She held my son's hand and said, "Don't worry, it will be all right." Everyone else ignored him. Sure, the doctors were busy with his body. It would have been merciful if he had been unconscious. They had important things to do. They cared only about his chest and belly. Not about the little boy who was in fear. Yes, he was a man, but at such a vulnerable moment, he was reduced to a little boy. I saw no sign of the slightest bit of human kindness. My son and I were irritants. Your team would have preferred for me to be gone and for him to be quiet. Eventually they got their wish. Dr. Stone, as head of surgery, perhaps as a parent yourself, do you not feel some obligation to have your staff comfort the patient? Would the patient not be better off with less anxiety, less fright? My son's last conscious memory will be of people ignoring him. My last memory of him will be of my little boy, watching in terror as his mother is escorted out of the room. It is the graven image I will carry to my own deathbed. The fact that people were attentive to his body does not compensate for their ignoring his being.*

This narrative illuminates the significance of not only "doing for" the body, but of also attending to the person through "being with" them. "Doing for" the body is necessary and important, especially in critical care situations. However, "being with" the person or family is equally necessary.

Rather than considering "doing for" and "being with" as two different things, nurses can consider them to be interrelated aspects of effective nursing care. More than a few things are always happening in every care interaction. A student nurse reflects about a care experience with a person having difficulty speaking after a stroke:

The [student] understood that the patient was upset during her morning care. Through patience and a willingness to spend time with the patient, the [student] was able to make a connection with her. She learned that the sponge used to clean the patient's teeth was not "minty" enough and she wrote [in her reflective journal]:

> *Although the conversation took a while because of my difficulty understanding her, I finally understood how it meant a lot to her if I would clean her mouth thoroughly. After I finished with her teeth she expressed how she felt much better and how she could taste the mint. Through her facial expression I was able to see how much she appreciated my time in trying to understand her and thoroughly cleaning her teeth and mouth. I felt I was making a difference in this patient's life even though it was very minor compared to the difficulties she was going through with her stroke." (Idzcak, 2007, p 70)*

The student realized what this woman needed—taking the time to be with her helped the student nurse better understand exactly what was needed, both "doing" and "being" actions.

Connecting With Persons and Their Families

Family nurses use both "doing for" and "being with" during family interactions. Nurses can "be with" individuals and families at the first meeting. Use eye contact as introductions are made. As questions about the person's current condition are asked, nurses listen carefully to responses and address unique needs. A meeting might occur because "doing for" is needed, but the nurse's presence or "being with" can change levels of satisfaction with what occurred.

Observing Nonverbal Cues

Nurses make better connections when they have a "being with" presence. Assessments and careful observations help nurses collect needed information. The nurse notes things that provide clues to needs beyond the biophysical. Is the person grimacing or do they have a flat affect? Are they calm or chaotic? Are significant family members present? Do family members ask questions that show concern? Although hearing oral responses is important, observing nonverbal cues is equally important. Nurses who have spent time "being with" those seeking care are more apt to be aware of nonverbal cues (Fig. 13.2). The nurse can adjust care based on cues and provide more personal care. The nurse might make a proposal (e.g., try sitting up instead of lying down). Or, the nurse might question: Besides medicines, what else has been helpful in relieving pain?

Assessing Personal and Family Needs

Family nurses accompany individuals and families through illness experiences to assure that things they value are addressed. Here are some questions the nurse might ask:

- What does this illness experience mean to you and your family?
- Is the person seeking care the family's primary breadwinner or does he or she play certain vital roles in the family?
- Will a significant monetary loss occur because of the situation at hand?

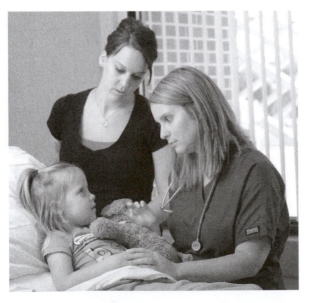

FIGURE 13-2 Nurses need to be aware of nonverbal cues.

- How long will this situation exist?
- Do the person and family understand the diagnosis and treatment?
- Is this a recurrence of a progressive disease that causes future concerns?
- What is your family's previous experience with illness, suffering, and healing?
- Does the treatment require lengthy time away from family, work, school, or other tasks?

When nurses ask questions about family needs, they better discern specific concerns. Nurses who *think family* know that addressing the specific needs of a family unit is the hallmark of family-focused nursing practice.

Providing Intentional Care

Nurses who *think family* are intentional in the care provided. They consider these things:

- What is the goal of this interaction?
- What is the most important thing that needs to be given attention?
- Is the priority to tell, show, or do? ("doing for")
- Is the priority to listen, notice, or respond? ("being with")

The nurse uses "doing for" and "being with" as intentional actions. Family-focused care requires both. Thinking about "doing for" and "being with" is important because what the nurse does and how it is done make a difference (Karlsson & Bergbom, 2010). People need human connections that affirm their humanity. Those interactions can occur while the nurse is giving other care. For instance, if the family shows interest in what is being done, the nurse can use this as a teachable moment. Thinking family shows genuine care as questions are asked. Commendations are given when family effectively demonstrates techniques. Nurses use their presence to guide, coach, and support.

Ways of Caring

Caring is an expected standard of nursing practice (American Association of Colleges of Nursing, 2008). Caring behaviors need to be used with family units, peers, and other health care team members.

"Doing for" and "being with" are two expressions of caring. "Doing for" is often seen as an instrumental behavior of caring. "Being with" is an expressive caring behavior. Florence Nightingale taught us first about caring. In her book *Notes on Nursing* (1859), she wrote of her frustration with nursing:

> . . . nursing has been limited to signify little more than the administration of medicine and the application of poultices. It [nursing] ought to signify the proper use of fresh air, light, warmth, cleanliness, quiet and the proper selection and administration of diet—all at the least expense of vital power to the patient. . . the very elements of nursing are all but unknown. (Nightingale, 1992, p 6)

Nightingale thought nursing was more than "doing for" patients; it requires care for the whole.

During the 1960s and 1970s, nursing moved away from emphasizing caring in favor of being more "scientific." Emphasis was placed on the physical sciences and psychomotor skills. In 1985, Jean Watson published her caring theory and encouraged nurses to recognize that caring is an essential aspect of nursing care. Consumers of nursing services want and need caring practices. Caring is a way to be in relationship with self, others, and the broader environment. The care experience cannot be separated from family, culture, community, and society (Watson & Foster, 2003).

Practicing nurses are expert role models who can provide first-person accounts to help our understanding of being healthy and being ill (Benner & Wrubel, 1989). These ideas made critical differences for persons and families. Note three ways nurses with expert family care skills care for persons in critical care units:

- Ensure that the family can be with the patient.
- Provide the family with information and support.
- Encourage family involvement in caregiving activities.

During the 1990s, the nursing literature said much about nursing's caring role. Nursing is informed caring for the well-being of others and this caring preserves human dignity and well-being (Swanson, 1993). For example, an infant and a new mother have many needed care areas (e.g., physiology, developmental, neurobehavioral, mother's beliefs, values, and understanding) (Swanson,1993). Nurses use caring techniques and knowledge in subtle ways. For example, a newborn intensive care unit nurse places a pacifier in a preterm infant's mouth before diapering. The nurse realizes that non-nutritive sucking is a self-soothing and oxygen-conserving infant self-care behavior. Nurses sense that an infant's overall well-being needs attention. They use caring ethics that treat the child as a person whose self-soothing abilities matter. Nurses apply their personal self-knowledge as they realize how they would wish to be treated if in the infant's position. Swanson's caring theory described five caring processes (Box 13.2).

Caring is one of nursing's four core values along with diversity, integrity, and excellence (National League for Nursing [NLN], 2010). Caring is a significant and necessary quality for nursing practice. The NLN (2007) defines caring as "promoting health, healing and hope in response to the human condition." Not only do nurses care for individuals, families, and communities, but they also need to care for each other and themselves. A tool that can be used by nurses to care for themselves and one another is the Commitment to My Coworkers pledge from Creative Health Care Management (Box 13.3). The goal is that the group accepts the commitment as the unit's working philosophy. The caring commitment has behavioral expectations. It provides personal ways for staff to address one another. It can help establish positive relationships in a healthy work environment.

BOX 13-2

Kristen Swanson: Five Caring Processes

1. Maintaining beliefs: Basic to nurse caring is an orientation of a "fundamental belief in persons and their capacity to make it through events and transitions and face a future with meaning" (Swanson, 1993, p 354).
2. Knowing: The nurse strives to "understand events as they have meaning in the life of the other." It "involves avoiding assumptions, centering on the one(s) cared for, thoroughly assessing all aspects of the client's condition and reality, and ultimately, engaging the self or personhood of the nurse and client in a caring transaction" (Swanson, 1993, p 355).
3. Being with: Being emotionally present to the other. Practices include being there, enduring, listening, attending, disclosing, and not burdening.
4. Doing for: Examples of doing for include both psychomotor activities and emotional support.
5. Enabling: The nurse enables the other to practice self-care. Enabling is defined as "facilitating the other's passage through life transitions and unfamiliar events" (Swanson, 1993, p 356).

> ## BOX 13-3
> ### Commitment to My Coworkers
>
> As your coworker with a shared goal of providing excellent nursing care to our patients, I commit to the following:
>
> - I will accept responsibility for establishing and maintaining healthy interpersonal relationships with you and every member of this staff. I will talk to you promptly if I am having a problem with you. The only time I will discuss it with another person is when I need advice or help in deciding how to communicate with you appropriately.
> - I will establish and maintain a relationship of functional trust with you and every member of this staff. My relationships with each of you will be equally respectful, regardless of job titles or levels of educational preparation.
> - I will not engage in the "3Bs" (bickering, back-biting, and blaming) and will ask you not to as well.
> - I will not complain about another team member and ask you not to as well. If I hear you doing so I will ask you to talk to that person.
> - I will accept you as you are today, forgiving past problems and ask you to do the same with me.
> - I will be committed to finding solutions to problems, rather than complaining about them or blaming someone for them, and ask you to do the same.
> - I will affirm your contribution to quality patient care.
> - I will remember that neither of us is perfect, and that human errors are opportunities, not for shame or guilt but for forgiveness and growth.
>
> _____
>
> Compiled by Marie Manthey; used with permission of Creative Health Care Management.

Caring and Nurse-Family Relationships

Caring for the family is challenging, complex, and multifaceted (Benner et al, 1999; Jeon, 2004; Ward-Griffin & McKeever, 2000). It is an interdependent activity. Both the family and the nurse must actively participate as they work together to build a therapeutic relationship. Nurses who *think family* recognize that the nurse must build the relationship and purposefully move with the family toward mutuality (Jeon, 2004). Mutuality involves collaboration, empathy, interdependence, equality, and reciprocal trust between the nurse and the caregiver (Jeon, 2004). When nurses share positive family experience stories with peers, others can transform beliefs and learn ways family care can improve outcomes. When nurses know what families need and expect when their loved ones seek health care services, they can practice and become competent family nurses. Families of critically ill persons have many needs (e.g., information, assurance, presence, support), but their greatest need is to be an integral part of the illness experience (Eggenberger & Nelms, 2007). Nurses who *think family* recognize how important it is to validate the importance of family in their loved one's care (Jeon, 2004).

Caring for Families in the Community

Financial costs have moved many health care services to shorter institutional stays and more care delivered at home by the family unit. Today, 85% of elder care is provided at home by family members—usually wives, daughters, or daughters-in-law (Ward-Griffin & McKeever, 2000). The U.S population has reached about 309 million people with expectations that it will grow to almost 440 million persons by 2050 (Shrestha & Heisler, 2011). In 1950, the older population made up 8.1% of the population, but that number will reach 20.2% in

2050 when one in five persons will be age 65 or older. Better medical practices, technologies, and medicines mean the baby-boom population will live longer and possibly be healthier, but their chronic illnesses and disabilities still need to be managed at home.

Many in this generation will live with family or independently in communities rather than in care facilities. Home situations are less predictable and nurses who *think family* are aware of risks and member concerns. Families have rules for the ways things get done and family nurses know that they have less control in a family's home and they are ready to work within family rules and values. Four distinct yet interconnected types of relationships are important in caring for frail elderly persons and others in their homes based on the amount of care required (Ward-Griffin & McKeever, 2000):

- Nurse-helper—The nurse gives and coordinates the majority of care; family members provide support.
- Worker-worker—The nurse teaches the family and helps the family members take increased responsibility for care based on their competence and skills.
- Manager-worker—The nurse gradually transitions from providing direct care to monitoring the family caregivers' skills and coping.
- Nurse-patient—Family caregivers need supportive care owing to caregiver burdens.

Relationships Between Community Nurses and Families

Considerable tension can occur in nursing relationships because of (1) unclear expectations between the community nurse and the family caregiver, and (2) an increased amount of physical, emotional, and intellectual labor care transferred from the nurse to family caregivers (Ward-Griffin & McKeever, 2000). Nurses who *think family* consider the potential caregiver role strain of providing 24-hours-a-day care and help find ways to increase support. Community mental health nurses who worked with families of older people suffering from depression found that use of therapeutic relationships improved quality of life for the families (Jeon, 2004). Nurses who form sensitive and caring relationships have also reported increased satisfaction in their practice (Wright & Leahey, 1999).

Barriers to Caring and Nurse-Family Relationships

Many things can be barriers to providing family care and developing therapeutic relationships. Some barriers are intrinsic barriers and belong to the nurse (e.g., attitudes, beliefs, assumptions). Others are extrinsic (e.g., information, technology, hospital systems)—they come from outside the nurse.

Intrinsic Barriers to Caring and Individual-Nurse-Family Relationships

Intrinsic barriers include multitasking, time concerns, belief that caring cannot be learned, lack of preparation or knowledge, assumptions, and fear of emotional pain, unmanaged anxieties, and burnout.

Multitasking

Millennial learners (born 1980–1999) embrace multitasking, often making it hard to focus on one thing. Quiet contemplation and critical reflection that characterize "being with" must be intentionally cultivated so that multitasking does not become a barrier (de Ruiter & Demma, 2011; Pardue & Morgan, 2008). Nurses can cultivate a contemplative attitude by reflecting on care experiences. Responding to questions in writing is useful; here are some ideas (Idczak, 2007):

- Describe an interaction (positive and negative) you had with a family today.
- What thoughts or emotions did you have while you were in the interaction?
- Describe how you experienced yourself during the interaction.
- Describe the emotions you noticed during the individual and family interaction.
- What things about this time seem most important?
- What other thoughts or feelings do you want to share?

Reflecting about experiences generates insights about self and others. Reflection is a way that nurses who have been mostly focused on "doing for" tasks can realize their need for engagement with individuals and families (Bail, 2007). Reflecting can help one think about better ways to "be with" individuals and their families.

Concerns About Time

A stressful barrier that prevents nurses from developing individual-nurse-family relationships is the belief that there is no time to care. Some think "being with" takes extra time. Nurses who *think family* know that caring is an attitude, a way of being or interacting, and doesn't always take more time. For instance, dressing changes take a certain amount of time, regardless of the caring or noncaring attitude by the nurse. Looking like one is pressed for time and hurried might be perceived as a lack of care. Both nonverbal or verbal cues are important. Nurses who *think family* are mindful that how they are "doing for" individuals and families expresses whether they are "being with" them. Dr. Cristina Garcia Vivar is a Spanish nurse studying ways families care for their dependent members (Box 13.4).

The Belief That Caring Cannot Be Learned and a Lack of Preparation

Another barrier is thinking that caring cannot be learned. Caring can be cultivated; students and experienced nurses can practice and learn caring behaviors. One study identified instrumental and noninstrumental caring factors as important (Palese et al, 2011). Instrumental

---

BOX 13-4

Family Tree

Cristina G. Vivar, PhD, MSc, RN (Spain)

Cristina Garcia Vivar, PhD, MSc, RN, is a nursing professor at the Faculty of Nursing, University of Navarra, Spain, and serves as the Assistant Director of the Department of Community and Maternal and Child Health Care. As a graduate student of Dr. Dorothy Whyte at the University of Edinburgh, Dr. Vivar developed a keen interest in family nursing, which led her to conduct her doctoral research with families experiencing cancer recurrence. Her current program of research focuses on families caring for a dependent relative. In Spain, nursing first became integrated into universities in 1997 with a 3-year diploma degree. This has recently expanded to include bachelor, master's, and doctoral degrees. Dr. Vivar has helped move family nursing in Spain forward through many initiatives, including organizing family nursing courses for practicing nurses; teaching family nursing courses to undergraduate and postgraduate students; supervising doctoral students conducting research in family nursing; and presenting her research in family nursing at seminars and at national and international conferences. In her current research, funded by the Spanish Ministry of Education, Dr. Vivar is examining the effectiveness of an educational intervention in Family Systems Nursing (using the Calgary Family Assessment and Intervention Models) with practicing nurses as a way to prepare more nurses to care for families in Spain.

caring is described as knowledge and skills. Patients ranked these acts as the most frequent caring behaviors used. However, the same individuals said that what gives them the greatest satisfaction with nursing care is "positive connectedness." These noninstrumental actions involved "being with" and include spending time, helping them understand, being patient, and involving them in care.

People must feel safe with others before positive connections can be made—a shared humanity with another person (Storr, 2010). For example, when personal thoughts, feelings, fears, and hopes are shared, one becomes vulnerable. Students can plan "being with" in ways similar to preparing for doing technical skills. First, review what has been learned about therapeutic communication and family connections. Next, identify positive and negative responses that might occur in a particular situation. Anticipate a variety of possible responses. Practice can help nurses recognize biases, assumptions, values, beliefs, and attitudes about situations and make needed adjustments. Reflection about experiences can transform nursing practice.

Assumptions

A major barrier to thinking family is a "know it all" attitude. If one appears arrogant or "not present," it is unlikely that others will want to share personal thoughts or feelings. Family-focused nurses explore needs of specific family units in tailored plans of care. Nurses listen to their needs and questions before a plan is made and then the plan is made cooperatively. Nurses need answers to questions such as these:

- What is the family's current level of well-being?
- What is important to this family that relates to the goal of well-being?
- What are the most important things needed at this particular time?
- How can I best learn what is most needed in this situation?

Use of active listening skills will help the nurse to notice and attend to what the family views as most important. Effective listening requires the nurse to be sensitive to personal bias that may influence what is noticed or observed about the family and the things individuals and family members verbalize. Preconceived notions, expectations, and ideas that say families should act in particular ways can interfere with or become barriers to the open stance necessary for family-focused care.

Identifying Personal Assumptions

All nurses have assumptions that shape what and how they notice things around them. Becoming aware of personal thoughts, bias, and prejudices can limit the negative effect of using them in practice (Johns, 1996).

Assumptions are our taken-for-granted beliefs about the world and our place within it; they seem so obvious to us as not to need to be stated explicitly. Assumptions give meaning and purpose to who we are and what we do. In many ways, we are our assumptions. So much of what we think, say, and do is based on assumptions about how the world should work and what counts as appropriate, moral action within it. . . . Ideas and actions that we regard as commonsense conventional wisdom are often based on uncritically accepted assumptions. . . . Critical thinking, at its core, is the process of hunting down and checking these assumptions. (Brookfield, 2005, pp 49–50)

Discovering one's assumptions involves reflection. What guides decisions, actions, and choices related to a particular situation? What can be done to check the accuracy of assumptions? How could one learn whether ideas are true or not? Try looking at the situation from another perspective. Imagine another possible viewpoint or explanation. What might happen if you had a different assumption? Knowing oneself and cultivating authentic caring relationships means assumptions are evaluated. Take a look at the Family Circle case study in Box 13.5, then review the questions and reflect on ways a family-focused caring nurse would respond.

Fear of Personal Emotional Pain and Unmanaged Anxieties

Nurses may be uncertain about what to say in response to those who express fears or concerns about death (Haraldsdottir, 2011). Fear of the emotional pain linked with suffering can be a barrier. However, family interactions provide excellent opportunities to develop confidence and overcome fears (Idczak, 2007; James & Chapman, 2009/2010). At end-of-life care or other critical times, nurses may think they are unprepared to know what to say or do. Previous life experiences influence responses.Those who have difficulty with personal distress or sorrow may shy away from others but those who have wrestled with loss or grief can use their experiences to offer empathy.

Being with an individual or family at end of life can be difficult. Using reminiscing to explore life experiences can be very useful at these times. One of this book's editors recalls a spontaneous review with six adult grandchildren as they stood around their grandmother's bedside for several hours while she was dying. The shared stories and

---

BOX 13-5

Family Circle

Jason, a married middle-aged father of three grade-school-age children, has decided to move his mother into the guest room in his home. Over the past few months, Jason has observed that his mother is having increased difficulty in her ability to care for herself in her home. She has been having trouble managing her multiple medication regimen and has had increased difficulty with mobility. She has become frail since the death of his father 1 year ago. Jason is afraid she will fall and have no one there to help. He expects his two siblings would be happy to contribute financially to help offset the expense of needed home modifications. He thinks they would rather pay for things like safety rails in the bathrooms and other miscellaneous expenses of the move, rather than see her move to a nursing home. He knows that his mother is happier living with family than with strangers and thinks she gets better care from family members. She could develop a closer relationship with their grandchildren and would want to contribute to child care when needed. This arrangement would allow him to fulfill his family obligation to care for her, just as his mom cared for him as a child. Besides, he does not think he could ever live down the guilt that he would experience if he put his mother in a nursing home.

1. What assumptions—explicit and implicit—do you think Jason is operating under in this situation? List as many as you can, then compare your list with that of a peer.
2. Of the assumptions you've listed, which ones could Jason check by simple research and inquiry? What things would he need to do?
3. Give an alternate interpretation of this scenario—a version of what is happening that is consistent with the events described, but that you think Jason would disagree with.
4. What barriers do you perceive for yourself as a nurse cultivating a family-based caring relationship in this home-care situation?
5. As a nurse in this home-care situation, discuss in a small group how you could enhance relationship-based care through "doing for" this family.
6. As a nurse in this home-care situation, discuss in a small group how you could enhance relationship-based care through "being with" this family.
7. Discuss the new thoughts this chapter has offered you in caring for this family.
8. Discuss the new thoughts from this chapter you have learned about caring for yourself as a nurse and a person.

memories about their grandmother caused them to laugh and cry together. The nurse was present, but in the background. If hearing is the last sense to go, then this grandmother faced her dying encircled by love knowing her life was important to her granddaughters.

Nurses might believe that a cheerful and upbeat attitude is better than engaging in the emotional experience. They sometimes think that treating critical situations as if they were normal is the best approach, but that is rarely the case (Haraldsdottir, 2011). Individuals and families appreciate sensitive responses to their unique personal needs. They often need someone to "be with" them during difficult times, even if this means sitting silently or using touch as a signal of care. If nurses compartmentalize or wall off their feelings, it could be that they block the reciprocity needed for a deeply caring relationship (Gerow et al, 2010).

Fear of Burnout

Nurses may also fear that caring too much will cause them to "burn out." However, research about nurses' experiences shows the opposite to be true—engaging with individuals and families is viewed as meaningful (Gerow et al, 2010; Johnston & Scholler-Jaquish, 2007). Nurses who believe they make a difference tend to be more satisfied with their work and have more positive responses when human connections are made (James & Chapman, 2009/2010). A nursing student wrote a reflection that said:

> The nursing internship enhanced my understanding about what it means to be a nurse by doing hands on nursing work full-time. Now, I really grasp that nursing is fundamentally caring for someone. The way my mind works, I always think about nursing as treating patients with highly skilled medical interventions. Diagnostics. Assessments. All that jazz. But a nurse performs so many functions of care. Whether it is administering medication or answering a call light to grab a patient something to drink. A nurse is so many things: a hybrid of a medical professional, a teacher, a hotel concierge, and so on. It is not so much the highly trained skills that patients appreciate, it is the things you do on instinct, your bedside manner that makes the biggest difference to a patient.

Note how this student's experience involves "doing for" and "being with" persons. This student understands that how one does things—one's "bedside manner"—is what truly makes a difference for individual and family experience. Another student writes:

> Despite all of the technical skills in nursing, the one part of nursing care that has inspired me the most has been the patient-to-nurse interaction. Just listening to patients' stories, giving them the love, support, and care they need, has been an incredible experience. I find it amazing how many people share their life story. People trust us, as nurses, and they can open up and share how they are feeling. I've been touched by so many people, young and old, and this has made me a more loving and compassionate person.

This reflection illuminates how nursing students learn the "being with" of nursing; they become self-aware and develop identity as a nurse and a person (Idczak, 2007). Human connections help nurses know they make a difference and affirm that nursing is a good career choice.

Extrinsic Barriers to Caring and Individual-Nurse-Family Relationships

Extrinsic barriers to caring and the individual-nurse-family relationships include outcomes-based work, understaffing, the use of technology, cultural or social barriers, modeled incivility, lack of cultural competence, and labeling.

Outcomes-Based Work

An extrinsic barrier to caring is the demand for task-based work. The value of nurses as employees is often measured in tasks completed and outcome achievement. Emphasis on priority setting keeps nurses focused on tasks and "doing for." Prioritization aims to improve efficiency and avoid errors. These goals are often measured by spending less time or money and using fewer staff members while ensuring safety, competency, and regulatory compliance.

In the current outcomes-based context, caring and "being with" those seeking care often seems less important because that work is less visible and difficult to measure or quantify. Its critical importance is often overlooked. "Doing for" can be measured. Stress on "doing for" might explain why students view physically based caring behaviors (e.g., patient monitoring, completing delegated tasks) as most important (Khademian & Vizeshfar, 2007). "Being with" often occurs in isolated settings and is less easily observed by others or counted as work done.

Health care organizations use tools to measure outcomes. Press Ganey is a company that works with health care organizations to help them innovate and become high-performance organizations (Press Ganey Associates, 2012). Performance is based on the collection and analysis of data to assess patient satisfaction. Their philosophy says that if positive patient experiences are provided, then positive clinical and financial outcomes will follow. High Press Ganey scores are viewed as a reflection of excellence in health care delivery. Press Ganey scores are widely accepted but they only measure perception of nursing care activities that are customer service oriented (e.g., respectfulness, giving clear directions, length of wait time for service). These fail to capture the important relational outcomes of individual-nurse-family relationships.

Understaffing

Understaffing can also be a barrier to caring or "being with" because it places demands on the nurses' time. Inadequate staffing is stressful and distracts from fully meeting less visible needs. The Magnet hospital movement, a recognition program run by the American Nurses Credentialing Center (2012), distinguishes nursing excellence. The program somewhat addresses the low staffing barrier by recognizing that appropriate staffing—with a highly educated staff—makes differences. Adequate staff improves outcomes, work satisfaction, and the likelihood of staying employed in nursing.

The Use of Technology

Technology can also be a barrier to "being with" others. Care providers focused on computers, digital screens, or equipment may pay less attention to care recipients, so care seekers think their needs and questions are less important. If communication via text messages or Facebook is preferred over face-to-face interactions, the value of personal relationships can be unknown, forgotten, or minimized.

Cultural or Social Barriers

Nurses may have personal or familial experiences that interfere with caring behaviors. Some families are less communicative or less demonstrably affectionate. If one has not experienced caring family relationships or seen caring behaviors modeled, it may be hard for them to use them. Educational practices can also be a deterrent. If competition among students rather than cooperation is promoted, introverted students might choose to be less visible or isolate themselves. Students compete to access specific clinical experiences, attain a job, or move up the ladder. Students who lack family experiences with valued caring relationships might avoid "being with" others (Young, Hayden-Miles, & Brown, 2010).

Modeled Incivility

Another extrinsic barrier is incivility. Students who see teachers as autocrats, dictatorial, or uncivil may mimic similar behavior in clinical practice (Clark & Davis Kenaley, 2011). How can students learn caring in an uncaring environment? Nursing actions should incorporate others, promote work as partners, employ coordinated efforts, and use collaborative environments. Academic incivility (e.g., rudeness, being discourteous) is behavior that disrupts the teaching-learning process (Feldman, 2001). Horizontal violence describes the phenomenon of nurses' disrespect for each other. All forms of incivility are barriers to caring, regardless of where it occurs.

Lack of Cultural Competence

Not understanding cultural differences can be a barrier to family-focused caring. Cultural constructs of cultural awareness, humility, knowledge, skill, and desire were discussed in Chapter 6. Knowledge about cultural differences can be institution based and is an ongoing learning process. Cultural competence implies:

- The nurse understands diverse worldviews, avoids stereotyping and misapplying scientific knowledge, and applies knowledge so care quality and health outcomes are improved (Fernandez & Fernandez, 2012).
- Nurses have cultural beliefs, practices, and flexibility that are respectful of others. Their actions involve listening, learning about unique qualities and situations, and providing care that supports health behaviors and eliminates barriers (Fernandez & Fernandez, 2012).

The Practice of Labeling

Labels for persons or families (e.g., the colon resection in room 308, a fresh open heart, overinvolved, demanding) erect barriers to caring. Labeling depersonalizes and causes nurses to be distant and detached (Barry & Purnell, 2008; Ironside, Diekelmann, & Hirschmann, 2005). Applying labels may influence the attention given or the ways things are heard. Labels project interpretations or meanings that might be false. Respect implies acceptance without labels. It is important not to label people by their disease (e.g., using the term diabetic instead of person with diabetes) and consider the household and community needs that influence their care needs (Box 13.6).

"Doing For" and "Being With" Means Knowing Oneself

Self-knowing or self-care are prerequisites to therapeutic relationships. One needs to identify and understand personal emotions. Knowing oneself is fundamental to maintaining personal health, empathizing with others, and having effective therapeutic relationships. Knowing oneself is developed through reflective self-discovery (Box 13.7).

Becoming a Reflective Practitioner

Reflecting on one's practice experience is a hallmark of being a professional (Schon, 1983). It is an essential skill that helps nurses connect previous learning and experience with current actions and outcomes. Reflection helps one construct meaning from experiences, interpret events, and identify important factors in complex situations. It can help one understand and make sense of experiences and events. Reviewing situations can increase

BOX 13-6

Evidence-Based Family Nursing

Diabetes: A Family Matter

The Family Health Model (FHM) was used to devise a plan for a toolkit that could be used in the Appalachian region of the United States to prevent type 2 diabetes and its complications. This most rural area follows the Appalachian Mountains from north to south, and includes 420 counties and parts of 13 states; only West Virginia is included in its entirety. Although type 2 diabetes is known to be preventable and manageable, it continues to spread across the nation and world. This region is recognized as part of what is called the "diabetes belt," and the disease is of epidemic proportions in a largely Caucasian population. This area has a disproportionate level of poverty and its associated problems compared to the rest of the nation. Theory was used to guide thinking about the research conducted as part of this focused work and to think about the consequences and needs of people living with risks for type 2 diabetes in this region. The contextual, functional, and structural domains of the FHM proved useful for thinking about the complex interactions faced by families as they live with and try to manage the disease in their homes and social settings in their communities (Denham, 2003). As family members live in their households, they share established routines and habits that can place members at risk for this disease. This region's high rates of obesity and physical inactivity are just two social factors that put rural residents at risk. The spread of type 2 diabetes is occurring at increasingly younger ages, and disease complications are widespread. Over many years, numerous research studies were conducted to learn more about this regional problem and to better understand the family experience of living with the disease. The toolkit devised uses community volunteers to promote healthy lifestyles, increase knowledge about the importance of active living, and spread knowledge about the disease. A variety of materials were created (e.g., a brochure series, plays, films, fotonovellas, activities) to spread culturally sensitive messages to rural Appalachian residents. An evaluation project and other research that has studied parts of this toolkit has shown that it is culturally sensitive for use with the target audience. The toolkit, Diabetes: A Family Matter and the Family Health Model, can be viewed online at <www.diabetesfamily.net>.

Source: Denham, S. A. (2011). Diabetes: A family matter. In E. K. Svavarsdottir & H. Jonsdottir (Eds.), *Family nursing in action* (pp 309–332). Reykjavik, Iceland: University of Iceland Press.

BOX 13-7

Questions for Self-Discovery

These questions offer some guidance for personal self-reflection and thinking about your relationships with peers, coworkers, and other professionals. Reflection can help nurses prepare to *think family* and offer family-focused care. Reflect on answers to these questions to better understand yourself:

- How do I feel cared for?
- How do I express my care for others?
- What are the areas of myself that do not feel nurtured?
- How do I replenish myself?
- How does self-replenishment relate to the leadership service of others?
- What makes me happy?
- What are my personal routines and rituals for letting go of work/obligations at the end of the day?
- Am I growing healthier in body, mind, and spirit?
- Am I helping others to grow professionally?

Source: Pipe, T. B., & Borst, J. J. (2009). Mindful leadership as healing practice: Nurturing self to serve others. *International Journal for Human Caring, 13*(2), 35–39.

awareness of personal patterns or experiences and reveal how single events are part of a whole. One's perspective is only one of many possible ways to see a situation. Nurses can examine perceptions as they reflect on experiences and this learning has the potential to transform one's practice.

Reflection can be cultivated and nurtured. As the nurse reviews what went right or wrong, what is and is not known get clearer. These viewpoints offer new ways to consider how to do things differently next time. Reflecting on good and bad experiences can prevent repeating similar mistakes. It is a way to identify things that really matter in nursing practice. Use the following questions to guide your reflections:

- What confused, surprised, or worried me today?
- What do I now understand for the first time?
- What am I still wondering about or questioning?
- Who did I disagree with today and why?
- What did I do today that makes me proud?
- In what ways did I practice "doing for" and "being with" today?

These questions can stimulate reflective thinking, a process (i.e., noticing, interpreting, responding, reflecting) important for thinking like a nurse (Tanner, 2006).

Nurses engage in public reflection all the time as they give reports at shift changes. When stories are shared about challenging, standout, or memorable experiences, reflection occurs. Reviewing stories can help nurses make sense of complex situations. They can help one ask questions and rehearse behaviors for doing things differently next time. Debriefings following a critical incident, a clinical experience, or a simulation scenario are reflective experiences. As participants talk about what did and did not happen, listeners see situations differently. Ideas can be reconstructed in meaningful ways. These kinds of activities enable lifelong learning, earmarks of the professional nurse (Fig. 13.3).

Taking Care of Oneself

The work of nursing—caring for others—demands that nurses stay fit. Physical, mental, emotional, and spiritual fitness are all important. Nurses cannot help anyone beyond where they themselves are at a particular point. Self-esteem must be maintained at a

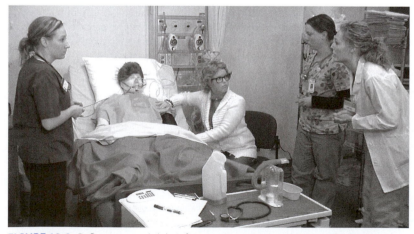

FIGURE 13-3 Reflections and debriefing are important experiences for nurses.

healthy level. Virginia Satir (1988) in her classic book, *The New Peoplemaking*, talks about the importance for those in helping professions to maintain a full "pot of self-esteem." Nurses need to understand what it takes to fill the "pot" as well as what depletes it. Use of reflection throughout a career can help nurses stay in tune with things and check their caring-potential temperature.

Doing a Personal Assessment

It is possible to be a member of a caring profession and neglect oneself. Self-care needs to be intentional, just like caring for others. It might mean conducting a personal inventory, taking stock of one's physical and emotional temperature. This may be as simple as asking oneself, Do I feel rested? Did I get enough sleep last night to keep me energized for the day or do I need to be gentle with my expectations for myself today? Am I eating healthy? Am I exercising? Do I have good work-family balance? Do I maintain healthy relationships? Taking stock also means knowing one's strengths so they can be built upon and limitations so they can be strengthened. What energizes me and makes me feel good about myself? Questions about what characterizes one's inner source of energy or happiness are useful (Box 13.8). Lack of self-care can impede or threaten one's ability to care for others.

Regular reflection about self-care helps develop the awareness needed to be a caring person (Wilson & Grams, 2007). A nurse involved in a structured self-care assessment noted: "When I care for myself, I ultimately help others. My cup is filled so I can fill other cups" (Wilson & Grams, 2007, p 19). The nurse who regularly cares for self embraces caring as a way of being. Another nurse stated, "Caring as a way of being rather than doing has been a new way of thinking. . . . I believe that being caring encompasses doing caring" (Wilson & Grams, p 19).

Developing Self-Care Goals

Following a personal assessment, self-care goals, along with strategies to meet identified goals, can be developed (Wilson & Grams, 2007). This step helps develop positive ways to care for self. Finding a positive role model or a clinical mentor can help in developing effective coping skills. Some nurses use faith and spirituality as ways to manage grief, stress, or emotional upheaval in order to strengthen themselves (Gerow et al, 2010). Personal caring rituals can be used—small acts of doing for others can ground everyday nursing

---

BOX 13-8

Questions for Exploring Sources of Strength, Meaning, and Joy

Questions such as the following can provide useful direction for personal reflections:

- What brought me to nursing/health care?
- What brings me strength?
- What/who inspires me?
- Where do I find joy and meaning?
- What legacy do I hope to leave with my leadership influence?
- What rituals can I build into my daily routine that will help me remember my connection with self and source?

Source: Pipe, T. B., & Borst, J. J. (2009). Mindful leadership as healing practice: Nurturing self to serve others. *International Journal for Human Caring, 13*(2), 35–39.

practice. One can be comforted by doing familiar tasks, things that can involve "doing for" and "being with." Each nurse needs to find favorite ways to care for mind, body, spirit, and relationships as intentional care for self (Brown, 2009). A simple way to care for self might involve being mindful: "Whatever I do first, that's what gets done." This statement reflects the realization that life is busy and complex—people get pulled in many directions. Whatever one chooses to do first in the day may be the only guaranteed thing done that day. It illuminates the importance of setting priorities when doing for oneself. For example, taking a walk first thing in the morning ensures that exercise is accomplished and reflective time occurs. Pick one's "first things" wisely—be intentional; it may be all one can do that day.

Slowing Down

Being busy is a hallmark of contemporary nursing practice (Olson, 2009). But being busy or looking busy often precludes engaging others in meaningful ways. Clearing a space for authentic relating with others—that is, without pretenses of any kind—is an attitude. Slowing down the busyness of daily living opens a space for anticipatory thinking—or, thinking about what might be coming next—and reflecting that characterizes expert nursing practice. One practical way to reduce one's busyness is to simply pause before saying "yes" to a request or agreeing to a new project. "Let me think about this for a bit—I'll get back to you" is all that needs to be said initially. This reply provides the freedom to fully examine one's reaction to the new activity—rather than saying "yes" out of habit. Pausing allows time for a cost-benefit analysis to be done before taking on more work.

Learning to slow down can be particularly challenging. E-mail, instant messaging, pagers, cell phones, and other emerging technologies seem to demand immediate response. Communication in health care is often high stakes, time sensitive, and centers on the preservation of life, health, and human dignity (Pipe & Borst, 2009). Being mindful in practice can help nurses attend to what is happening, being present in the moment. Mindfulness is paying attention and slowing down to pay attention, to consider being given a clinical nursing assignment with many unknowns and uncertainties. Mindfulness means avoiding automatic responses and stopping to take a breath and organize a plan. Mindfulness (e.g., aliveness, self-awareness, self-control) can be developed through training (Scheick, 2011). Breathing exercises, meditation, and yoga are approaches to practicing mindfulness. These actions can help reduce stress, increase healing, and relieve suffering.

Developing an Aesthetic Attitude

Aesthetics involves paying attention to the things that move one emotionally—things that are beautiful, thought provoking, or personally satisfying. Aesthetics reflects the art of nursing—recognizing and holding dear the human experience of illness, health, and healing (Leight, 2002). Cultivating this appreciation implies grasping the full scope of human potential while being open to new possibilities. Paying attention to human experience means seeing the person and not a diagnosis. Developing an aesthetic attitude requires listening to intuition, an inner voice about what matters (Barry & Purnell, 2008). This reflection may occur when obtaining a health history, debriefing after a critical incident, or reading a qualitative report that describes a particular phenomenon or social process. Photos, film, paintings, sculpture, poetry, music, and other art forms tell stories that can be reflected upon and interpreted. What is the artist trying to say about what matters in the experience of being human? Developing one's creative self may feel risky to the nurse grounded in science or caught up in the tasks of "doing for" individuals and families. Nurses need aesthetics; this reflection is the nourishment that inspires and helps connect with core beliefs (Box 13.9).

BOX 13-9

Aesthetic Reflection

On the Web, find an image of the painting by Frida Kahlo entitled *The Broken Column* or one by Rufino Tamayo entitled *The Family*. You can enter the artists' names and painting titles into the search engine. While viewing the image, think about these questions and suggestions:

- If you could tell a story about the person/people in this painting, what would you say?
- What does this painting tell about being human?
- What one word would you use to describe this painting? Why?
- What feelings does this painting evoke in you?
- What do you think the title of this painting means?
- Describe any emotions this painting evokes.
- What do you think the artist is trying to say in this painting?
- What does this painting say to you personally?

Chapter Summary

The core of nursing work is caring—in this instance, family-focused caring. Caring relationships are essential to professional nursing practice and require personal strength. Nurses might find caring relationships challenging when personal experiences conflict with what is met in practice. Nurses can develop the inner strength needed to watch families struggle with issues. They can learn ways to support them as they handle unfamiliar situations. Nurses can use intentionally focused efforts to build skills and confidence for working with family units. Nurses who *think family* use their roles to provide safe and competent care as they "do for" and "be with" others. Family nurses collaborate with family unit members as they establish new life patterns or make sense of critical and unexpected life events. Nurses can use self-care actions to prepare them to "do for" and "be with" those to whom they give care.

REFERENCES

American Association of Colleges of Nursing. (2008). *Essentials for baccalaureate education.* Washington, DC: Author.

American Nurses Credentialing Center. (2012). Program overview. Retrieved from American Nurses Credentialing Center Web site: http://nursecredentialing.org/Magnet/ProgramOverview.aspx

Bail, K. S. (2007). Engaging nurses in patient care: Clinical reflection by a student nurse. *Contemporary Nurse, 25,* 156–162.

Barry, C. D., & Purnell, M. J. (2008). Uncovering meaning through the aesthetic turn: A pedagogy of caring. *International Journal for Human Caring, 12*(2), 19–23.

Benner, P., Hooper-Kyriakidis, P., & Stannard, D. (1999). *Clinical wisdom and interventions in critical care: A thinking-in-action approach.* Philadelphia: W. B. Saunders.

Benner, P., & Wrubel, J. (1989). *The primacy of caring: Stress and coping in health and illness.* Menlo Park, CA: Addison-Wesley.

Brookfield, S. D. (2005). Overcoming impostorship, cultural suicide, and lost innocence: Implications for teaching critical thinking in the community college. *New Directions for Community Colleges, 130*(Summer), 49–57.

Brown, C. J. (2009). Self-renewal in nursing leadership: The lived experience of caring for self. *Journal of Holistic Nursing, 27,* 75–84. doi:10.1177/0898010108330802

Clark, C. M., & Davis Kenaley, B. L. (2011). Faculty empowerment of students to foster civility in nursing education: A merging of two conceptual models. *Nursing Outlook, 59,* 158–165.

Coetzee, M. (2004). Learning to nurse children: Towards a model for nursing students. *Journal of Advanced Nursing, 47*(6), 639–648.

Denham, S. A. (2003). *Family health: A framework for nursing.* Philadelphia: F. A. Davis.

Denham, S. A. (2011). Diabetes: A family matter. In E. K. Svavarsdottir and H. Jonsdottir (Eds.), *Family nursing in action* (pp 309–332). Reykjavik, Iceland: University of Iceland Press.

de Ruiter, H. P., & Demma, J. M. (2011). Nursing: The skill and art of being in a society of multi-tasking. *Creative Nursing, 17*(1), 25–29. doi:10.1891/1078-4535.17.1.25

Eggenberger, S. K., and Nelms, T. (2007). Being family: The family experience when an adult member is hospitalized with a critical illness. *Journal of Clinical Nursing, 16*, 1618–1628.

Feldman, L. J. (2001). Classroom civility is another of our instructor responsibilities. *College Teaching, 49*, 137–140.

Fernandez, V., & Fernandez, K. (2012). Transcultural nursing: Cultural competence. Retrieved January 23, 2012 from Transcultural Nursing Web site: http://www.culturediversity.org/cultcomp.htm

Gerow, L., Conejo, P., Alonzo, A., Davis, N., Rodgers, S., & Williams Domian, E. (2010). Creating a curtain of protection: Nurses' experiences of grief following patient death. *Journal of Nursing Scholarship, 42*, 122–129. doi:10.1111/j.1547-5069.2010.01343.x

Haraldsdottir, E. (2011). The constraints of the ordinary: "Being with" in the context of end-of-life nursing care. *International Journal of Palliative Nursing, 17*(5), 245–250.

Hartrick Doane, G. A. (2002). Beyond behavioral skills to human-involved processes: Relational nursing practice and interpretive pedagogy. *Journal of Nursing Education, 41*, 400–404.

Henderson, V. (1991). *The nature of nursing: A definition and its implications for practice, research, and education. Reflections after 25 years.* New York: National League for Nursing.

Idczak, S. E. (2007). I am a nurse: Nursing students learn the art and science of nursing. *Nursing Education Perspectives, 28*(2), 66–71.

Ironside, P. M., Diekelmann, N., & Hirschmann, M. (2005). Students' voices: Listening to their experiences in practice education. *Journal of Nursing Education, 44*, 49–52.

James, A., & Chapman, Y. (2009/2010). Preceptors and patients—the power of two: Nursing student experiences on their first acute clinical placement. *Contemporary Nurse, 34*(1), 34–47.

Jeon, Y-H. (2004). Shaping mutuality: Nurse-family caregiver interactions in caring for older people with depression. *International Journal of Mental Health Nursing, 13*, 126–134.

Johns, C. (1996). Visualizing and realizing caring in practice through guided reflection. *Journal of Advanced Nursing, 24*, 1135–1143.

Johnston, N. E., & Scholler-Jaquish, A. (Eds.). (2007). *Meaning in suffering: Caring practices in the health professions. Interpretive studies in healthcare and the human sciences* (Vol. 6). Madison: University of Wisconsin Press.

Karlsson, M., & Bergbom, I. (2010). Being cared for and not being cared for—A hermeneutical interpretation of an autobiography. *International Journal for Human Caring, 14*(1), 58–65.

Khademian, Z., & Vizeshfar, F. (2007). Nursing students' perceptions of the importance of caring behaviors. *Journal of Advanced Nursing, 61*(4), 456–462. doi:10.1111/j.1365-2648.2007.04509.x

Leight, S. B. (2002). Starry night: Using story to inform aesthetic knowing in women's health nursing. *Journal of Advanced Nursing, 37*(1), 108–114.

National League for Nursing. (2007). NLN core values. Retrieved from National League for Nursing Web site: http://www.nln.org/aboutnln/corevalues.htm

National League for Nursing. (2010). *Outcomes and competencies for graduates of practical/vocational, diploma, associate degree, baccalaureate, master's practice doctorate, and research doctorate programs in nursing.* New York: Author.

Nightingale, F. (1992). *Notes on nursing: What it is and what it is not.* Commemorative edition. Philadelphia: J. B. Lippincott.

Olson, M. E. (2009). The "millennials": First year in practice. *Nursing Outlook, 57*, 10–17. doi:10.1016/j.outlook.2008.06.001

Palese, A., Tomietto, M., Suhonen, R., Efstathiou, G., Tsangari, H., Merkouris, A., & Papastavrou, E. (2011). Surgical patient satisfaction as an outcome of nurses' caring behaviors: A descriptive and correlational study in six European countries. *Journal of Nursing Scholarship, 43*, 341–350. doi:10.1111/j.1547-5069.2011.01413.x

Pardue, K. T., & Morgan, P. (2008). Millennials considered: A new generation, new approaches, and implications for nursing education. *Nursing Education Perspectives, 29*(2), 74–79.

Pipe, T. B., & Borst, J. J. (2009). Mindful leadership as healing practice: Nurturing self to serve others. *International Journal for Human Caring, 13*(2), 35–39.

Press Ganey Associates. (2012). Our mission. Retrieved from Press Ganey Web site: http://www.pressganey.com/aboutUs/ourMission.aspx

Satir, V. (1988). *The new peoplemaking.* Mountain View, CA: Science and Behavior Books.

Scheick, D. M. (2011). Developing self-aware mindfulness to manage countertransference in the nurse-client relationship: A developmental and evaluation study. *Journal of Professional Nursing, 27*(2), 114–123. doi:10.1016/j.profnurs.2010.10.005

Schon, D. A. (1983). *The reflective practitioner: How professionals think in action.* New York: Basic Books.

Shrestha, L. B., & Heisler, E. J. (2011). The changing demographic profile of the United States. Congressional Research Service #7-5700, CBS Report for Congress. Retrieved February 27, 2012 from http://www.fas.org/sgp/crs/misc/RL32701.pdf

Storr, G. B. (2010). Learning how to effectively connect with patients through low-tech simulation scenarios. *International Journal for Human Caring, 14*(2), 36–40.

Swanson, K. M. (1993). Nursing as informed caring for the well-being of others. *Image: Journal of Nursing Scholarship, 25*(4), 352–357.

Tanner, C. (2006). Thinking like a nurse: A research-based model of clinical judgment in nursing. *Journal of Nursing Education, 45*(6), 204–211.

Verghese, A. (2009). *Cutting for stone.* New York: Vintage Books.

Ward-Griffin, C., & McKeever, P. (2000). Relationships between nurses and family caregivers: Partners in care? *Advances in Nursing Science 22*(3), 89–103.

Watson, J. (1985). *Nursing: Human science and human care.* New York: National League for Nursing.

Watson, J., & Foster, R. (2003). The Attending Nurse Caring Model®: Integrating theory, evidence and advanced caring-healing therapeutics for transforming professional practice. *Journal of Clinical Nursing, 12,* 360–365.

Wilson, C. B., & Grams, K. (2007). Reflective journaling and self-care: The experience of MSN students in a course on caring. *International Journal for Human Caring, 11*(1), 16–21.

Wright, L. M., & Leahey, M. (1999). Maximizing time, minimizing suffering: The 15-minute (or less) family interview. *Journal of Family Nursing, 5,* 259–274. doi: 10.1177/107484079900500302

Young, P., Hayden-Miles, M., & Brown, P. (2010). Narrative pedagogy. In L. Caputi (Ed.), *Teaching nursing: The art and science* (2nd ed., Vol. 2, pp 804–836). Glen Ellyn, IL: College of DuPage Press.

CHAPTER 14

Family-Focused Nursing Actions

Sandra K. Eggenberger • Wendy Looman

CHAPTER OBJECTIVES

1. Explain core processes from nursing and family perspectives.
2. Describe relationships among family, family context, core processes, and family-focused nursing practices.
3. Discuss ways core processes are linked to health.
4. Identify ways nurses can use core processes to design nursing actions.
5. Describe family-focused nursing actions that lead to quality care outcomes.

CHAPTER CONCEPTS

- Caregiving
- Cathexis
- Celebration
- Change
- Communication
- Connection
- Coordination
- Core processes
- Family meetings
- Nursing actions

Introduction

In family-focused nursing practice, care involves intentional actions, family partnerships, and thinking family. Although actions are often specifically targeted to fulfill individual needs, they aim to optimize family health. Family nursing is holistic care for family units regardless of the nursing action being implemented. The Family Health Model (Denham, 2003) describes core family processes as part of the functional domain. Core processes attend to ways family members interact; they are potential areas of strengths. These processes are also linked with wellness, health, prevention, illness, care management, and other related needs. The seven core family processes—communication, caregiving, cathexis, celebration, change, connectedness, and coordination—are used to guide assessment, nursing actions, and outcome evaluation. Core processes are central to individual and family health.

Nurses who *think family* use the individual-nurse-family partnership to identify goals and plan actions directly linked to safe, therapeutic, and quality care outcomes. Nurses use core family processes to identify strengths, address health concerns, minimize health risks, and maximize health potentials (Denham, 2003) so they can identify and design strategic actions for family unit needs. Nurses who *think family* know that health and illness can never be separated from the daily lives in shared family households. This chapter describes ways nurses use core processes to empower and support family units as they strive for member and family health. Relevant nursing actions and evidence related to each of the core process are presented.

Family-Focused Nursing Actions

Even when the family is not physically present, the family remains a significant force in the lives of persons seeking health or illness care. Therefore, family nursing actions are critical to all health and illness outcomes. The nurse can still *think family* even when focusing on individual needs. Individual care is directed toward the family unit because current evidence shows strong links between individual and family health (Kaakinen, Harmon Hanson, & Denham, 2010; Weihs, Fisher, & Baird, 2002). However, more research aimed at development, testing, implementing, and evaluating the effectiveness of nursing actions with the family unit is needed (Chesla, 2010).

The Family Health Model focuses on core family processes and provides a framework to plan, guide, and evaluate nursing actions (Denham, 2003). Delivering competent, safe, and quality care demands nursing actions that guide and evaluate progress toward individual and family goals. Action implies doing and influencing (Abate, 2002).

Nursing is a practice discipline and actions must be skillfully completed using relational and scientific elements (Chinn, 2008; Dahnke & Dreher, 2011). Effective family-focused nursing care considers the unique nature, experience, strengths, challenges, and needs of family units (Almasri et al, 2011; Siminoff, Wilson-Genderson, & Baker, 2010). These actions consider the family's beliefs, values, patterns, functioning, and culture (Kaakinen, Gedaly-Duff, Coehlo, & Harmon Hanson, 2010; Pavlish & Pharris, 2012).

Delivering Family-Focused Nursing Actions

When planning, delivering, and evaluating care, nurses have an obligation to partner with a family about the course of actions to be taken (American Nurses Association, 2001). Several elements of a nursing action need to be considered. First, who is the recipient of the nursing action? Is the action aimed specifically toward unique persons or the family unit as a whole? Even in a situation in which the nurse is focused on an individual's acute care needs, there is still the opportunity to address and meet the needs of multiple household members (Fig. 14.1). Nurses can communicate with ill persons or arrange a family meeting to resolve caregiving decisions. At times the family unit is the direct care recipient, such as when a family is negotiating end-of-life care.

Second, nursing actions address the variable of concern or what can be influenced. What elements of the family's experience, strengths, and needs are or are not being met? Do the nursing actions aim to increase family communication or ease suffering? Does the action focus on anxiety about caring for an ill or dying member? Communication must be clear and directed at the need.

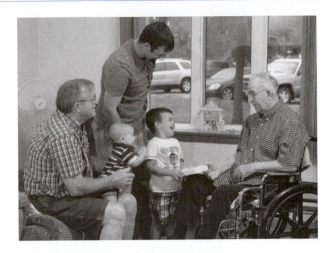

FIGURE 14-1 Multiple family members have various needs for nursing care.

Third, consider the setting. Does the nursing action take place in an acute care hospital, a clinic, or the family's home? What factors need to be addressed in this setting? What coordination needs to occur among care settings with multiple medical providers? Care needs influence the direction of nursing actions and nurses' skills influence the effectiveness of the care delivered (Nelms & Eggenberger, 2010; Newman, 2008). Does the nurse intentionally include the family in care?

Care Models to Guide Nursing Actions

Evidence that family-focused nursing actions can improve health and illness outcomes exists, but family interventions still need to be fully developed and used in nursing practice (Chesla, 2010; Duhamel, 2010). A variety of models that address family nursing actions exist. Earlier in this text (Chapter 7), four particular models to guide nursing practice were discussed: the Illness Beliefs Model, Calgary Family Intervention Model, Family Health System Model, and Family Management Style Framework. The Illness Beliefs Model focuses on strengthening and facilitating beliefs and challenging constraining ones (Wright & Bell, 2009). The Calgary Family Intervention Model (CFIM) focuses on cognitive, affective, or behavioral domains of family functioning (Wright & Leahey, 2012). The CFIM suggests that interventions to promote, improve, or sustain family functioning should be offered (Wright & Leahey, 2013). The Family Health System (FHS) Model describes family realms of development, interaction, coping, integrity, and health processes, and suggests nursing actions in these areas (Anderson & Tomlinson, 1992). The Family Management Style Framework (FMSF) explains ways families respond to enduring children's chronic illness by examining the component of definition of the situation, management behaviors, and perceived consequences (Knafl, Deatrick & Havill, 2012).

Nursing Actions Focused on Family Core Processes

Family interviews are nursing actions that provide nurses with the opportunity to better understand members and household concerns in the initial and ongoing assessments (Nelms & Eggenberger, 2010; Wright & Leahey, 2013). Exploration of family processes during these assessments can be used to intentionally plan tailored interventions that are designed to meet unique family unit needs. Directing nursing care to family processes facilitates a partnership to support family units as goals are set, plans are developed, and actions taken to identify strengths and concerns (Denham, 2003).

Core Family Processes

Core family processes provide ways to approach families and assist them to plan for needed changes. Process implies a course of action, series of changes, and progress (Abate, 2002). Families live their lives differently as they face health problems, manage illnesses, and work to prevent diseases or complications (Rolland & Walsh, 2005). On-going interactions among household members influence well-being and family health (Denham, 2003). If a parent experiences an acute illness it may disrupt prior patterns and roles and may create conflict. Chronic conditions can challenge members' abilities and stretch their limits. Nurses can assist families in developing plans, understanding responses, planning for the future, and managing needs (Chesla, 2010; Kaakinen et al, 2010; Segrin & Flora, 2011).

Core Processes—A Framework for Nursing Actions

Family processes can be disrupted when illness or a crisis strikes, and core processes can help guide assessment and suggest areas for nursing actions that can help (Denham, 2003). Figure 14.2 shows a range of nursing actions that can be used with families; each of these actions may be appropriate in different situations and in support of the various core processes. Figure 14.3 depicts linkages of nursing action, core processes, and targeted care outcomes for family units (Denham, 2003). Figure 14.4 identifies collaborative relationships for provision of coordinated care.

Nurses who *think family* consider the location and type of family household, as well as the neighborhood and community, which can influence planning, implementation, and

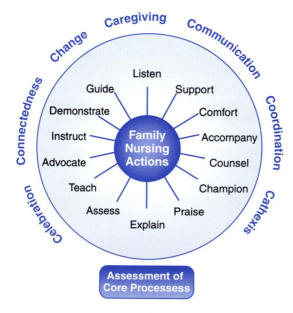

Nurses assess core processes of indviduals and family units, and then use nursing actions to plan, implement, and evaluate care.

FIGURE 14-2 Nursing actions, and core processes.

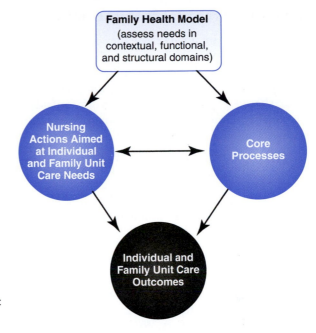

FIGURE 14-3 The Family Health Model: family needs and care outcomes.

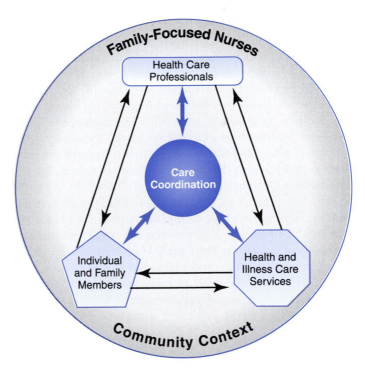

FIGURE 14-4 Nursing actions in care coordination.

evaluation of care. Family-focused nursing actions view the core processes of the family system within the community and societal systems. Although time is not depicted in Figure 14.4, it is considered as its passing means development, social, and political changes that affect care needs. The nurse can use a framework of core family processes to identify family strengths and incorporate these into the plan for care, set goals, and evaluate outcomes. The individual-nurse-family partnership is used to set goals and plan ways to achieve them.

Using Core Processes to Meet Complex Care Needs

Core processes are not discrete; they are connected to the life surrounding the family. Family units have complex interactions with the larger community. Core processes can be used to understand ways particular families respond to life experiences and daily life that affect family health. Nurses who *think family* know family members live interdependent lives, with shared experiences linked to life outside their household boundaries. Although personality, motivation, genetics, and other factors influence lives, these factors are bound to environmental factors often beyond their control. Family-focused nurses understand that continuity of care reaches beyond the walls of health care settings. Change is certain in families with multiple transitions, but they are still a family. However, the meanings of these transitions to the family must be considered when planning nursing actions. A nurse's challenge is to help families identify solutions they value and offer support that empowers them to adjust to change and make needed changes in their own world.

Intentional Nursing Actions to Guide Core Family Processes

Core family processes provide ideas about ways family nurses can assist family units to attain, maintain, and regain health and manage illness experiences. Nurses act as advocates, guides, coaches, teachers, coordinators, counselors, and evaluators (Hamric, Spross, & Harmon Hanson, 2009; Kaakinen, 2010). Intentional actions are necessary to address care needs. An ecological point of view can guide intentional thinking and acting to address needs in a complex world. Family nurses know that effective actions are singularly focused but must address the complexity that surrounds interactions. Family connections beyond household boundaries and within the community create potential threats and supports. Social and political realms might seem outside the family, yet they may intensify threats and strengthen supports linked with health and illness. An ecological perspective helps one see community linkages, and social networks are windows to risks and strengths. Core processes address broad factors associated with individual and family health.

Nurses who *think family* use evidence to support actions. Living with illness, maintaining health, or preventing disease are not singular actions, but involve complicated family system interactions with social and institutional networks. As nurses identify health in relationship to the family unit's past, present, and future, core processes offer a framework for addressing needs. They inform the planning, development, and evaluation of nursing actions that meet a breadth of health and illness experiences across the life span. Table 14.1 lists the core processes suggested by the Family Health Model (Denham, 2003) and provides examples of assessments, actions, and evaluation strategies to be used in nursing practice. Interview questions, family dialogue, and conversations are used during assessment and care. This intentional nursing action invites reflection, relationship development, and inquiry. Use of core processes suggests goals or outcomes to evaluate as care is planned.

Case Introduction

This chapter refers to the Zimanske family, previously introduced in Chapter 11 as a family experiencing chronic illness. The family includes Michael, diagnosed with Schimke immune-osseous dysplasia (SIOD) at age 7, a sibling named Jessica, and parents Theresa and Don. This family experienced an unexpected journey filled with times of uncertainty and struggles. An obscure diagnosis was followed by years of illness and multiple acute exacerbations requiring hospitalization. The family experienced other member illnesses during this time. Throughout this section of the chapter content related to the core process

TABLE 14-1	Core Family Process: Assessment and Family-Focused Nursing Action		
CORE FAMILY PROCESS	**FAMILY NURSING ASSESSMENT**	**FAMILY-FOCUSED NURSING ACTION**	**EVALUATION**
Cathexis	Create and discuss a family genogram and ecomap with family members. Explore a family's emotional connections. Sample question: Can you tell me how your family members are linked to each other? This must be difficult for your family to see your son and brother's condition constantly deteriorating.	Discuss the differences in ways family members view health and illness experiences and the influence on the emotional bonds. Allow time for reflection on family connections (Moules, Thirsk, & Bell, 2006). Discuss aspects of grief using intergenerational perspectives (O'Leary, Warland, & Parker, 2011). Explore the ongoing nature of grief.	Knowledge of family structure, function, and relationships are evident to health care providers. Family begins to explore their relationships and influence on health promotion, maintenance, and illness care.
Communication	How would you describe your family's communication about this illness? In what ways does your family's communication influence health?	Arrange a family meeting focused on developing individual understandings about needs and coping of the family unit. Guide family discussion of family needs. Explore with the family data collected during creation of the genogram and ecomap.	Family members express improved comprehension of beliefs about illness, coping, emotions, responses, and communication. Family members describe communication patterns that support health. Families set goals for improving communication.
Caregiving	What type of care does your family member require from your family? Can you describe how your family cares for members? What is the most difficult part of caring for your family member? What is the most positive element of caring for your family member?	Identify member roles in providing care for the ill individual. Describe support needed for family caregiving roles. Find ways family can access needed resources. Commend members for strengths in caregiving roles. Identify priority concerns related to caregiving roles in the family.	Concerns about priority areas of caregiving identified are resolved. Family members are building on strengths in caregiving roles.

Continued

TABLE 14-1	*Core Family Process: Assessment and Family-Focused Nursing Action—cont'd*		
CORE FAMILY PROCESS	**FAMILY NURSING ASSESSMENT**	**FAMILY-FOCUSED NURSING ACTION**	**EVALUATION**
	How can I most help you as you care for your ill family member?	Help family communicate about stress and strain of caregiving.	
Celebration	Tell me the ways your family enjoys spending time together? What are times that you enjoy being together? How does your family usually celebrate a holiday? What changes do you foresee will need to occur so that your family can enjoy special time together?	Identify possible ways family can continue valued family traditions. Create a list of celebrations that can still occur and note needed modifications. Consider options for new activities to share in the future.	Family's celebrations, rituals, and routines are viewed as meaningful. Family activities are viewed as special and valued times.
Change	Can you describe the most difficult change you and your family will need to make as a result of this chronic illness? Describe concerns about family routines that will need to change.	Identify family beliefs that support healthy changes (Wright & Bell, 2009). Coach ways to move toward positive health changes (Hamric, Hanson, Tracy, & O'Grady, 2014). Commend strengths (Wright & Leahey, 2013).	Family members identify specific steps to making needed changes. Family members discuss ways conflicts can be negotiated Arrangements are made for needed changes.
Connections	Examine social connections in the ecomap developed with the family. What ways are you involved with the community? Tell me about your relationships with your health care providers. How do your social networks provide needed support?	Provide information about local support services or groups. Discuss ways family can fulfill family roles and responsibilities and still care for self. Identify ways members can access supports (e.g., church, friends, social networks). Explore ways the Internet can be used to link with those experiencing a similar condition.	Family members maintain caring relationships that provide needed support. Individuals have adequate personal time each week. Respite care is arranged through a network of neighbors and other friends.

TABLE 14-1	Core Family Process: Assessment and Family-Focused Nursing Action—cont'd		
CORE FAMILY PROCESS	**FAMILY NURSING ASSESSMENT**	**FAMILY-FOCUSED NURSING ACTION**	**EVALUATION**
Coordination	How does your family work together to coordinate care for your family member? What are the biggest struggles that your family experiences as you try to coordinate available services with needs?	Identify available community resources that can support the family. Provide a list of social agencies where additional care services might be accessed. Contact health care provider(s) about a referral to social services for needs in the home.	Family members develop a schedule that identifies who will regularly perform various tasks. The nurses, social worker, and family arrange for needed home services.

will be introduced with quotes from the family providing the opportunity to apply the knowledge. This case illustrates ways nurses can use core processes to facilitate family-ocused nursing actions. The narratives are linked with core family processes to demonstrate family needs and nursing actions.

Cathexis: Core Family Process

Cathexis is "the emotional bond that develops between individuals and family as members invest emotional and psychic energy into loved ones" (Denham, 2003, p 125). This term is a useful way to understand the attachment that develops among family members. Bonds are often expressed as warmth, care, love, and regard—factors that promote family health (Denham, 2003). Childhood attachments continue into adulthood and throughout family life act as driving forces for family functioning and routines (Wood, Klebba, & Miller, 2000). Family members depend on one another for emotional, physical, and economic support (Denham, 2003).

Cathexis refers to family members' invested efforts in one another as they rely on and care for one another. Decathexis is the disconnecting or disentangling needed when a family member grieves the loss of a close attachment following death or other loss (Denham, 2003; Rando, 1984). Decathexis occurs as those left alone learn to separate their lives from persons or things once essential in life. Grief experts suggest loss is an evolving disconnection from the deceased that allows the family to continue life without a person (Moules, Simonson, Fleiszer, Prins, & Glasgow, 2007; Moules, Simonson, Prins, Angus, & Bell, 2004). Decathexis causes separation and interrupts attachments. Divorce or diseases that affect a member's proximity and personhood (e.g., Alzheimer's disease) create needs for decathexis. Cathexis is about strengthening attachments and relationships for the good of individual members and the family unit.

Cathexis as a Family-Focused Nursing Action

Commitment and attachment are central to family life with bonds developing as members are added to the family unit (Boss, Doherty, LaRossa, Schumm, & Steinmetz, 1993). The nurse can use an understanding of cathexis to support healthy family bonds. For example, after a child is born, nurses support bonding between parent and newborn and teach skills to care for and protect the baby. Children and adults need similar bonding in their shared lives to influence health. Commitment among family members in particular and across family units varies. An individual's health affects the family unit and family health affects individual members (Kaakinen et al., 2010). Emotional bonds unite families and strong committed support is a foundation to build upon. These bonds are threatened when disruptions and conflicts occur and during times of stress and illness (Eggenberger & Nelms, 2007; Siminoff et al., 2010). Box 14.1 describes a program of research that addresses the individual-nurse-family partnership.

Nurses can focus on cathexis during transitions and changes surrounding illness, severe stress, or death (Moules, Thirsk, & Bell, 2006; O'Leary, Warland, & Parker, 2011). Box 14.2 identifies potential concerns linked with the cathexis process—commitment, loss, grief, chronic sorrow, and ambiguous loss—which are areas for identifying nursing actions. Grief and loss are expected life aspects, but are difficult for most people. Chronic sorrow lacks a predictable end and can occur when living with a disability or an increasingly worsening chronic illness. This sorrow occurs with childhood problems and also with older persons' caregivers (Burke, Eakes, & Hainsworth, 1999; Moules et al., 2007; Zerwekh, 2006). Ambiguous loss occurs with physical or psychological absence or if a body is missing because of a natural disaster (Boss, 2006; Garwick, Detzer, & Boss, 1994). Loss triggers needs for family members to cling together; hence, cathexis or drawing together often needs to occur.

BOX 14-1

Evidence-Based Family Nursing Practice

Living with advanced lung disease can be a challenging experience for individuals and their family members, an area of care not often addressed in the literature. Treatment often occurs as episodic and isolated events focused on individual needs; rarely is chronic obstructive pulmonary disease (COPD) viewed as a family event. Individual's symptoms of breathing difficulties, fatigue, malnutrition, anxiety, and depression are likely to increase over time. Costs to families such as caregiver burden and increased care expenditures are reasons this is a serious chronic condition. An outpatient clinic at Landspitali University Hospital in Reykjavik, Iceland, uses a nurse clinic for persons with breathing problems. The focus is on the unmet health care needs of individuals and family members. A holistic approach and collaborative partnership occur between the family unit and health professionals. A nursing partnership framework is used to focus on the entirety of health-related problems to foster possibilities. Through a relational dialogue, areas of family involvement, living with symptoms, and access to health care are addressed. The dialogue allowed meanings to emerge that were then acted upon. Nurses focused on positive regard, building trust, and respect for personal values and ways of being. As all think together, whatever emerges as the concerns becomes the focus of the care. Using both quantitative and qualitative research methods, the number of hospitalizations showed about an 80% decrease. Individuals reported a more satisfactory quality of life and a decrease in symptoms caused by the disease. Families gained greater capacity to manage the disease at home as they better understood the disease and the consequences of actions and gained independence in care decisions. Nurses established trusting relationships that enabled more coherent actions to be taken. Health professionals became more accessible and interactions more meaningful.

Source: Ingadottir, T., & Jonsdottir, H. (2010). Partnership-based nursing practice for people with chronic obstructive pulmonary disease and their families: Influences on health-related quality of life and hospital admissions. *Journal of Clinical Nursing, 19*(19/20), 2795–2805. doi:10.1111/j.1365-2702.2010.03303.x

BOX 14-2

Phenomena Related to Cathexis

Family commitment and affiliation: Bonds develop between family members and unit.

- Family transitions may require committed supports for health and illness care (Meleis, 2010).

Loss: Family loses an attachment to a person or object through life-changing and family experience.

- Grief involves working to incorporate loss into life and move forward.
- Complicated loss may suggest need for referral to family support services (Holtslander & McMillan, 2011; Moules, Simonson, Fleiszer, Prins, & Glasgow, 2007; Worden, 2009).

Chronic sorrow: Ongoing emotional response that ebbs and flows when a functional loss occurs in oneself or another attached person

- Recurring and pervasive loss with no predictable end triggered by events that remind one of the continuous gap between what might have been and realities faced
- Often triggered by events that remind one of the continuous gap between what might have been and realities faced (Eakes, 1993; Eakes, Burke, & Hainsworth, 1998; Isaakson & Ahlstrom, 2008; Lindgren, Burke, Hainsworth, & Eakes, 1992; Melvin & Heater, 2004; Moules et al, 2007).

Ambiguous loss: Absence of a person either physically or psychologically

- Examples of physical absence could be a war causing a family member's death, divorce in the family, or child's death. Psychological absence can be a family member's depression or neurological disorder, such as Alzheimer's disease (Boss, 2006).

Case Study Application: Family Illness and Cathexis

Throughout Michael's chronic illness, the Zimanske family experienced needs and concerns linked with cathexis. The family was strongly connected at the time of diagnosis and during illness, but members lived independent lives and a shared journey with chronic illness. Chronic sorrow was a recurring part of their lives each time Michael faced a critical change. As he moved from walking to a scooter to a wheelchair to attend school they faced grief and sorrow. Theresa struggled to keep Michael in school to be with friends and normalize life. Family members had continuous losses as the disease progressed. Life was a roller-coaster with remissions interrupted by exacerbations. Nursing actions to address chronic sorrow would have been useful throughout the illness and even after his death. The Zimanskes lived with the unending nature of the illness, emotional pain, and loss over time. Even after Michael's death, anniversaries were reminders of hopes and dreams unfulfilled. Some families bond more closely together as they share experiences known only to them. Sometimes conflicts and internal stress develop because individuals pull away as they grieve differently. Cathexis is about coming together as a family to strengthen bonds, stretch capacities, and make use of limited resources.

THERESA: "Our family had a strong emotional attachment to each other and the family. Michael's illness was a grief process over time. We were mad and angry about the diagnosis. It was hard to hear that my son was chronically ill and would die. Jessica, Michael's sister, had a big role in the illness and her bonds with Michael were strong. Yet, nurses often consider the parents with an ill child, but not the sibling. When I was diagnosed with breast cancer I was forced to think about myself and what my possible loss could mean for the family."

Table 14.2 identifies aspects of cathexis, areas of strengths, and potential concerns that often emerge in family life. Focused nursing actions and possible evaluation methods are proposed. Family assessments are actions that help the nurse and the family gain understandings of family strengths and find ways to build on those strengths.

TABLE 14-2   *Potential Areas of Focus in Cathexis*

NURSING ASSESSMENT	FAMILY-FOCUSED NURSING ACTION	EVALUATION
Commitment and affiliation within the family unit and individual members: Explore genogram and ecomap to identify strengths and needs related to family bonds.	Recognize cultural and individual variations in the view of family commitment (Giger & Davidhizar, 2007). Help family to develop skills and techniques that facilitate attachment and commitment (Veltri, 2010). Observe and praise behaviors of warmth and care that develop between parents and children, new members of a family, and societal networks (Davidson, London, & Ladewig, 2012).	Bonds within and outside the family unit develop that promote health of members and family unit. Members and family unit function to address needs linked with activities of daily living and meeting goals.
Loss: Use assessment techniques that invite family dialogue and nurse-family conversation.	Explore changes in family dynamics and relationships during times of transitions with additions or changes in family members (Meleis, 2010). Recognize cultural and individual variations in the view of loss for each family (Shaefer, 2010). Invite family members to express grief, and listen to the answer of each family member (Shaefer, 2010). Provide accurate information about the death, loss, and grief (Shaefer, 2010). Acknowledge and discuss family members' various forms of coping with the loss and encourage family members to talk with each other (Segrin & Flora, 2011). Statements such as: "I am so sorry for your loss. This must be a difficult experience for you and your family." Questions such as: "How can I help you?" Then, listen to the answer of each family member (Shaefer, 2010). Assist family in grief work though efforts such as finding meaning in the experience (Moules, Simonson, Gleiszer, Prins, & Glagow, 2007). As appropriate, refer family members to needed and available resources (McDaniel, Campbell, Hepworth, & Lorenz, 2005).	Individuals and family experience losses, but manage in ways that support health and well-being of all members. Individuals understand that grief processes may differ, but look for ways to communicate needs and concerns to each other.
Chronic sorrow: Assess chronic sorrow using instrument such as Chronic Sorrow Questionnaire (Burke, 1989). Therapeutic communication, such as: Tell me about you, your family, and this illness.	Validate the presence of chronic sorrow with the family and provide reassurance of the normality of this reaction (Bettle & Latimer, 2009; Isaakson & Ahlstrom, 2008). Assist family members in recognizing and building on existing strengths (Bettle & Latimer, 2009).	Individuals and family recognize problems associated with chronic sorrow and develop strategies to effectively manage problems.
Ambiguous loss: Explore family's perception of loss.	Assist family as they attempt to find meaning in loss (Boss, 2006). Guide individual family members and the family in planning the future (Boss, 2006). Assist family members as they identify individual and family past strengths and develop sources of support (Boss, 2006).	Individuals and family express understandings about the meanings of loss and identify specific ways to manage uncertainties over time.

Communication: Core Family Process

Family communication is a continuous, complex, and changing process that affects the mental and physical well-being of individuals and family units (Segrin & Flora, 2011; Weihs et al, 2002). As a core process, communication is used to interact around needs related to health and illness. Communication patterns are shaped in families by their unique histories, life experiences, and current events. Family systems form different communication patterns as individual, dyadic, and triadic forms influence family routines and rituals (Denham, 2003; Segrin & Flora, 2011). Mutually supportive member relationships and clear direct communication about an illness and its management can contribute to individual and family health (Denham, 2003; Weihs et al, 2002).

The complex nature of family communication emerges from the extensive relationships and influencing factors within the family unit and beyond. Ongoing interactions among family members and their extended network can be continual communication challenges. Social networks can act as strengths or threats. Interactions with nurses and health care professionals during times of illness bring additional layers of complexity to communication. Families also must grapple with competing messages received from the media, community, and political milieu. Multiple networks of formal and informal communication confront families daily.

Case Study Application: Communication Among Family Members

Family communication patterns are worthy of attention during illness experiences. Some families have continuous open dialogue about health and illness. Other families manage silently with little attention given to health or illness. Although people do not speak everything on their minds, lack of shared concerns about health or illness can make changes difficult. Usual forms of communication can intensify during times of crisis or stress. Communication can become a strength to build upon, while some techniques can cause conflict and be disruptive (Segrin & Flora, 2011). Effective or ineffective communication not only influences member relationships, but also influences abilities to interact with health providers around health and illness. For example, family communication filled with criticism and blame can lead to hostility and discord, creating more individual or family health risks (Weihs et al, 2002). Silence and avoidance about an illness can contribute to suffering, turmoil, and disagreements (Wittenberg-Lyles, Goldsmith, Ragan, & Sanchez-Reilly, 2012; Zhang & Siminoff, 2003). Nurses who *think family* know the importance of discourse to facilitate meaningful conversations around health, illness, and caring actions. Families experiencing illnesses and related challenges can be additionally burdened with ineffective communication to manage existing problems or needs.

THERESA: "With seven brothers and sisters in my family it can be a challenge to communicate, but we put everything on the table. We had open and honest discussions about what was happening and going to happen. My husband's family had a different style of communication that made it difficult for our extended families to manage and deal with Michael's illness."

Clear communication between families and nurses is critical to health and illness experiences. Members experience emotions, navigate the health care system, manage multiple concerns linked with illness, and learn necessary actions linked with disease self-management (Chesla, 2010; Clabots, 2012). Nurses who *think family* invite questions and communicate to:

- Ensure that consistent messages are delivered and understood.
- Deliver a constant exchange of relevant and timely information.
- Acknowledge the individual and family unit experience of health and illness.

Nurses who *think family* aim to build trusting individual-nurse-family partnerships. A caring nursing presence acknowledges family difficulties, advocates for members, and guides supportive communication as members wrestle with time uncertainty, distress, and decisions (Agard & Maindal, 2009; Sveinbjarnardottir, Svavarsdottir, & Hrafnkelsson, 2012).

Listening and Responding to the Family Story

Nurses need to be present, listen, and communicate with those seeking care for health and illness. Nurses can help break silences and use communication to guide decisions, learn new information, and resolve conflicts related tohealth and illness management (Segrin & Flora, 2011; Zhang & Siminoff, 2003). Effective family communication can be protective, support resilience, and decrease difficulties of managing illness (Black & Lobo, 2008). Constructive and purposeful communication is needed for collaborative individual-nurse-family relationships.

THERESA: "It seemed that health care providers wanted to act independently. They often seemed to have the belief that they did not need to include the family. We had care conferences and meetings when there was a crisis. It would have been so helpful to be more proactive and meet as a family with care providers. It would have been helpful to have a nurse who could help us talk and plan because they were the most consistent persons providing Michael's care. They could have provided us with information and guided us in the dialogue and decisions."

The nurse can use the core process of communication to help families develop, understand, and learn protective communication methods rather than criticism and conflict (Weihs et al, 2002). Interventions that promote direct communication, foster emotional expression, and assist a family to deal with loss and conflict can improve care outcomes (Chesla, 2010; Weihs et al, 2002). Nursing actions focused on communication and relationships have improved outcomes compared to usual care that may not focus on this process (Chesla, 2010).

THERESA: "At times it seemed that the providers wanted to put the burden on the family to say the words they don't want to say. We were often left crying in the waiting room with no nurse present to listen or help my family talk to each other. We need a nurse to help share the burden and help us say the words."

Families involved in the care and support of their family member with illness have improved recovery (Black, Boore, & Parahoo, 2011). The family's perception of nurse support, collaboration, and respect is increased with good communication (Mitchell, Chaboyer, Burmeister, & Foster, 2009). When nurses invite family to participate in family member care, the flow of information and communication is easier, family members believe they receive greater support, and are more satisfied with care (Roberti & Fitzpatrick, 2010). Table 14.3 examines concerns that often emerge around communication.

Caregiving: Core Family Process

Children, adults, and the aged all have caregiving needs. The unique illness management tasks and caregiving skills are not always inherent in the family, but often need to be taught and learned. Some caregiving arises as family bonds generate strong attachments that encourage a milieu of protective watchfulness and attention to development, health and illness (Carr, 2014; Denham, 2003). As a core process, nurses can use caregiving to address wellness, health promotion, prevention, and care management for acute episodic, chronic, or debilitating conditions. Many families welcome adding children and assume caregiving tasks to guide healthy development into adulthood. Ideally, families socialize members to practice healthy behaviors and interact in ways that serve member, family, and societal needs. Wellness, health promotion, and disease prevention are closely tied to family health routines and caregiving. A family experiencing an acute illness or chronic condition often needs to acquire caregiving skills and knowledge (Hsiao & Van Riper, 2010; Li & Loke, 2013). An acute illness suggests needs for caregiving tasks (Boyoung, Fleischmann, Howie-Esquivel, Stotts & Dracup, 2011; Kamban

TABLE 14-3	*Potential Areas of Focus in Communication*	
NURSING ASSESSMENT	**FAMILY-FOCUSED NURSING ACTIONS**	**EVALUATION**
Identify the following: • Family communication strengths • Disruptions in family communication • Ability to engage in useful communication that meets needs of individual and the family • Whether communication supports individual and family unit needs Use therapeutic questioning, such as: "Tell me about the ways your family has effectively solved problems in the past." "In the past, when your family has faced troubles, what kinds of things worked best as you tried to resolve the problems?"	Promote family dialogue to continually exchange information, and convey emotions that protect and support family (LeGrow & Rossen, 2005; Nelms & Eggenberger, 2010). Explore past family communication patterns and compare with current ones (Segrin & Flora, 2011). Educate family members about the importance of communication and explain ways it can positively influence health and illness. Coach family members in effective communication that fosters resiliency, using clarity, open emotional expressions, and collaborative problem solving (Black & Lobo, 2008). Facilitate family negotiation to solve problems and resolve conflicts (Black & Lobo, 2008).	Family members' communication patterns help them solve problems, make decisions, and promote well-being of family unit members. Communication is effectively used to identify meaningful goals and negotiate differences to achieve goals.

& Svavarsdottir, 2013). Chronic conditions require watchful attention, learning new skills, or modifying family health routines (Davis, Gilliss, Deshefy-Longhi, Chestnutt, & Molloy, 2011; McGhan, Loeb, Baney, & Penrod, 2013).

Caregiving in Chronic Illness

Caregiving roles linked with chronic conditions are long-term requirements. More family caregivers are needed (Pierce & Lutz, 2013; University of Michigan Health System, 2006) to care for a growing portion of society:

- Growing numbers of adults over 65 years of age are living with multiple chronic illnesses.
- Approximately 15% to 18% of children are now living with chronic conditions.
- Over one-third of young adults already suffer from a chronic condition.

These statistics mean families need to take on roles as informal caregiving systems with regular responsibilities for assisting members. Caregiving demands can be needs for emotional support or actual assistance (Pierce & Lutz, 2013). New family roles might need to be learned, personal care services provided, concerns linked with employment resolved, care for an ill member provided, and other family household needs addressed (Pierce & Lutz, 2013; Siminoff et al, 2010). As health and illness transitions occur new caregiving roles are needed. Caregiving strain and burden are often related to the stress, struggles, and conflicted feelings about caregiving roles (Hunt, 2003). The strain and burden of prolonged caregiving can result in caregiver depression and increased mortality risk (Bastawrous, 2012; Perkins et al, 2013; Pierce & Lutz, 2013; Siminoff et al, 2010). Nurses who *think family* realize the core process of caregiving requires intentional thoughts and actions so nursing actions guide a family in planning and delivering caregiving.

Case Study Application: Family Caregiving Experience

The Zimanske family worked together. Theresa changed jobs so she could work near the school so Michael could continue attending. She became his transportation and closest care provider. As a family unit, they jointly cared for Michael and reached out to friends and support systems. Yet, they still needed support as caregivers. They wanted nurses to demonstrate understanding about the strains of caregiving experiences. The years of demands were not easy. The family needed nurses to recognize their stress and the burden of continuous caregiving demands and responsibilities.

THERESA: "I recall one situation where I had taken Michael to a clinic appointment. I had no time to shower, care for myself, and I was struggling. I needed support in my caregiving role. The next day a nurse called me to make a follow-up check. She asked, 'And how are you doing? Yesterday I noticed that you were tired. This must be difficult for you.' It was important for a nurse to check on me and follow up. I wanted nurses to try to walk in my shoes for just a moment. I appreciated that telephone follow-up and concerns for me as the caregiving mother."

Nurses in all care settings can strengthen caregivers' abilities as they provide necessary care for members. Family-focused nurses address caregiving, encourage and support family caring, and help them meet concerns that surface in caring for members (Couture, Ducharme, Lamontagne, 2012; Lubkin & Larsen, 2013). Nursing actions start with listening and observing. Regardless of the practice setting, thinking family implies focusing actions on development of caregiving capacities (Pierce & Lutz, 2013). Family-focused nurses empower, enable, equip, and prepare families. Boxes 14.3 and 14.4 highlight the contributions of faculty committed to developing the practice of nurses with families.

Family-focused nursing actions enable families to identify and mobilize strengths and resources to manage care situations, satisfy members' needs, and sustain usual family life as much as possible (Cleek, Wofsy, Boyd-Franklin, Mundy, & Howell, 2012; Pierce & Lutz, 2013). Nursing actions to build confidence are often more effective than merely focusing on education; self-confidence in new caregiver skills is necessary (Couture et al, 2012). Actions tailored and responsive to needs of family units produce the best care outcomes (Williams & Bakitas, 2012). Table 14.4 identifies the core process of caregiving and provides examples of assessment, nursing actions, and evaluation.

BOX 14-3

Family Tree

Dorothy Whyte, BA, PhD, RN, RCN, HV, RNT (Scotland, United Kingdom)

Dorothy Whyte, BA, PhD, RN, RCN, HV, RNT, was enrolled in a doctoral program in the Department of Nursing Studies, Edinburgh University, Scotland, when she learned about the First International Family Nursing Conference scheduled in Calgary, Alberta, Canada, in 1988. Her attendance at this landmark conference greatly influenced her writing and thinking about families. Her doctoral research, completed in 1990, focused on chronic illness in children. In her subsequent role as a faculty member at Edinburgh University, she developed the first family nursing course. In 1997, she edited the book *Explorations in Family Nursing*. Through the use of case studies written by her students and colleagues, she demonstrated the relevance of family nursing in the United Kingdom. Dr. Whyte and her colleagues co-developed the Family Nursing Network Scotland [FNNS] in 1997. The aim of this network is to support clinical nursing, education, and research with families. Until her retirement from Edinburgh University in 1999, Dr. Whyte supervised and mentored master's and doctoral family nursing students from the United Kingdom and other European countries. Her influence continues to be felt and acknowledged by these former students who are now providing significant leadership in family nursing in their countries.

BOX 14-4

Family Tree

Kazuko Suzuki, DSN, PHN, RN (Japan)

Dr. Suzuki has made the growth of family nursing in Japan a key priority and believes this has been her most important life work. Her foundational leadership at Chiba University and Tokai University was especially significant in the development of family nursing in Japan. Tokai University was the second university in Japan to offer master's level preparation for clinical nurse specialists in family nursing. Dr. Suzuki taught family nursing for 5 years at Chiba University and for 11 years at Tokai University where she mentored a large number of clinical nurse specialists in family nursing. She continued this teaching focus at Tokai University until her retirement in 2008. In 1995, Dr. Suzuki coauthored (with Hiroko Watanabe) the first textbook in Japan on family nursing titled *Family Nursing: Theory and Practice* (Japan Nursing Association Publishing Company), which has now been published its fourth edition. She served as a board member of the Japanese Association for Research in Family Nursing (JARFN) from its beginning in 1994 and was the second president (2004–2007). In 2011, Dr. Suzuki was awarded an Innovative Contribution to Family Nursing Award from the *Journal of Family Nursing* at the 10th International Family Nursing Conference in Kyoto, Japan.

TABLE 14-4	*Potential Areas of Focus in Caregiving*	
FAMILY ASSESSMENT	**FAMILY-FOCUSED NURSING ACTIONS**	**EVALUATION**
Health maintenance and disease prevention	Educate about health maintenance and teach illness prevention. Identify and mobilize family strengths. Consider cultural differences and expectations linked with caregiving tasks.	Family promotes emotional and physical health for all members.
Available family resources and networks	Explore resources of family and community. Discuss with family the potential ways to access networks.	Family has maximized use of available resources for health of all members.
Difficulties adjusting to caregiving trajectories such as: • Assuming the caregiving role • Seeking formal care assistance • Leaving the role	Provide information in a variety of forms. Build family caregiver confidence (Pierce & Lutz, 2013). Support family presence and vigilance as appropriate (Carr & Clarke, 1997).	Family is confident and empowered with caregiving roles and transitions (Pierce & Lutz, 2013).
Caregiver stress, strain and burden Assess using caregiver burden and strain measures (Rodakowski, Skidmore, Rogers, & Schulz, 2012).	Help caregiver gain access to services. Obtain respite care. Arrange phone conference with family members and health care providers. Provide access to Internet chats. Provide caregiving Web sites.	Family accesses resources and recognizes strengths and limitations as caregivers.
Shifting family roles	Explore past, current, and changing family roles with caregiving.	Family adjusts to changes in family roles and coordinates changes.

Celebration: Core Family Process

Almost everyone loves a celebration, but it is not usually the first thing on nurses' minds when they think of health or illness. The core process of celebration points to unifying family events with positively shared family meanings to commemorate (Denham, 2003). Celebrations, traditions, and rituals are tied to belonging, and they contribute to family identity and integrity (Denham, 2003). Family rituals often include celebrations that can generate family healing as members connect, empower one another, and decrease stresses of daily life and illness (Moriarty & Wagner, 2004). Children's birthday celebrations are an example of family rituals that are often repeated multiple times throughout the evolving family's life and have potential to contribute to family well-being and family connections (Lee, Katras, & Bauer, 2009). A ritual such as a birthday celebration may be unique among families. Families tend to view celebrations positively and when an event is not celebrated as usual stress or even grief might occur. Family ritual as a shared time to promote close relationships is a prominent aspect of resilient families (Black & Lobo, 2008; Walsh, 2003). Nurses who *think family* know some celebrations are valued and take note of special times and facilitate and encourage the family's observance of those special events.

Case Study Application: Celebration

Nurses do not always think about family celebrations in nursing roles. Yet, a family's times of sharing together are valued and provide a reprieve from life's struggles. Taking time away from stressful needs can help preserve family resiliency. Nurses can encourage families to share stories about past celebrations and describe the value or meanings of events and their cultural and religious significance.

   THERESA: "At 10 years old, Michael's favorite holiday was Halloween. He was hospitalized on Halloween and stressed about not being able to go to school. Even though he was isolated, nurses figured out a way that kids from his class could connect with him to celebrate the holiday. School friends came in their costumes. The nurses even came in costumes and they helped him dress up for Halloween. This meant a great deal to Michael and our family."

   Nurses can assist families to find ways to continue celebrations despite barriers. Families can benefit from community resources such as the mission of the Make-A-Wish Foundation to create celebratory events that enrich the lives of children who have life-threatening medical conditions. Children with diabetes may be able to attend a diabetes camp and gain confidence, knowledge, and skills as they join with other children at camp events. Nurses can use actions to help families construct new celebrations or modify old ones in response to an illness or other life transition (Denham, 2003).

Change: Core Family Process

Change is a constant element of family life with ongoing alterations in the family social systems and larger environments (Denham, 2003; Wright & Leahey, 2013). Change, as a core process, can be defined as the dynamic family process that requires alteration or modification, redirection of attentions or resources, or substitutions (Denham, 2003). Needs for change come in unexpected and unpredictable forms that can be demanding to the family. Developmental changes occur throughout life as family members grow and develop, but when an unknown situation or uncertainty surfaces, preparation for change can be limited. Life events such as death, war, unemployment, or serious illness in one family member can initiate changes affecting the family unit (Wright & Leahey, 2013).

Individual changes due to health or illness often require changes in others and precipitate significant transitional needs (Meleis, 2010). Nurses who *think family* assist members as they face, manage, and engineer the uneasy stressors that accompany change. Individual-nurse-family relationships can assist family units by sorting out the implications of abrupt alterations, teaching new things, coaching in lifestyle changes, or counseling about options and choices.

Health behavior changes in a family often are a key to prevention and management of illness (Shumaker, Ockene, & Riekert, 2009). For example, tobacco use, unhealthy diets, and physical inactivity play roles in causation and progression of chronic disease (United States Department of Health and Human Services, 2012). Objectives to increase life quality and not just years of life aim to eliminate health disparities and improve lifestyle behaviors (United States Department of Health and Human Services, 2012). Nurses have a responsibility to help create a context for some anticipated changes (Wright & Bell, 2009; Wright & Leahey, 2013). Family units exist within a social system and physical environment linked to change, some of which cannot be controlled by them (Denham, 2003). Thus, nursing actions can assist family members in attending to household concerns as adjustments to change are needed.

Nurses use teaching, coaching, and collaboration to facilitate changes that support health and illness (Hamric, Hanson, Tracy, & O'Grady, 2014; Wright & Leahey, 2013). Providing and exchanging useful information is a critical first step in addressing change. Families often need someone to listen as they face changes. They need to be guided to solve problems or adopt new routines. Nurses can support health-promoting changes through actions that build confidence and empower (Pierce & Lutz, 2013). Empowering provides information, skills, and resources to manage circumstances and needed changes (Hulme, 1999; Pierce & Lutz, 2013).

Managing change requires skill to navigate through conflicts and resistance and emerge with successful outcomes (Mason & Butler, 2010). This is not easy for families or nurses. It takes time, practice, and support when failure occurs. Motivational interviewing is useful in identifying and altering behaviors (Mason & Butler, 2010; Rollnick, Miller, & Butler, 2008) through several actions:

- Ask questions, be curious.
- Listen and understand the family's desires for change.
- Guide the family by suggesting options.
- Plan and take actions aligned with family values.
- Create confidence and empower the family.

Nurses need to understand and be sensitive to family concerns linked with change. Education and interventions linked with emotions and relationships need attention.

Case Study Application: Change

Change can occur quickly or over time; it is not usually a particular one-time event (Mason & Butler, 2010). Stages of change—precontemplation, contemplation, preparation, action, maintenance, and termination—are viewed as places where people are as they confront needs for change (Prochaska, Johnson, & Lee, 2009). Precontemplation refers to the time when the individual is not intending to change; contemplation is when the person intends to change in the next 6 months. Preparation is when action is expected in the immediate future and action includes modifications. Maintenance is when an individual is likely to continue the change. Termination of the change process occurs when the person will not return to unhealthy ways.

Nurses can help families identify the stage at which members are in readiness to change. Different nursing actions are needed at each stage. The first critical step is assessing where individuals and families are in the change process. Most people need to know the benefits of change and the risks associated with not changing. Nurses can provide positive supports regardless of where persons are in readiness to change. Nurses who *think family* recognize that nursing actions to address change depend upon readiness to change and other family factors.

Inviting change through therapeutic communication is central to family nursing practice (Wright & Bell, 2009). Respecting beliefs and managing constraining beliefs sets the stage for nursing actions and supports (Wright & Bell, 2009). Family members need skills to solve problems and resolve difficult situations.

THERESA: "Michael's illness kept changing. It would have been helpful to know what change may be next. Every family is different. Our family needed help to redesign our vision of family life. It's an evolution and process that takes repeated conversations. Our family was often in disbelief about what was happening around us. Our emotions, visions, and dreams had not caught up with the changes. We needed guidance in how to deal with the countless changes in Michael, our family, and each of our own lives."

Goals

When change is needed, the individual-nurse-family relationship provides ways to collaborate and partner as goals are set and strategies developed. Nurses assist families by asking questions and then working with them to set specific goals tied to a needed change and develop strategies or actions to accomplish that change. The actions should be measurable.

- Who—Who in the family do we need to involve?
- What—What needs to be accomplished by the individuals or the family unit? Does the nursing action fit this family?
- When—By what time/date can the family accomplish this?
- Where—Where does this need to be addressed? Is it something to do at home, school, or work?
- Which—Which barriers, constraints and resources need to be addressed by the family?
- Why—Why is this change necessary? What are the benefits if the family meets the goal? What are the risks if they fail to meet goal?
- How—How does the family view this change? How do individual family members influence this change?

A goal has specific criteria to measure progress. Focusing on whether a goal is attainable assists the nurse and family to realistically consider capacity to attain it. What are the member attitudes, abilities, skills, and family resource factors? Goals are set to be accomplished and measured within a particular timeframe. What barriers need to be overcome? What resources are needed? Goal achievement requires nursing actions that fit family needs (Wright & Leahey, 2013). Family beliefs, values, roles, member processes, and culture need to be considered (Bulecheck & McCloskey, 1992). Family nurses respect unique beliefs and partner to attain optimal health outcomes as changes are managed (Table 14.5).

Connection: Core Family Process

Connection, another core process, refers to bonds and links among family members, the family as a system, and systems external to the family household. Connections occur among relational bonds, commitments, and resources. Connections may be simple, as in a shared music interest or a biological relationship to a grandparent. Connections can also be complex, as in the network of multiple members in a blended family and various resources linked to the family system or particular members (Fig. 14.5). For example, a

TABLE 14-5	*Potential Areas of Focus in Change*	
ASSESSMENT	**FAMILY-FOCUSED NURSING ACTIONS**	**EVALUATION**
Engage in a family conversation that encourages family members to tell their story and invites reflection on beliefs about health and illness (Wright & Bell, 2009). Assess context of the family that influences health (e.g., cultural influences, social environment) (Schneider & Stokols, 2009).	Create collaborative relationship with family. Explore illness beliefs, strengthen facilitative beliefs, challenge constraining beliefs (Wright & Bell, 2009). Listen and understand family's reason for making or not making changes. Increase family awareness of need for change. Identify supports for change. Set goals and identify strategies for making the change. Establish a timetable for making changes.	Family sets goals. Family engages in planned strategies that facilitate meeting goals. Changes are made and goals are accomplished.

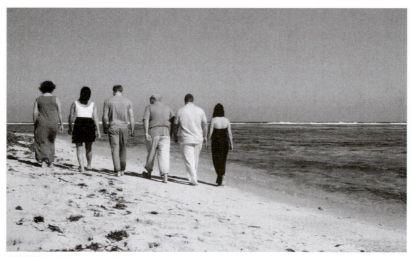

FIGURE 14-5 Family connections.

child from an earlier relationship might be covered under a different health insurance plan from other family members. Connection sometimes varies among members in a single household. Connections within a family can be strengthened or weakened over time. Boundaries between family systems and ecological environments influence some family connections. For instance, if family members believe they should be self-sufficient in managing problems, they may be reluctant to seek help from outsiders. This could limit their access to available resources. On the other hand, a family with open boundaries might pursue every resource possible.

In the Family Health Model (Denham, 2003), connections are described as ways individuals are committed to and linked through interests, values, roles, and identities. Social ties are potential resources linked to positive health outcomes (Giordano, Bjork, & Lindström, 2012; Looman, 2006). For example, neighborhood characteristics such as attachment and informal social control are linked with mothers' parenting mastery (Carpiano & Kimbro, 2012). Living in a neighborhood where social connections are strong may help families access supportive networks and needed resources.

A study of Swedish families indicated that high degrees of family, school, and neighborhood connectedness facilitated higher levels of child well-being (Eriksson, Hochwolder, Carlsund, & Sellström, 2012). Connectedness was measured using responses to such cues as "You can trust people around here" and "People say 'hello' and often stop to talk to each other on the street" (Eriksson et al, 2012). Trusting attitudes and friendly neighbors affect individual and family health. If trust and social connections are interconnected, stronger social networks help families use relationships to access resources (Giordano et al, 2012). Table 14.6 provides direction for assessment, nursing actions, and evaluations linked with connection.

Case Study Application: Genograms and Ecomaps Provide Connections

Connections can be health promoting. Nurses can use knowledge about community resources to help families access resources. Tools discussed earlier in the book, such as genograms and ecomaps, can be used to assess family connections. Genograms provide a picture of the family and related health risks. An ecomap is a snapshot of social relationships that can help identify potential resources (Rempel, Neufeld, & Kushner, 2007; Wright & Leahey, 2013).

TABLE 14-6	*Potential Areas of Focus in Connection*	
NURSING ASSESSMENT	**FAMILY-FOCUSED NURSING ACTIONS**	**EVALUATION**
Create and discuss a family genogram with members of the family.	Ask family members to share in the process of creating the genogram. Identify actual and potential sources of support from extended family members. Identify any barriers or threats that need attention. Engage the family in a discussion of ways family members facilitate or create barriers to connections within and outside the family.	Family members share perceptions about the family structure, roles, and connections within and across generations. Goals and a plan of action are generated.
Create and discuss the family's ecomap	Identify sources of support, through social network connections and links to supportive resources over time. Identify any barriers or threats that need attention. Discuss existing connections as potential, but untapped resources. Explore shared perceptions and meanings about connections. Identify supports outside the family boundaries.	Family members identify existing resources and potential connections to needed resources for support that promotes health and manages illness. Goals and a plans of action are generated.

Used interactively, the genogram, a graphic representations of information about family, usually over at least three generations, can aid thinking about family as a system connected to the larger world (McGoldrick, Gerson, & Petry, 2008). The genogram can identify ways members are connected legally, emotionally, socially, and genetically. Discussions can lead to learning about member roles and values. This is a nonthreatening way to ask questions about member connections or relationships and identify ways members interact with one another (McGoldrick et al, 2008). A completed genogram offers a tangible map of the family story. It may reveal connections to resources that may not have been recalled before the exercise.

Creating an ecomap, a graphic representation of social networks and bonds within them, can generate dialogue as information about key sources of support is gathered (Hartman, 1995). Sources include kin, friends, support groups, schools, religious affiliations, employers, and professionals (Rempel et al, 2007). The ecomap can be used to discuss strengths and directions of relationships. The ecomap creation may reveal strong or weaker connections and help discern boundaries that exist between members and systems external to the family household.

Creating a genogram and ecomap with the Zimanske family provided nurses with broader historical data and information about social contexts. For example, extended family members played important roles in the Zimanske family's life. Theresa had a large number of siblings and several living nearby in a rural farming area and they were instrumental supports and willing to stay with Michael or offer assistance as needed, including emotional supports. Faith-based activities played important roles in the family's social and spiritual lives. Their church affiliation linked them to caring congregants over many years. Their faith connected them to a higher power to trust and seek spiritual guidance during the long illness. Nurses knew the information on the Zimanske family genogram and ecomap. "We became human . . . we began connecting as human beings rather than as doctor-patient," explained Teresa. Theresa believed that these tools helped nurses provide their family more effective care.

Coordination: Core Family Process

Coordination, as a core process, refers to cooperative sharing of resources, skills, abilities, and information within and outside the family. There are several purposes of coordination:

- Use time and other resources wisely.
- Optimize efforts to achieve individual and family health.
- Achieve individual and family goals.

Coordination involves decisions about daily activities, routines, networking with support systems, and negotiating a satisfactory balance between available resources and needs of individuals and the family unit. Coordination is important to the promotion of care maintenance for wellness, prevention, illness, disease, or disability.

Family coordination includes participation, organization, focalization, and affective contact (Fivaz-Depeursinge & Corboz-Warnery, 1999; Lavadera, 2011). These factors address the following:

- Participation is the ability of family members to interact and not exclude certain members in shared activities.
- Organization is clear communication that honors members' roles in a family activity. It is what helps a family complete needed tasks.
- Focalization is the ability to focus attentions as activities are carried out.
- Affective contact pertains to members encouraging and appreciating everyone's contribution and promoting fun and harmony during activities.

Coordination involves members' unique processes, communicating, respecting roles, paying attention to goals, and recognition of member contributions.

Coordination entails cooperative sharing of resources, skills, abilities, and information within the family and exchanges with larger contextual systems (Denham, 2003). Working together and sharing resources can optimize health potentials and goal accomplishment. Effective coordination is often a silent and unrecognized family strength because it occurs without overt negotiation or discussion (Denham, 2003). Lack of family cooperation is a problem when activities and behaviors are not effective in meeting goals, lead to disputes or stress, and are unaddressed. For example, schedules may be disrupted when a parent is hospitalized because of an automobile accident. This interferes with usual coordination of meal preparation, child care, or transportation. This disruption may manifest itself as a crisis of time management for others and lead to unexpected stress. A teenager may be asked to assume a role of child care and rebel when it interferes with plans. Nurses who *think family* assess family routines and identify disruptions. What coordination needs to occur to help this family organize? Table 14.7 identifies some areas for assessment, nursing actions, and areas to evaluate in the coordination process.

Case Study Application: Coordination

Coordination assists family members by enabling them to work in unity and share resources, skills, abilities, and information. Begin with assessment of the family's collective awareness of needs and resources linked to a specific situation. Do family members agree or disagree on the problem and what is needed? An acutely ill father is being discharged after a lengthy hospitalization. Do the spouse, teen children, and extended family agree about the family's most pressing needs? The coordination process suggests nursing actions that assist the family unit in the following:

- Recognize and include needs of all members.
- Communicate and respect roles.
- Attend to family unit stress, concerns, and frustrations.
- Appreciate the contributions of each member.
- Identify available resources, shared goals.
- Include all in shared decision making.

In the Zimanske family, Michael had many lengthy hospitalizations, including one in which he received a kidney transplant from a family member. Coordination as a core family process required each family member to recognize and include others in the preparation for discharge after transplant. Although not all members were physically present when Michael was discharged, the process considered the concerns of various member needs during the recuperation phase, such as Jessica's social needs and Theresa and Don's work schedules, so there would always be a caregiver present. It also included the needs of Michael's aunt, the kidney donor, who would be simultaneously recovering at a different home. Nurses who *think family* recognize that coordination involves support, roles, relationships, resources, threats, and balanced attention to individual and family needs in addition to the skills and information needed to ensure safe physical care.

Coordination as a family process is important for health promotion and during times of stress. In a study of healthy dual-income families, findings indicated "busy families lead lives where more than half of all activities unfold as non-routine," and "family members do not have perfect knowledge of each other's routines (Davidoff, Zimmerman, & Dey, 2010, p 2469). The families studied were not ill, but were leading

TABLE 14-7	*Potential Areas of Focus in Coordination*	
NURSING ASSESSMENT	**FAMILY-FOCUSED NURSING ACTIONS**	**EVALUATION**
Identification and collective awareness of needs	Encourage family members to verbalize perceived needs. Offer guidance in naming needs family member express that might be implied, but not spoken.	Family members have a shared understanding of individual and collective family unit needs. The family names one or more current needs that were previously implied.
Identification and collective awareness of resources	Facilitate identification and "cataloging" of available resources, skills, abilities, and information. Commend families and individuals when resources, skills, and abilities are apparent.	Family members identify a set of resources available to satisfy identified needs. Families identify and call upon existing strengths as resources.
Identification of family goals	Assist the family to identify goals for health or illness management and move toward consensus.	Family members have a shared understanding of goals to achieve. Resources are coordinated to meet identified needs.
Cooperation	Offer guidance in negotiations. Assist family to coordinate resources to meet member and family unit needs.	Family members are willing to "give and take" and share. Family is adapting as needed to manage changing needs for support and resources.
Decision making	Facilitate decision making by listening. Reflect on problem identification that needs resolution. Prioritize needs.	Family members prioritize needs, act on decisions, resolve problems, and meet individual and family unit needs.

typical lives as a busy family. Theresa described her family's experience during this transplant as "stress times a million." Stability of routines is important in family lives and the adaptation of new behaviors can be stressful (Denham, 2003). Stressful events require families to negotiate unfamiliar situations and coordinate or share in needed changes. Box 14.5 provides a case to explore family processes and family-focused nursing actions.

BOX 14-5

Family Circle

Maria Sanchez is a 78-year-old woman who has lived alone in a small rural community in the Midwest. Maria's husband is deceased and her three adult children live on the east and west coasts. Maria has been independent since her husband's death 10 years ago, but recently her eldest son James has noticed she seems forgetful when he calls. He decides to fly home for a visit. When he arrives, he notices that she keeps leaving the stove on and seems unable to safely drive to get groceries. She says she has not been feeling good and has little appetite. A few days later, Maria becomes seriously ill. James takes her to the hospital and she is admitted with pneumonia. She is eating little and has a temperature of 101°F. Maria asks the nurses if she is going to get to return home soon. She is on intravenous antibiotics, but is not improving. James contacts his sister, and the nurse caring for Maria in the room hears their conversation as she cares for the other person in the room. James tells his sister that she is going to have to come be with their mother. He tells her that he has to return to his business. His sister Sarah says she has no one to watch the children and cannot leave them. The nurse hears James say they that it would be useless to call their brother Peter because he can hardly take care of himself.

General Questions:

- What is the nurse's responsibility in taking care of Maria Sanchez?
- What concerns will the nurse have for Maria's discharge?
- What do you think the nurse might do after she hears this conversation?

Family-Focused Questions:

- What family nursing actions might the nurse consider for this family?
- Using family-focused actions, what core family processes might be concerns in this situation?
- Consider the opportunities that family-focused nursing actions might create compared to individual-focused actions.

Core Processes and Family Meetings

Family nursing places families at the center of nursing actions. A nurse-led family meeting is a specific nursing action that includes the family unit and provides opportunities to hear and address needs and concerns. Core processes are part of a toolbox of ideas to approach nursing care for families. Family meetings can be used to communicate with the family, make decisions, or identify strategies to resolve pending problems. Most families value time to meet with a nurse who will guide, mentor, and inform them about illness management, care treatments, and behavior changes (Hamric et al., 2014 McDaniel et al., 2005). Nurses may need to initiate these meetings because many families have not had a previous experience with them and, therefore, would not request them.

Family meetings are a time when nurses can directly target family processes, member concerns, and support needs. Bringing a family together has healing potential and can ease family suffering and distress (Legrow & Rossen, 2005; Wiegand, 2006; Wright & Leahey, 2013). The therapeutic nature of a family meeting allows questions, exploration of family beliefs, and relationship building (Nelms & Eggenberger, 2010). These meetings have the potential to decrease frustrating confrontation, misunderstandings, and family dissatisfaction (Nelms & Eggenberger, 2010; Hannon, O'Reilly, Bennett, Breen, & Lawlor, 2012). Table 14.8 describes purposes, strategies, and potential outcomes of family meetings. These meetings need to be inclusive and welcome all interested members. Dialogue to support understanding is encouraged, directions are identified, and guidance offered to improve care outcomes. Family meetings facilitate family processes and communication with the health care team (Box 14.6).

TABLE 14-8	*Purpose, Strategy, and Outcomes of Family Meetings*	
PURPOSE	**STRATEGIES FOR FAMILY-FOCUSED NURSING ACTIONS**	**OUTCOMES**
Share and exchange information.	Provide consistent communication with family and interprofessional team. Create a comfortable and welcoming atmosphere.	Informed family with increased trust.
Encourage healthy patterns of communication.	Model communication facilitative techniques to family members. Help individuals to share ideas. Respect beliefs; avoid stereotypes and assumptions.	Open, honest, respectful family communication during stress of illness experience. Respectful understandings of differences and consensus among family members (Wiegand, 2006).
Identify family beliefs that influence health.	Clarify individual and family unit beliefs. Identify facilitating and constraining beliefs (Wright & Bell, 2009).	Move toward facilitating beliefs.
Facilitate understandings of individual family members' thinking.	Direct attention to individuals during the meeting. Strive for consensus. Use negotiation as a tactic for resolving conflicts.	Family members acknowledge the needs and concerns of other members.

BOX 14-6

Research Evidence About Family Meetings

Selected research findings about the benefits of family meetings:

Arranging family participation in the nursing home setting is a way to improve the well-being of the older adult resident while maintaining the family's ongoing participation in the care of their loved ones (Dijkstra, 2007).

Including family caregivers of clients living with cancer in psychoeducational interventions has been found to alleviate caregiver distress (Doorenbos et al, 2007).

Involving parents of children with diabetes in interventions increases parents' knowledge and supports coping with the illness (Chesla, 2010).

Developing skills through interventions that improve family relations while managing a chronic illness demonstrates improved outcomes, such as a decrease in family members' anxiety, depression, and sense of illness burden, when compared to usual care (Chesla, 2010).

Providing quality end-of-life care in hospital settings requires the involvement of family, and family conferences are a way to facilitate decision making with end-of-life issues (Fineberg, Kawashima, & Asch, 2011; Wiegand, 2006).

Participating in family meetings that aim to attend to spiritual and psychosocial needs can be a potentially useful intervention according to patients, family members, and staff in a palliative care setting; however, strategies to overcome implementation barriers are needed (Tan et al., 2011).

Facilitating family meetings at predetermined scheduled times in the acute care setting can minimize the uncertainty and distress of the family experience (LeGrow & Rossen, 2005; Nelms & Eggenberger, 2010).

Arranging conferences with families in primary care settings provides the best outcomes for patient and moves the family and provider toward common understandings (McDaniel et al., 2005).

Case Study Application: Family Meetings

Conducting family meetings requires careful planning and implementation. Nurses often rely on someone like the chaplain, social worker, or physician to lead these meetings and manage family dynamics. Although others might participate in a family meeting, it is often the nurse who has the greater understanding of the family needs and works with them most closely. Nurses familiar with family situations and who have some relationship with the family are likely the best ones to lead family meetings. As the meeting begins, identify the purpose of the meeting and goals to address. Set a time limit so the family will know how long you will be available. Do not overestimate what might be accomplished, but recognize that even brief conversations with a family can have a positive influence on the family (Halldórsdóttir & Svavarsdóttir, 2012; Svavarsdottir & Sigurdardottir, 2013) and family meetings can be beneficial to patients and families (Tan, Wilson, Olver, & Barton, 2011).

THERESA: "I asked for family meetings, but they only occurred when we had a crisis event. It would have been helpful to be more proactive. The registered nurses would have been great conveners of family meetings because they knew Michael and us so well. Family meetings could have helped us think, talk and share our concerns."

Nurses can use family meetings to:

- Listen and understand the family experience.
- Integrate their knowledge or expertise linked to illness and treatments with the family's experiential expertise of the individual who is ill and each other.
- Identify the emotional issues or care barriers and facilitate action plans.

Box 14.7 describes some strategies to use for successful family meetings.

BOX 14-7

Successful Communication Through Family Meetings

Before conducting a family meeting, the nurse can use the following steps to address the needs of those taking part:

- Consider the purpose and what needs to be accomplished through the family meeting.
- Identify and invite all family members who need to be present; consider privacy needs as members are included.
- Provide quiet environment with room for family members.
- Arrange a time that is convenient for the majority of family members.
- Identify the health care team members who need to be present.
- Provide ample time for opportunity to listen to family members.
- Plan for the need to begin, maintain, and terminate the meeting with appropriate statements and actions.

Chapter Summary

Family-focused nurses intentionally place the family unit in the center of practice and treat them as the unit of care. The core processes from the Family Health Model (Denham, 2003) provide guides for nurses' actions with families. Core processes of communication, caregiving, cathexis, celebration, change, connectedness, and coordination are guides for intentional nursing actions. Therapeutic conversations and family meetings bring nurses and families together so they can collaborate through individual-nurse-family partnerships to satisfy unique needs,, consider choices of action, resolve problems, and make decisions. Nurses who *think family* recognize family processes are central to family life and require nursing actions that recognize areas of concern and strength.

REFERENCES

Abate, F. R. (Ed.). (2002). *Oxford American dictionary of current English*. New York: Oxford University Press.

Agard, S. S., & Maindal, H. T. (2009). Interacting with relatives in intensive care units: Nurses' perceptions of a challenging task. *Nursing in Critical Care, 14*(5), 264–272.

Almasri, N. A., Palisano, R. J., Dunst, C. J., Chiarello, L. A., O'Neil, M. E., & Polansky, M. (2011). Determinants of needs of families of children and youth with cerebral palsy. *Children's Health Care, 40*(2), 130–154.

American Nurses Association (ANA). (2001). *Code of ethics for nurses with interpretative statements*. Silver Spring, MD: Author.

Anderson, K. A., & Tomlinson, P. S. (1992). The family health system as an emerging paradigmatic view for nursing. *Image: Journal of Nursing Scholarship, 24*, 57–63.

Bastawrous, M. (2012). Caregiver burden—A critical discussion. *International Journal of Nursing Studies, 49*(11), 431–441.

Benzies, K., & Mychasiuk, R. (2009). Fostering family resiliency: A review of the key protective factors. *Child and Family Social Work, 14*, 103–114.

Bettle, A. M. E., & Latimer, M. (2009). Maternal coping and adaptation: A case study examination of chronic sorrow in caring for an adolescent with a progressive neurodegenerative disease. *Canadian Journal of Neuroscience Nursing, 31*(4), 15–21.

Black, K., & Lobo. M. J. (2008). A conceptual review of family resilience factors. *Journal of Family Nursing, 14*(10), 33–55.

Black, P., Boore, J. R. P., & Parahoo, K. (2011). The effect of nurse-faciliated family participation in the psychological care of the critically ill patient. *Journal of Advanced Nursing, 67*(5), 1091–1101. doi:10.1111/j.1365-2648.2010.05558.x

Boss, P. G. (2006). *Loss, trauma, and resilience: Therapeutic work with ambiguous loss*. New York: Norton.

Boss, P. G., Doherty, W. J., LaRossa, W. R, Schumm, W. R., & Steinmetz , S. K. (Eds.). (1993). *Sourcebook of family theories and methods: A contextual approach* (pp 651–672). New York: Plenum.

Boyoung, H., Fleischmann, K. E., Howie-Esquivel, J., Stotts, N. A., & Dracup, K. (2011). Caregiving for patients with heart failure: Impact on patients' families. *American Journal of Critical Care, 20*(6), 431–442. doi:10.4037/ajcc2011472

Bulecheck, G. M., & McCloskey, J. (1992). *Nursing interventions: Essential nursing treatments* (2nd ed.). Philadelphia: W. B. Saunders.

Burke M. L., Eakes, G. G., & Hainsworth, M. A. (1999). Milestones of chronic sorrow: Perspective of chronically ill and bereaved persons and family caregivers. *Journal of Family Nursing, 5*, 374–387.

Carpiano, R. M., & Kimbro, R. T. (2012). Neighborhood social capital, parenting strain, and personal mastery among female primary caregivers of children. *Journal of Health and Social Behavior, 53*(2), 232–247. doi:10.1177/0022146512445899

Carr, J. M. (2014). A middle range theory of family vigilance. *MEDSURG Nursing*, 23(4), 251–255.

Carr, J. M., & Clarke P. (1997). Development of the concept of family vigilance. *Western Journal of Nursing Research*, 19(6), 726–739.

Chesla, C. (2010). Do family interventions improve health? *Journal of Family Nursing*, 16(4), 355–377. doi:10.1177/1074840710383145

Clabots, S. (2012). Strategies to help initiate and maintain the end-of-life discussion with patients and family members. *MedSurg Nursing*, 21(4), 197–203.

Cleek, E. N., Wofsy, M., Boyd-Franklin, N., Mundy, B., & Howell, T. J. (2012). The family empowerment program: An interdisciplinary approach to working with multi-stressed urban families. *Family Process*, 51(2), 207–217. doi:10.1111/j.1545-5300.2012.01392.x

Chinn, P. (2008). The discipline of nursing. *Advances in Nursing Science*, 31(1), 1.

Couture, M., Ducharme, F., & Lamontagne, J. (2012). The role of health care professionals in the decision-making process of family caregivers regarding placement of a cognitively impaired elderly relative. *Home Health Care Management & Practice*, 24, 283–291.

Dahnke, M. D., & Dreher, H. M., (2011). *Philosophy of science for nursing practice: Concepts and application*. New York: Springer.

Davidoff, S., Zimmerman, J., & Dey, A. K. (2010). How routine learners can support family coordination. Paper presented at the *Proceedings of the 28th International Conference on Human Factors in Computing Systems*, pp 2461–2470.

Davidson, M. R., London, M. O., & Ladewig, P. A. (2012). *Olds' maternal-newborn nursing and women's health across the lifespan* (9th ed.). Upper Saddle River, NJ: Pearson Prentice Hall.

Davis, L. L, Gilliss, C. L., Deshefy-Longhi, T., Chestnutt, D. H., & Molloy, M. (2011). The nature and scope of stressful spousal caregiving relationships. *Journal of Family Nursing*, 17(2), 224–240.

Denham, S. (2003). *Family health: A framework for nursing*. (2003). Philadelphia: F. A. Davis.

Dijkstra, A. (2007). Family participation in care plan meetings: Promoting a collaborative organizational culture in nursing homes. *Journal of Gerontological Nursing*, 4, 22–31.

Doorenbos, A. Z., Given, B., Given, C. W., Wyatt, G., Gift, A., Rahbar, M., & Jeon, S. (2007). The influence of end-of-life cancer care on caregivers. *Research in Nursing and Health*, 30(3), 270–281.

Doran, G. T. (1981). There's a S. M. A. R. T. way to write management goals and objectives. *Management Review* (AMA Forum), 70(11), 35–36.

Duhamel, F. (2010). Implementing family nursing: How do we translate knowledge into clinical practice? Part II: The evolution of 20 years of teaching, research, and practice to a center of excellence in family nursing. *Journal of Family Nursing*, 16(10), 8–25.

Eakes, G. (1993). Chronic sorrow: A response to living with cancer. *Oncology Nursing Forum*, 20, 1327–1334.

Eakes, G., Burke, M. L., & Hainsworth, M. A. (1998). Middle-range theory of chronic sorrow. *Image: Journal of Nursing Scholarship* 30, 179–184.

Eggenberger, S. (2011, June 25). Psychometric testing of the family nurse presence (FNP) instrument among family members in critical care: Making visible the importance of understanding, connecting, including, and listening for nurses. Presentation at the 10th International Family Nursing Conference. Kyoto, Japan.

Eggenberger, S. (2012). The science of nursing actions. Presentation at Minnesota State University, Mankato School of Nursing.

Eggenberger, S. K., Meiers, S. J., Krumwiede, N. K., Bliesmer, M., & Earle, P. (2011). Family reintegration: A family health promoting process in chronic illness. *Journal of Nursing and Health Care of Chronic Illness*, 3, 283–292.

Eggenberger, S. K., & Nelms, T. (2007). Being family: The family experience when an adult member is hospitalized with a critical illness. *Journal of Clinical Nursing*, 16, 1618–1628.

Eriksson, U., Hochwolder, J., Carlsund, A., & Sellström, E. (2012). Health outcomes among Swedish children: The role of social capital in the family, school and neighbourhood. *Acta Paediatrica*, 101(5), 513–517. doi:10.1111/j.1651-2227.2011.02579.x

Fineberg, I. C., Kawashima, M., & Asch, S. M. (2011). Communication with families facing life-threatening illness: A research-based model for family conferences. *Journal of Palliative Medicine*, 14(4), 421–427. doi:http://dx.doi.org/10.1089/jpm.2010.0436

Fivaz-Depeursinge, E., & Corboz-Warnery, A. (1999). *The primary triangle: A developmental systems view of fathers, mothers, and infants*. New York: Basic Books.

Garwick, A. W., Detzer, D., & Boss, P. A. (1994). Family perceptions of living with Alzheimer's. *Family Process, 33*(3), 327–340. doi:10.1111/j.1545-5300.1994.00327.x

Giger, J. N., & Davidhizar, R. (2007). Promoting culturally appropriate interventions among vulnerable populations. *Annual Review of Nursing Research, 25*, 293–316.

Giordano, G., Bjork, J., & Lindström, M. (2012). Social capital and self-rated health—A study of temporal (causal) relationships. *Social Science Medicine, 75*(2), 340–348. doi:10.1016/j.socscimed.2012.03.011

Halldórsdóttir, B. S., & Svavarsdóttir, E. (2012). Purposeful therapeutic conversations: Are they effective for families of individuals with COPD: A quasi-experimental study. *Nordic Journal of Nursing Research and Clinical Studies / Vård I Norden, 32*(1), 48–51.

Hamric, A. B., Hanson, C. M., Tracy, M. F., & O'Grady, E. T. (2014). *Advanced practice nursing: An integrative approach* (5th ed.). St. Louis: W. B. Saunders.

Hamric, A. B., Spross, J. A., & Harmon Hanson, S. M. (2009). *Advanced practice nursing: An integrative approach* (4th ed.). St. Louis: W. B. Saunders.

Hannon, B., O'Reilly, V., Bennett, K., Breen, K., & Lawlor, P. G. (2012). Meeting the family: Measuring effectiveness of family meetings in a specialist inpatient palliative care unit. *Palliative and Supportive Care, 10*(1), 43–49.

Hartman, A. (1995). Diagrammatic assessment of family relationships. *Families in Society, the Journal of Contemporary Human Services, 76*(2), 111–122.

Holtslander, L. F., & McMillan, S. C. (2011). Depressive symptoms, grief, and complicated grief among family caregivers of patients with advanced cancer three months into bereavement. *Oncology Nursing Forum 38*(1), 60–65.

Hsiao, C. Y., & Van Riper, M. (2010). Research on caregiving in Chinese families living with mental illness: A critical review. *Journal of Family Nursing, 16*(1), 68–100. doi:10.1177/1074840709358405

Hulme, P. A. (1999). Family empowerment: A nursing intervention with suggested outcomes for families of children with a chronic health condition. *Journal of Family Nursing, 5*(1), 33–50.

Hunt, C. (2003). Concepts in caregiver research. *Journal of Nursing Scholarship, 35*(1), 27–32. doi:10.1111/j.1547-5069.2003.00027.x

Ingadottir, T., & Jonsdottir, H. (2010). Partnership-based nursing practice for people with chronic obstructive pulmonary disease and their families: Influences on health-related quality of life and hospital admissions. *Journal of Clinical Nursing, 19*(19/20), 2795–2805. doi:10.1111/j.1365-2702.2010.03303.x

Isaakson, A. K., & Ahlstrom, G. (2008). Managing chronic sorrow: Experiences of patients with multiple sclerosis. *Journal of Neuroscience Nursing, 40*(3), 180–191.

Kaakinen, J. R. (2010). Family nursing process: Family nursing assessment models. In J. R. Kaakinen, V. Gedaly-Duff, E. P. Coehlo, & S. M. Harmon Hanson (Eds.), *Family health care nursing: Theory, practice and research* (4th ed.). Philadelphia: F. A. Davis.

Kaakinen, J. R., Gedaly-Duff, V., Coehlo, E. P., & Harmon Hanson, S. M. (Eds.). (2010). *Family health care nursing: Theory, practice, and research* (4th ed.). Philadelphia: F. A. Davis.

Kaakinen, J. R., Harmon Hanson, S. M., & Denham, S. A. (2010). Family health care nursing: An introduction. In J. R. Kaakinen, V. Gedaly-Duff, D. P. Coehlo, & S. M. Harmon Hanson (Eds.), *Family health care nursing: Theory, practice and research* (4th ed.). Philadelphia: F. A. Davis.

Kamban, S. W., & Svavarsdottir, E. K. (2013). Does a therapeutic conversation intervention in an acute paediatric setting make a difference for families of children with bronchiolitis caused by respiratory syncytial virus (RSV)? *Journal of Clinical Nursing, 22*, 2723–2733. doi:10.1111/j.1365-2702.2012.04330.x

Kean, S. (2010). The experience of ambiguous loss in families of brain injured ICU patients. *Nursing in Critical Care, 15*(2), 66–75.

Knafl, K., & Deatrick, J. (1990). Family management behaviors: Concept synthesis. *Journal of Pediatric Nursing, 5*, 15–22.

Knafl, K. A., Deatrick, J. A., & Havill, N. L. (2012). Continued development of the family management style framework. *Journal of Family Nursing, 18*(1), 11–34. doi:10.1177/1074840711427294

Lavadera, A. L. (2011). Assessing family coordination in divorced families. *American Journal of Family Therapy, 39*(4), 277. doi:10.1080/01926187.2010.539479

Lee, J., Katras, M. J., & Bauer, J. W. (2009). Children's birthday celebrations from the lived experiences of low-income rural mothers. *Journal of Family Issues, 30*(4), 532–553.

Legrow, K., & Rossen, B. E. (2005). Development of professional practice based on a family systems nursing framework: Nurses' and families' experiences. *Journal of Family Nursing, 11*(1), 38–58.

Li, Q. P., Mak, Y. W., & Loke, A. Y. (2013). Spouses' experience of caregiving for cancer patients: A literature review. *International Nursing Review, 60*(2), 178–187. doi:10.1111/inr.12000

Lindgren, L., Burke, M., Hainsworth, M., & Eakes, G. (1992). Chronic sorrow: A lifespan concept. *Scholarly Inquiry for Nursing Practice, 6*, 27–40.

Looman, W. (2006). Development and testing of the Social Capital Scale for families of children with special health care needs. *Research in Nursing and Health, 29*(4), 325–336.

Lubkin, I. M., & Larsen, P. D. (2013). *Chronic illness: Impact and interventions* (8th ed.). Burlington, MA: Jones & Barlett.

Mason, P., & Butler, C. C. (2010). *Health behavior change: A guide for practitioners* (2nd ed.). Edinburgh: Elsevier.

McGhan, G., Loeb, S. J., Baney, B., & Penrod, J. (2013). End-of-life caregiving. *Journal of Gerontological Nursing, 39*(6), 45–54. doi:10.3928/00989134-20130402-01

McDaniel, S. H., Campbell, T. L., Hepworth, J., & Lorenz, A. (2005). *Family-oriented primary care* (2nd ed.). New York: Springer.

McGoldrick, M., Gerson, R., & Petry, S. (2008). *Genograms: Assessment and intervention* (3rd ed.). New York: Norton.

Meleis, A. I. (Ed.). (2010). *Transitions theory: Middle range and situation—Specific theories in nursing research and practice.* New York: Springer.

Meleis, A. I. (2012). *Theoretical nursing: Development and progress* (5th ed.). Philadelphia: Wolters Kluwer Health.

Melvin, C. S., & Heater, B. S. (2004). Suffering and chronic sorrow: Characteristics and a paradigm for nursing interventions. *International Journal for Human Caring, 8*(2), 41–47.

Mitchell, M., Chaboyer, W., Burmeister, E., & Foster, M. (2009). Positive effects of a nursing intervention on family-centered care in adult critical care. *American Journal of Critical Care, 18*(6), 543–553.

Moriarty, P. H., & Wagner, L. D. (2004). Family rituals that provide meaning for single-parent families. *Journal of Family Nursing, 10*(2), 190–210.

Moules, N. J., Simonson, K., Fleiszer, A., Prins, M., & Glasgow, B. (2007). The soul of sorrow work: Grief and therapeutic interventions with families. *Journal of Family Nursing, 13*(1), 117–141.

Moules, N. J., Simonson, K., Prins, M., Angus, P., & Bell, J. M. (2004). Making room for grief: Walking backwards and living forward. *Nursing Inquiry, 11*(2), 99–107.

Moules, N. J., Thirsk, L. M., & Bell. J. M. (2006). A Christmas without memories: Beliefs about grief and mother—A clinical case analysis. *Journal of Family Nursing, 12* (4), 426–441. doi: 10.1177/1074840706294244

Nelms, T. P., & Eggenberger, S. K. (2010). Essence of the family critical illness experience and family meetings. *Journal of Family Nursing, 16*(4), 462–486.

Newman, M. A. (2008). *Transforming presence: The difference that nursing makes.* Philadelphia: F. A. Davis.

O'Leary, J., Warland, J., & Parker, L. (2011). Bereaved parents' perception of the grandparents' reactions after perinatal loss and in the pregnancy that follows. *Journal of Family Nursing, 17*(3), 330–356.

Pavlish, C. P., & Pharris, M. D. (2012). *Community-based collaborative action research: A nursing approach.* Sudbury, MA: Jones & Bartlett.

Perkins, M., Howard, V. J., Wadley, V. G., Crowe, M., Safford, M. M., Haley, W. E., . . . Roth, D. L. (2013). Caregiving strain and all-cause mortality: Evidence from the REGARDS study. *The Journal of Gerontology: Psychological Sciences and Social Sciences, 68*(4), 504–512. Epub 2012 Oct 2. doi: 10.1093/geronb/gbs084

Pierce, L. L., & Lutz, B. J. (2013). Family caregiving. In I. M. Lubkin & P. D. Larsen (Eds.), *Chronic illness: Impact and intervention.* Burlington, MA: Jones & Bartlett.

Prochaska, J. O., Johnson, S., & Lee, P. (2009). The transtheoretical model of behavior change. In S. A. Shumaker, J. K. Ockene, & K. A. Riekert (Eds.), *The handbook of health behavior change* (3rd ed.). New York: Springer.

Rando, T. A. (1984). Random notes: The patient is not a dirty word. *Family Systems Medicine, 3*, 230–233.

Rempel, G., Neufeld, A., & Kushner, K. (2007). Interactive use of genograms and ecomaps in family caregiving research. *Journal of Family Nursing, 13*(4), 403–419. doi:10.1177/1074840707307917

Richardson, J. B., & Brakle, M. V. (2011). A qualitative study of relationships among parenting strategies, social capital, the juvenile justice system, and mental health care for at-risk African American male youth. *Journal of Correctional Health Care, 17*(4), 319–328. doi: 10.1177/1078345811413081

Roberti, S. M., & Fitzpatrick, J. F. (2010). Assessing family satisfaction with care of critically ill patients: A pilot study. *Critical Care Nurse, 30*(6), 18–26. doi: 10.4037/ccn/2010448

Robinson, C. A., & Wright, L. M. (1995). Family nursing interventions: What families say makes a difference. *Journal of Family Nursing, 1*, 327–345.

Rodakowski, J., Skidmore, E. R., Rogers, J. C., & Schulz, R. (2012). Role of social support in predicting caregiver burden. *Archives of Physical Medicine Rehabilitation, 93*(12), 2229–2236.

Rolland, J. S., & Walsh, F. (2005). Systemic training for health care professionals: The Chicago Center for Family Health approach. *Family Process, 44*(5), 283–301.

Rollnick, S., Miller, W. R., & Butler, C. (2008). *Motivational interviewing in health care: Helping patients change behavior*. New York: Guilford Press.

Rook, D. W. (1985). The ritual dimension of consumer behavior. *Journal of Consumer Research 12*, 251–264.

Roos, S. (2002). *Chronic sorrow: A living loss*. New York: Brunner-Routledge.

Schneider, M., & Stokols, D. (2009). Multilevel theories of behavior change: A social ecological framework. In S. A. Shumaker, J. K. Ockene, & K. A. Riekert (Eds.), *The handbook of health behavior change* (3rd ed.). New York: Springer.

Segrin, C., & Flora, J. (2011). *Family communication*. Mahwah, NJ: Lawrence Erlbaum Associates.

Shaefer, S. (2010). Perinatal loss and support strategies for diverse cultures: Discussion paper. *Neonatal, Paediatric and Child Health Nursing, 13*(1), 14–17.

Shumaker, S. A., Ockene, J. K., & Riekert, K. A. (2009). *The handbook of health behavior change* (3rd ed.). New York: Springer.

Siminoff, L. A., Wilson-Genderson, M., & Baker, S., Jr. (2010). Depressive symptoms in lung cancer patients and their family caregivers and the influence of family environment. *Psycho-Oncology, 19*(12), 1285–1293. doi:10.1002/pon.1696

Svavarsdottir, E. K., & Sigurdardottir, A. (2013). Benefits of a brief therapeutic conversation intervention for families of children and adolescents in active cancer treatment. *Clinical Journal of Oncology Nursing, 17*E, 346–357. doi:10.1188/13.ONF.E346-E357

Sveinbjarnardottir, E. K., Svavarsdottir, E. K., & Hrafnkelsson, B. (2012). Psychometric development of the Iceland Expressive Family Functioning Questionnaire (ICEFFQ). *Journal of Family Nursing, 18*(3):353–377. doi:10.1177/1074840712449204

Tan, H., Wilson, A., Olver, I., & Barton, C. (2011). The family meeting addressing spiritual and psychosocial needs in a palliative care setting: Usefulness and challenges to implementation. *Progress in Palliative Care, 19*(2), 66–72. doi:10.1179/1743291X11Y.0000000001

Tomlinson, P. S., Peden-McAlpine, C., & Sherman, S. (2011). A family systems nursing intervention model for paediatric health crisis. *Journal of Advanced Nursing, 68*(3), 705–714. doi: 10.1111/j.1365-2648.2011.05825.x

United States Department of Health and Human Services. (2012). Healthy people 2020. Retrieved on December 21, 2012 from http://www.healthypeople.gov/2020/default.aspx

University of Michigan Health System. (2006). *Children with chronic health conditions*. Ann Arbor, MI: Author. Retrieved March 2, 2013 from http://www.med.umich.edu/yourchild/topics/chronic.htm

Veltri, L. (2010). Family nursing with childbearing families. In J. R. Kaakinen, V. Gedaly-Duff, D. P. Coehlo, & S. M. Harmon Hanson (Eds.), *Family health care nursing: Theory, practice and research* (4th ed.). Philadelphia: F. A. Davis.

Walsh, F. (2003). Family resilience: A framework for clinical practice. *Family Process, 42*, 1–18.

Weihs, K., Fisher, L., & Baird, M. (2002). Families, health and behavior: A section of the Commissioned Report by the Committee on Health and Behavior: Research, Practice and Policy. *Families, Systems and Health, 20*(1), 7–46.

Weiss, R. S. (1974). The provisions of social relationships. In Z. Rubin (Ed.), *Doing unto others* (pp 17–26). Englewood Cliffs, NJ: Prentice Hall.

Wiegand, D. L. M. (2006). Withdrawal of life-sustaining therapy after sudden, unexpected life-threatening illness or injury: Interactions between patients' families, health care providers, and the healthcare system. *American Journal of Critical Care, 15*(2), 178–187.

Williams, A., & Bakitas, M. (2012). Cancer family caregivers: A new direction for interventions. *Journal of Palliative Medicine, 15*(7), 775–783. doi:10.1089/jpm.2012.0046

Wittenberg-Lyles, E., Goldsmith, J., Ragan, S. L., & Sanchez-Reilly, S. (2012). Dying with comfort: Family illness narratives and early palliative care. *Journal of Social Work in End-of-Life and Palliative Care, 8*(2), 202–203.

Wood, B. L., Klebba, K. B., & Miller, B. D. (2000). Evolving the family biobehavioral model: The fit of attachment. *Family Process, 39*(3), 319–344.

Wood, B. L., Klebba, K. B., & Miller, B. D. (2002). Evolving the biobehavioral family model: The fit of attachment. In Boss, P. G. (Ed.), *Family stress: Classic and contemporary readings.* Thousand Oaks, CA: Sage.

Worden, J. W. (2009). *Grief counseling and grief therapy: A handbook for the mental health practitioner* (4th ed.). New York: Springer.

Wright, L. M., & Bell, J. M. (2009). *Beliefs and illness: A model for healing.* Calgary, Alberta, Canada: 4th Floor Press.

Wright, L. M., & Leahy, M. (2013). *Nurses and families: A guide to family assessment and intervention.* Philadelphia: F. A. Davis.

Zerwekh, J. V. (2006). *Nursing care at the end of life: Palliative care for patients and families.* Philadelphia: F. A. Davis.

Zhang, A. Y., & Siminoff, L. A. (2003). Silence and cancer: Why do families and patients fail to communicate. *Health Communication, 15*(4), 415–429.

CHAPTER 15

Teaching Family Members Supportive Care

Sharon A. Denham • Sandra Eggenberger

CHAPTER OBJECTIVES

1. Define the family support construct.
2. Describe family needs for support to meet wellness, health promotion, care maintenance, and disease management throughout the life course.
3. Compare the benefits of various forms of support with various health and illness needs.
4. Identify intentional nursing actions that effectively provide family support during different health and illness experiences.

CHAPTER CONCEPTS

- Caregiver burden
- Compassion fatigue
- Coordinated care
- Discharge planning
- Emotional support
- Family health routines
- Informational support
- Instrumental support
- Intentional support
- Nurse support
- Organizational support
- Resources
- Respite care
- Spiritual support
- Support
- Support groups

Introduction

The term *support* is used often, but has many meanings. It might be a column or beam that braces an architectural structure. Technical support may mean the repair person who comes to fix an appliance, such as a computer when your hard drive crashes. In the world of politics, support might be a form of advocacy provided by lobbyists. Support can be linked with state initiatives like child support, support groups, or even financial support. In medical care, we speak of life supports to assist critically ill persons. Support also implies caregiving for a person in need. This chapter identifies the ways nurses who *think family* can provide supportive family care and describes many aspects and forms of support needed by individuals and families when health or illness is the concern.

Nursing Care and Supportive Actions

Nurses often ask about the availability of support. When asked, most respond with an affirmative answer. Conversation often goes like this: "Do you have support when you go home?" The individual responds, "Oh yes, I have my family." End of discussion! When a person says they have support most nurses stop talking and move on to a different topic. Usually, no further assessment about specific care needs occurs.

Defining Support

Support can be viewed as informational, instrumental or provisional, emotional and relational, resources, organizational, and social (Schaffer, 2004). Nurses most often address some informational and educational supports during times of stress, illness, and symptom management (Trecartin & Carroll, 2011). Informational or educational support refers to instructions or teaching provided for care management. Instrumental or provisional support refers to the tangible goods, resources, and services that families need (House, 1981). Emotional support involves things like feeling loved, admired, or heard and focuses on relational aspects (Norbeck, 1981). Appraisal support refers to affirming actions (Kahn & Antonucci, 1980). Other kinds of support can also be considered. For example, social support that comes from family and friend networks and the community environments can include tangible things like resources and supplies, but organizational and community networks also offer a variety of services to ease a burden (Looman, 2006).

Nurses and Delivery of Support

Nurses generally need to go deeper with communications about support and ask more follow-up questions to clarify what families understand about support. What kind of support are you referring to and what do people think you mean? These two interpretations can be very different. Is what is available what is specifically needed? Assumptions that individuals or families are fully aware of the degree or types of support needed can be mistaken. Nurses who *think family* give thoughtful explanations. Out of curiosity, they ask powerful questions. The purpose is to ensure that the family is prepared to self-manage a health condition in the family household.

An example of a powerful question might be: "What do you expect will happen when you get home?" Generally, people speak of positive outcomes they expect. They talk about hopes. People can underestimate the type and quantity of help they might need in achieving their hopes, overestimate their capabilities, or underestimate the barriers they will face. It is hard to know what is going to happen if you have not previously experienced it. Just asking if support is available is usually the wrong question.

Rather than asking if support is available, the nurse asks what they will need at home to manage: What kinds of things will you need when you get home? What is it going to take to achieve your goals? Who is going to be there to . . .? As things are discussed, nurses who *think family* describe care, treatments, medications, and resources needed. The nurse might say, "Your doctor has ordered physical therapy for 6 weeks, you will start on Monday. Because you are not able to drive, who will be able to transport you?" Many people do not obtain physical therapy because they can't get there!

Nurses can check to see what questions still need answers. What is the level of confidence linked with changing dressings? If the person cannot reach or see a surgical incision, then who will assist with dressing changes and observing signs of healing? If the person is blind, how will she identify her medications so she can take them safely? Individual-nurse-family partnerships for support imply that household needs are understood in relationship to pre-scribed medical care and self-management needs. If support is fragmented, then the family is not empowered. How will persons independently do self-care without professional as-sistance? What are the safety concerns linked with the family household? Nurses who *think family* guide conversations about anticipated needs and monitor responses. Families are experts about their home and lives. They know what is needed, but may not say unless a trusted relationship has been formed (Fig. 15.1).

Family Conversations Around Support

In health care settings, even when needed support is limited or totally unavailable, people often still say, "Yes, we have what we need." But they might not fully understand exactly what they need. Some may think "Families should take care of their own and not ask for outside help" and be unwilling to expose their frailties or needs. Some may believe that a family does not expose troubles to outsiders, so they are hesitant to disclose their true needs. Those who value strong individualism may be hesitant and unwilling to expose their vulnerability. Pride can prevent them from admitting they need help or lack resources.

Asking "Do you have support at home?" is not the best question to ask. A different helping approach may be more effective and usually begins with establishing a trusting re-lationship before asking about support. Most people need to sense a sincerity of concern before they openly expose themselves and their needs. For example, you might start by ex-plaining the kinds of things that will be needed following a hospital discharge. Describe needed care requirements, treatments to be provided, special equipment needs, and the kinds of caregiver time demands usually expected with a similar condition.

Here is an example of a therapeutic conversation about support. "I know you will be going home in a few days. Most people who have had a condition like yours have some difficulty doing some personal or hygiene care for the first 3 to 5 days. You might need some assistance getting a bath and going to the bathroom at home. How easy will it be for you to get from your bed to the bathroom?" If this person must climb stairs or will be alone some of the time, you could suggest durable medical equipment and mention safety concerns. Ask if a family member is available to assist with meal preparation before explaining the prescribed diet. This person might need specific instructions and need to talk with the dietitian. Discuss the new medicines ordered for home use and see if the per-son knows what side effects to watch for when taking the medicines. You might ask if there

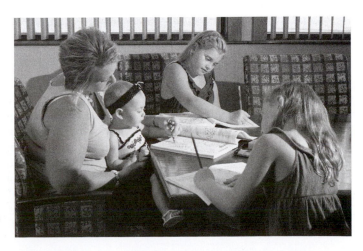

FIGURE 15-1 Nurses are able to provide support for families.

is any problem paying for prescriptions. If the person seems uncertain, then this might be a good time to consult a pharmacist to see if there are other options if this drug is expensive or suggest a generic substitute. Ask if the person knows what to do when he gets home and describe things to do if problems arise. Obtaining family information can reveal some of the realities and risks the person may have to deal with and gives him a chance to discuss specific support needs. Nurses who *think family* realize that knowing and addressing the unique family household needs can help avoid future problems and ensure that adequate forms of support are available.

Using Individual-Nurse-Family Relationships to Provide Support

Nurses who value family caring actions provide information and emotional support (Robinson, Pesut, & Bottorff, 2012). Nurses usually can help individuals and families return to their household equipped to manage their concerns. Nurses who *think family* empower those in their care and provide reassurance as they help families figure out what they need and how to get it and provide the information and guidance they need to be prepared.

Nurses help families of chronically ill persons learn best ways to assist and encourage by recognizing and praising caregiving actions (Chesla, 2010; Wright & Leahey, 2012). A nurse supports a man whose spouse is diagnosed with multiple sclerosis (MS) by curiously listening to his concerns. Before giving expert instructions, the nurse uses powerful questions: What is troubling you most at this time? What would best help you attend to this need? The nurse might think he needs medical equipment at home or is worried about activities of daily living. The nurse might be surprised when he sharply replies, "I am so frustrated with this disease. It has changed our sex life and she won't talk about it." Topics not often discussed might be high on the list of worries for those living with serious medical conditions.

What should this nurse do in this situation? The nurse might be uncomfortable discussing sexual relationships, but knows that loss of nerve function, fatigue, muscle spasms, loss of bladder control, and other things can interfere with sexual functions. The nurse might say, "You should talk to your doctor about this when she comes in." Or the nurse could be silent, listen, and then say, "I can sense you are troubled. What do you think your wife might be feeling?" Using an open-ended question invites conversation. The nurse might just listen and say little. Maybe he might say to the man, "I know this must be difficult. Do you want to brainstorm some ideas about the ways to discuss this with her?" The nurse might tell him about a MS support group that he could join, provide information about a therapist that might help, or suggest that he let his wife know that he still deeply loves her and desires her closeness.

Community Support

Extended family and close friends are often key sources of support—but coworkers, religious or community members, and professional caregivers also provide supports (Almasri et al., 2011; Haggman-Laitila, Tanninen, & Pietila, 2010). In some critical situations, caregiving resources beyond what the family can provide might be needed. For example, a child or adult with a severe disability or a family caring for a member at the end of life might need around-the-clock assistance. Nurses can offer some suggestions, but might enlist a social worker to locate help and coordinate around-the-clock care. Hospice experience with individuals living alone saw corps of neighbors and church friends create around-the-clock caregiver networks. Network members can do a variety of things such as provide transportation, listen, be available, provide a safe atmosphere, and share information (Benzies & Mychasiuk, 2008). Nurses who *think family* are gatekeepers to

---

BOX 15-1

Family Tree

Hiroko Watanabe, MS, RN (Japan)

Hiroko Watanabe, MS, RN, has had a sustained focus and national influence on family nursing in Japan. She was the first faculty member of Family Nursing at Chiba University, where she started the first undergraduate level course in Family Nursing. She has published more than 10 textbooks about the Watanabe Family Assessment Model, and her textbook coauthored with Dr. Suzuki on family nursing, *Family Nursing Theory and Practice*, is known and used in all nursing schools in Japan. She is the Chief Editor (with Dr. Sayumi Nojima) of the *Japanese Journal of Family Nursing*. She gives over 100 family nursing lectures each year all over Japan. Ms. Watanabe has also served as a board member of the Japanese Association for Research in Family Nursing (JARFN) for many years.

---

support networks. It is important to remember that families with other cultures or ethnicities may have different values around support and may need to be communicated with differently (Box 15.1).

Types of Support

Not everyone needs the same types of support. Social support can be useful with mental and physical health and help with adjustments to daily life. However, the most beneficial social support matches the need. Actions are not helpful if support is unwanted or provided in wrong ways. People offer different forms of support. Differences between perceived needed support and received support occur. Received support is what the recipient believes has been given; perceived support is what the support giver thinks he does. In families, conflicts arise when intended actions are perceived as inadequate by the recipient.

Gender often influences differences in the types of support needed and given. Women are often more engaged in social networks and more comfortable giving emotional support. It is similar to nurturing roles they often assume. Men might be slower to offer emotional support, but quick to provide instrumental support. Several years ago a gentleman participating in a focus group listened to another man talk about the ways his wife helped him manage his diabetes. Well into the discussion, he said, "I would like your wife to talk with mine. I never get that kind of help at home." Remember that, although some attributes are generally ascribed to one gender, people are different, so assess each individual before making assumptions. Identify what forms of support are needed.

Instrumental Support

Instrumental support is linked with necessary tasks but can range from simple, such as picking up medicine from the pharmacy occasionally, to demanding, such as helping someone with toileting around the clock, regularly preparing meals, or assisting with daily bathing. It might also include making arrangements for home assistive devices such as hand rails for getting in and out of the tub or a special shower chair. Or it may entail helping a person with a disability or mental illness to pay bills, run errands, or do household chores.

Instrumental supports contributes to health and enables persons to recover or live. A longitudinal data study of 4,211 families discovered that neighborhood disadvantage means mothers with young children have less instrumental support, especially financial assistance, from family and friends (Turney & Harknett, 2010). Geographical location of households makes a difference in the support available, as can social class. Research has shown that those in a higher social class with a mobility disability had more instrumental support than those in a lower social class (Nilsson, Avlund, & Lund, 2010). Sometimes individuals need short-term or temporary support, such as during recuperation. At other times it is for a long term. Instrumental support is tangible service that contributes to meeting distinct needs, a concrete form of social support to assist others. Provisional support might have emotional attachments and be perceived as helpful and caring (Semmer et al., 2008). If instrumental support needs go on too long, then such support can become burdensome to families.

Informational Support

Informational support is providing facts, figures, or other information to guide behaviors, suggest actions, and supply ideas about managing a particular situation. Informational support can be linked to tangible resources and visible services, such as finding a community support group for a family with a substance abuse problem. Informational support can be advice, guidance, or written or oral instruction. Family nurses identify the kinds of information needed because individuals and families differ widely. Thus, needs for the same medical diagnosis will differ. Box 15.2 provides ideas to consider when thinking about needed informational support.

Assessment, planning, intervention, monitoring, and evaluating techniques are linked with informational support. To plan for effective information support, it is essential to identify communication barriers and remember that family members not physically present

---

BOX 15-2

Questions About Informational Support for Nurses

Never ask, "Do you have any questions?" Families often do not know what questions to ask. Rather, approach the situation with more open-ended questions. Consider what knowledge and skills are brought into the current situation and what can be added to what is already known:

- Have you ever done anything like this before?
- What will this look like at home?
- What things are most worrisome to you?
- What kinds of concerns do you have about what needs to be done at home?
- Sometimes people are nervous about care needs. What things are you most concerned about?
- What is the most important thing that you have learned so far?

When delivering informational support or education to individuals and family members, here are some questions to reflect upon:

- Is the information provided accurate?
- What does the individual need to know to best promote health or manage an illness condition?
- What is the best way to provide the educational information?
- When is the best time to communicate the educational information?
- How can the appropriate family members best be included in information sessions?
- Are there any low literacy or health literacy concerns?
- What cultural considerations should be taken into account when providing information?
- Can some forms of technology be used in providing ongoing information?
- How will future questions get answered with accurate information in a timely way?
- What media forms can be used to aid understandings about health and illness?
- What different understandings and knowledge do family members bring to the situation?

may also need information. Using circular questions may help identify more specific needs. Using teach-back or return demonstration methods helps to ensure understanding.

Do not underestimate the power of media and social networks in information sharing. Information abounds, but whether it is accurate or delivered in timely ways can be critical. Family nurses can play bigger roles in ensuring that information to support health, prevent adverse outcomes, and manage care is delivered effectively. In what ways can nurses advocate for information needs to better support household management of individual and family health? Are there technologies that can be used to provide the right information at the right time?

Medical Treatments

A primary concern of informational support is to prevent adverse care outcomes. People living with a chronic condition might spend a maximum of 1 to 2 hours a year talking with a physician or nurse about their care. The hours in a year (24 hours a day, 7 days a week for 365 days) amount to 8,760 hours. If you subtract 2 hours spent getting medical instructions, families are left with 8,758 hours every year trying to figure out what to do. Who do they call when help is needed, questions arise, or confusion occurs? Current care systems often fail to provide ongoing informational support. In the household, family and others influence care. What information is needed? How can this be provided in clearer and more useful ways?

Special emphasis is needed when it comes to teaching accurately about prescribed medical treatments and medications so that errors are avoided. Handing someone a prescription for medications is not enough. Family units need clear explanations about purpose, administration, side effects, benefits, drug interactions, use of over-the-counter drugs, costs, and adverse responses with foods. They need to know what side effects should trigger a visit to their doctor or emergency department. They need a place to go to have questions answered. Family-focused nurses realize that medications alone may not meet all needs.

Medication errors are costly, often preventable, and all too common. The American Geriatric Society 2012 Beers Criteria Update Expert Panel advises use of their criteria to improve outcomes in older persons. A systematic evidence-based review of the literature was used to identify effects of various medications on older adults. The Beers Criteria identify actions of potentially inappropriate medications to avoid with elderly persons. In some medications the high risks outweigh the benefits. One needs to take special care with older persons as well as with those who are very young.

Emotional Support

Emotional support is critical to health, abilities to cope, and positive psychological states of belonging and security, but some persons are hesitant to share private or personal information (Cassel, 1976; Cohen, Gottlieb, & Underwood, 2001; Schaffer, 2004). Receiving emotional support involves the experience of feeling respected, admired, or loved (Norbeck, 1981). Emotional support gives encouragement, reassurance, acceptance, and respect (Schaffer, 2004). Giving or receiving emotional support does not come natural to everyone. Even nurses can be uncomfortable giving emotional support because they become vulnerable. Thinking family means emotions are aligned with the human condition and always exist. Giving emotional support is not a recipe to follow, but might involve being present, listening, touching, or offering kind words.

Families are interdependent systems; their are strengthened by their emotional bonds and support they provide one another. Determining the nature of family connectedness could suggest that some emotional support is needed from outside the family or for the whole family unit, not just an ill member (Cray, 2012; Schaffer, 2004; Scharpe, 2012; Sveinbjarnardottir, Svavarsdottir, & Hrafnkelsson, 2012).

Offering Emotional Support

Family nurses offer emotional support for illness needs, areas of stress, coping with suffering, and referrals for counseling (McCubbin & McCubbin, 1996; Wacharasin, 2010). They can use therapeutic communication and teach relationship skills to families (Box 15.3). Emotional support can be companionship, care that brings a sense of belonging, being part of a group, or having social significance. Companionship is having another caring person present and not being alone. It might mean being part of a social network or having a shared interest. For children, emotional support most often comes from the parents, but throughout a lifetime types of companionship needs and emotional bonds can change.

Nurses offer emotional support during the time that family units are managing serious acute illness and making end-of-life decisions (Couture, Ducharme, & Lamontagne, 2012; Wiegand, Deatrick, & Knafl, 2008). Therapeutic relationships include families in care of individual members as family needs are recognized as important in health or illness situations (Cray, 2012). Nurses serve as family advocates as they strive to understand the impact of the medical diagnosis. A welcoming caring environment purposefully addresses family needs and invites them to participate in family member care (Svavarsdottir, 2008). Cray (2012) developed a family comfort intervention that includes five components:

- Welcome the family to the unit.
- Provide information.
- Invite the family to the setting.
- Provide specific directions.
- Listen to the family as an expert in care.

A comfort intervention has great potential to provide the family emotional support.

Spiritual Support

For some, spiritual or religious beliefs are among the most powerful beliefs an individual or family holds (Wright, 2005). Although limited, nursing research shows positive relationships between religion and spirituality with health outcomes (Wright, 2008). Family nurses can

---

BOX 15-3

Providing Emotional Support

Nurses can provide emotional support in many ways:

1. Comforting family in ways that are meaningful to family
2. Encouraging family to share experiences and listen to family members
3. Acting responsibly to include family and meet family's expectations
4. Providing realistic reassurance to family
5. Being reliable with actions
6. Offering guidance and direction to the family
7. Including the family members when planning, sharing, and acting

For further discussion, see Bulecheck & McCloskey, 1992, p 328; Couture, Ducharme, & Lamontagne, 2012; Edvardsson, Sandman, & Rasmussen, 2006; Kolcaba, 2003; Weiss, 1976.

support ways for those beliefs to empower families and manage illness. Asking questions and listening to families' beliefs and practices is a good way to begin, and developing a trusted relationships helps families feel more comfortable sharing their beliefs with nurses. You might notice religious or spiritual symbols that the family has visible to begin a conversation about the influence of their beliefs on the situation.

Nurses meet people in the midst of the uncertainty surrounding crisis and change, sometimes at the most devastating points in life. They ask questions that nurses just cannot answer; all they can do is be present. Why me? Why us? What does a situation mean? The search for meaning is often an individual journey, a lonely path. What are nurses' roles as individuals and families grapple with emotional pain, chaos, and uncertainty?

Religion and Spirituality

The term *spirituality* is derived from the Latin word *spiritus* referring to breath, vital spirit, or soul (Burkhardt & Nagai-Jacobson, 1994). Spirituality is experienced in the context of relationships with sacred sources, nature, others, and self. Spiritual needs are related to finding meaning in suffering and illness, affirming connections, and forming a relationship to peace, courage, and trust (Wright, 2005). Cultures and belief systems mean spirituality has unique perspectives. A holistic nursing framework defines three spiritual characteristics (Dossey, 1997; Dossey & Keegan, 2013; Wright, 2005):

• Unfolding the mystery of life's meaning
• Inner strength and meanings
• Harmonious interconnections among self, environment, and a higher power

Nurses use this framework to offer spiritual support. It is a way to explore meanings, search for inner strengths, and connect to things beyond oneself.

Religion and spirituality provide support, yet often nurses lack confidence in dealing with subjective dimensions of human existence (McSherry & Jamieson, 2011). Religion and spirituality are not synonymous. Religion generally refers to an organized system of beliefs and practices shared by a group (Wright, 2005). The shared values and beliefs center on a divine entity. Rituals and celebrations focus on religious values. If religious support is needed, then it is appropriate to seek a chaplain or pastoral referral. Nurses can assist the family with contacts if needed. Nurses don't know about all religions, but they can use curious inquiry to learn about practices, rituals, or dietary implications, especially those that have meaning to the individual and family. You might need to explore religious beliefs about what foods can be eaten, how food is prepared, and other practices that are viewed as part of healing and wholeness.

Arthur Kleinman, a distinguished professor of anthropology at Harvard University, has investigated questions about what really matters. He thinks about relationships between health, illness narratives, moral life, caregiving, human values, or spirituality. He offers questions a nurse might ask of self and others:

• How does family see the illness problem and solution?
• What worries you the most?
• What do you fear most about the illness?

As nurses recognize needs for spiritual support, some might fear ways to respond. Spiritual support is generally not given in answers or advice, but as presence and tolerance for unanswerable questions. Nurses who *think family* listen to uncomfortable questions, hear the uncertainty, and endure the anguish as they collaborate with individuals and families (Fig. 15.2).

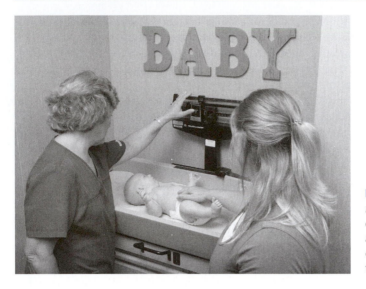

FIGURE 15-2 Nurses who *think family* listen to uncomfortable questions, hear the uncertainty, and endure the anguish as they collaborate with individuals and families.

Organizational Support

Organizational support involves examining a system, such as individual, family, health care organization, or community, to see what supports are needed. Nurses who *think family* recognize that community agencies and other organizations provide support. Several types of organizations can provide support:

- Federal or state agencies that assist with some illnesses—Medicaid, Medicare, Maternal and Child Health Bureau
- National condition-related groups—American Heart Association, American Cancer Society, American Diabetes Association, and others
- Volunteer organizations—faith or civic groups, Salvation Army, food pantries
- Outpatient services—home health agencies, hospice, and public health
- Individuals within larger systems—social worker, chaplain, dietitian

Organizational support can be structural relationships, but can also have relational elements within the system (Gutierrez, Candela, & Carver, 2012). System support includes educational opportunities, financial services, decision making, policies, and leadership to guide, coach, and serve. An organization can help solve problems, offer guidance, and use team strengths.

Nurses who *think family* ask questions like: What is the fit between the family and organizational system? Organizational support means resources are available to encourage, fortify, or undergird specific needs. Nurses can be trusted advocates within organizational systems. Advocacy is derived from the Latin word *advocatus* and it means pleading the cause of another. As organizational representatives, nurses provide support for family needs (Meiers & Brauer, 2008).

Instruments of Support

A living will and a durable power of attorney for health care might be viewed as organizational supports. In some states, these documents are combined into a single form. A durable power of attorney identifies an individual to manage financial affairs, make health care decisions, or conduct other business if the person is incapacitated. A general durable power of attorney allows an individual to conduct legal actions but a limited durable power of attorney covers specific events, like selling property or making health care decisions.

A durable power of attorney for health care appoints someone trusted as a health care agent. They make health care decisions and ensure wishes of the designee are followed. Living wills are written statements that detail the care desired if an individual is incapacitated. It bears no relationship to a conventional will or living trust used to leave property at death. A living will is strictly a way to identify health care preferences. It can say a great deal about the kind of health care services individuals want.

Purposes of Support

Support is associated with health and illness and includes the ways resources are supplied, services provided, and information accessed. Support suggests helping to bear responsibility or assist with burden management. Families might be prepared for usual needs, but struggle with prolonged responsibility (Elliott, Burgio, & DeCoster, 2010; Denham, 2003). Extended supports require large expenditures of resources and personal energy. Family nurses assist with coordinated care as transfers from one setting to another occur, including moving from acute care to the family household. Support requires assessment and intentional planning (Table 15.1).

TABLE 15-1	*Examples of Family Support Needs*
TYPES OF SUPPORT	**EXAMPLES OF SUPPORT NEEDS**
Instrumental support	• Food, clothing, and shelter • Financial resources • Transportation • Help with errands and tasks
Information support	• Facts about the diagnosis • Instructions for prescribed medications • Abilities to perform needed treatments • Directions on dietary changes • Follow-up visits • Things to observe for and report • What to do in an emergency
Companion support	• Friendship • Someone to share activities • Make days meaningful • Provide a sense of belonging • Caregiving
Emotional support	• Trust • Relationship • Manage threats and uncertainties • Presence of a listening person or network
Spiritual support	• Answer questions • Search for meaning • Moral understandings • Valued connectedness to something bigger than self
Organizational support	• Peer groups • Support groups • Educational conferences • Problem-solving processes

Influence of Support on Health

It is generally assumed that when support is available positive health outcomes are likely. However, few research studies have identified causal links between social support and health outcomes (Schaffer, 2004). Recent nursing studies from around the globe suggest that family nursing interventions that address educational, emotional, relational, and social support do have positive family outcomes (Chesla, 2010; Svavarsdottir, Tryggvadottir, & Sigurdardottir, 2012; Wacharasin, 2010). A literature review completed in Finland examined family nursing intervention studies and found that emotional support was a key element in family nursing (Mattila, Leino, Paavilainen, & Åstedt-Kurki, 2009). Table 15.2 identifies two models to explain influences of support on health.

Intentional Supportive Actions

Nurses regularly provide support, but it is especially important for family education to be intentional and personalized to fit unique situations. Intentional action implies deliberation and purposeful planning to fulfill expressed needs. Support vested in needs of others and not merely serving nurses' purposes is most useful.

Families with dependent children or adult members unable to provide independent self-care rely upon many types of support. Nurses who *think family* act intentionally and assess those needs to determine the supports that will be most effective. Based on culture, literacy, disease condition, and family household, what is needed? What does the family yet need to know? Has the timing of medication delivery been explained? What should the family do in emergencies? Does the family know what defines an emergency? See Box 15.4 to consider different ideas about using social support to support health.

To effectively offer the best support for medical concerns, it is essential to determine what is already known and where specific needs are. A usual focus of nurses is providing medical information and sometimes that can be hard. If a condition has been longstanding, information needed might not be about managing the disease, but rather preventing complications or supporting some aspect of organization in the family household.

TABLE 15-2	*Comparison of Models of Social Support and Health*
STRESS-BUFFERING MODEL	**MAIN EFFECT MODEL**
This model suggests support resources strengthen the ability to manage stressful situations.	This model suggests social support directly influences health.
The nurse may develop a comforting protective relationship with a family who is enduring a critical illness or preparing to provide care to a chronically ill family member.	The nurse provides information that introduces reasons to adopt healthier lifestyle behaviors.
The nurse provides emotional support, information, and connections to resources that assist a family to positively respond to stressful situations.	The nurse encourages actions that motivate family members to set goals.
The nurse's actions create a buffering situation and provide support so the family can better manage.	The nurse could lead a family meeting and bring family members together to develop goals, communicate about problems that need to be resolved, and make decisions in a protective and connecting social context.

Source: Adapted from findings of Cohen, S., Gottlieb, B. H., & Underwood, L. G. (2001). Social relationships and health: Challenges for measurement and intervention. *Advances in Mind-Body Medicine, 17*, 129–141.

Nurses can waste valuable time repeating information the family already knows. Find out what is known and what is unclear, and provide that information. Needs might not be about the medical care, but the financial costs or accessibility of medications or treatments. A household family member might have a prescription drug abuse problem that creates continual chaos in the home. If this person is to be discharged with prescriptions for pain management, what intentional actions should the nurse take?

Nurses use deliberate and thoughtful actions to address assessed needs. Therapeutic empathic relationships weigh real needs against agency or institutional ones. Ask what their concerns are: As you plan to go home, what concerns you the most? Who in your family is most bothered by what is happening? What additional supports are most needed at your home? What is most troubling about living with this condition? Help family members set goals, identify strategies to take, and decide how outcomes will be measured. Box 15.4 provides a case you can use to consider various support needs.

Making Life Changes

Illness is a family matter that causes a range of responses and concerns that need attention (Chesla, 2010; Denham, 2003; Wright & Bell, 2009; Wright & Leahey, 2012). When something extraordinary happens, family life can get disrupted and changes can have far-reaching

---

BOX 15-4

Family Support

Several years ago, Kimberly was diagnosed with type 1 diabetes at the age of 11 years. As a single parent, she gave birth to a daughter by a cesarean section at the age of 21 years after a difficult pregnancy and years of progressing diabetes-related complications from poor self-management (e.g., neuropathy, Charcot's syndrome, vision changes, depression). As an adult of 32 years, she lost her vision and suffered kidney failure simultaneously. At the time of diagnosis, her mother, continually at her bedside, was largely ignored. Finally, when the doctor shared the diagnosis and proclaimed things were under control, he gave only brief information about her condition and provided two rather large books about kidney failure and what to expect. "Read these," he said, "and let me know if you have any questions." He exited and was never seen again. Kimberly was in a medical crisis and was hospitalized for about 3 months. Nurses and others continually came and went from the room day after day and week after week, but very few ever offered information unless asked some specific question. Questions often received a terse inconsiderate response with no sense of therapeutic communication offered. Although Kimberly's caregiving needs would be great after discharge, no formal education was ever offered. She went home with gastroparesis, blind, on kidney dialysis, and frightened. After 5.5 years on dialysis, she received a kidney transplant and was started on immunosuppressive drugs. At 46 years of age, Kim lives with her sister as her caregiver. She has a history of cardiac disease (i.e., myocardial infarction, four stents, hypertension), chronic pain, a bipolar diagnosis, severe Charcot's foot that makes walking even short distances difficult, and limited social interaction. She is currently on 17 different medications that she takes several times daily and is continuously busy seeing various specialists.

Questions to Consider:

- What kinds of support do you think might have been useful for Kimberly during different periods of her life?
- What kinds of support do you think might have been useful for Kimberly's family members during different periods of her life?
- What might a family nurse do to ease the burden for Kimberly and her family?

effects. Sometimes those situations cause communication issues among family members. As roles change, stressful decisions about household chores, transportation, or finances might need to occur. Families are not always well prepared to address these changes. Nurses can help families with member communication. They can partner with them to identify pros and cons of actions and suggest other options.

Disruptions in Family Health Routines

When health concerns or attempts to achieve a healthier lifestyle disrupt usual routine, families often struggle to find ways to best change their usual life patterns. Needed changes are not always easy to make. Those changes require not only the will to change but also accepting the results or disruptions made in usual daily life. Families may not know what questions to ask, who to ask, or where to find needed supports. Family units often need help planning actions and coping, critical areas in behavior change (Sniehotta, Schwarzer, Scholz, & Schuz, 2005). Nurses might think about support with discharge plans from acute care, but be less aware of needs in ambulatory care settings. Nurses who *think family* know support is valuable for family household members and understand the types of support most effective regardless of the problem (Box 15.5).

If the family doesn't value the potential positive outcomes of change, it is unlikely that change will happen. They need to know reasons for the change and implications of changing and not changing. They need to be committed to overcome the difficulty of making those changes. The stages of change or what is often called the transtheoretical model (Prochaska & Velicer, 1997), discussed in Chapter 14, suggests that most at-risk people barely spend 40% of their time thinking about change, 40% of people spend some time thinking about change in sincere ways, and only 20% of them actually get ready to take action (Prochaska & Velicer, 1997). Many are not ready to take action when given a diagnosis and a medical regimen to follow. A family unit must value a change and believe it is needed before making efforts. As a family nurse, how can you best assist people to move along a continuum of readiness to change?

Nurses' Roles in Family Support

In addition to providing care instructions for medical concerns, nurses can offer others forms of support:

- Coach about wellness plans and goal setting for the family unit.
- Discuss health promotion and help locate resources.
- Teach about illness and disease prevention, safety, managing medical care.
- Identify family health routines and suggest strategies for change.
- Set times for follow-up and stress its importance.
- Provide reasons to adhere to the prescribed medical regimen.

BOX 15-5
Important Steps for Successful Change
Actions leading to desired changes essentially require these elements: • Intentions to act   • Abilities to overcome obstacles to action   • Commitment to be persistent and consistent in behaviors over time   • Social network supporting the action *or* collaboration with a social network

Effective family nurses pay attention to readiness to change, availability of resources, and family capacities to fulfill member needs. Nurses who *think family* realize that not understanding family needs or assuming the family knows more than they do can negatively influence outcomes. Effective nurse interactions address needed support that sometimes gets forgotten.

Family Perspectives

If families do not understand the information and lack support, they may be ill prepared to provide effective care once the discharged member returns to the family household. When people do not value or understand how to self-manage prescribed treatments, they are unlikely to take steps that result in desired medical outcomes. Complicated care can be overwhelming and create family conflicts. Nurses who *think family* offer guidance to overcome these problems without judgment. Labeling persons who haven't managed conditions as nonadherent, noncompliant, or even dysfunctional is an ineffective way to support positive changes. Who *think family* realize that most people are usually doing the best they can given their circumstances. Nurses must be sensitive to the ways they communicate needs for change.

Adherence

Adherence or nonadherence can be linked to the value of support the individual and family have received. Adherence implies that individuals follow a prescribed treatment plan as an active participant (Vuckovich, 2010). Individuals are told many things by different health care professionals at different care settings over long periods of time and sometimes the information they receive is conflicting. To ensure the best adherence or compliance to prescribed treatments, nurses need to ensure that families have needed information and supports (Box 15.6). Whether they can adhere to or comply with a treatment plan is linked to factors such as lifestyle, stresses, time management, organizational abilities, resources, and religious beliefs. Family nurses know members balance multiple concerns. The nurse's role is to provide support not judgment!

BOX 15-6

Family Tree

Rutja Phuphaibul, DNSc, RN (Thailand)

Rutja Phuphaibul, DNSc, RN, is a Professor at the Ramathibodi School of Nursing, Faculty of Medicine, Ramathibodi Hospital, Thailand. She has also served as the Chair of the doctoral program (International Program) in Nursing, Mahidol University, in Bangkok. She credits her doctoral education at the Department of Family Health Nursing, University of California, San Francisco (1981–1984) with providing her an excellent foundation to become a family nursing leader in her country. In 1987, she and her colleagues at Khon Kaen University established the first master's program in family nursing in Thailand. Dr. Phuphaibul published the first family nursing textbook in the Thai language: *Family Nursing: Theoretical Perspective and Its Application*. The book is now in its fourth edition. Her family nursing research has focused on Thai family tasks development, which includes the study of families with infants, toddlers, school-age children, and adolescents. In 2001, her research accomplishments were recognized by the Okura Foundation, the Nurses Association of Thailand, and she received an award from the Nursing Council in Thailand in 2003. In 2007, she was honored with an Innovative Contribution to Family Nursing Award by the *Journal of Family Nursing* at the Eighth International Family Nursing Conference in Bangkok, Thailand.

Discharge Planning

Family care needs are seldom well documented. In acute care, family may not be involved until the point of discharge. It is imperative to create new ways to identify and address family unit care needs before discharge regardless of the care setting. Nurses who *think family* consider likely care needs as persons move from one care setting to another, including living at home. Most time is spent at home, the place where most care is received. Discharge needs to include the following:

- Individual and family capacity to manage care when professionals are not available
- Available and well-supported caregivers
- Family strengths to build upon and plans to overcome threats
- Clear understandings of medications and treatments at home
- Reasons for various forms of medical follow-up and what to do when concerns arise
- Ways needed supports will be obtained
- Clear instructions, skills for care, and where to access more information

It may also be effective to call persons and families after they return home to provide additional support or provide more information that they didn't realize they needed to help reduce hospital readmissions (Kind et al., 2012). Calls to ensure people come to scheduled medical appointments have been useful. However, use of communication methods through e-mail, smartphones, and digital devices may improve connections and provide necessary information between visits. Communication and care aligned with support and empowerment are needed at the household level to ensure optimal outcomes. Healthy or unhealthy lifestyles are learned and practiced in family households. More attention needs to be paid to making positive changes to improve possibilities that desired outcomes will be achieved (Box 15.7).

BOX 15-7

Providing Family-Focused Support

Nurses can provide family-focused support in many ways:

- Assist parents with instructions for care of newborns, young children, and teens.
- Educate pregnant mothers about the benefits of breastfeeding.
- Instruct the parents of a child newly diagnosed with asthma or chronic condition about concerns to address in the home.
- Give information to a caregiver about Alzheimer's disease concerning safety and disease progression.
- Educate an adult and her family members about care for a chronic illness and help them make intentional plans, set goals, and acquire needed resources.
- Help a family manage grief and loss after the death of a loved one.
- Share information needed when a family member needs rehabilitation and discuss implications this will have on the family.
- Praise a family for their caregiving actions and accomplishments in management of a chronic illness.
- Talk with families about areas in which they might need support or see potential conflicts.
- Lead family discussions in which members share concerns, needs, and coordinate plans.

Assist a family to access community networks that provide respite services, support groups, or group educational sessions for individuals and family members.

Coordinated Care

Coordinated care to satisfy varied needs is most effective if the circle of care extends beyond care providers, systems, or agencies. Standardized methods and systemic improvements for priority household needs require critical attention. Over a decade ago an Institute of Medicine (2001) report identified priority areas for care improvement:

- Stay healthy (preventive care).
- Get better (acute care).
- Live with an illness (chronic care).
- Address the end-of-life care needs (palliative care).

When coordinated care systems are inadequate, they do not meet the unique needs of families. New systems to more effectively fulfill family needs are necessary for health promotion and effective management of chronic conditions.

Coordinated care must be holistic and include multiple care practitioners, community resources, and family households. In an ideal world, what do you think well-coordinated care that meets real needs of family units would look like? Although the family assumes the larger burden for meeting individual care needs, they are often poorly prepared. Nurses who *think family* focus on addressing what families truly need to provide when clinicians are not present. Coordinated care takes into consideration wellness and prevention and ensures that the specific areas of support needed are addressed. Box 15.8 provides questions for reflection.

Meeting Family Support Needs

Nurses who *think family* wisely assess situations and identify ways to encourage and empower for:

- Management or prevention of other illness events
- Steps to take in returning to usual activities of daily life
- Strategies for creating new health routines
- Self-care for those doing caregiving tasks

Family Unity

The family is an entity assumed to be valued by individuals, but some families have severe and irreconcilable member differences and conflicts. Not all members value the same thing.

BOX 15-8

Reflective Questions to Determine Support Needs

- What does this person need at home?
- Do this person and family fully understand the actions to be taken at home?
- Do this person and family understand how to do what is prescribed?
- What kinds of resources do family members need in the home?
- Who will assist with self-care activities at home?
- What do emotional responses about this illness experience and future needs imply?
- What medications, assistance, or resources does the family need help accessing?
- Is this person and family well prepared to do what is needed at home?
- Are needed professional and community resources accessible?
- What questions still need answers to best manage the care needs?

Not all family members always communicate well with one another. Disagreements and arguments occur even in the most caring families. When some family members experience a loss of control they become terrified, frightened, or enraged. Others are capable, resourceful, and willing to take charge. Some think others are not doing their part. Thus, nurses who *think family* consider the uniqueness of family units and some basic guidelines that can guide family support (Box 15.9).

Nurses often have only a brief time to identify potential risks and supports needed by individuals within a family, and information gathered might come in small fragmented bits. In some situations, what the nurse learns may be only the tip of an iceberg with most concerns hidden from view. Suppose the support is needed in a household by a person who has had an acute condition but is also a veteran, has a severe disability, and is suffering from post-traumatic stress disorder (PTSD). What happens if the doorways in the family home are not big enough to accommodate a wheelchair? Certainly, the family's needs will be quite complex. Suppose violence or child abuse has occurred. There are critical care, legal, and policy concerns to address. What if the individual receiving care was treated for acute pancreatitis and is an alcoholic or a family member abuses street drugs? An elderly couple has an aging son with Down syndrome or an older spouse cares for his mate with Alzheimer's disease? What implications do these things have on families? What safety issues need to be resolved?

Thinking family encourages the nurse to just listen to what is said but also what is not said. A skilled family nurse asks questions, reflects on implications, and partners with the family unit to ensure the best support possible considering a host of issues in both the home and the community. When working with family health issues in community settings, advocacy has to do with prevention, advocacy, and policy. Nurses also use advocacy to support individuals in agency settings. A nurse working in a state or federal prison system might find himself needing to advocate for an inmate's medical care needs, or inform family of critical concerns. Support also has environmental perspectives. A community health nurse works with local residents to identify ways to make their community safe and support healthier lives.

Creating Action Plans to Support Families

As nurses *think family*, they intentionally collaborate and plan with families to identify reasonable steps that, if followed, will achieve goals. Planning entails specific care needs. Ask "What troubles you most as you think about your condition?" The nurse and family work together to address the concern.

BOX 15-9

Guidelines for Provision of Family Support

The Family Preservation and Support Services Program Act of 1993 suggests some guidelines about family support:

- It should be family driven and have a true partnership established, regardless of who are viewed as members.
- It should be comprehensive, flexible, and individualized to meet specific literacy, cultural, and valued needs.
- It should build on strengths and empower the individual and family members.
- It should include prevention and care coordination.
- It should use available formal and informal types of support.
- It should increase confidence and competence.
- It should enhance the health of all family members and the family unit.

BOX 15-10

Social Support Case Study

Carol is a 44-year-old woman with two children, Jonathan, 8 years old, and Sarah, 6 years old. James, her husband, works in the local automotive factory. Both participate in athletic, school, and church activities. Carol does the transportation, home care, and child care. Carol stated, "My children are my primary focus. They are involved in school and our church. I work part-time as a receptionist in a marketing office." She has no adverse medical history, but has experienced numbness and weakness over the past month. She has visited the primary care clinic twice with no definitive diagnosis and is anxious about her condition. She asked the nurse: "What could be wrong with me? This is more than a virus, but they are not telling me. I am confused about what is taking so long to figure out." Recent symptoms include fatigue and visual problems. A complete diagnostic evaluation including a magnetic resonance imaging (MRI) scan of the brain and spinal cord and cerebrospinal fluid examination have been done. Finally, she was diagnosed with multiple sclerosis. She spoke with the nurse: "I wish my husband was here. I don't know how I am going to handle this. How bad is this going to get? Is it just going to keep getting worse?" Her parents visited for a time following her diagnosis. Carol was started on several medicines including an antidepressant to help her manage. Carol's mother accompanied her to follow-up visits where she presents with increased difficulty climbing stairs at home. Carol says, "I don't want to worry my parents. They are already anxious about my diagnosis. I don't know how I am going to manage my children's activities. I don't want them to miss games or school activities." She is hospitalized for more neurological evaluation and medication regimen treatments. Carol is discharged after 2 days with a change in medications. During the discharge James looks concerned. In the hallway he tells the nurse that he is overwhelmed and fearful about what all this means. This terrible disease had caused his mother's death.

Compare patient-focused and family-focused care. Consider the diagnosis and think about the family illness experience. How might nursing actions differ in this case?

Traditional Questions:

1. What do you view as Carol's educational needs at the time of discharge?
2. What discharge coordination needs require the nurse's attention?
3. What specific instructions would you give Carol at discharge?

Family-Focused Questions:

1. If the nurse is thinking family, how would education and information exchange with this family occur?
2. What coordinated care needs to be done during the discharge to meet family household needs?
3. What community support networks might the nurse suggest?

Family Example of Needed Supports

This example takes into account interacting needs of household members. Mr. Jamisen, a 38-year-old man, recently suffered a myocardial infarction and spent several days in an intensive care unit (ICU). He has been told repeatedly that his condition is serious and he must make lifestyle changes. The dietitian discussed dietary changes. A physical therapist spoke with him about needs to increase physical activity, and he is scheduled to attend cardiac rehabilitation classes next week. His doctor said he needs to reduce his weight by 6%. He has smoked a pack of cigarettes a day for 25 years and must quit. He has several new medications and must monitor his blood pressure closely. He must rest for a few days and then gradually increase activity. He has to miss work for the next 6 weeks. He has follow-up visits with his cardiologist and family physician. The doctor wants him to join a heart healthy program sponsored by the hospital and to bring a family member. Doing these activities means a 45-minute drive each way from his home. Now *think family* and make a list of issues that might be troubling Mr. Jamisen. What concerns do you think his family has? If you were preparing for his discharge, what supportive actions might he need? What might his family need? What things should a family nurse assess?

Suppose that before discharge you discovered that Mr. Jamisen does not understand his dietary changes and he has tried to quit smoking before but was not able to do it because his wife also smokes. He wants to return to work right away because when he does not work, his family has no income. He has some health insurance, but is not sure that it is enough to cover these hospital bills. He doubts it will pay for cardiac rehabilitation. He is not sure he can pay for his medicines. He works hard, but his paycheck is inadequate to cover bills. He has been saving money to buy his son baseball cleats and a glove for his upcoming birthday. He is worried that his libido will not return and does not know what problems this will cause in his marriage. No one has talked to him about any of these things. You are the nurse caring for him. Create an action plan to address his needs. Box 15.10, on the previous page, offers a case study about Carol and her family's care needs, take time to consider the questions.

Nursing Actions to Support Care Needs

The nurse assigned to Mr. Jamisen has been speaking with him about returning home. She senses his anxiety and lack of ease with making changes. She suggests that his wife come in early the next morning before discharge so that they can work together and create an action plan. His nurse can see that he is overwhelmed. The nurse assists them in setting meaningful realistic goals and they work together to develop an action plan for change (Box 15.11). She reviews the kinds of informational, instrumental, resource, emotional, and appraisal support for actions.

Some families have difficulty following prescribed medical orders. Table 15.3 provides examples for actions related to the Jamisen family's dietary routines. Note the ideas for changing dietary routines. Keep in mind that the Jamisen family also has other areas of concern. Dietary routines are extensive and involve more than just Mr. Jamisen. In fact, most routines involve interactions of multiple members and perhaps persons outside the household. In Mr. Jamisen's case, changes involve his wife and three school-age active children. Other life changes involve extended family, close friends, neighbors, his employer,

---

BOX 15-11

Potential Family Challenges Following a Myocardial Infarction

A person who has recently suffered a myocardial infarction is likely to be discharged home with many medical management care needs, but other needs might require various other forms of support. Here are some examples of individual or family concerns that might need some different forms of support:

- Dietary changes (e.g., budget, shopping, label reading, nutrition, portion size)
- Physical activity (e.g., plan for beginning, buddy system, safety information)
- Tobacco (e.g., smoke reduction or stopping plan, supports for changing habits)
- Sexuality (e.g., fears, information, education, answers to questions)
- Employment (e.g., time off work, physical limitations, financial concerns)
- Medications (e.g., costs, insurance, knowledge about side effects and interactions)
- Physical therapy (e.g., transportation, costs, anxieties, personal motivation)

Family-focused nurses identify what forms of support might be needed to address these challenges (e.g., emotional, instrumental, informational, resource, spirituality).

TABLE 15-3	*Action Planning for Dietary Changes*					
TYPE OF ACTION	**SUPPORT NEEDED**	**WHO IS INVOLVED?**	**WHEN WILL IT OCCUR?**	**WHERE WILL IT OCCUR?**	**WHAT IS NEEDED?**	**WHAT IS TO BE ACHIEVED?**
Meal planning	Information Appraisal	Wife	Weekly	Home	Time to plan the week's menus: Who else will be involved in the planning? When will this be done?	More nutritious meals (e.g., more vegetables and fruits; fewer sugary drinks and processed foods; choose healthy snacks)
Shopping	Information Emotional	Wife and husband	Weekly	Local grocery and farmer's market	Identify a weekly food budget allowance based upon family needs to budget for other things besides food.	Spend an agreed-upon budgeted amount, but purchase more nutritious foods and fewer snack items. Learn to read labels. Avoid extra stops at the store to pick up items and avoid spontaneous purchases.
Cooking	Information Appraisal	Wife and other family members	Daily	Home	Allow time for meal preparation, use better organizational skills, and gain access to healthy recipes.	Fewer meals are eaten outside the home, less processed food is eaten, and portion sizes are considered.
Breakfast	Information Appraisal	Family	Daily	Home	Healthy items are available for breakfast and time for breakfast is allowed in the mornings.	Healthier start for all family members, avoid purchasing items outside home, consume fewer high-sugar and high-fat content food items.

Continued

TABLE 15-3   *Action Planning for Dietary Changes—cont'd*

ACTION	TYPE OF SUPPORT NEEDED	WHO IS INVOLVED?	WHEN WILL IT OCCUR?	WHERE WILL IT OCCUR?	WHAT IS NEEDED?	WHAT IS TO BE ACHIEVED?
Daily lunches	Information Appraisal	Whole family	5 days a week	Planning when shopping and preparing other meals (e.g., ways to use leftovers).	Purchase healthy lunch items, prepare lunches the night before work or school days.	Consume healthy lunches that include at least one fruit and vegetable.
Evening meals with family	Emotional Appraisal	Whole family	At least 4 to 5 times weekly	Home	Family members commit to personal schedule changes; family works together to cook meals, some meal preparation done on weekends.	Family time for conversation and sharing activities; meals high in nutrition; refrain from eating fast food for dinner.
Reduce snacking	Emotional Resource	Whole family, extended family, and close friends	Daily	Home and outside the home	Plan for some physical activity during the day; limit screen time to no more than 2 hours daily, and identify active hobbies.	Mr. Jamisen to lose 10 pounds over next 3 months; more active lifestyle; and no snacking after 7 p.m. or when watching TV.
Limit eating outside the home	Emotional Resource	Whole family	Daily	Home	Plan ahead for nights children have afterschool activities.	Save money for a special family fun activity; develop healthier family routines.

and others. Nurses who *think family* realize that achieving wellness and managing an illness take huge family resources.

Nurses who *think family* know discharge planning begins long before a person leaves the acute care center. Ongoing discussions about care and family needs occur throughout the stay. His nurse spoke with Mr. Jamisen's wife about care needed each day when she visited. Mr. Jamisen and his family have many areas of change to address. It is overwhelming! In Chapter 4, motivational interviewing was described; review those ideas again. Think about how you could use this with Mr. Jamisen. Say, "I know your doctor and others have talked with you about changes. It is good to form a plan for how you can make them. The changes are important because they can help you prevent another heart attack. As you think ahead, what are your biggest challenges?" Suggest making a list of things to speak with his family about. Setting some goals and developing an action plan can help (Table 15.3). Address the two biggest concerns. Gaining control in one life area can offer a sense of accomplishment that equips one to manage other areas. If Mr. Jamisen and his wife have specific plans, they will be better prepared to make changes (Table 15.4). Conversations like this may feel uneasy at first, but they get easier with practice.

Helping Families Manage Care Needs

Family transitions often create stress, anxiety, and uncertainty. Families socially construct lives they view as normal. Things like developmental stages, personality or cultural traits, values, sociocultural patterns or traditions, and other environmental factors need to be considered. Readiness to change is a conversation family nurses also need to have with family members. Different families require different approaches. Table 15.5 provides some specific challenges the Jamisen family might face as they alter dietary routines. Think about ways you can help this family avoid potential trouble spots.

Family Household Needs

Appraisal can be used to address a breadth of potential needs from varied perspectives. Although families share some traits, quick judgments, bias, or stereotypes can lead to erroneous assumptions. Box 15.12 suggests potential areas for support. Nurses who *think family* are careful about the ways they approach sensitive subjects, but they do not avoid topics just because they are uncomfortable. The family nurse curiously inquires with

TABLE 15-4	*Stages of Change*
CHANGE STAGE	**BEHAVIORS**
Precontemplation	Not yet acknowledging a problem behavior exists
Contemplation	Acknowledging there is a problem, but not prepared to make a change
Preparation	Getting ready to change
Action	Beginning to change behaviors
Maintenance	Maintaining the behavior change over time
Relapse	Returning to old behaviors and failing to maintain new changes

Source: Prochaska, J. O., Norcross, J. C., & DiClemente, C. C. (1994). *Changing for good: The revolutionary program that explains the six stages of change and teaches you how to free yourself from bad habits.* New York: Morrow.

TABLE 15-5   Challenges in Managing Dietary Changes

FAMILY STRESSOR	AREAS OF CONCERN	WAYS TO REDUCE POTENTIAL STRESSORS	POSITIVE COPING MECHANISMS	WAYS TO GIVE SUPPORT
Unhealthy snacking in evenings can create potential disagreements within the family.	• Children used to sugary treats may resist change. • Wife might not see why she has to change habits. • He refuses to make dietary changes. • Food is used as a comfort measure.	• Involve family in some active things during evenings. • Discuss risks involved with not making needed changes. • Discuss ways family can be healthier.	• Stop buying less healthy food items. • Keep healthy snacks readily available. • Plan more active nightly activities with all family members involved. • Limit screen time.	• Wife plans meals and uses shopping list. • Family assists by prepackaging healthy snacks. • A family contract identifies ways members will support one another. • Children identify ways to encourage father.
Mr. Jamisen suffers from depression linked with his medical condition that impacts other family members.	• Eating when sad or frustrated. • Too much time spent sitting and watching TV when home. • Forgets to take prescribed medications.	• Identify actions to substitute for eating and prevent depression. • Create a plan to get more physical activity daily. • Discuss ways to monitor whether medications are taken daily.	• Choose healthier snacks. • Work on a hobby or start a new one. • Use a daily medication box prepared each week.	• Family will walk and be more active together. • Decrease screen time and share new hobby with older son. • Wife will fill medication box weekly and daughter will check daily that medications are taken.
Temptations with food at work when Mr. Jamisen returns.	• Peers bring in doughnuts daily. • Seeing other people eat fast food adds temptation. • Go with buddies for a beer after work three to four times a week.	• Avoid break room in mornings. • Use part of break time to get some activity before or after lunch. • Decrease the number of times out with buddies and plan other activities.	• Bring coffee from home in a thermos, avoid break room. • Eat a nutritious lunch. • Plan activities with children.	• Find a friend with a similar illness condition or one who is health conscious. • Identify a work buddy who is willing to walk at lunch. • Ask family members to help overcome the challenges.
General dislike of fruits and vegetables and Mr. Jamisen's excessive beer drinking trouble the family.	• Prefers meat and potatoes. • Has never tried many different foods. • Has refused to eat differently in the past. • Consumes several bottles of beer in evenings and more over the weekend.	• Keep some favorite foods, but eat them less often. • Set goal to try one new fruit and vegetable each week. • Find new recipes to try. • Discuss what happens if you do not change. • Identify ways to reduce beer drinking.	• Cook smaller amounts and have fewer leftovers. • Have a family contest for who can find the best recipe for the vegetable of the week. • Read about ways to prevent disease complications.	• Family spends time on weekends cooking together. • Mr. Jamisen will challenge his son to a vegetable cooking contest. • Family discusses risks of not changing habits. • Identify ways to spend money saved from reduced beer consumption.

BOX 15-12

Reflections About Potential Support Needs

As nurses *think family* and conduct support appraisals or assessments, they do some personal reflection and engage family members in topics that can help identify support needs. Engaging individuals and family members in conversations with questions like the following can offer important insights and help develop action and coping plans:

- What is the family's prior experience with caregiving? Have they coped well?
- What has been difficult or stressful for them in the past?
- What kinds of things have helped before? What are their strengths?
- What does the family foresee as their greatest needs? What do they fear the most?
- Are those in the family who will be caregivers comfortable with needed changes?
- How will the family access resources that seem to be lacking?
- What community resources are are available for the family?

genuine care: "What areas will cause your family the most difficulty? What resources might be hard for you to obtain? Do you see areas where help you need might not be easily available?" Family nurses avoid know-it-all attitudes, are careful to not be condescending, do not act in ways that cause people to be defensive, and know ways to sensitively encourage sharing of vulnerabilities.

Creating a Checklist

Create a systematic checklist of things to consider with each family. At first this can be a written list you keep in your pocket, but you can commit it to memory as you gain expertise with family conversations. Identify what is absolutely necessary to discuss and what is optional. The result might be tasks, responsibilities, and organizational concerns. Say, "I see you have six areas of concern on your list. Can you tell me what is most important?" Discussing everything in depth is impossible. So use your time to cover areas of greatest concern. In the Jamisen family, members need to know the critical signs to watch for that indicate problems. They need to know the most important care aspects to follow. They need to know where to go to get answers to questions and what to do for an emergency. Two months later other concerns are likely to be more prominent.

Using a systematic process like creating a checklist to identify potential support needs can be completed with every person and help in coordinating care needs. Perceptions based upon family appearance, abilities to articulate concerns, and health insurance availability can overlook true needs. Exhaustion, worry, and fears may not be readily visible. A home visit and observation of an orderly environment may fail to disclose underlying tensions and animosity between members. How will care be managed at home? Are two people needed to transfer or is one enough? Who will be available to help at night? Will caregivers get adequate rest? How will medications be administered safely at home to a person with a cognitive disorder? Can the family afford to rent needed equipment? Will they purchase and correctly use the prescribed drugs? Are they aware of side effects? What happens if the family refuses to help? Has a visiting nurse service been arranged? Does the family know what to expect? Who will drive to radiation treatments for the next 5 weeks? Families can use help sorting through the many things that accompany changes in health and illness.

Nurses who *think family* recognize that long-term stress and burdens wear on even the most willing caregivers. Sometimes families are reluctant to expose their worries in front of the person needing care. Will the family need respite care? Will it be available? Is adequate support available for a long-term condition? If the person is aphasic and has paralysis on one side, does the caregiver know how to help them dress? It is not unusual for anger or frustration to occur. How does the family manage then? Nurses who *think family* understand that helping families think through and answer questions can avoid later problems. These conversations might seem like interruptions to the task of orientations of nursing practice, but these actions influence care outcomes and satisfaction.

Support From Family Caregivers

It is estimated that about one in five households provide informal care to an adult with caregiving lasting from months to decades (Pierce & Lutz, 2013). Caregiving includes direct care, emotional support, and management for both in- and out-of-home activities, finances, and transportation (Levine, Reinhard, Feinberg, Albert, & Hart, 2003). Numerous stresses over time may result in caregiver burden, strain, or compassion fatigue (Clark & Diamond, 2010; Del-Pino-Casado, Frias-Fri'as-Osuna, Palomino-Moral, & Pancorbo-Hidalgo, 2011; Empeno, Raming, Irwin, Nelesen, & Lloyd, 2011). Caregiver burden has been linked to depression (Clark & Diamond, 2010), stress (Bastawrous, 2013), and other adverse psychological and physical health effects (Clark & Diamond, 2010). It can result in physical, psychological, spiritual, and social exhaustion (Lynch & Lobo, 2012; Potter et al., 2010). Therefore, support for caregivers is important. Nurses can assist persons to locate support groups or respite care, and encourage honest sharing and communication with one another (Popejoy, 2011). Nurses who *think family* help members listen to member needs, encourage families to seek supports when needed, and show them where they can get answers to pressing needs.

Balancing Complex Family Needs

When thinking about family support, it is important to ask two questions: "What does the individual need? What do family caregivers or supporters need?" Families have traditions that includes rituals, routines, and family health routines; some are planned and others evolve (Denham, 2003). Change can cause a sense of uneasiness. Changes often involve decisions and adjustments that families might not choose or want. Thus, what the nurse might view as an ordinary transfer to a nursing home is a tumultuous tragedy for a family managing guilt because they had promised this would never occur.

Families often have to choose among multiple household priorities. Life has many needs and electing one thing and forfeiting another is difficult. A family with a teetering household balance can crash with uncertain consequences. The choice to have an elective surgery can be wrought with upheaval. Suppose the family is already dealing with member problems, what happens if a new critical diagnosis is given for a member? It is possible that layers of stress can totally overwhelm them. Before judging a family's caregiving approach, family nurses try to understand the challenges they face.

Family Health Routines

In the Family Health Model, the idea of structure is used to describe the ways family members use beliefs, values, attitudes, information, knowledge, resources, prior experiences, and other things to structure, form, or create behaviors that influence health and illness (Denham, 2003). The discussion of family health routines provides ways to discuss usual health practices. When change is needed, new routines are constructed and old ones deconstructed. For instance, health routines linked with personal hygiene are often rooted in teachings received as children. They have a deep-seated nature that tends to be consistent throughout life. If routines are altered, making adjustments can be difficult. Toilet training turns out to be a big deal in most families. Having adults applauding your success of uri-nating or defecating in a toilet rather than diaper or underwear is an important celebration. As toddlers we are proud of ourselves and value the praise received. Mission impossible becomes a rewarded event, but what happens when underwear is soiled as an adult. What happens if a colostomy is needed, or urinary incontinence or loss of bowel control occurs as we age? Interrupted routines cause great distress. Suppose this is more complicated by the need for an adult daughter to attend to her aging father. Routines around sexuality are also alarming. How could a family nurse assist with needed routine changes?

Nurses can use family health routines to assess current practices and plan needed changes. If an individual needs to alter routines, the change will likely affect others in the household. Support to change family health routines seldom happens easily. Comfortable behaviors must be replaced. For this reason, coordinated care is essential. Table 15.6 iden-tifies the six categories of family health routines in the Family Health Model: self-care, safety and prevention, mental health behaviors, family care, illness care, and member care-giving (Denham, 2003). Assessment of family routines can suggest ways to set goals, make decisions, plan actions, and identify where support is needed. Family members can discuss not only their own personal routines but also those of others in a household. Families know who does what, where, when, and how. Involving multiple members in discussions about health routines can be useful in identifying priorities and planning change strategies.

Readiness to Change

An important aspect about change is timing. When change is needed, not everyone is ready to adapt at the same time. Seldom will everyone be at the same stage of readiness for change. Trying to change can turn into anarchy and rebellion! Change is a process. It takes time, thoughtfulness, and commitment. Listening to a family is critical at all stages of change (Mason & Butler, 2010). Remember, changes that are made must be sustained over time. Change seldom occurs in linear or consistent ways. Big change can occur in a single person or in a single behavior, but other routines can be ignored. For example, a person might be willing to increase physical activity, but refuse to consume more green vegetables. Gaps are often seen between good intentions, actions, and results. Change is not easy, but it can be facilitated by a family nurse who asks, informs, reassures, listens, and empowers.

Family Support Groups

Support groups can help families manage emotional and physical health situations. Family members report that support groups provide empathy and enhance their abilities to deal with emotions, gain experiential knowledge, and obtain peer support (Munn-Giddings & McVicar, 2006). The benefits of group participation for those with a psychiatric condition include in-creased disease knowledge, reduced burden and distress, increased abilities to manage daily life, and enhanced social support (Chien & Norman, 2009). Palliative care support groups are a positive experience for family members as they help with information and provide as-surance about the adequacy of care being given (Henriksson, Benzein, Ternestedt, & Ander-shed, 2011). Caregiving can be lonely and frustrating. Box 15.13 provides evidence about the positive outcomes that can be achieved through individual-nurse-family partnerships. Care-givers gain strength when they understand they are not alone and that others contend with similar things. Family members who attend support groups in hospital settings during acute illness have reported positive experiences (Henriksson & Andershed, 2007). Participation dur-ing a serious illness provides emotional support, and the relationships formed help members endure the stress of hospitalization (Scharpe, 2012). It can be comforting to share stories with group members and get reassurance from those with similar fears and vulnerabilities

TABLE 15-6	*Family Health Routines*

FAMILY HEALTH ROUTINE	ASPECTS OF THE ROUTINE	ROUTINE DESCRIPTION
Self-care routines	Dietary • Hygiene • Sleep-rest habits • Physical activity and exercise • Gender and sexuality	Patterned behaviors linked with usual activities of daily living experienced across the life course.
Safety and prevention	• Health promotion • Disease prevention • Tobacco use • Abuse and violence • Alcohol and substance abuse • Wrongful use of prescription drugs • Immunizations	Routines pertain to health protection, disease prevention, avoidance of participation in high-risk behaviors, and prevention of unintended injuries across the life course.
Mental health behaviors	• Self-esteem and self-worth • Personal integrity • Work and play • Coping with stressors	Routines are linked with having a valued and meaningful personal life.
Family care	• Family fun (e.g., relaxation actions, hobbies, vacations) • Celebrations, traditions, and special times • Spiritual and religious practices • Sense of humor • Pets	Routines include activities, traditions, behaviors, and special celebrations that provide for a meaningful life, shared pleasure or enjoyment, and happiness for multiple members.
Illness care	• Decision making about medical consultation • Use of health care services • Follow up with prescribed treatments • Use of alternative therapies • Use of over-the-counter medications, herbs, and vitamins	Routines are linked with various ways members make decisions related to illness or disease care needs; choose when, where, and how to use services or treatments to manage an illness or disease; and ways chosen to respond to medical directives or health information.
Member caregiving	• Health teaching (i.e., health promotion; disease management) • Caregiving roles and responsibilities • Provision of illness care • Supportive member interactions	Routines are ways family members provide care to one another across the life course; ways children, youth, and others are socialized to participate in health ideals, health-promoting actions, and illness care; and ways members provide support to one another for development and maintenance of individual health routines.

Source: Adapted from Denham, S. A. (2003). *Family health: A framework for nursing.* Philadelphia: F. A. Davis.

(Scharpe, 2012). Support groups help participants with direction as information is exchanged and decisions shared. Groups offer time to reflect about experiences, loss, and grief. Nurses who *think family* encourage individual and family participation.

Supports for Family Nurses

Compassion fatigue in nurses is a phenomenon described in the literature, a situation that sometimes accompanies caring (Figley, 2002). Exhaustion can happen when caring for those in stressful, difficult and troubling situations. Therefore, it is important to also attend to personal and professional health. To be able to give support to others, nurses also need support. Forms of support needed will likely differ throughout nursing careers. Nurses born and trained in different nations will likely need supports as they adapt to working in a foreign care system. Nurses moving from staff to administrative jobs might require supports as they transition to new positions.

BOX 15-13
Evidence-Based Family Nursing Practice

Chronic obstructive pulmonary disease (COPD) is a serious disease largely focused on the person's distress, and often minimal attention is given to the family as they live with it. Living with advanced COPD is difficult and challenging for those with the disease and their family. When persons are met in health care settings, they are often treated as if this is a one-time event, a pathophysiological condition, and only episodic needs are addressed. The breadth of the symptoms, seriousness of the disease, and associated family needs are rarely addressed. A synthesis of research findings suggests that when family nurses form partnerships with families and other health professionals, illness outcomes are improved. The development of a hospital-based nursing practice partnership was tested using dialogue with each patient admission involved: (a) family involvement, (b) symptoms and care needs, and (c) reliable and timely access to health care services. A prospective and retrospective intervention study evaluated the effectiveness of the partnership and qualitative studies were used to study the meaning and experience of the partnership. The three studies demonstrated significant enhancement of the health status of individuals and family members. Outcomes from the intervention study demonstrated 80% decrease in hospital admissions, improved quality of life, improved use of inhaler medications, and decreased anxiety, depression, and malnutrition. The qualitative study found that families (a) had greater knowledge about the disease and ways to manage it, (b) increased capacity to provide needed supports, and (c) acted more independently. These partnerships created trusting relationships that helped family members work together. Using a nonprescriptive dialogue, the nurse attends to things of concern to the individual and family. Medical management in technocratic institutions presents barriers to the development of effective partnerships that need to be overcome. Individual and family dialogue provided insight into real needs and gave information about the best ways to assist them to manage problems. More needs to be known about ways to develop and maintain coordinated care for persons with COPD when care is multidisciplinary, interinstitutional, and largely home based. Additional study is needed to identify ways partnerships that include the individual, nurse, and family can optimize the care outcomes for those with COPD.

Source: Jonsdottir, H., & Ingadottir, T. S. (2011). Nursing practice partnership with families living with advanced lung disease. In E. K. Svavarsdottir & H. Jonsdottir (Eds.), *Family nursing in action*. Reykjavik, Iceland: University of Iceland Press.

Personal religious and cultural understandings vary, and tolerance for differences is not always discussed. However, nurses have a moral obligation to provide the same quality care to all persons regardless of their race, ethnicity, sexual orientation, or gender identity. Gay, lesbian, bisexual, and transgendered (GLBT) nurses might need supports. Although many GLBT persons are employed in nursing, they are largely invisible and perhaps only known to close friends (Stephany, 1992). GLBT persons should have the same rights and protection from discrimination as all other employees (Bartlett, Warner, & King, 2002). Nurses not identifying as GLBT might experience discomfort when caring for someone with a different gender identity. The Gay and Lesbian Medical Association, founded in 1981, has a mission to ensure equality in health care for GLBT individuals and health care providers. It is useful for nurses to recognize that status in same-gender partnerships or unions is treated differently throughout the United States. However, attitudes, social policies, and laws are changing quickly.

Students just graduating from a formal educational setting as a registered nurse can find great challenges as they transition from the classroom to clinical settings. Moving from a school assignment of two patients with a teacher nearby can be radically different from a full assignment and answering to a charge nurse or supervisor. As a student, one can go to a faculty member or a peer for clarification or explanation. However, once employed, where to turn for support can be unclear. Some senior people can be intimidating, but many are supportive. Job orientation provides explanations about organizational structure, but nurses need to know who to go to for support. Preceptors are available for a time to answer questions, advise, and can assist with adjustment or transition into the workforce.

Newly employed nurses usually work with more experienced persons. Informal support systems are useful, but new nurses may be slow in locating an encouraging circle of coworkers. Noting persons who reached out to you when you are hired can sometimes indicate who might be a source of future support. Personalities and forms of interactions differ. For instance, extroverted persons may be outgoing and welcome you to the work unit. Novice nurses need not be fearful of engaging quieter persons or those seeming more distant. Persons more introverted may be less forward and seem more guarded, but they could be the best persons to seek out for answers to questions and provide support. If you work in a large facility, a formal support group for nurses might exist. If not, talk with others and see if one can be started. Colleagues and peers can provide some support, but mature nurses need to take some responsibility for their distinct needs.

Chapter Summary

Families provide support for members, but they need assistance to learn the best ways to manage health, care for illness, and make needed changes. *Thinking family* requires nurses to be adept in using various support approaches. Intentional assessment and planning will assist families so they can satisfy care needs in valued ways. Family nurses use collaborative partnership to identify goals, plan actions, and evaluate outcomes. Support must be given based on unique needs that take into account family processes, household qualities, and availability of needed resources. Individual-nurse-family partnerships can be used to improve health outcomes, strengthen a family's support, and assist in making changes that promote individual and family health. Outcome measurement can be used to measure the success of efforts provided.

REFERENCES

Alicke M. (1985). Global self-evaluation as determined by the desirability and controllability of trait adjectives. *Journal of Personality and Social Psychology, 49,* 1621–1630.

Almasri, N., Palisano, R. J., Dunst, C., Chiarello, L. A., O'Neil, M. E., & Polanksy, M. (2012). Profiles of family needs of children and youth with cerebral palsy. *Child Care Health Development, 38*(6), 798–806.

American Geriatrics Society 2012 Beers Criteria Update Expert Panel. (2012). American Geriatrics Society updated Beers Criteria for potentially inappropriate medication use in older adults. *Journal of the American Geriatrics Society, 60*(4), 616–631.

Bartlett, A., Warner, J., & King, M. (2002). Gay and lesbian special interest group. *The Psychiatrist, 26,* 437–438.

Bastawrous, M. (2013). Caregiver burden—A critical discussion. *International Journal of Nursing Studies, 50*(3), 431–441.

Benzies, K., & Mychasiuk, R. (2008). Fostering family resiliency: A review of the key protective factors. *Child and Family Social Work, 14,* 103–114.

Black, K., & Lobo, M. (2008). A conceptual review of family resilience factors. *Journal of Family Nursing, 14*(10) 33–55. doi:10.1177/10748407312237

Brookfield, S. (2009). The concept of critical reflection: Promises and contradictions. *European Journal of Social Work, 12*(3), 293–304.

Brown, J. D. (2012). Understanding the better than average effect: Motives (still) matter. *Personality and Social Psychology Bulletin, 38*(2), 209–219.

Brown, M. A. (1986). Social support during pregnancy: A unidimensional or multidimensional concept? *Nursing Research, 35*(1), 4–9.

Bulecheck, G. M., & McCloskey, J. (1992). *Nursing interventions: Essential nursing treatments* (2nd ed.). Philadelphia: W. B. Saunders.

Burkhardt, M. A., & Nagai-Jacobson, M. G. (1994). Reawakening spirit in clinical practice. *Journal of Holistic Nursing, 12*(1), 9–21.

Cassel, J. (1976). The contributions of the social environment to host resistance. *American Journal of Epidemiology, 104*(2), 107–123.

Chesla, C. (2010). Do family interventions improve health? *Journal of Family Nursing, 16*(4), 355–377.

Chien, W. T., & Norman, I. (2009). The effectiveness and active ingredients of mutual support groups for family caregivers of people with psychotic disorders: A literature review. *International Journal of Nursing Studies, 46*(12), 1604–1623.

Clark, M. C., & Diamond, P. M. (2010). Depression in family caregivers of elders: A theoretical model of caregiver burden, sociotropy, and autonomy. *Research in Nursing and Health, 33*(1), 20–34.

Clark, P. C. (2002). Effects of individual and family hardiness on caregiver depression and fatigue. *Research in Nursing and Health, 25*(1), 37–48.

Cohen, S., Gottlieb, B. H., & Underwood, L. G. (2001). Social relationships and health: Challenges for measurement and intervention. *Advances in Mind-Body Medicine, 17,* 129–141.

Couture, M., Ducharme, F., & Lamontagne, J. (2012). The role of health care professionals in the decision-making process of family caregivers regarding placement of a cognitively impaired elderly relative. *Home Health Care Management & Practice, 24,* 283–291.

Cray, N. M. (2012). Family centered comfort intervention in the post-operative neurosurgical general care unit. Unpublished master's thesis. Minnesota State University, Mankato, MN.

Del-Pino-Casado, R., Frias-Fri'as-Osuna, A., Palomino-Moral, P. A., & Pancorbo-Hidalgo, P. L. (2011). Coping and subjective burden in caregivers of older relatives: A quantitative systematic review. *Journal of Advanced Nursing, 67*(11), 2311–2322. doi:10.1111/j.1365-2648.2011.05725.x

Denham, S. A. (2003). *Family health: A framework for nursing.* Philadelphia: F. A. Davis.

Dossey, B. M. (1997). *Core curriculum for holistic nursing.* Gaithersburg, MD: Aspen Publishers.

Dossey, B. M., & Keegan, L. (2013). *Holistic nursing: A handbook for practice* (6th ed.). Burlington, MA: Jones & Barlett.

Edvardsson, D., Sandman, P. O., & Rasmussen, B. (2006). Caring or uncaring-meanings of being in an oncology environment. *Journal of Advanced Nursing, 55*(2), 188–197.

Elliott, A. F., Burgio, L. D., & DeCoster, J. (2010). Enhancing caregiver health: Findings from the resources for enhancing Alzheimer's caregiver health II intervention. *Journal of American Geriatrics Society, 58,* 30–37.

Empeno, J., Raming, N. T. J., Irwin, S., Nelesen, R., & Lloyd, L. S. (2011). The hospice caregiver support project: Providing support to reduce caregiver stress. *Journal of Palliative Medicine, 14*(5), 593–597.

Figley, C. R. (2002). Compassion fatigue: Psychotherapists' chronic lack of self care. *Journal of Clinical Psychology, 58*(11), 1433–1441.

Guether, C. L., & Alicke, M. D. (2010). Deconstructing the better-than-average effect. *Journal of Personal Social Psychology, 99*(5), 755–770.

Gutierrez, A. P., Candela, L. L., & Carver, L. (2012). The structural relationships between organizational commitment, global job satisfaction, developmental experiences, work values, organizational support, and person-organization fit among nursing faculty. *Journal of Advanced Nursing, 68,* 1601–1614. doi:10.1111/j.1365-2648.2012.05990.x

Haggman-Laitila, A., Tanninen, H. M., & Pietila, A. M. (2010). Effectiveness of resource-enhancing family-oriented intervention. *Journal of Clinical Nursing, 19*(17), 2500–2510.

Henriksson, A., & Andershed, B. (2007). A support group programmed for relatives during the late palliative phase. *International Journal of Palliative Nursing, 13*(4), 175–183.

Henriksson, A., Benzein, E., Ternestedt, B., & Andershed, B. (2011). Meeting needs of family members with life-threatening illness: A support group program during ongoing palliative care. *Palliative and Supportive Care, 9,* 263–271.

Hilbert, G. A. (1990). Measuring social support in chronic illness. In O. L. Strickland & C. F. Waltz (Eds.), *Measurement of nursing outcomes* (pp. 79–95). New York: Springer.

House, J. S. (1981). Work stress and social support. Englewood Cliffs, NJ: Prentice Hall.

Hupcey, J. E. (1998). Clarifying the social support theory-research linkage. *Journal of Advanced Nursing, 27*(6), 1231–1241.

Institute of Medicine. (2001). Priority areas for national action: Transforming health care quality. Washington, DC: Agency for Healthcare Research and Quality. Retrieved September 25, 2012 from http://www.ahrq.gov/qual/iompriorities.htm

Jonsdottir, H., & Ingadottir, T. S. (2011). Nursing practice partnership with families living with advanced lung disease. In E. K. Svavarsdottir & H. Jonsdottir (Eds.), *Family nursing in action.* Reykjavik, Iceland: University of Iceland Press.

Kahn, R. L., & Antonucci, T. C. (1980). Convoys over the life course. Attachment, roles, and social support. In P. B. Baltes & O. G. Brim (Eds.), *Life-span development and behavior* (pp 254–283). New York: Academic Press.

Kind, A. J. H., Jensen, L., Barczi, S., Bridges, A., Kordahl, R., Smith, M. A., & Asthana, S. (2012). Low-cost transitional care with nurse managers making mostly phone contact with patients cut rehospitalization at a VA hospital. *Health Affairs, 31*(12), 2659–2668.

Kolcaba, K. (2003). *Comfort theory and practice: A vision for holistic health care and research.* New York: Springer.

Langford, C. P. H., Bowsher, J., Maloney, J. P., & Lillis, P. P. (1997). Social support: A conceptual analysis. *Journal of Advanced Nursing, 25*(1) 95–100.

Levine, C., Reinhard, S. C., Feinberg, L. F., Albert, S., & Hart, A. (2003). Family caregivers on the job: Moving beyond ADLs and IADLS. *Generations, 27*(4), 17–23.

Looman, W. S. (2006). Development and testing of the social capital scale for families of children with special health care needs. *Research in Nursing and Health, 29,* 325–336.

Lynch, S. H., & Lobo, M. L. (2012). Compassion fatigue in family caregivers: A Wilsonian concept analysis. *Journal of Advanced Nursing, 68*(9), 2125–2134.

Mason, P., & Butler, C. C. (2010). *Health behavior change: A guide for practitioners* (2nd ed.). Edinburgh: Elsevier Ltd.

Mattila, E., Leino, K., Paavilainen, E., & Åstedt-Kurki, P. (2009). Nursing intervention studies on patients and family members: A systematic literature review. *Scandinavian Journal of Caring Sciences, 23*(3), 611–622. doi:10.1111/ju.1471-6712.2008.00652.x

McCubbin, M. A., & McCubbin, H. I. (1996). Resiliency in families: A conceptual model of family adjustment and adaptation in response to stress and crises. In H. I. McCubbin, A. I. Thompson,

& M. A. McCubbin (Eds.), *Family assessment: Resiliency, coping and adaptation* (pp 1–64). Madison: University of Wisconsin Press.

McSherry, W., & Jamieson, S. (2011). Nurses knowledge and attitudes: An online survey of nurses' perceptions of spirituality and spiritual care. *Journal of Clinical Nursing, 20*(11–12), 1757–1767.

Meiers, S. J., & Brauer, D. (2008). Existential caring in the family health experience: A proposed conceptualization. *Scandinavian Journal Caring Science, 22,* 110–117.

Munn-Giddings, C., & McVicar, A. (2006). Self-help groups as mutual support: What do carers value? *Health and Social Care in the Community, 15*(1), 26–34.

Nelms, T. P., & Eggenberger, S. K. (2010). Essence of the family critical illness experience and family meetings. *Journal of Family Nursing, 16*(4), 462–486.

Nilsson, C. J., Avlund, K., & Lund, R. (2010). Mobility disability in midlife: A longitudinal study of the role of anticipated instrumental support and social class. *Archives of Gerontology and Geriatrics, 51*(2), 152–158.

Norbeck, J. S. (1981). Social support: A model for clinical research and application. *Advances in Nursing Science, 3*(4), 43–59.

Norbeck, J. S., Lindsey, A. M., & Carrieri V. L. (1983). Further development of the Norbeck social support questionnaire: Normative data validity testing. *Nursing Research, 32*(1), 4–9.

Pierce, L. L., & Lutz, B. J. (2013). Family caregiving. In I. M. Lubkin & P. D. Larsen (Eds.), *Chronic illness: Impact and intervention.* Burlington, MA: Jones & Bartlett.

Popejoy, L. L. (2011). Complexity of family caregiving and discharge planning. *Journal of Family Nursing, 17,* 61–81.

Potter, P., Deshields, T., Divanbeigi, J., Berger, J., Cipriano, D., Norris, L., & Olsen, S. (2010). Compassion fatigue and burnout: Prevalence among oncology nurses. *Clinical Journal of Oncology Nursing, 14*(5), 56–62.

Prochaska, J. O., & Velicer, W. F. (1997). The Transtheoretical Model of behavior change. *American Journal of Health Promotion, 12*(1), 38–48.

Prochaska, J. O., Norcross, J. C., & DiClemente, C. C. (1994). *Changing for good: The revolutionary program that explains the six stages of change and teaches you how to free yourself from bad habits.* New York: W. Morrow.

Robinson, C. A., Pesut, B., & Bottorff, J. L. (2012). Supporting rural family palliative. *Journal of Family Nursing, 18*(4), 467–490. doi:10.1177/1074840712462065

Schaffer, M. A. (2004). Social support. In S. J. Peterson & T. S. Bredow (Eds.), *Middle range theories.* Philadelphia: Lippincott, Williams & Wilkins.

Scharpe, B. (2012). The family experience of participating in an intensive care unit support group. Unpublished Master's thesis. Minnesota State University, Mankato, MN.

Semmer, N. K., Elfering, A., Jacobshagen, N., Perrot, T., Beehr, T. A., & Boos, N. (2008). The emotional meaning of instrumental social support. *International Journal of Stress Management, 15*(3), 235–251.

Sherwood, P. R., Given, B. A., Given, C. W., Sikorskii, A., You, M., & Prince, J. (2012). The impact of a problem-solving intervention on increasing caregiver assistance and improving caregiver health. *Supportive Care in Cancer, 20*(9), 1937–1947.

Sniehotta, F. F., Schwarzer, R., Scholz, U., & Schuz, B. (2005). Action planning and coping planning for long-term lifestyle change: Theory and assessment. *European Journal of Social Psychology, 35*(4), 565–576.

Stephany, T. M. (1992). Promoting mental health: Lesbian support groups. *Journal of Psychosocial Nursing Mental Health Services, 30*(2), 35–38.

Stewart, M. J. (1989). Social support instruments created by nurse investigators. *Nursing Research, 38*(5), 268–275.

Svavarsdottir, E. K. (2008). Excellence in nursing: A model for implementing Family Systems Nursing in nursing practice at an institutional level in Iceland. *Journal of Family Nursing, 14,* 456–468. doi:10.1177/1074840708328123

Svavarsdottir, E. K., & Rayens, M. K. (2005). Hardiness in families of young children with asthma. *Journal of Advanced Nursing, 50*(4), 381–390.

Svavarsdottir, E. K., Tryggvadottir, G. B., & Sigurdardottir, A. O. (2012). Knowledge translation in family nursing: Does a short-term therapeutic conversation intervention benefit families of children and adolescents in a hospital setting? Findings from the Landspitali University hospital family nursing implementation project. *Journal of Family Nursing, 18*(3), 303–327.

Sveinbjarnardottir, E. K., Svavarsdottir, E. K., & Hrafnkelsson, B. (2012). Psychometric development of the Iceland-Family Perceived Support Questionnaire (ICE-FPSQ). *Journal of Family Nursing, 18*(3), 328–352.

Tilden, V. P., Nelson, C. A., & May, B. A. (1990). The IPR inventory: Development and psychometric characteristics. *Nursing Research, 39*(6), 337–343.

Trecartin, K., & Carroll, D. L. (2011). Nursing interventions for family members waiting during cardiac procedures. *Clinical Nursing Research, 20*(3), 263–275.

Turney, K., & Harknett, K. (2010). Neighborhood disadvantage, residential stability, and perceptions of instrumental support among new mothers. *Journal of Family Issues, 31*(4), 499–524.

Vuckovich, P. K. (2010). Compliance versus adherence in serious and persistent mental illness. *Nursing Ethics, 17*(1), 77–85.

Wacharasin, C. (2010). Families suffering with HIV/AIDS: What family nursing interventions are useful to promote healing? *Journal of Family Nursing, 16*, 302. doi:10.1177/1074840710376774

Weinert, C. (1988). Measuring social support: Revision and further development of the personal resource questionnaire. In O. L. Strickland & C. F. Waltz (Eds.), *Measurement of nursing outcomes* (pp. 309–327). New York: Springer.

Weiss, R. (1976). Transition states and other stressful situation: Their nature and programs for their management. In G. Caplan & M. Killiea (Eds.), *Support systems and mutual help: Multidisciplinary explorations* (pp. 213–232). New York: Grune & Stratton.

Werner, J. S., & Frost, M. H. (2000). *Stress and coping: State of the science and implications for nursing theory, research, and practice 1991–1995*. Glenview, IL: Midwest Nursing Research Society.

Werner, J. S., Frost, M. H., & Orth, K. S. (2000). Stressors and health outcomes: Synthesis of nursing research, 1991–1995. In J. S. Werner & M. H. Frost (Eds.), *Stress and coping: State of the science and implications for nursing theory, research, and practice 1991–1995* (pp. 9–55). Glenview, IL: Midwest Nursing Research Society.

Wiegand, D. L. M. (2006). Withdrawal of life-sustaining therapy after sudden, unexpected life-threatening illness or injury: Interactions between patients' families, health care providers, and the healthcare system. *American Journal of Critical Care, 15*(2), 178–187.

Wiegand, D. L., Deatrick, J. A., & Knafl, K. (2008). Family management styles related to withdrawal of life-sustaining therapy from adults who are acutely ill or injured. *Journal of Family Nursing, 14*(1), 16–32.

Wright, L. M. (2005). *Spirituality, suffering and illness: Ideas for healing*. Philadelphia: F. A. Davis.

Wright, L. M. (2008). Softening suffering through spiritual care practices: One possibility for healing families. *Journal of Family Nursing, 14*(4), 394–411.

Wright, L. M., & Bell, J. M. (2009). *Beliefs and illness: A model for healing*. Calgary, Alberta, Canada: 4th Floor Press.

Wright, L. M., & Leahy, M. (2012). *Nurses and families: A guide to family assessment and intervention*. Philadelphia: F. A. Davis.

INDEX